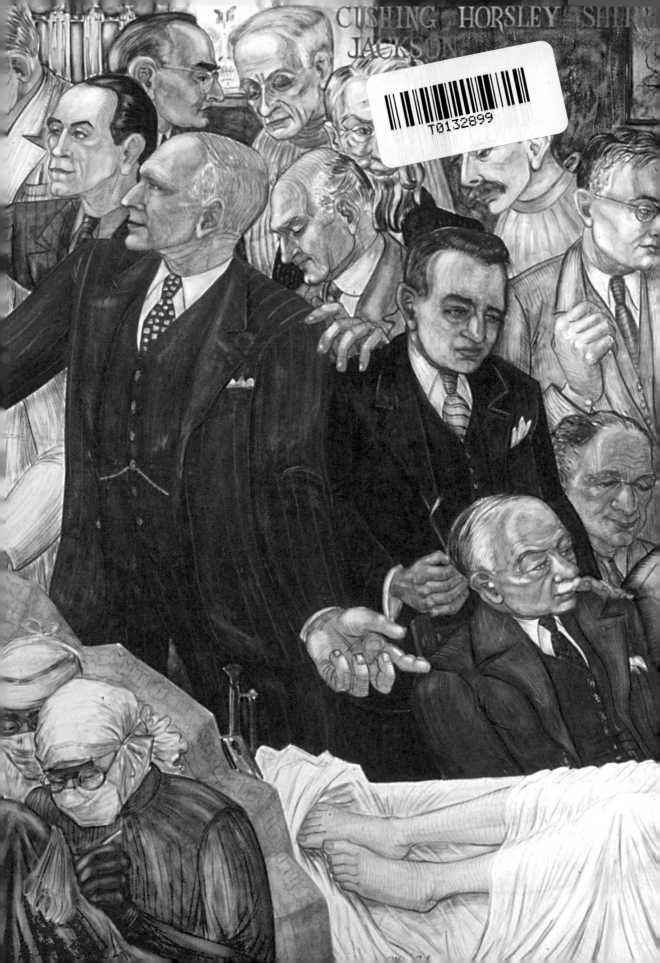

CUSHING   HORSLEY   SHER

JACKSON

The Wounded Brain Healed

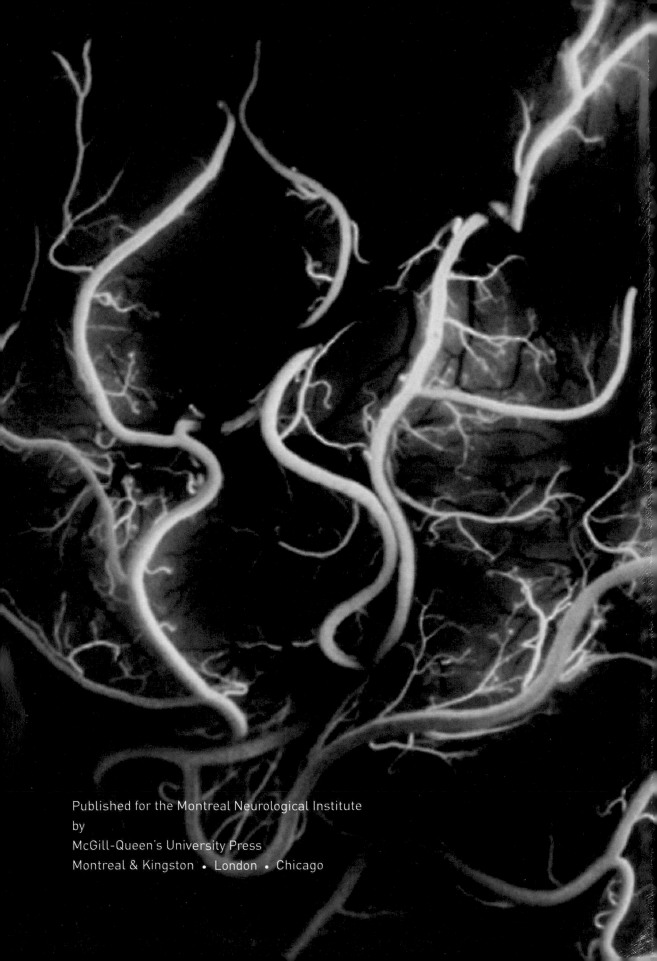

Published for the Montreal Neurological Institute
by
McGill-Queen's University Press
Montreal & Kingston • London • Chicago

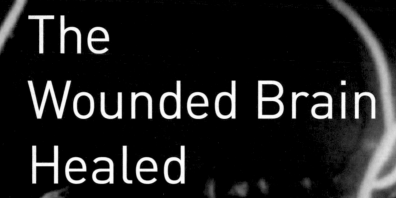

The
Wounded Brain
Healed

The Golden Age of the
Montreal Neurological Institute
1934–1984

WILLIAM FEINDEL AND RICHARD LEBLANC

ISBN 978-0-7735-4637-0 (cloth)
ISBN 978-0-7735-9816-4 (ePDF)

Legal deposit second quarter 2016
Bibliothèque nationale du Québec

Printed in Canada on acid-free paper

McGill-Queen's University Press acknowledges the support of the Canada Council for the Arts for our publishing program. We also acknowledge the financial support of the Government of Canada through the Canada Book Fund for our publishing activities.

Library and Archives Canada Cataloguing in Publication

Feindel, William, 1918–2014, author
The wounded brain healed : the golden age of the Montreal Neurological Institute, 1934–1984 / William Feindel and Richard Leblanc.

Includes bibliographical references and index.
Issued in print and electronic formats.
ISBN 978-0-7735-4637-0 (bound). – ISBN 978-0-7735-9816-4 (ePDF)

1. Montreal Neurological Institute – History. 2. Research institutes – Québec (Province) – Montréal – History. 3. Brain – Research – Québec (Province) – Montréal – History. 4. Brain – Diseases – Patients –Care– Québec (Province) – Montréal–History. 5. Neurosciences – Research – Québec (Province) – Montréal–History. I. Leblanc, Richard, 1949–, author II. Title.

RC339.C3F44 2016   612.8'09   C2015-908107-6
                                            C2015-908108-4

Contents

Contributors / ix

Acknowledgments / xi

Foreword / xiii

Prologue

1 Wilder Penfield: His Journey to Montreal / 3
WILLIAM FEINDEL AND ELIZABETH MALONEY

2 Towards a New Venture / 18
WILLIAM FEINDEL AND ELIZABETH MALONEY

Part One

The Sub-Department of Neurosurgery at the Royal Victoria Hospital,
1928–1933

3 Otfrid Foerster and the Surgical Treatment of Epilepsy / 29

4 The Royal Victoria Hospital / 40

5 The First Research Program at the Royal Victoria Hospital:
A Vasomotor Mechanism of Focal Epilepsy / 64

Part Two

The First Director, 1934–1959

6 The Founding of the Montreal Neurological Institute / 79

7 The First Year and the Second / 97

8 Elvidge, McNaughton, and Jasper / 114

9 Rumours of War / 129

10 "Cry 'Havoc' and let slip the dogs of war" / 144

11 Home Front / 157

12 Life at the Institute / 169

13 Valour / 178

14 The Postwar Period / 193

15 *The Cerebral Cortex of Man* / 205

16 Incisural Sclerosis / 222

17 Bridging Two Solitudes / 232

18 The New Half-Century / 239

19 The MNI and the National Institutes of Health / 250

20 The McConnell Wing / 257

21 William Feindel's Departure / 270

22 Neuropsychology at the MNI / 279

23 A Tribute to William Cone / 297

24 Melancholia: 4 May 1959 / 302

Part Three

The Second Director, 1960–1972

25 Twenty-Five Years on University Street / 309

26 Theodore Rasmussen / 321

27 Penfield in Russia / 333

28 Penfield in China / 341

29 Red Cerebral Veins / 347

30 Herbert Jasper's Departure / 360

31 A Rainbow of African Violets / 374

Part Four

The Third Director, 1972–1984

32 A Fair Trial Followed by a Hanging / 389

33 *Ars Longa* / 400

34 *Vita Brevis*, 5 April 1976 / 412

35 The Third Foundation / 415

36 The Last Half-Decade / 423

Epilogue: The Boy from Bridgewater / 437

Themes

1 Building the Institute / 441

ANNMARIE ADAMS AND WILLIAM FEINDEL

2 Neurochemistry at the MNI / 459

HANNA M. PAPPIUS

3 Multiple Sclerosis: Care and Research at the MNI / 498

JACK ANTEL AND WILLIAM SHEREMATA

4 William Howard Feindel and the Origins of Neurosurgery
in Saskatchewan / 506

MARTHA RIESBERRY

Appendices

Appendix 1 Japanese Chapter of the MNI, 1955–1984 / 512

Appendix 2 Fellows Day Lecturers, 1957–1984 / 514

Appendix 3 Hughlings Jackson Lecturers, 1935–1984 / 516

Notes / 521

Index / 613

Contributors

Annmarie Adams, BA, MArch, PhD, FRAIC, William C. Macdonald Professor and former director of the School of Architecture, McGill University

Jack P. Antel, MD, director, Neuroimmunological Diseases Research Group, Montreal Neurological Institute and Hospital; professor, Department of Neurology and Neurosurgery, McGill University

Helmut Bernhard, medical photographer, scientific illustrator, Neuro Media Services, Montreal Neurological Institute and Hospital

William Howard Feindel, OC, GOQ, MD, CM, DPhil, FRCSC, director emeritus, Montreal Neurological Institute

Richard Leblanc, BA, MSc, MD, FRCSC, physician scientist, Montreal Neurological Institute; professor, Department of Neurology and Neuro-surgery, McGill University

Elizabeth Maloney, BA, MLIS, writer, editor, and research librarian, Montreal

Hanna Maria Pappius, PhD, professor, Department of Neurology and Neuro-surgery, Montreal Neurological Institute and Hospital, McGill University

Martha Riesberry, BSc, MD, CCFP, rural physician, instructor, Michener Institute for Applied Health Sciences

William A. Sheremata, MD, University of Miami Hospital

Ivan Woods, MD, senior neurologist, Montreal Neurological Institute and Hospital; associate professor, Department of Neurology and Neurosurgery, McGill University

Acknowledgments

This book would have never reached the printing press were it not for the unwavering support and generosity of Norah Nasser Al-Manquor and Mrs Sawsun A.A. Abudulwahab, which allowed this project to move forward following Dr Feindel's passing. We are also pleased to acknowledge generous donations from the J.W. McConnell Family Foundation. No institution has a more loyal friend. We are most grateful to Mrs Ann McCain-Evans, the family and friends of Brenda McHardy, and the Class of 1945 of the Faculty of Medicine of McGill University for their generous support. Dr Guy Rouleau, director of the Montreal Neurological Institute and Hospital; Dr Viviane Poupon, executive director, Partnerships and Strategic Initiatives; Mr Zahoor Chughtai, director, Administration and Finance; and Michael Peccho, executive director, External Affairs Office, whose support allowed this project to continue at a most critical time are gratefully acknowledged. We are also grateful to the Department of Neurosurgery at the Montreal Neurological Institute and Hospital, and individual members of the MNI staff who generously supported our project. We also wish to express our gratitude to the Osler Library of the History of Medicine, McGill University, its staff, and Director Christopher Lyons, for facilitating access to the Wilder Penfield Archives.

Dr Feindel gathered a talented staff to help with this project, and we are pleased to acknowledge Mr Duncan Cowie, Mr Matthew Garsia, Mrs Elizabeth Maloney, and Mrs Pamela Miller. Special thanks are owed to Mrs Ann Watson, who met every challenge with poise and grace.

The cheerful cooperation of Mr Marcus Arts and the staff of the Neuro Media Services are also greatly appreciated. Special thanks are directed to Mr Helmut Bernhard, photographer and medical illustrator, whose help was invaluable in retrieving archival photographs and photographing new images for inclusion in our book. We are also grateful to Mr Bernhard for allowing us to publish the touching anecdote that he generously provided.

I am grateful to Jason R. Karamchandani, neuropathologist and director of Experimental Neuropathology, Montreal Neurological Institute and Hospital, McGill University, for reviewing some of Dr Cone's original histology slides; to Robert Nitsch, professor and director, Institute for Microscopic Anatomy and Neurobiology, Johann Wolfgang Goethe-Universität Frankfurt am Main, for his translation of some of Foerster's comments into English; to Dr Barry G.W. Arnason, James Nelson & Anna Louise Raymond Professor of Neurology, University of Chicago, for his reminiscence of multiple sclerosis research at the MNI; and to Dr Mark C. Preul, director, Neurosurgery Research Laboratory, Barrow Neurological Institute at St-Joseph's Hospital and Medical Center, Phoenix, Arizona, for productive discussions.

My special thanks go to the Feindel family, Mrs Faith Lyman Feindel, Anna, Chris, Janet, Michael, and Patricia, who placed their trust in me at the most difficult of times. Finally, many thanks are due to Dr Kathleen F. Knowles for a critical reading of the manuscript and for blocking wobbly metaphors.

Opposite: Lobby ceiling of the Montreal Neurological Institute. The aphorism in the ribbon encircling the ram's head reads, "But I have seen a severely wounded brain heal." The photograph first appeared in W. Penfield, "The Significance of the Montreal Neurological Institute," *Neurological Biographies and Addresses Foundation Volume* (London: Oxford University Press, 1936).

Foreword

I have seen the wounded brain heal.
– Galen

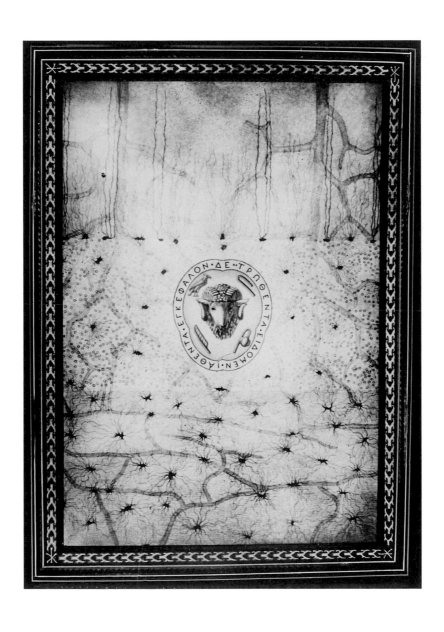

On the ceiling of the Montreal Neurological Institute's lobby there appears a ram's head surrounded by pictographs of a vulture, a length of folded linen, effluent, and a flowering reed, all encircled by a ribbon of Greek letters. The ram's head represents Aries, the astrological symbol that presides over the brain, and the symbols around Aries are Egyptian hieroglyphs from the Edwin Smith papyrus that, in the composite, are the earliest written representation of the brain.[1] The epigraph first appeared as a comment by the physician Galen on Hippocrates, who had written that a wound to the head is always fatal. Galen, however, wrote in the margin of his book of Hippocratic aphorisms, "But I have seen a severely wounded brain heal."[2]

It is not by chance that Galen's observation came to be at the centre of the Montreal Neurological Institute's welcoming alcove. Wilder Penfield had been taken aback when asked, "What goes on in the brain. How does it heal?"[3] That question took Penfield to Madrid, first to learn the techniques of staining brain cells with silver and gold salts, then to study brain wounds.[4] The question thus answered by his own microscopic observations, Penfield set upon his life's goal, to heal the wounded brain.

Prologue

It is usually true that a man who will make a good leader is the man
to whom a small group of younger men are loyal.
– Penfield

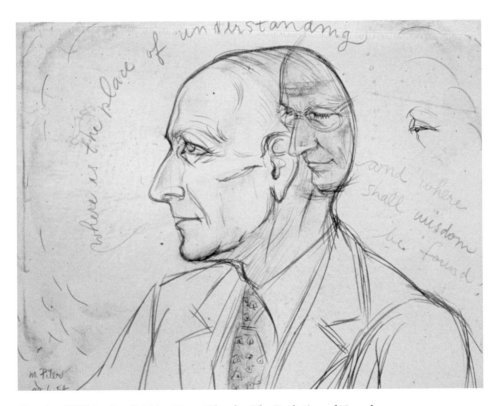

Sketch of Wilder Penfield by Mary Filer for *The Evolution of Neurology*, 1953.
(MNI Archives)

1

Wilder Penfield: His Journey to Montreal

WILLIAM FEINDEL AND ELIZABETH MALONEY

PRINCETON

On the evening of 12 January 1928 in New York City, Wilder Penfield left the Laboratory of Neurocytology at the Presbyterian Hospital, took a cab to Grand Central Terminal, and boarded the Delaware and Hudson's overnight train to Montreal. The *Montreal Limited* meandered north through the Hudson River Valley, past the Adirondack Mountains, along Lake Champlain, and into Canada, a scenic route even in winter, when the sheer rock faces lining the mountainous landscape are glazed with ice. At night, and under a waning moon, our traveller would have seen shimmers of light across the clearings. In the prepared mind of the scientist, an unexpected illumination could point to the resolution of an idea, but it could also become a trail-mark for future travellers. From early research in his medical training, Penfield was drawn to explore the landscape of the brain, guided by mentors who prepared the way and encouraged his venture. Like the pioneers who had blazed through the countryside, he was now answering a call for a new direction in Canadian neurosurgery, one that he hoped would lead him to solve some of the brain's greatest mysteries.

In the early twentieth century, defining and treating illnesses of the brain was a solitary pursuit. Few medical graduates were interested in neurology, and neurosurgery was what Penfield described to his mother as a "terrible profession,"[5] more than likely to lead to a patient's death. By 1928, and at the age of thirty-seven, Penfield had already made a name for himself in the relatively new field of neurological surgery. During the past six years in New York at the Presbyterian Hospital, he had gained responsibility for neurosurgery and had begun research on the pathology of the nervous system. His wife, Helen Kermott Penfield, and their four children were comfortably settled in the New York suburb of Riverdale, and after a long financial struggle for the family while he studied medicine and then brain surgery, his salary was finally increasing steadily. Nevertheless, his role as a neurosurgeon at the new Neurological Institute was uncertain, and there was no laboratory there for him to continue his research. Edward Archibald's invitation to come to Montreal offered the possibility of combining the study and treatment of brain illnesses on his own terms.

On the overnight *Montreal Limited*, Penfield might well have pondered how he had arrived at this defining moment in his life. Wilder Graves Penfield, the youngest of three children, was born on 26 January 1891, to Charles Samuel Penfield and Jean Jefferson. Shortly after their marriage in 1880, Charles Penfield developed a debilitating ailment that Wilder later surmised was chronic appendicitis. Advised that the only cure was "under canvas," Charles travelled alone by train to Montana, where he easily adapted to outdoor survival in the western wilderness. For a time, the cure was successful and Charles started a medical practice in Spokane Falls, Washington, but he continued to return to the woods, setting up his tent away from his responsibilities to his family and patients.[6]

In 1903, Jean Jefferson Penfield left Charles and Spokane, taking the children to her parents' home in Hudson, Wisconsin.[7] Jean was her son's faithful advisor and confidante. For over thirty years, Wilder sent her a weekly report of his thoughts and activities, and "she understood me completely, at every stage and [gave] me everything I needed, in sympathy and love."[8] When he was thirteen, Wilder's mother heard a Rhodes Scholar speak about his experiences at Oxford University, and she decided this would be "just the thing" for her son. As Penfield remembered, "In order to win this three-year scholarship, all I had to do, during the next eight years, was to make myself into an 'all-round' scholar and athlete and leader."[9] To that end, Jean Penfield put much of her energy into providing Wilder with a solid, Rhodes-worthy education. She founded the Galahad School, a private boarding school that aimed for high academic standards and sports training that would prepare talented pupils like Wilder for university. Princeton was chosen as the next major step on Wilder's path to Oxford. He and his mother believed that his chances to become a Rhodes candidate might fare better in New Jersey, which had fewer colleges and competitors.[10]

Jean, a strict Presbyterian, also directed Wilder's early religious education, ensuring that he continually studied biblical passages for meditation, even when he was away at summer camp. Wilder took her guidance in stride: "I'll try and do all that God and you want me to do," he wrote to his mother.[11] Over the years, he developed a deep commitment to his faith, along with the precept to do good in the world. Wilder did consider entering the ministry but changed his mind after meeting prospective seminarians at Princeton whose goals were more temporal than spiritual.[12]

Wilder's letters home during his four years at Princeton hardly indicated his future direction as a neuroscientist. After an uneasy start socially, Princeton gradually became his world, so that by junior year, he was a member of several clubs, a keen wrestler, football player, faithful varsity team supporter, and a popular man on campus. Before entering his final year, when he had to consider a future occupation, he became more serious about his studies, observing that "social and athletic success would leave nothing behind but the ashes of a fierce little fire."[13] Although reluctant to follow medicine, imagining that his father's undesirable traits might be hereditary, he knew that he wanted to continue with postgraduate work: "There was so much to learn … and beyond the learning, there was truth unguessed and yet to be discovered. There was work for me to carry out, and that work could only be on this same higher level, somewhere in the world. I wondered whether it was too late for me to change, to do better work and to move from the commonplace toward true excellence along some highway of the mind."[14]

The one academic subject at Princeton that gained more than the required attention for Penfield was biology. The popular biology course was taught by the chair of the department, the eminent biologist and zoologist Professor Edwin Grant Conklin.[15]

As a student, Conklin had entered Johns Hopkins University in 1888, just as work was being completed on a new medical facility, part of the generous endowment from the progressive American financier Johns Hopkins. A few years earlier, pathologist William H. Welch[16] and physiologist H. Newell Martin[17] were hired to organize and direct the hospital's laboratories, "where scientists could work on the frontiers of pathology, well funded, appreciated, left alone, just as in Germany."[18] Welch helped recruit the other founding physicians of the Johns Hopkins Hospital: William Osler, William Stewart Halsted, and Howard Kelly.[19] It was in this energetic atmosphere that Edwin Conklin found his vocation as a scientist.[20] When Conklin was hired at Princeton in 1910, "one of the largest and most complete laboratories for biology and geology in the country"[21] had just been built at Guyot Hall. Wilder Penfield was the beneficiary of these new facilities, as well as Conklin's extensive training under Osler and Welch's stewardship at Johns Hopkins. Conklin's enthusiasm for discovery under the microscope, uncovering "mysteries of human things,"[22] so impressed Penfield that he realized he wanted to study medicine: "How directly one would be helping human beings in medical research and how satisfying it would be to treat the sick yourself."[23]

As Penfield was beginning to plan his future in medicine, medical education in North America was undergoing a significant change. In the early twentieth century, the two major philanthropic organizations, the Carnegie Foundation and the Rockefeller Institute, were concerned about the slow pace of attempts to prevent and cure infectious diseases, in spite of the proliferation of medical schools that in 1907 numbered 155 across North America.[24] The Carnegie Foundation commissioned Abraham Flexner to conduct a survey of medical training in the United States and Canada and to write a report, published in 1910.[25] The outcome of Flexner's report was that Carnegie and Rockefeller, two critical donors, reviewed their funding of medical schools and hospitals and subsequently supported only those that met high standards. On a positive note, Flexner rated Johns Hopkins Hospital and Dispensary at the top, with the laboratory facilities for scientific research "in every respect unexcelled."[26] If Penfield was looking to continue exploration under the microscope, Johns Hopkins offered the best facilities in the country, largely because of the work of William Osler.

In spite of this new motivation, Penfield was not entirely certain about his choice of medicine as a career; above all, he was haunted by memories of his father's failure. It was during this period of indecision that Penfield came to know John Grier Hibben.[27] In her inimitable way, Jean Penfield wrote to the president of Princeton, asking him to advise her son. Hibben, perhaps recalling his own mother's efforts to provide a good education for her son after his father had died during the Civil War, replied, "I have been particularly drawn to your boy and feel that he has the gifts of mind and of temperament which will make his life a power for good."[28] Penfield thus had the attention of someone with experience and influence to approve his plan to attend Oxford as a Rhodes Scholar after graduation, followed by medical school at Johns Hopkins.[29]

Penfield's attempts to obtain the Rhodes Scholarship, however, were more difficult than he had anticipated. Although he had passed the preliminary Rhodes exam in his sophomore year, without being accepted as a candidate,[30] he felt he was well prepared to merit the scholarship in his senior year. In the end, the committee granted the scholarship to the other finalist, with the assurance from the secretary of the Rhodes Trust that if Penfield applied the next year, he would be the successful candidate. To reach this stage for which he had prepared throughout his teenage and early adult years, and not obtain the award, was a bitter blow. Penfield didn't think he would apply again, "because I was just mad at being thrown down twice."[31]

The Rhodes rejection meant that Penfield would have to find other means of funding his medical education, and ensure that at least he would have a place at his preferred medical school. With Hibben's introduction, Penfield approached John Finney, Halstead's assistant at Hopkins,[32] about a possible intervention to treat Princeton's baseball team mascot, a devoted young fan named Hughie Golden. Hughie's dwarf-like appearance displayed the symptoms of a hormone deficiency that Professor Conklin had described in his biology course. Penfield contacted Finney when the Princeton Tigers were on the road at Baltimore, and Finney invited him and Hughie to the Finney home. While it was concluded that nothing could change Hughie's situation, Finney recognized Penfield's compassion for the health of the child and his interest in probing the source of the medical problem. He offered Penfield a summer job tutoring his four children at the family's summer home on Little Fish Island, off Chester, Nova Scotia. In this idyllic setting, referred by the local residents as "Mrs Finney's Hat," Penfield kept the children occupied with activities and water sports. He also spent his evenings with Finney, and as he told his mother, "a chance to know [him] was too good to miss."[33] A few months later, Finney wrote Penfield a letter of introduction to Sir William Osler, then Regius Professor of Medicine at Oxford University.

After his summer with the Finneys, Penfield continued to earn money for his medical education, teaching German at the Galahad School and coaching football. By October 1913, with encouragement from his mother, Penfield thought he would try again for the Rhodes, "unless a coaching job should come my way."[34] In December, he heard from the Rhodes Committee that he would be offered the scholarship beginning in September 1914. At last he had received the prize that he and his mother had pursued for so many years. But war was declared in July, and travelling to England to study didn't seem to be a practical plan. After attempting late applications to Harvard and Johns Hopkins without success, Penfield was accepted at the College of Physicians and Surgeons in New York. He also became engaged to Helen Kermott, a teacher from his hometown of Hudson.[35] Later in the fall, however, Penfield received a note from another Rhodes Scholar telling him that with most of the male students away at war, the atmosphere for learning couldn't be better, and he requested a January 1915 admission to Oxford.[36]

OXFORD

Penfield still intended to apply to Johns Hopkins University Medical School, seeing the Rhodes Scholarship as a way of paying for two years of required pre-clinical study, equivalent to the first two of four years at Johns Hopkins. As he told the dons when he arrived at Merton College, he wasn't really interested in obtaining his Oxford BA, which would normally take three years, but he did want to do the required medical courses in two years. To his surprise, they refused. Penfield had Finney's letter of introduction to William Osler, and he

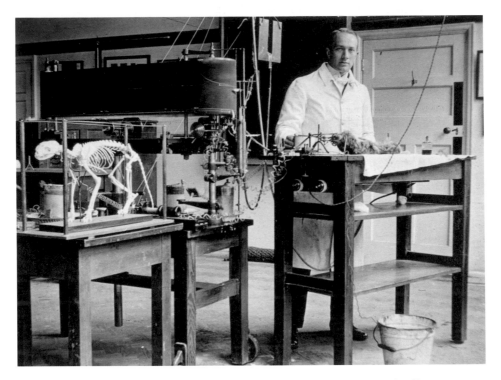

Figure 1.1: Wilder Penfield in Sherrington's laboratory at Oxford, 1916. (William Feindel, "The Physiologist and the Neurosurgeon: The Enduring Influence of Charles Sherrington on the Career of Wilder Penfield," *Brain* 130 [2007]: 2760)

thought he should at least try to ask his help to change the scope of the scholarship. He presented himself at the Oslers' home, appropriately named "The Open Arms," and Lady Osler invited him to come for tea.

Sir William Osler, the most renowned physician and medical writer of his day, had graduated from McGill Medical School in 1872. After two more years of study in London, Berlin, and Vienna, he returned to McGill where, at age twenty-five, he was named professor of the Institutes of Medicine, charged with teaching medical students how to use a microscope.[37] Also appointed as pathologist to the Montreal General Hospital, he performed and recorded almost a thousand autopsy examinations during the next decade. The experience formed the solid foundation of his later fame as an astute diagnostician, erudite teacher, and popular author. His bibliography listed more than 1,400 works, with 200 articles written on neurology alone.[38] He became a vigorous advocate for the emerging special field of neurosurgery.

As Osler's accomplishments grew, he attracted the attention of prestigious universities, each trying to woo him away from McGill. In 1884, he joined the

School of Medicine of the University of Pennsylvania in Philadelphia, the old-est medical school in America, where he proposed reforms to the way medi-cine was taught. Five years later, he became the first professor of medicine and physician-in-chief at the newly opened Johns Hopkins Hospital in Baltimore. Osler taught his students at the bedside in the Edinburgh tradition, offering a practical, caring, and hands-on approach to healing, which helped to change the face of medical education in America. After a decade, he became increas-ingly active in teaching and writing, as well as consulting, lecturing, and at-tending meetings of medical, scientific, and librarian societies, some of which he organized. One of Osler's great contributions while at Johns Hopkins was his incomparable textbook, *The Principles and Practice of Medicine*,[39] first pub-lished in 1892, "at once a monument to the achievements of nineteenth-century scientific medicine and a gateway to the twentieth century."[40] Written for practitioners and students of medicine, it quickly became a bestseller, and for more than a half century, influenced generations of physicians through its sixteen editions.[41]

In August 1904, Osler was offered the Regius Professorship of Medicine at Oxford, which was less demanding than his work at Hopkins. During the next fifteen years at Oxford his reputation grew even further, and he became the leading personality of his time in the practice, teaching, and art of medicine. He took particular interest in students like Penfield who were beginning to explore possibilities for their future in medicine. After listening to Penfield's argument for cutting short the usual three-year Oxford program of study, Sir William made arrangements for Penfield to take a course in anatomy at Edinburgh Uni-versity during the summer vacation so that he could complete the courses needed for his BA in two years.

Wilder Penfield entered Mob Quad, the medieval section of Merton College that had been student quarters for the distinguished seventeenth-century physicians Thomas Willis and William Harvey. He enrolled in the course of mammalian physiology directed by the newly elected Waynflete Chair of Phys-iology at Oxford, Professor Charles Sherrington.[42] Sherrington had spent the previous fifteen years as Holt Professor of Physiology at University College, Liverpool, where his research on the nervous system attracted international attention. Medical students such as Harvey Cushing, who became the foremost neurosurgeon in America, made the detour to Liverpool to spend time observ-ing in Sherrington's laboratory during their postgraduate visits to European medical centres.[43]

When Sherrington was appointed to Oxford, war had been declared, and most young British men had put aside their education in order to volunteer for military service. His physiology class in January 1915 was "decimated, but for three physically unfit men, three women and the three American Rhodes Scholars,"[44] including Penfield. It was an opportunity for them to have personal tutoring and follow the detailed course of experiments that Sherrington had developed over the years for physiological study.

Sherrington's laboratory course on mammalian physiology was a highly organized series of twenty-one exercises performed over the Oxford term of study, proceeding from introductory lessons on using equipment and preparing the specimens, to the complex preparations expected of the experienced researcher. These exercises were of great value to Penfield, as he learned how to gently handle living tissues, to use fine surgical dissection instruments, and to maintain the vital function of the experimental animals. An illustration of Penfield's work on arterial pressure was selected to accompany one of the experiments[45] when the *Practical Exercises* were published as a manual after the war.[46] Throughout the manual, Sherrington annotated each set of instructions with extensive bibliographic references to previous studies, dating from the seventeenth century. As he stated in the preface, he included the historical notes "to enable the student best to assess for himself the intellectual cost and value of the observations he is repeating."[47] Sherrington's superior approach to research, defining its worthiness in the development of medical knowledge, inspired Penfield to continue investigating the workings of the brain: "I came to realize that here in the nervous system was the great unexplored field – the undiscovered country where the mystery of the mind of man might someday be explained."[48]

An unexpected turn of events during the spring vacation of 1916 found Penfield spending two weeks as a guest of Sir William and Lady Osler at the Open Arms. He was crossing the English Channel in the SS *Sussex* en route to France for the second time to volunteer as a wound dresser in a Red Cross hospital when a torpedo from a German submarine blew off the ship's bow. Thrown into the air and landing hard on the remainder of the deck, he badly injured his knee. He was rescued, but not before experiencing the intense fear that he was about to die before he could accomplish all that he hoped.[49] Penfield's convalescence was kindly arranged by the Oslers, and he was able to closely observe Sir William as he prepared talks, visited patients, and entertained friends and students. His was a model for the family and professional life that Penfield envisioned for himself. Remembering this influential period in his life, he wrote, "If I summon before me my highest ideals of men and medicine, I find them sprung from the spirit of Osler."[50]

HOPKINS

Penfield and the two other American Rhodes Scholars, Wilburt Davison and Emile Holman, graduated from Sherrington's physiology class, received their BAs, and were admitted to Johns Hopkins for two years of clinical training, supported by Osler's letters of reference. During the summer of 1917, Penfield married Helen Kermott, and a few days after the wedding, they sailed for France to volunteer at the Red Cross Military Hospital. There he met his friend and mentor John Finney, who was setting up the medical unit for the newly-arrived US contingent. He advised Penfield to return to Baltimore and finish his medical degree: "Your country needs well-trained doctors more than it does orderlies in the Army Medical Corps."[51]

In his last trimester at Johns Hopkins, Penfield felt privileged to contribute to the war effort by working in Professor William Howell's physiology laboratory on research into the effects of shell shock on soldiers. He also did a separate independent study, examining microscopic sections of specimens removed from patients during surgery, and writing up his descriptions and diagnoses, verifying his results with the departmental findings. He was learning pathology on his own. As he wrote, "There is no one to instruct me."[52]

After graduating from Johns Hopkins in June 1918, Penfield obtained a surgical internship for six months at the Peter Bent Brigham Hospital in Boston, where Harvey Cushing was chief of surgery. Cushing had graduated from Harvard Medical School in 1896 and was William Halsted's assistant resident in surgery at Johns Hopkins for four years before spending time abroad with Theodor Kocher and William Horsley, as well as Charles Sherrington.[53] As an observer, Penfield made detailed notes and drawings of Cushing's techniques, adding his own commentary about how he might change the surgical intervention. Penfield and Cushing became close friends over the years, writing letters to consult each other on difficult cases, exchanging slides, and referring patients whose illness required a particular specialization. Penfield "held an abiding respect for Cushing and regarded him as his main mentor in neurosurgery."[54] Although Cushing offered him a place as an assistant on his service, Penfield had already decided to return to Oxford for the third year of his Rhodes Scholarship and continue his physiological research in Sherrington's laboratory: "I wanted to know all that was known about the human brain, neuropathology, neuroanatomy, and neurocytology. Then I would learn clinical neurology and finally go on to the operative technique of neurosurgery."[55]

Penfield arrived in England with Helen and their two children in December 1919 and was welcomed by his former professor. Sherrington's election as president of the Royal Society of London meant that he would not spend a lot of time with Penfield in the laboratory, but he was continually available for consultation. Penfield called at the Osler home, but it was enshrouded in sadness: Sir William and Lady Osler's only son, Revere, had been killed on the battlefield near the end of the war, and it was a tremendous loss, from which Sir William never recovered. He contracted pneumonia after visiting a patient and passed away on 29 December 1919. Penfield attended the memorial service, thinking of his friend and mentor as "one of my heroes," who would always be with him.[56]

During his graduate work at Oxford, Penfield carried out two projects. First was a study of the Golgi apparatus of the nerve cells located in the anterior horn of the spinal cord that control muscle contraction. Following transection of the sciatic nerve, he noted changes in the Golgi apparatus, characterized by its eccentric displacement and retispersion in the nerve cell body. For this research, which was published in *Brain*,[57] Penfield received his Oxford BSc.

A more extensive project, a detailed study of spinal reflexes in the chronic as well as the acute decerebrate animal, was carried out with Cuthbert Bazett and also reported at length in *Brain*.[58] Sherrington had used the decerebrate preparation since 1898, during his Liverpool period, but most of his studies had been in the acute stage after decerebration. It was a tour de force for Bazett and Penfield to keep their animals surviving for as long as three weeks. Their results added to the understanding of how the lower part of the brain reacts after head injury, and how human brain mechanisms relate to consciousness.

These two research projects in the Sherrington laboratory epitomized Penfield's later career; he would become an expert neurocytologist and neuropathologist on the one hand, and on the other, a neurosurgeon well-versed in the fundamentals of the nervous system.[59] In a tribute to Sherrington many years later, Penfield noted, "It was not the example of Horsley or Cushing that led me into surgery of the nervous system. It was the inspiration of Sherrington. He was, so it seemed to me from the first, a surgical physiologist, and I hoped then to become a physiological surgeon."[60]

After the Rhodes Scholarship funding finished, Penfield was able to continue his graduate work on a Beit Memorial Research Fellowship, obtained through Sherrington, with references from Gordon Holmes and Harvey Cushing. He spent six months at the National Hospital for Paralysis and Epileptics, Queen Square, London, where he was fortunate to come under the influence of outstanding clinical teachers. Among them were Godwin Greenfield, with whom he studied neuropathology, and Gordon Holmes, the neuroanatomist and neurologist who became a teacher, advisor, and close friend.[61] He then went to London in 1903 and became an assistant house physician at Queen Square under Hughlings Jackson, whose view of clinical investigation was that it was necessarily linked to pathology – "A practitioner must not be a pathologist only, although unless he be a pathologist, he cannot be a good practitioner."[62] In addition to working with Holmes, Penfield also assisted the neurosurgeon Percy Sargent, a student of Sir Victor Horsley, the father of British neurosurgery. This was Penfield's first exposure to brain surgery in the operating room. Sargent's rapid, skilful resection of a skull tumour prompted Penfield to review a series of similar cases, some operated on by Horsley, and this study became the basis for Penfield's first neurosurgical publication.[63]

At the end of his time in London and Oxford, Penfield and his family set sail for New York in May 1921. He had received a job offer in Detroit at the Henry Ford Hospital, but at the interview he discovered that laboratory research by physicians was not encouraged there. While visiting friends and former teachers in Boston and New York, he heard that Allen Whipple had an opening at the Presbyterian Hospital.

COLUMBIA

Allen Whipple had been appointed to the surgical staff of New York's Presbyterian Hospital in 1921. He was recognized as an upcoming leader in American surgery, known for developing techniques for surgery on the gall bladder and pancreas, and influential in American surgical education. Whipple offered Penfield his ideal job, "exactly as I would have wished for if I had Aladdin's lamp":[64] a university appointment, a guaranteed income, opportunity to take general training with senior members of the surgical team and to manage any neurosurgical cases himself, the chance to teach residents and students, to oversee neurological autopsies, and to pursue his research in pathology. He was also able to travel and visit established neurosurgeons to learn their surgical rituals – Walter Dandy in Baltimore, Charles Frazier in Philadelphia, and Harvey Cushing in Boston.[65]

As Penfield's surgical skill steadily improved, he began to take a special interest in epilepsy. William Clarke, the surgical pathologist at the New York College of Physicians and Surgeons, prompted his research plans. Clarke suggested that Penfield study experimental brain wounds at different intervals by examining glial cells under the microscope. After months of work, Penfield had only mediocre results. The cell-staining techniques available in Clarke's laboratory were inadequate and showed the cells only "in ghostly outline … It was said that they nourished and supported the neurons but no one could see what they were doing and I could not tell how they might be changing while the brain recovered from injury. Perhaps if I could demonstrate these cells clearly I might understand the healing process in the brain and discover why a healing scar is followed so often by epilepsy."[66] Penfield recalled that Sherrington had suggested that he learn the staining techniques using silver and gold salts developed by Santiago Ramón y Cajal[67] and his collaborator, Pio del Río-Hortega. Allen Whipple generously supported Penfield's quixotic request for study leave in Spain. He secured funds from Mrs Isabel Stillman Rockefeller, the mother of one of his patients, as well as donations from his surgical colleagues to underwrite the trip for him, his wife, and family to spend six months in Madrid and France. While in Spain, Penfield worked with del Río-Ortega, from whom he learned the metallic techniques for staining glial cells, and with whom he made perhaps his most significant discovery, the oligodendrocyte.[68] It is also with del Río-Hortega that Penfield identified the meningocerebral cicatrix.[69] After Penfield's study trip, Whipple put him in full charge of neurosurgery at the Presbyterian Hospital. In addition, he was asked by Walter Palmer, director of Medical Services, to see patients with neurological problems on the medical wards. He became responsible for reporting the neuropathology of autopsy cases and of the neurosurgical specimens sent from Charles Elsberg's operations at the Neurological Institute of New York. He also acquired an assistant, William Cone, a graduate of Iowa Medical School, who had come to the laboratories of the Presbyterian on a National Research Council Fellowship; he too was keenly interested in brain pathology and neurosurgery.

To meet Penfield's needs for research, a room in one of the hospital towers was rebuilt to create a laboratory of neurocytology, along the design of the Spanish laboratories, with the provision of a technician and secretary. Another gift from Mrs Isabel Stillman Rockefeller covered the cost of this laboratory for the next three years.[70] Penfield and Cone worked effectively as complementary partners on the wards, in the operating room, and in the laboratory. Their situation seemed solidly established and their future appeared promising. Transfer of the patients and staff of the old Presbyterian Hospital to the new medical complex now under construction uptown was planned to take place in March 1928. To this would be added a new building for the Neurological Institute, scheduled to open in March 1929. But in those plans lay Penfield's main cause for concern. He had previously tried to work at the New York Neurological Institute, but had been frustrated by the lack of research laboratories. In addition, the real situation, as Penfield later explained it, was that he could not accept dictation from the institute's chief neurosurgeon,

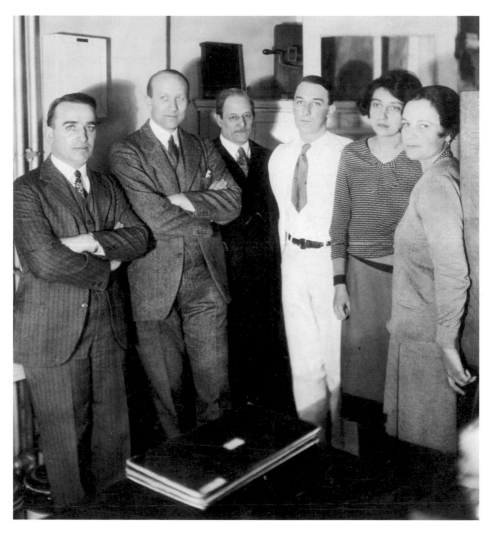

Figure 1.2: The Department of Neuropathology at Columbia, 1927: (*left to right*) Cone; Penfield; Laidlaw; Deery; a technician; and, Gourday, secretary. (Wilder Penfield Archive)

Charles Elsberg, or the chief neurologist, Frederick Tilney, both of whom dominated the field of these specialities. Elsberg, in particular, a graduate in medicine from Columbia University who had been the first chief of neurological surgery at the institute since 1909 and became its director in 1927, evidently held a firm hand over the future plans for the new institute, and Penfield felt left out of this planning process. He understood well that the Neurological and Neurosurgical Service, as well as the neuropathological laboratories, that he and Cone had worked so hard to develop at the Presbyterian Hospital, would be absorbed into the new Neurological Institute. And next in

line to succeed Elsberg as director of the Neurosurgical Service at the new
institute was Byron Stookey, four years senior to Penfield. A soundly competent clinical surgeon, Stookey had worked with the British surgeons during the
war, then since 1919 he had practised neurosurgery at the Bellevue Hospital
and the institute.

This was Penfield's situation in June 1927 when he unexpectedly received
a letter from Edward Archibald of Montreal, asking whether he would consider taking charge of neurosurgery at the Royal Victoria Hospital and McGill
University:

> Dear Dr Penfield,
> I am looking for a man to come up to Montreal and do neurological sur-
> gery. Such a man would have a practically independent service in the
> Royal Victoria Hospital, and would also have a University appointment.
> There would be no particular salary, but it could be practically guaran-
> teed that all the private work of this nature in the Hospital would go to
> him. The field is open; there is nobody else doing it in Montreal, except
> one of the juniors at the General Hospital, who is also a general surgeon.
> The Medical Board of the Royal Victoria Hospital is supporting me
> unanimously, as also the Board of Trustees.
>   I am writing to ask whether you would consider a position of this
> sort. I have been doing this work up to the present, but I am anxious to
> devote myself more to lung surgery, and I would turn over to you every-
> thing in neurological surgery that came my way, and I know that all the
> others of the staff would do the same … I would be glad to run down for
> a day or two to New York and see you, preferably on a day when you
> could show me some operating.[71]

Archibald visited New York on 25 June 1927 and watched Penfield and Cone
remove an acoustic neuroma. Then Archibald and Penfield exchanged ideas
over a very long lunch, and Archibald described his aim to strengthen McGill's
surgical department. Penfield explained his ambitious plans for neurosurgery,
and he was charmed and inspired by Archibald and attracted by his depiction
of Montreal, "this great bilingual city." But he made it clear to Archibald from
the outset that he would not come to Montreal simply to practise neurosurgery
but to build up a team to develop a neurological clinic and to continue neuropathological research.

In a letter to Archibald, Penfield itemized the requirements, which included
the segregation of beds for neurosurgical patients, a clinical intern and a research fellow in neurosurgery, academic standing for neurosurgery equal to that

for neurology, association with both the Royal Victoria and Montreal General Hospitals, an examining room with diagnostic equipment and the vital part of the clinic, the laboratory of neuropathology, "where the Staff of Neurology and Neurosurgery could work together with common interests and mutual benefit," like the Neurocytology Laboratory in New York. The laboratory would need equipment and a budget. He also requested a guarantee for his own income of $10,000 yearly for five years (less than he was then making in New York). He required a further safeguard, inasmuch as there was no chief surgeon at the RVH, that if a chief other than Archibald was appointed, no change in the organization of the neurosurgical clinic could be made without a year's notice. If the arrangements for scientific work and the guarantee of his income could be assured, Penfield concluded, "I very much want to accept an invitation to Montreal."[72] After discussing the offer with Bill Cone, Penfield added Cone's salary to the list of requirements.

Archibald wrote on 9 August that he would meet the conditions in Penfield's outline; this would require agreement between the faculty and the hospitals and the garnering of the necessary funds. In a reply of 16 September, Penfield noted, "I am anxious to know the outcome of the committee meetings as I find an unsettled state of mind hard to bear." And he added, "You paint a rather alluring future in Montreal which I should like to believe possible." He expected to hear from Archibald "in the next week or two," but by the end of October, Archibald reported that so far he had no support for the laboratory expenses or for the salary of Dr Cone. In early January 1928, having given up all expectation of Montreal, Penfield began to prepare for the move up to the new Columbia University Medical Center, where Elsberg had made him feel that "he *might* have a place for me"[73] at the Neurological Institute of New York.

Then, on 10 January 1928, Archibald sent a telegram asking if Penfield could come to Montreal for a day of discussion. Two evenings later, the *Montreal Limited* sped through the darkness to its destination, and as the winter light broke through the morning fog on the river, Wilder Penfield sensed that he was beginning a new journey after a long preparation, but it was one for which he was ready. When the train arrived at the majestic Windsor Station, Penfield stepped out onto the freshly fallen snow and reached for the outstretched hand of Edward Archibald, who was waiting for him on the platform.

2

Towards a New Venture

WILLIAM FEINDEL AND ELIZABETH MALONEY

MCGILL AND THE ROCKEFELLERS

When Wilder Penfield and Edward Archibald arranged to meet in Montreal on a cold day in January 1928, both knew what they hoped to gain from the visit. They had been corresponding for several months since Archibald's initial interview with Penfield in New York, and his subsequent invitation to consider taking over the neurosurgical clinic at Montreal's Royal Victoria Hospital. Along with his academic role as chairman of the Department of Surgery, Archibald was responsible for neurosurgery at the RVH, but he had become more interested in pursuing thoracic research, and he wanted to centre his surgical expertise in that specialty. His background and training in neurosurgery, as well as a reference from his friend, Archibald Malloch, the medical historian and close friend of Sir William Osler, led him to consider Penfield as the ideal candidate to replace him.

His visit to New York to observe Penfield remove a brain tumour, and their long talk afterwards, during which both men outlined their hopes for creating a solid neurosurgical practice, convinced Archibald that Penfield was the right man for the job. As he later wrote to Penfield, "If you do come, I expect that ten years from now the hub of surgical neurology, in this continent, will be transferred from Boston [where Harvey Cushing was the surgeon-in-chief] to Montreal."[1]

Archibald understood that the key to Penfield's accepting the Montreal position was to secure laboratory space for neurological research in close proximity to the neurosurgical clinic. "Neurosurgery must go hand-in-hand with neurology," Penfield had written to him. "The ideal relationship seems to me to be that the neurosurgeon should be a neurologist by interest and training, a surgeon by profession."[2] Combining surgical expertise with dedicated laboratory research was exactly the direction that the dean of the Faculty of Medicine,

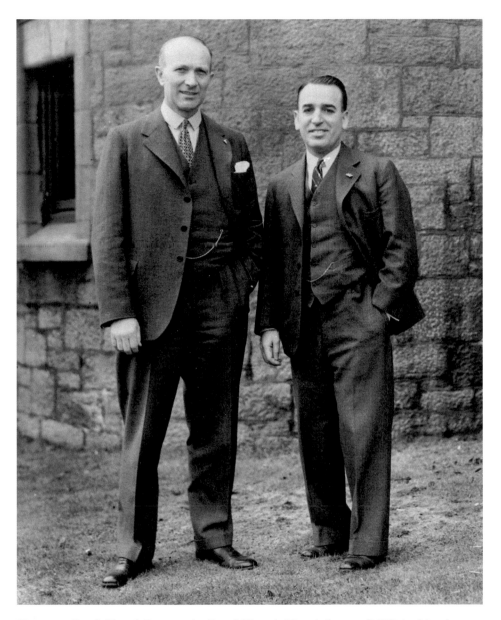

Figure 2.1: Penfield and Cone at the Royal Victoria Hospital, 1928. (MNI Archives)

Charles F. Martin, was planning in his reform of the medical education program that had been in place for twenty years at McGill.

Like Archibald, Charles Martin was a graduate of McGill. He received his medical degree in 1892 and then studied in Germany under the pathologist Johannes Orth,[3] before becoming a staff member at the RVH. Seven years later, he was named professor of medicine at McGill and physician-in-chief at the

RVH and was considered one of the most brilliant clinical teachers of his day.[4] During the First World War he served with the McGill Surgical Unit in Boulogne, where Herbert S. Birkett, Archibald, Jonathan Meakins, John McCrae, Campbell Howard, and Colin Russel, among others, worked closely together to treat wounded soldiers. After the war, their loyal team spirit was evident in planning the future of McGill medicine.

As chairman of the Education Committee of the medical faculty, Martin had ideas for making significant changes in the way medicine was taught at McGill and practised in the hospital's clinics. While he was in London at the end of the war, he had the opportunity to seek Sir William Osler's opinion about a reorganization of the clinical services, including the development of a research unit that would improve McGill's future as a centre of progressive medical education.[5] Osler had been proposing changes to medical education for many years, and he was a very enthusiastic supporter of Martin's plans.[6] In particular, Osler proposed the appointment of full-time, salaried professors and teaching assistants to operate the university clinics. Osler's plan was eventually adopted by the Faculty of Medicine and laid the groundwork for McGill's later success in combining teaching and research with clinical practice. As for funding to achieve this goal, "an appeal should be made to the public," and also to the Rockefeller Foundation, which had been very generous in supporting medical schools in the United States. A month later, while he was on vacation in Jersey, Osler sent a letter to John D. Rockefeller Jr, which began, "Do you think the Board would help the establishment at Montreal of up-to-date medical & surgical clinics?"[7] This letter proved to be a catalyst for bringing about major donations to McGill from the Rockefeller Foundation.

Osler was already well known and respected by the Rockefellers. "It was [his] popular textbook of 1892, *The Principles and Practice of Medicine*,[8] that instigated Frederick Gates to persuade John D. Rockefeller, Sr to direct his immense fortune to medical research."[9] Gates, Rockefeller's close advisor and "architect of John D. Rockefeller Sr's philanthropic plan,"[10] had read Osler's book "from beginning to end with absorbing interest and with a medical dictionary at my side." The result was the founding of the Rockefeller Institute for Medical Research, chaired by William H. Welch, Osler's colleague and co-founder of Johns Hopkins Hospital. As Gates described these events to Osler, he added, "You might be gratified to know of an incidental and perhaps to you quite unexpected good which your valuable work has wrought."[11] Osler replied the next day, "I have been greatly interested in the Rockefeller Institute, and feel sure that good results will come of it." He then pointed out the shortcomings of research and teaching in North American medical schools, explaining that "there is an increasing difficulty in getting the best sorts of men to devote themselves to scientific work. One serious problem is the limited number of positions with which living salaries are attached."[12]

In 1907, the Medical Building at McGill was destroyed by fire. Osler, then at Oxford, wrote to Gates to ask if the Rockefellers could help, but the response was far from forthcoming.[13] John D. Rockefeller Jr himself replied to Osler, regretting that the General Education Board could not fund McGill because its New York charter permitted grants only within the United States.[14] However, Osler's letter evoked a debate that led to the formation of a committee, chaired by William Welch, which recommended expansion of the board's interests to a wider mandate to aid medical education and preventive medicine. Thus, Osler's request stimulated much consideration and expert consultation that resulted in the incorporation of the Rockefeller Foundation in 1913 "to promote the well-being of mankind throughout the world."[15] In light of these connections, Osler turned again to the Rockefellers, this time to help establish "up-to-date Medical and Surgical Clinics"[16] for McGill. On Christmas Day 1919, John D. Rockefeller Sr announced another gift of $100 million to the Rockefeller Foundation, intending this donation "for the promotion of medical education and public health in different parts of the world."[17] And in making the gift, Rockefeller specifically expressed an interest in Canadian medical education. Unfortunately, Osler would never hear of McGill's good fortune. Unable to shake off a persisting lung infection that had plagued him through the fall, Osler died at Oxford on the afternoon of 29 December 1919.

Between March and July of 1920, the Rockefeller Foundation's representatives George Vincent and Richard Pearce made four visits to Montreal.[18] Aware that the Rockefeller Foundation encouraged their funding institutions to provide matching funds from private and government sources, Chancellor Edward Beatty assured Vincent that $900,000 to construct new buildings for physiology, pathology, and psychiatry could be raised by McGill. On this basis, and a report by Richard Pearce, the executive committee of the Rockefeller Foundation Board adopted a resolution to pledge $1,000,000 to McGill to serve as a general endowment for the Faculty of Medicine.

Meanwhile, General Sir Arthur Currie, newly appointed principal of McGill, had been busy shoring up the university's finances. Formerly commanding officer of the Canadian Corps in France during the First World War, Currie brought to McGill the outstanding gifts of organization and energy that he had displayed so brilliantly on the battlefields of Europe. During his first six months in office, together with some members of the board of governors, he visited alumni across Canada and the United States in a highly successful fundraising campaign to mark McGill's centenary. Within two days of receiving the Rockefeller letter of 23 November 1920, Currie wrote the secretary of the foundation that $6,321,511 had been raised or pledged.[19]

On 5 October 1922, Sir Arthur Currie presided over the formal opening of the new wing of the Biological Building to house botany, zoology, biochemistry, physiology, and pharmacology, equipped for pre-clinical laboratories. The construction heralded the first stage of a Rockefeller-McGill program for a sweeping reorganization of the medical school. Present at the opening were Sir Charles Sherrington, president of the Royal Society of London, and Harvey Cushing, then in the midst of writing his Pulitzer Prize–winning opus, *The Life of Sir William Osler*. Both spoke eloquently about the future of medical education, and Sherrington paid tribute to the high humanitarian aims of the Rockefeller Foundation.[20]

In his discussions with the Rockefeller Foundation, Charles Martin emphasized that an essential part of medical educational reform at McGill was to create a university clinic. Pearce agreed that it would be supported by the foundation, providing that the clinic was managed by Jonathan Meakins.[21] Meakins, a McGill graduate, was the professor of therapeutics at the University of Edinburgh. In 1919, he set up an innovative biological laboratory at Edinburgh, which combined academic and clinical medicine, providing for the routine needs of the clinical staff and performing clinical research. "In effect, Meakins' laboratory served not so much as a means of promoting collaboration between clinicians and academics, but rather as a site at which scientists could gain access to clinical material for the pursuit of their own relatively abstract research programs."[22] Meakins's project drew the attention of Richard Pearce as the kind of program that the Rockefeller Foundation wanted to fund. It provided Meakins with a full-time salary, and his university clinic would be supported annually through a grant.[23] Meakins returned to Montreal in 1924, and was named chair of medicine, physician-in-chief of the RVH, and director of the McGill University Clinic. As his colleague Peter T. Macklem later wrote, "Dr Meakins more than fulfilled his mandate to establish clinical research at the RVH. He wrested control of clinical laboratory services away from the Department of Pathology, so the clinical biochemistry and hematology laboratories became part of the Department of Medicine, and provided the department with an extremely valuable research infrastructure. This extraordinary accomplishment made the RVH almost unique in the world."[24]

PENFIELD AND MCGILL

These years of putting the medical education reforms in place, as well as the founding of the university clinic, created an energetic environment that Archibald believed would appeal to Penfield. Archibald and Martin had worked incessantly behind the scenes to assure support from the medical staff at the hospital and the university, as well as to obtain the promise of funding for the new neurosurgery position from patrons in the community. The day of Penfield's visit had been carefully planned: Archibald would meet Penfield's overnight train at Windsor Station and take him to his Westmount home for breakfast. At the hospital, Martin and Meakins would join them in the operating theatre, where Penfield would perform a pneumoencephalogram and give a lecture on the diagnosis of brain tumours. A visit to Horst Oertel's Pathological Institute was also scheduled, where they would discuss Penfield's laboratory needs for his research, before heading to lunch at the stately Mount Royal Club. Later in the afternoon, they would have tea with Sir Vincent Meredith, formidable president of the RVH. Penfield would then take the evening train back to New York. But not everything went as smoothly as Martin and Archibald had expected. The demonstration caused stress to the patient, so it had to be postponed and be completed by a resident. More importantly, Horst Oertel was less than enthusiastic about having Penfield share his laboratory space. Meakins and Archibald knew this to be a key issue: without the ability "to go back and forth quickly from laboratory to operating table,"[25] there would be no reason for Penfield to come to Montreal.

From his own experience in developing a long-term research process, Meakins understood that Penfield's decision to take the position rested on whether he could continue the neurological investigations he had begun at the Presbyterian Hospital. He quickly offered to rearrange his university clinic so that Penfield and his research staff would have three small rooms in which to work. He told Penfield, "I'm ready to do this because you say you hope to serve the future of medical neurology as well as surgical neurology."[26] They toured the busy laboratory facilities, and as Penfield later wrote, "I was content at once. To be crowded, I realized was nothing. The advantage of working in such an environment of quality and scientific excellence was everything."[27]

Lunch in Penfield's honour at the Mount Royal Club was a success. The warm hospitality of the guests reminded Penfield of his time at Oxford, and he had a sense "of being at home with men I liked."[28] Penfield and Archibald walked up from the club along Peel Street, which was brilliant with banks of new snow. There was a last meeting, one that Archibald was dreading, with Sir Vincent Meredith, who, in his position as president of the RVH, had continuously raised barriers to Archibald's prospective appointment as surgeon-in-chief. He had been given the impression that Archibald was "too occupied with research"[29] to take on administrative duties. Sir Vincent was not in good health, however, and Penfield rightly predicted that he would not have a major role in overseeing the hospital's activities for very long.

In spite of the unexpected insight into the politics and power at McGill and the RVH, the day ended positively, and Penfield agreed to accept the position, later recalling that as he and Archibald walked down the steep hill from the hospital, the winter sunset cast a golden light on the great buildings of Montreal below them. "This beauty," he wrote, "seemed to me a promise, for great things in the years to come."[30]

On the train back to New York after his Montreal visit, Penfield had another sleepless night, looking out at the darkness and wondering if he had made the right decision. It was an enormous commitment, not only for his own future and that of his family, but also to Archibald, Martin, and Meakins, who all believed that he could develop a strong neurosurgery department at the RVH. He reasoned that he could carry on at the New York Presbyterian Hospital at a certain level, but he also knew that he did not have enough experience to fully understand how to effectively treat an injured brain. Arriving at the Yonkers Station near his home in Riverdale, Penfield saw hope in the sunrise that carried its brilliance from the previous day's promise. During the next few days, while he and Helen absorbed the meaning of the move, Penfield wrote to Charles Martin asking if it was safe to "burn my bridges." Martin's reply was "Burn your bridges."[31]

It was not easy for Penfield, or for William Cone, who agreed to accompany him, to quietly move away from New York. Both were offered prestigious jobs to stay at the Presbyterian Hospital. Cone was promised his own laboratory, and for awhile Penfield believed he would lose his closest colleague in neurological research to the newly built Neurological Institute of New York. Penfield had initially suggested to Edward Archibald that he take the opportunity to travel and study in Europe before beginning work at the RVH.[32] The deciding factor was a case referred to him by a friend of his former professor of surgical pathology at the New York College of Physicians and Surgeons, William Clarke. At the time, Clarke encouraged Penfield to intensify his research on the brain, asking him some pointed questions: "What goes on in the brain? How does it heal? What is the cause of epilepsy?"[33] The patient had suffered severe epileptic seizures after a fall. Penfield had operated and was "forced to remove more than half of the right frontal lobe, a very radical procedure. But that is what I did."[34] The surgery seemed to be successful, but Penfield could not predict what the outcome would be for the patient, and it troubled him. By chance, a colleague mentioned a neurological surgeon in Germany who was treating epileptic cases with success. Penfield immediately planned a six-month sabbatical to study and observe in Otfrid Foerster's neurological clinic in Germany.

PART ONE

The Sub-Department of Neurosurgery at the Royal Victoria Hospital, 1928–1933

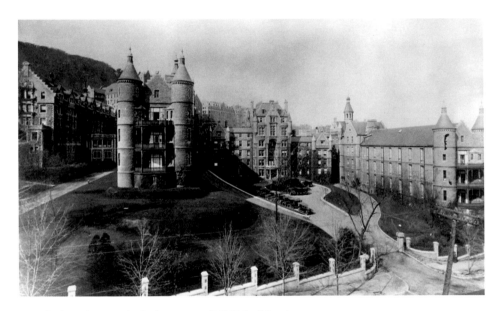

Royal Victoria Hospital, circa 1928. (MNI Archives)

3

Otfrid Foerster and the Surgical Treatment of Epilepsy

If you would be a surgeon, follow the army.
– Hippocrates

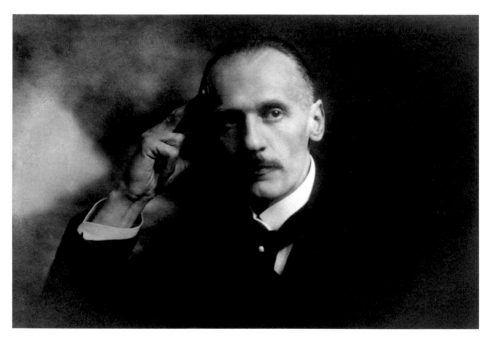

Figure 3.1: Otfrid Foerster. (MNI Archives)

Otfried Foerster was born in 1873 in Breslau, in the province of Silesia, the easternmost part of Germany. As a young man, Otfried, who would change his name to the less Teutonic Otfrid, was educated in the arts and in the classics of Western civilization by his father, a professor of philology and of archeology.[1] Foerster learned to speak ancient Greek and Latin, French, English, and Italian. As befits a realist living in a disputed area on the Germano-Polish frontier, he also learned Polish and Russian.[2] The latter served Foerster well later in his career when he was called upon in 1922 by the newly formed Union of Soviet Socialist Republics to attend Lenin, who was slowly dying from a stroke.[3]

After a brief interest in the natural sciences, Foerster set his sail on the great uncharted sea of neurology. He obtained his medical degree in 1897 at the age of twenty-four, and at the suggestion of his teacher, Karl Wernicke, he travelled to Paris, London, and Heiden, Switzerland, to complete his medical training in neurology.[4] His primary goal was to study the anatomy of the brain with Jules Dejerine, but while in Paris he also studied with Pierre Marie and Joseph Babinski.[5] From Paris, Foerster travelled to England, where he visited David Ferrier's laboratory at a time when Ferrier was studying the localization of motor function of the brain in a variety of animals, including the great apes. Through the influence of the great French clinicians and the pioneering British experimenters, Foerster honed the two great skills that characterized him as a physician-scientist: remarkable powers of observation, and the application of insights gained in the laboratory to the care of his patients.

At the end of his European travels, Foerster made the first of his four trips to the United States, to popularize a new treatment for tabes dorsalis, a syphilitic infection of the spinal cord, on which he had worked with Heinrich Frenkel in Switzerland.[6] It was on this trip that he met John D. Rockefeller, whose foundation would later play such a great part in Foerster's and Penfield's careers.

Foerster's initial experiments in cerebral localization were performed in a laboratory in his cellar and financed by his clinical practice. Later, when he was allocated research space in a hospital, his laboratory – where he studied the fragments of damaged brain that he had removed during surgery – consisted of a counter behind a partition in a hallway, between patient beds.[7] It was in such settings that Foerster made his great contribution to the surgical treatment of epilepsy.

Foerster became a neurosurgeon not by choice but by necessity and perhaps out of desperation, when, at the age of forty-three, as a consultant neurologist to the Sixth Army Corps in Breslau, during a shortage of qualified surgeons, he was called upon to operate on soldiers with spinal injuries.[8] At the end of the Great War, Foerster saw many who had fallen in battle, struck down by head wounds, only to become prey to uncontrollable epileptic attacks. Wartime head wounds, if not fatal, are a formidable challenge for the surgeon, even today, and in 1914, they were a nightmare from which few awoke. Not only did one have to deal with the loss of brain substance produced by the shock wave of the missile, but the projectile carried with it hair, skin, and jagged bone fragments into the cranial cavity. More often than not, the wounds became purulent as infection set in. If the patient survived, there resulted a complex, disorganized scar, which Penfield referred to as the "meningocerebral cicatrix," which is highly epileptogenic.

THE MENINGOCEREBRAL CICATRIX

On 22 April 1928, Penfield wrote his mother, "Last Sunday came a telegram from Foerster to say he would operate on a case that I would be interested in, the next day. He did a splendid operation removing a 16-year-old gunshot wound scar from the brain. It had caused epilepsy and pulled the whole brain over in a way I had discussed in London last June.[9] He made it possible to get hold of some chemicals and I took the specimen for examination. During the next three or four days I worked hard at the tissue and succeeded in getting some very pretty stains of different kinds of glia cells. In such tissue lies hidden some of the secrets of epilepsy."[10]

Penfield's first significant contribution to neurosurgery was the description of the meningocerebral cicatrix (MCC), such as the one Foerster removed from his patient, with the great Spanish histologist Pío del Río-Hortega in 1927.[11] Using del Río-Hortega's gold and silver stains, Penfield observed that the MCC is composed of radially arranged strands of fibrous tissue. Abnormal blood vessels invade the region as the collagenous core thickens, solidifies, and contracts, causing a contraction of the injured area towards the site of entry.[12] This reaction is especially severe in the presence of infection:

> In large wounds with much brain destruction, and particularly in those where there is some degree of infection, the resultant gliosis and cicatricial contraction is many times increased … there is widespread fibroblastic growth and a network of collagen fibers is laid down so vigorous, dense and tangled that the contractile forces might well be considerable. The surrounding gliosis is equally vigorous. If such traction is exerted local movement of the brain is to be expected … The cortex may be pulled down toward the connective tissue core, and the white matter … can be seen to deviate toward the focus.[13]

Penfield goes on to state that Foerster had seen the effect of such a cicatrix on pneumoencephalography (PEG) – the insufflation of air into the fluid cavities of the brain – and thus identifying the site of the lesion.[14]

Penfield stressed that the meshwork of blood vessels entrapped within the cicatricial core anastomosed with the cortical blood vessels of the tissue around the offending scar.[15] This observation led Penfield to theorize that the progressive traction of the arteries encased within the scar on the surrounding cortical arterioles could result in vasoconstriction and focal ischemia, which would, in turn, produce an epileptic seizure. Thus, Penfield felt that the MCC was in itself sufficient to cause post-traumatic epilepsy: "Through this vascular scar is exerted, inevitably, an active pull upon the brain … This pull, and the plexus of newly formed vessels caught in it, provide in our opinion a mechanism very important in the aetiology of the focal epilepsy which results from a penetrating wound of the brain."[16]

The discovery of the MCC stimulated Penfield's interest in the surgical treatment of epilepsy, since he had identified a lesion that he could operate upon with the hope of a cure or at least of mitigation of a patient's seizures. It also stimulated his interest in cerebrovascular physiology and cerebral vasoreactivity that would prove to be fertile ground for research. Indeed, one of Penfield's first significant papers to come from Montreal, even before the MNI was formally inaugurated, was on vasodilator nerves, which he wrote with one of his first fellows, Jerzy Chorobski. But for now, Penfield was more interested in Foerster's approach in the surgical treatment of post-traumatic epilepsy.

"I DECIDED THAT I COULD DO NO WORSE"

As part of his approach to the treatment of epileptic patients, Foerster first obtained a detailed description of the seizure by interviewing the patient and his family. He then performed a meticulous physical examination. This information would provide clues to the site of the offending lesion. Foerster would often have his patient hyperventilate, which, in changing the balance between the oxygen and carbon dioxide concentrations in the brain, often produced a seizure, whose onset Foerster could observe to confirm his initial impression of the site of the epileptogenic lesion.[17] PEG provided final corroboration of the site of the scar. He then convinced a surgeon trained in another specialty to breach the calvarium and operate upon the brain so as to resect the scarred area.[18] Eventually, Foerster took up the scalpel himself, because, as he explained, "I have to make a diagnosis, I have to go with a patient to the operating room. I have to tell Mikulicz (a general surgeon) where to operate. I have to tell him what to do when he gets inside, and then the patients all died. I decided I could not do worse."[19]

Craniotomy – the surgical removal of a bone flap to expose the underlying brain – was, in Foerster's time, a formidable undertaking and was considered only in the direst of circumstances. In this mythic phase of neurosurgery, when neither the way in nor the way out was known, and before the importance of asepsis was realized, the surgical mortality was horrendous. In addition, there were no effective ways of arresting bleeding, which, if severe, could cause shock, even death from loss of blood. Heavy bleeding also flooded the operative field,

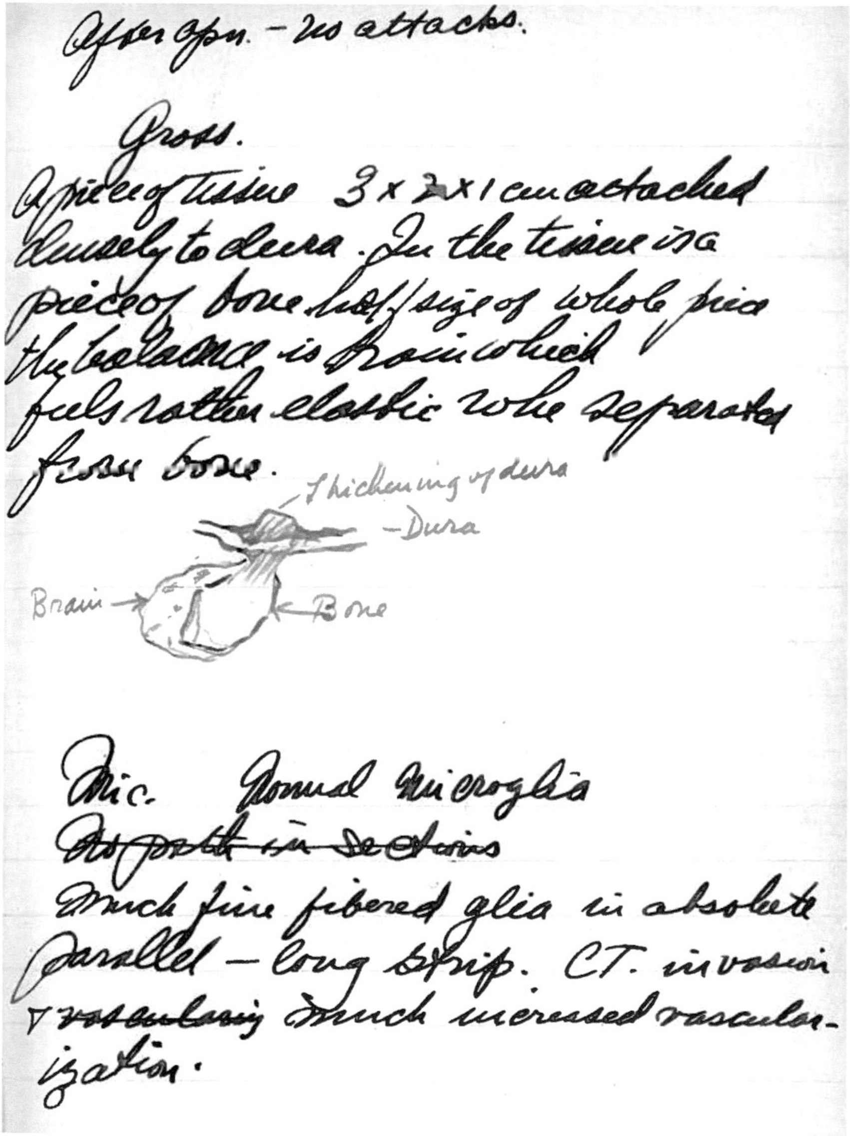

After opn. – no attacks.

Gross.

A piece of tissue 3 x 2 x 1 cm attached densely to dura. In the tissue is a piece of bone half size of whole piece the balance is brain which feels rotten elastic when separated from bone.

Thickening of dura

– Dura

Brain →

← Bone

Mic. Normal microglia
No path in sections
Much fine fibered glia in absolute parallel – long strip. CT. invasion & vascularity much increased vascularization.

Figure 3.2: A page from the notebook that Penfield kept in Breslau, depicting his sketch and description of a meningocerebral cicatrix. (McGill Archives)

obscuring the surgeon's view. Foerster's operative results, however, were good enough for patients to continue to come to him for relief. Eventually, brain surgeons also made their way to his clinic. All would comment on Foerster's gentleness when dealing with the cortex of the brain, but few would be kind in their assessment of his surgical abilities. Paul Bucy, the influential American neurosurgeon remembered "a small stooped man, asthenic in appearance …

amazingly alert mentally and very vivacious," a man who "operated under unbelievably difficult conditions and was a very crude surgeon."[20] To another observer, "it was quite obvious to one watching Foerster operate that he had not grown up in surgery ... Everything [in his operating room] seemed to be unusual and unsurgical."[21] It must have been a daunting sight to watch Foerster operate. The means at his disposal were rudimentary, and as Bucy noted, "one of the greatest deficiencies was the lack of adequate illumination. The only light he had came from a brass student light held in the hands of anyone that he could get to do so."[22]

Perhaps recalling his father's lectures in archaeology, Foerster, operating under local anesthesia, did not raise a bone flap as we would today, all of one piece, but rather he chipped away, bit by bit, at the skull until an opening of adequate size was produced. Nonetheless, as Zülch points out, with his "narrow and skilled hands ... Foerster was very subtle when he opened the dura mater, and his results were in his time surprisingly good because of his remarkable speed and manual dexterity and his superb understanding of the nervous system."[23]

It was in this darkened atmosphere that Foerster undertook the operative treatment of epileptic patients. His rationale was quite simply that there was a scar resulting from the original injury that, in Penfield's words, "exerted an evil influence" on the brain – what Penfield would later refer to as "nociferous cortex" – setting off a cascade of uncontrolled electrical activity leading to a seizure. Thus, with the passage of time and as his reputation grew, a steady stream of neurosurgeons came to Foerster's clinic, some to hold lights, most to be illuminated, all to be welcomed.

A GENTLE CURRENT APPLIED TO THE BRAIN

Foerster confirmed that the area that he proposed to excise was epileptogenic by gently tugging on the epileptogenic scar or by electrically stimulating the suspicious area and its surroundings, in an attempt to produce a seizure. The offending area would then be excised. With the advent of electroencephalography (EEG) in 1934, Foerster performed an electro-corticogram (ECoG) using small recording electrodes, gently applied to the surface of the exposed brain, to identify the epileptic focus, much as Penfield would but with more refined equipment.[24]

As he had observed Ferrier do in his laboratory, Foerster applied a gentle, low-voltage current to discrete points of the exposed cortex using a small, stimulating hand-held electrode, and observed which involuntary movement was

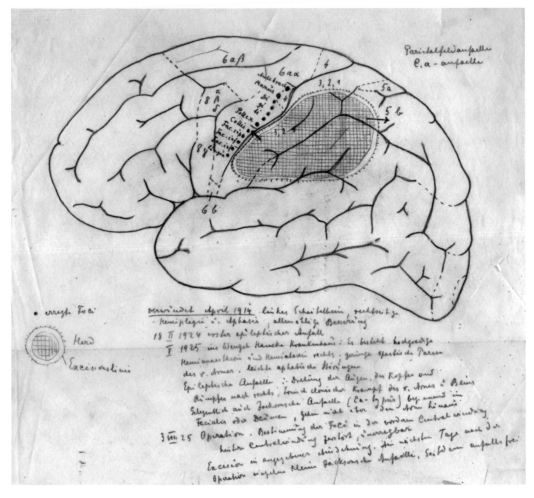

Figure 3.3: Foerster's brain map and notes on patient K., whose seizures originated from the parietal region. The notes and the map illustrating the results of stimulation to identify the motor strip and epileptogenic zone are typical of Foerster's clinical method, operative approach, and scientific contributions to neurophysiology. The arrow indicates a dot corresponding to the thumb area where stimulation produced a seizure (*erregte Foci*). The inner circle to the left indicates the epileptogenic area and the outer circle indicates the excision line. Forester's handwritten notes indicate that the patient sustained a wound to the right parietal bone in April 1914, which produced hemiplegia and aphasia that slowly improved. He experienced his first seizure ten years later, on 18 February 1924. Examination in May 1925 revealed pronounced right-sided hemi-anaesthesia and hemi-ataxia, slight spastic paresis of the right arm, and mild aphasia. Epileptic seizures consisted of turning of the eyes, head, and trunk to the right, and tonic-clonic spasms of the right arm and leg. There were occasional Jacksonian seizures involving the face or leg, which did not extend beyond the arm. The patient was operated upon on 3 August 1925. An epileptic focus was identified in the pre-central convolution. The post-central gyrus was scarred and unresponsive to electrical stimulation. The area indicated on the brain map was resected. There were a few Jacksonian seizures on the first post-operative day but the patient was seizure-free thereafter. (MNI Archives)

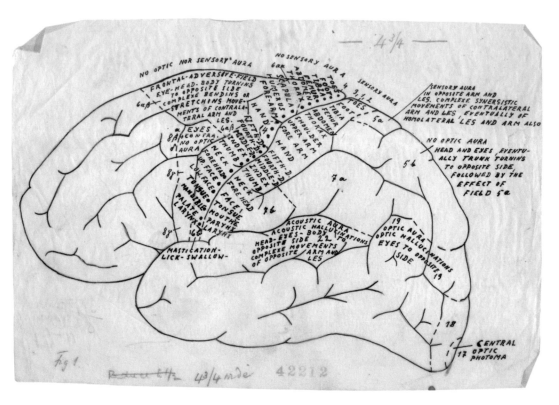

Figure 3.4: Penfield's tracing of Foerster's composite map where he has transcribed and translated Foerster's results of cortical stimulation from German to English. (Penfield Archives. The final illustration was published in O. Foerster and W. Penfield, "The Structural Basis of Traumatic Epilepsy and Results of Radical Operation," *Brain* 53 [1930]: 99–119)

produced or where a sensation was felt as a result of the stimulation.[25] These points were suitably marked, photographically recorded, and, most importantly, were considered verboten, a no-man's-land that he could not breach with his scalpel. In this way, not only did Foerster remove the offending tissue in individual patients, but he also produced one of the first, accurate sensorimotor brain maps. It is for this great contribution to the understanding of the human brain that Sherrington "regarded Foerster as worthy of the Nobel prize for presenting clinical neurology in its entirety on the basis of a comprehensive knowledge of the physiology of the nervous system."[26]

FOERSTER AND CÉCILE AND OSKAR VOGT

The pre-operative localization of the seizure focus, however, required more than clinical acumen. It required knowledge of the results obtained by the physiologist working in the laboratory. The importance of the collaboration between clinician and experimenter was highlighted by Penfield, who wrote apropos of operating on patients with post-traumatic epilepsy, "In the analysis of convulsion patterns it is necessary to borrow from the observations of the experimental physiologists."[27] The Vogts performed electrical stimulation on the brain of experimental animals, much as Foerster did in his patients, and the Vogts and Foerster compared their results to better understand the cortical structure–function relationship in animal and human. Igor Klatzo, the Vogts' student and later Penfield's fellow, has highlighted the benefits of Foerster and Vogt's collaboration: "A triumphant point of collaboration between the Vogts and Foerster on this subject was reached when, on the same day, they mailed from Berlin and Breslau separately accumulated charts containing marked points of cortical stimulation with description of observed physiological responses in primate and human brains, respectively. The comparisons of these independently obtained observations revealed a striking similarity between man and monkeys regarding the topographic patterns and close association between cytoarchitectonic substrate and type of an elicited response."[28] It is noteworthy that two of Penfield's most distinguished fellows, Igor Klatzo and Jerzy Olszewski, studied with Oskar Vogt before Penfield invited them to join him in Montreal.

A CLEAN, RADICAL REMOVAL

It was in this atmosphere of scientific rigour and collaboration that Penfield came to Breslau in 1928. During his stay, he studied the results of Foerster's approach in the treatment of epileptic patients and observed that seven out of ten patients operated on by Foerster were rendered free of epilepsy. Penfield used the techniques of staining brain cells with gold and silver that he had learned in Spain to compare the MCC that Foerster had removed with the almost imperceptible reaction produced by a meticulous surgical incision of the brain in laboratory animals. Penfield then concluded that the clean, surgical scar produced by the resection of the offending cicatrix would not trade one seizure pattern for another. Thus, Foerster and Penfield stated that, regarding the surgical treatment of epilepsy, "the important feature is that the removal is radical, clean, and directed towards the lesion responsible for the attacks," and

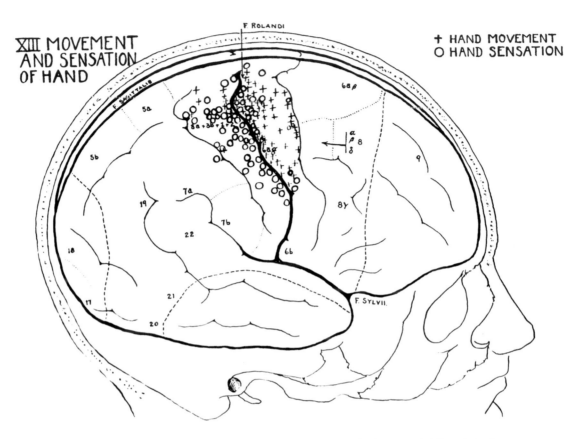

Figure 3.5: Results of sensorymotor stimulation overlaid on Penfield's original standardized brain map, from Edwin Boldrey's MSc thesis, "The Architectomic Subdivision of the Mammalian Cortex Including a Report of Electrical Stimulation of One Hundred and Five Human Cerebral Cortices," McGill University, 1936.

that the "radical, clean excision of a contracting scar does not result in scar reformation." More explicitly, after reviewing Foerster's huge experience and his own limited personal practice, Penfield concluded that "the results seem to justify radical excision of contracting areas and possibly of other foci. Such radical procedures must be preceded by careful study with scientific methods, and further safeguarded by an electrical exploration of the cortex under local anesthesia. With these precautions radical excision can be carried out without fear of removing innocent vital areas, and with the justifiable hope that the remaining comparatively normal brain thus free from tension or stimulation may no longer be subject to epileptic discharges, and its owner may be freed from the curse of epilepsy."[29]

It is this realization, the greatest advance to date in the care of epileptic patients, that Penfield, along with fine surgical instruments of German steel, brought from Breslau to the New World.

Foerster's last years were of sad decline. Out of favour, to his credit, with the National Socialists because of his attendance to Lenin and because of his wife's Jewish heritage, this man, who "wrote well and lectured brilliantly and lived for neurology,"[30] was forbidden to read anything but German scientific journals.[31] Stricken by tuberculosis, unable to work, Foerster and his wife took refuge in a Swiss sanatorium, where he died, on 15 June 1941. His wife joined him in death the following day.

"His mind was inductive, searching, and analytical, and he was untiring in the pursuit of truth, which led him in the end to lonely places."[32]

4

The Royal Victoria Hospital

The differences between the American and Canadian Medical profession
have little to do with science and much with tradition and background.
For me, to leave the one and enter the other is made easier by years of
medical study in Great Britain, and because of the fact that I can claim
as my teacher and friend, a great Canadian, Sir William Osler.
– Wilder Penfield[1]

THE ROYAL VICTORIA HOSPITAL

Upon their arrival in Montreal, Penfield and Cone constituted the Sub-Department of Neurosurgery within the Department of Surgery at the Royal Victoria Hospital. The Department of Surgery was under the chairmanship of Edward Archibald, one of the most respected and able surgeons in America at the time.[2] Neurosurgery had, however, been performed at the Royal Victoria Hospital before the arrival of Penfield and Cone. James Bell, the second head of surgery at the RVH, and his counterpart in medicine, James Stewart, had developed an interest in neurological diseases and had become de facto neurosurgeon and neurologist. Bell at first limited himself to operating upon patients who had sustained a head injury, but, with experience, he took on more elective cases. Bell taught his neurosurgical techniques to Edward Archibald, who was gradually assigned neurosurgical cases of his own.[3]

Archibald was born in Montreal in 1872 and graduated from McGill Medical School in 1896. Following graduation, Archibald travelled to Breslau, to the clinic of one of the giants of modern surgery, Jan Mikulicz-Radecki, where he came to believe that "advances in surgery could only come from research and familiarity with the basic sciences."[4] To better his skills in the treatment of neurological conditions amenable to surgery, Archibald spent three months at Queen Square, London, with Sir Victor Horsley in neurosurgery and with Sir William Gowers in neurology. Colin Russel had preceded Archibald at Queen Square and had written a paper on the somatotopic organization of the cerebral cortex and spinal cord with Horsley.[5] Russel

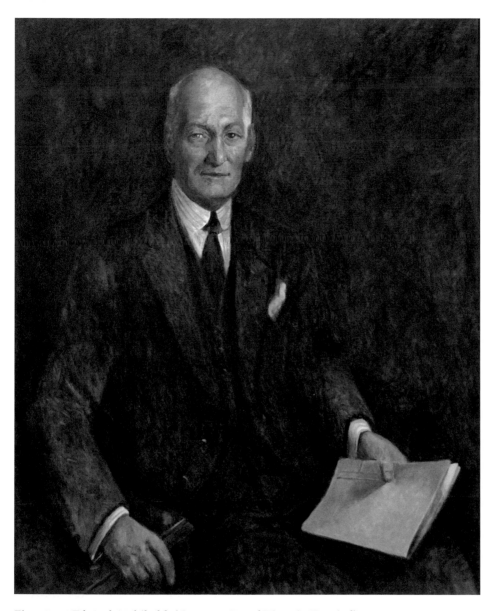

Figure 4.1: Edward Archibald. (Courtesy Royal Victoria Hospital)

became neurologist-in-chief at the RVH upon James Stewart's death in 1906.[6] In 1909 Russel wrote one of the first papers on the localization of psychical phenomena in temporal lobe epilepsy in a patient harbouring a tumour in the left mesial temporal structures. In so doing, Russel anticipated the interest of the institute in temporal lobe epilepsy and the role of the amygdala and hippocampus in its manifestations.[7]

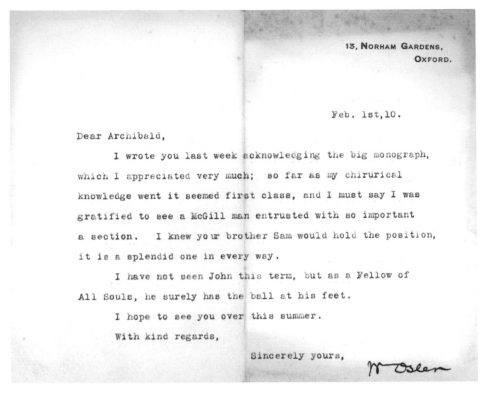

13, NORHAM GARDENS,
OXFORD.

Feb. 1st,10.

Dear Archibald,

I wrote you last week acknowledging the big monograph,
which I appreciated very much; so far as my chirurical
knowledge went it seemed first class, and I must say I was
gratified to see a McGill man entrusted with so important
a section. I knew your brother Sam would hold the position,
it is a splendid one in every way.

I have not seen John this term, but as a Fellow of
All Souls, he surely has the ball at his feet.

I hope to see you over this summer.

With kind regards,

Sincerely yours,

W Osler

Figure 4.2: Letter from Sir William Osler to Archibald, 1911, in appreciation for his *Surgical Affections and Wounds of the Head*. Sam Archibald, to whom Osler refers, was Edward's elder brother. (Edward Archibald Fond, Osler Library)

Relying heavily on the RVH's pathological museum, Archibald in 1908 published the wonderfully illustrated, 305-page monograph, *Surgical Affections and Wounds of the Head*, to rival Cushing's *Surgery of the Head* published the same year.[8] Archibald's monograph had wide distribution and was praised by his friend Sir William Osler.[9]

Later, in 1913, Archibald published a paper on ventricular puncture to relieve intracranial pressure in patients with a cerebral tumour.[10] Shortly thereafter, with the onset of the Great War, he joined the Canadian Expeditionary Corps and served in France. There, like Foerster on the other side of the wire, he gained considerable experience in the treatment of head injuries,[11] then returned from France in 1917. In recognition of his neurosurgical expertise, Archibald was invited in 1920 to be a founding member of the Society of Neurological Surgeons, the first neurosurgical society.

The Department of Surgery at the RVH was reorganized into two services in 1925. Both dealt with head injuries, while complex elective cases were sent to

Harvey Cushing in Boston. Archibald was dissatisfied with this situation, and in 1927 he proposed that the Royal Victoria Hospital establish a sub-department of neurosurgery, and sought advice of Archibald Malloch on a suitable candidate to head it. Malloch, "a medical historian and bibliophile … greatly influenced by Sir William Osler at Oxford … suggested Wilder Penfield, assistant director of neurosurgery at the Neurological Institute of New York."[12]

Archibald's knowledge of the major neurosurgical centres at the time, and his acquaintance with their directors, was invaluable in helping Penfield favour Montreal over others who had approached him, even as the summer months brought McGill to a standstill and no decision on Penfield's appointment was forthcoming. As Archibald wrote to Penfield on 9 August 1927,

I communicated through the Superintendent to the President, Sir Vincent Meredith, the substance of our talk and your general attitude, together with the information that you would not be available until next year. The President is, I think, sympathetic but merely repeated that the matter would have to be left to be got to during the summer. Things are, therefore, at a standstill for the moment, but I may say that I am quite determined that you shall come here. If you do I expect that ten years from now the hub of surgical neurology, in this continent, will be transferred from Boston to Montreal. There is nobody in Boston who can fill Cushing's shoes, and I shall expect at the very least that for the eastern half of the continent you will dispute the honours of the game with [Walter] Dandy [in Baltimore], with [Francis Clark] Grant [in Philladelphia] following as an indifferent third. Not one of them all, that I know of, is doing any fundamental work in histology, and scarcely anybody in physiology or experimental surgery. With your training along those lines you will repeat Cushing's career, and do better than he did along the experimental line.[13]

To makes matters worse for Archibald, Harvard made Penfield a tempting offer, which he relayed to Archibald on 10 November 1927:

Since I last wrote to you I have had several letters from Dr Quinby whom you know at the Brigham and I think I ought to tell you the content of these letters. Apparently they intend to organize a surgical unit similar to the medical unit which Dr Peabody had at that hospital. Dr Cobb also has a unit on full-time devoted to neurology at the same hospital. He tells me that I am being considered with one or two other men to head this unit. It would carry with it, of course, a professorship of surgery at Harvard and would involve a certain amount of surgical teaching.

There goes with the unit a budget of $30,000 ... .The chief drawback to the thing seems to me to be the fact that it carries with it some of the cares of general surgery which I should gladly avoid. On the other hand, the association with Cobb and also with Mallory would be very pleasant.[14]

Archibald responded on 14 November 1927, and put paid to Harvard:

My dear Penfield:

Your letter alarms me.

I don't think this unit at the City Hospital will be able to touch ours in the matter of opportunity for research. I assume that only a small part of this budget of $30,000 will go for neurological surgery, and I should imagine you would have very little teaching in your line, with Harvey Cushing in the same city, and occupying the position of senior professor. I am expecting that you will compete with Harvey Cushing in another city than Boston, where you might be more independent, and I feel perfectly certain that we can offer as big a source of material as can the B.C.H. [Boston City Hospital], considering that Cushing and [William Jason] Mixter are already so well established in that city. However, before the month is up I expect to have a definite statement ready for you, and I trust you will still be willing to come up here and see our people whenever I send you word.

Yours sincerely,

E. Archibald[15]

Archibald remained quite busy with neurosurgical cases throughout this period, and his enthusiasm at turning the neurosurgical service over to Penfield is almost palpable in a letter that he wrote to him on 18 June 1928: "I have on hand at the moment a gasserian ganglion, which I am to do tomorrow, and another case of tic [*douloureux*], possibly for alcohol [injection], a case of traumatic 7th nerve palsy, and a pituitary case with headache, one eye quite blind and a temporal blindness on the other side. Tomorrow I have to see a case of frontal tumour in the public ward. I have been trying to put off cases until fall, for you. The gassarian won't wait." And again, on 9 August, "I have, I think, two pituitary cases for you. We shall do our best to line up material."[16]

Archibald was true to his word and, from their arrival at the Royal Victoria in September 1928 to the end of December of that year, Penfield and Cone performed forty-nine theatre cases.

With the coming of Penfield and Cone, Archibald was freed of his neurosurgical responsibilities and could devote all of his time to his first love, thoracic surgery.[17] Anticipating the expansion of this discipline at the RVH, Archibald recruited Norman Bethune who, like Penfield, had arrived at the hospital in 1928. Bethune would become a hero of the Chinese Revolution, and Penfield alluded to a comradeship with him in order to facilitate his entry into the People's Republic of China in 1960.[18]

Edward Archibald died shortly before Christmas 1945. As befits one great academic surgeon reflecting on the passing of another, Penfield's eulogy of Archibald is heartfelt and generous:

> I cannot close this report without paying tribute to Canada's first neurosurgeon, Edward Archibald. … As a young man he was fascinated by the unexplored areas of surgery, and he chose to develop two non-existent special fields: surgery of the brain and surgery of the lung. Before long he had written a treatise on head injury in American Practice of Surgery, which was a classic in the first decade of the twentieth century.[19] But after becoming Professor of Surgery at McGill … he decided to restrict his work, and he therefore brought others to Montreal to take up neurosurgery. He handed over his practice, raised money for the support of the newcomers' laboratory, and enlisted the sympathetic assistance of Dean Martin. Thus it may be said that more than any other man, *he created neurosurgery here and laid the groundwork for the development of the Institute* … We mourn his passing and *acknowledge him as the founder of this school of neurosurgery.*[20]

THE SUB-DEPARTMENT OF NEUROSURGERY:
"A FEW FELLOWS AND A WOMAN OF FINE CHARACTER"

Madeleine Louise Ehret Ottman
The Sub-Department of Neurosurgery at the RVH was provided with neurosurgical instruments and a designated operating room, a nurse-anaesthetist, Mary Roach, and an operating room nurse, Kathleen Zwicker-Grier.[21] But a viable academic sub-department of neurosurgery also needed fellows who, while training in neurosurgery, would participate in research. And that required

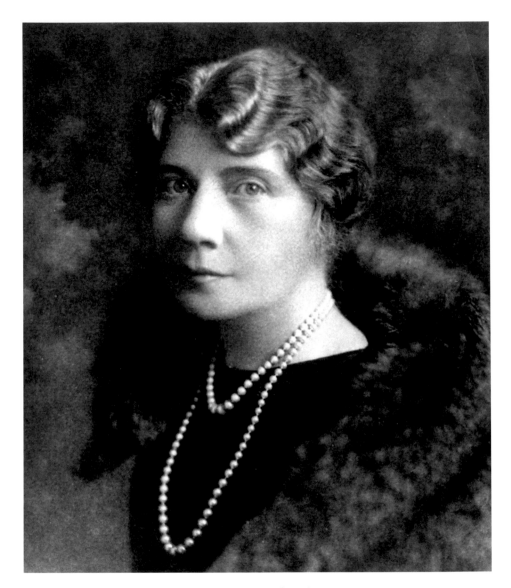

Figure 4.3: Madeleine Louise Ottman. (MNI Archives)

funding. The first to come forward with financial support for Penfield's academic activities in Montreal was Madeleine Ottman. Penfield first met Ottman in Breslau, where she was consulting with Foerster on behalf her son, suffering from epilepsy, and on whom Penfield eventually operated at the RVH. Madeleine Ottman made her gratitude to Wilder Penfield heart-warmingly clear and assured him of her continuing support in an undated, handwritten note:

Dear Dr Penfield,

It gives me great pleasure to be able to send you my check for $10,000 for research in epilepsy for this coming year. May it be of some little help to you, who are doing such outstanding, such real works for humanity in its great suffering. The next check for the same amount will be sent to you within the year. … I wish to take this opportunity to thank you from the very bottom of my heart for all your kindness to [redacted] and to me, and above all else for all you have done for [redacted] and your great care of him during his serious illness.

There are debts than can never be paid but I do want you to know that.[22]

Penfield wrote to her on 1 June 1929 on the impact of her altruism:

Dear Mrs Ottman

… The cheque for $10,000, which you have given us for research in epilepsy has just been turned over to the University to form "The Madeleine L. Ottman Fund for Research in Epilepsy." I doubt if it is possible for you to realize how much of a help this gift is. We do want to go forward in this research and it is quite a struggle. This will lift us over many of the difficulties and I hope that your generosity will bear fruit of which you will be proud.

Thank you so much.

Yours very sincerely,

WGP[23]

Madeleine Ottman died in 1930, but her death did not put an end to her generosity, as she left part of her estate for the continued support of Penfield's activities, a gift that Penfield acknowledged in a letter to her brother, dated 22 August 1930, in which he announces his plans for the Neurological Institute.

I thought that you might be interested to know of a move that we are planning to make at McGill. I have wanted very much to express some-how the gratitude which I feel to the memory of Mrs Ottman. For her generosity has made it possible for me to push ahead a great deal of re-search which otherwise would have been seriously handicapped.

We have created a fellowship of twenty-four hundred dollars yearly, to be taken from the money which she left, and to be used by a man who is working on one of the problems which lies before us in epilepsy. The fellowship will be called "The Madeleine Ehret Ottman Memorial Fellowship in Neurosurgery." It will appear in the University Calendar and in any publication which the Fellow may make he will sign himself "Madeleine Ehret Ottman Research Fellow" …

I wish that I could make some more eloquent gesture in appreciation of your sister's attitude, but I thought I would like to have you know that we have done this. This year there will be four younger men who have come here to work upon some aspects of our problem, who are being helped by smaller fellowships which are simply called "Neurosurgical Research Fellowships" but which also will be drawn from the money she gave us and from the money she bequeathed us when it shall be available.

I do not think I have met a woman in my practice with a stronger, finer character than that of Mrs Ottman. I would like to think that I could go through the terrible experience which she faced with the same quiet courage that she showed.

With best regards[24]

Without Madeleine Ottman's altruism and timely support the nascent MNI might have been still-born.[25]

Table 4.1
The Sub-Department of Neurosurgery Royal Victoria Hospital, 1928–32

Year	Attending surgeons	House surgeons
1928	Wilder G. Penfield	Arthur R. Elvidge
	William V. Cone	
1929	Wilder G. Penfield	Arthur R. Elvidge
	William V. Cone	James A. Brown
1930	Wilder G. Penfield	Arthur R. Elvidge
	William V. Cone	Earl Brewer
1931	Wilder G. Penfield	Thomas I. Hoen
	William V. Cone	Lyle Gage
	Arthur Elvidge	Arne Torkildsen
1932	Wilder G. Penfield	Joseph P. Evans
	William V. Cone	Wilbur Sprong

Source: RVH, *AR 1928–1932*.

Although Penfield's career was still in its early stage in 1928, he was nonetheless an experienced neurosurgeon who had made substantial contributions to neuropathology by his mastery of the histological techniques that he had learned from del Río-Hortega, and Cone was increasingly recognized as an insightful neuropathologist.[26] Thus, Penfield and Cone welcomed their first two fellows, Ottiwell Jones and Dorothy Russell.

Ottiwell Jones

Ottiwell Jones was already a neurosurgeon when he came to Montreal in 1928, having trained with Howard Naffziger of San Francisco, who had been a pupil of Cushing. Although not as well known as Dorothy Russell, Jones nonetheless made a significant contribution to neurosurgery in the two-burr-hole technique for the evacuation of subdural hematoma that is still used today and is often the first surgical procedure that a neurosurgical resident is allowed to perform.[27] Like Dorothy Russell, Jones came to Montreal to learn the Spanish techniques for staining glial cells. Like many fellows to come, Jones experienced Penfield's friendship and hospitality, as he relates in a biographical sketch: "[I] lived with Dr Penfield for days at a time, taking a regular Sunday morning walk with him, usually ending with tea at a friend's home."[28] Jones returned to San Francisco after his fellowship, where he had a very successful academic career.[29]

Dorothy Russell

Jones was soon joined by Dorothy Russell, a Rockefeller Fellow training in neuropathology. Born in Sydney, Australia, and educated in England, Russell graduated from the London Hospital Medical College in 1922. The neurosurgeon Hugh Cairns – who influenced so many MNI fellows, including William Feindel, Jerzy Chorobski, and Francis Schiller – encouraged Russell to consider a career in neuropathology, and she obtained a Rockefeller Scholarship to study the topic. She first went to Boston to learn the conventional techniques for the histological staining of neural tissue with Frank Burr Mallory at Harvard. While there, she caught the notice of Harvey Cushing, who wrote to Penfield on her behalf on 15 December 1928: "There is a Miss (Dr) Dorothy Russell who is working around here just now with Mallory – a friend and co-worker of Cairns who is going back to the London Hospital. She is counting on having a session with you if you can take her. I have not seen much of her, but like her greatly and recommend her warmly."[30] Thus, Dorothy Russell came to Montreal and learned the gold and silver techniques that Penfield had mastered in Spain.[31] Undoubtedly encouraged by the power of these techniques, Russell undertook the study

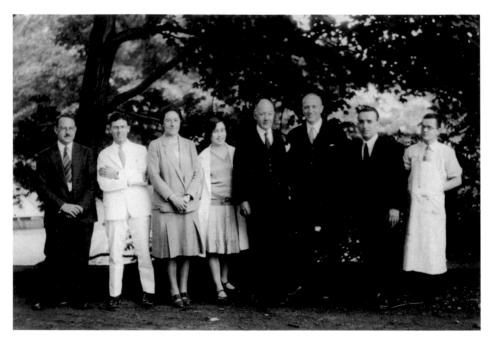

Figure 4.4: The Department of Neuropathology, Royal Victoria Hospital, McGill University, spring 1929: (*left to right*) Ottiwell Jones, University of California at San Francisco; Maurice Brophie, resident in neurology; Dorothy Russell, research fellow, London General Hospital, UK; Hope Lewis, secretary; Colin Russel, neurologist; Wilder Penfield; William Cone; Edward Dockrill, technician. (MNI Archives. See also Penfield, *No Man Alone*)

of microglia, with evident success.[32] Dorothy Russell returned to England in 1930, where she had a brilliant career, publishing two remarkable books, *Observations on the Pathology of Hydrocephalus* and, with Lucien Rubenstein, *Pathology of Tumours of the Nervous System*.[33] Russell would become *the* authority on the pathology of brain tumours. She remained a good friend of the MNI. She was a distinguished guest at the institute's inauguration ceremonies in 1934, and she was awarded a doctorate *honoris causa* from McGill University during events marking MNI's twenty-fifth anniversary.

Jonathan Meakins, the influential professor of medicine at McGill University, had provided Penfield and Cone with three rooms for laboratories, which they partitioned off into six smaller, separate spaces, referred to as "'Madrid cubicles,' equipped with workbench, sinks and shelves."[34] The support personnel included a technician, Edward Dockrill, a nurse, Catherine Dart, and a secretary, Hope Lewis, "who was the expert on train timetables and in correcting Penfield's spelling."[35] Dorothy Russell describes the working environment in

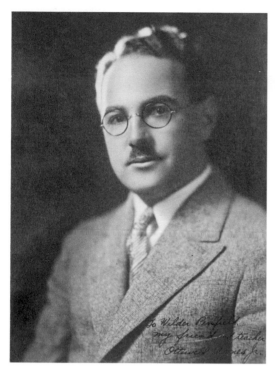
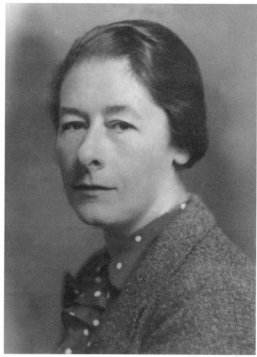

Figures 4.5 and 4.6: Ottiwell Jones and Dorothy Russell. (Penfield Archives)

these quaintly named cubicles: "We grappled with the metallic methods of the Spanish school, which gave us a slant on the embryology and evolution of glial cells. Bill Cone was enthusiastic about this and egged me on."[36]

Joseph Evans

The next fellow to come to Penfield and Cone was Joseph P. Evans, who was also the first recipient of the Ottman Research Fellowship in Epilepsy. Evans graduated from Harvard Medical School in 1929. Influenced by his contact with Harvey Cushing while at Harvard, Evans decided to pursue a career in neurological surgery and trained with Wilder Penfield and William Cone from 1929 to 1937. Evans was awarded the first MSc of the new Sub-Department of Neurosurgery at McGill in 1930 for his thesis "A Study of the Effects of Cerebral Wounds and Cerebral Excisions," and he received a doctorate, also from McGill, in 1937 for his dissertation "Study of Cerebral Cicatrix"[37] Joseph Evans had a noteworthy academic career and became the second of four consecutive MNI fellows to hold the position of head of Neurosurgery at the University of Chicago.

Jerzy Chorobski

The international character of the fellowship program under Penfield and Cone was firmly established in 1930 with the arrival of Jerzy Chorobski from the University of Warsaw as the second Ottman Research Fellow in Epilepsy, and Arne Torkildsen from the University of Oslo. Jerzy Chorobski had travelled widely in Europe and trained with Babinski before coming to Montreal. Chorobski worked with Penfield on the innervation of the cerebral vasculature, in a collaborative effort that included Henry Forbes and Stanley Cobb at Harvard. Penfield's relationship with Chorobski was unique and ran through the course of their lives and the life of the institute.

Arne Torkildsen

Arne Torkildsen was the second Continental fellow to join Penfied and Cone. He graduated from the University of Oslo in 1927. After a period of clinical practice, he found his way to Queen Square, to enhance his knowledge of neurology. Torkildsen came to the RVH in 1930 to work with Penfield and he stayed for four years, seeing the creation of the Montreal Neurological Institute at the end of his stay.[38] Torkildsen's study of the ventricular system was the most important project on which he worked while in Montreal.[39]

The demonstration of the ventricles by PEG left much to be desired, because it was difficult to fill all parts of the ventricles with air. Especially troublesome was the demonstration of the temporal horns – which Torkildsen refers to as the inferior horns – of the temporal lobes. So, despite the widespread use of diagnostic air studies, the exact shape and dimensions of the ventricles were conjectural. Torkildsen shed light on the anatomy of the ventricular system and on its relationship to the cerebral cortex. For this, he turned to a method that Leonardo da Vinci had devised to demonstrate the shape of the ventricles in cows. Leonardo gave instructions to "make two air holes in the horns of the great ventricles and insert melted wax by means of a syringe, making a hole in the ventricle of the memoria, and through this hole fill the three ventricles of the brain; and afterwards when the wax has set take away the brain and you will see the shape of the three ventricles exactly. But first insert thin tubes in the air holes in order that the air which is in these ventricles may escape and make way for the wax."[40] The brain substance was then removed and a wax casting of the ventricles remained.

As Torkildsen described his method, "The procedure has been to insert one "brain needle" in the anterior horn, one in the posterior and one in the inferior horn … The one in the anterior horn was used for injection of melted paraffin … the other two were used as outlets in order to allow the cerebrospinal fluid and air to escape … When the injected mass had solidified … the procedure was interrupted and dissection of the brain was undertaken. After the paraffin cast had been dissected free from the brain it was put in plaster of Paris … and after this had solidified it was heated sufficiently to melt away the paraffin. Then the empty cavity was filled with lead, [and] the plaster broken away."[41]

With these studies, Torkildsen shed light on the anatomy of the ventricular system and on its relationship to the cerebral cortex. He also demonstrated that there could be slight differences in the shape of the lateral ventricles, especially in the occipital and temporal horns, from one individual to the next. This finding would later be pertinent in the radiological assessment of cerebral dominance.

Following his stay in Montreal, Arne Torkildsen returned to Norway, where he established a department of neurosurgery reminiscent of the MNI. There, he applied the knowledge of the ventricular system that he acquired in Montreal, and achieved international fame for developing the first effective treatment of hydrocephalus, a condition that had been universally fatal.[42]

Isadore Tarlov

Americans were not disadvantaged with the coming of Europeans to the RVH. Isadore Tarlov, from Johns Hopkins University, and Lyle Gage, from the University of Pennsylvania, joined Chorobski and Torkildsen. Tarlov is reputed to have been Penfield's first resident at the MNI, but Cone had a greater influence on Tarlov's later career as a master of spinal surgery. Isadore Tarlov made significant contributions to our understanding of the spinal nerve roots and filum terminale during his time at the MNI, work for which he was awarded an MSc in 1932 for his thesis, "The Structure and Functional Relationship of the Cerebrospinal Nerve Root."[43] As a fellow in neuropathology, Isadore Tarlov, under the supervision of William Cone, reviewed the pathology slides of Penfield's sister Ruth, obtained from the resection of her frontal tumour performed by Harvey Cushing (see below). While in Montreal, Tarlov met his future wife, the artist and sculptor Fella Bechman, who designed a stained glass window for the McGill Chapel. From the MNI Tarlov went to Chicago, having obtained a fellowship to work with Percival Bailey. Tarlov was named professor and chairman of Neurosurgery at New York Medical College in 1940 and had a major impact on the treatment of spinal cord and peripheral nerve injuries.

Lyle Everett Gage

Lyle Everett Gage also obtained an MSc from McGill University for his thesis, "The Effects of Vasomotor Nerve Section on Experimental Epilepsy," while

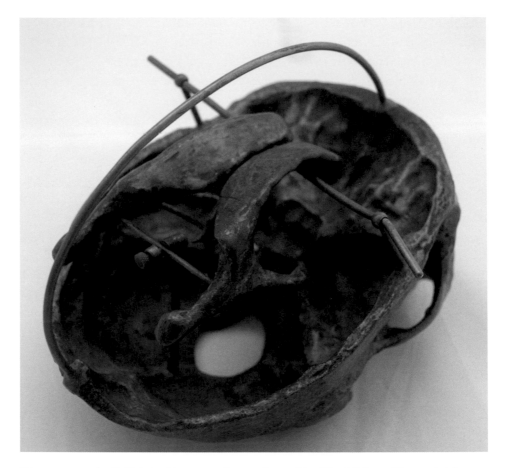

Figures 4.7 and 4.8: Original brass casting performed by Thorkildsen. The ventricles move left and right and swivel forwards and backwards to give a sense of their movement and shift in the presence of a mass lesion. The arc represents the distance from the skull to the ventricles. (Courtesy Roméo Ethier, MNI. Photographer Helmut Bernhard, MNI)

working with Penfield in 1931.[44] In 1933 Gage collaborated with Penfield on an important paper in which the results of cortical stimulation performed by Penfield himself are illustrated.[45] As such, it is a forerunner of the homunculus that was later described by Penfield and Boldrey and extensively elaborated upon by Penfield and Rasmussen.[46] Penfield seems to anticipate this development as he and Gage conclude their paper: "Electrical exploration of the cortex in conscious patients during craniotomy has given us unusual opportunity to study cerebral physiology, both normal and abnormal. Although some of our observations are of necessity incomplete, we have nevertheless recorded them in the expectation that they may be as useful to others as they have been to us in the study of cerebral localization."[47]

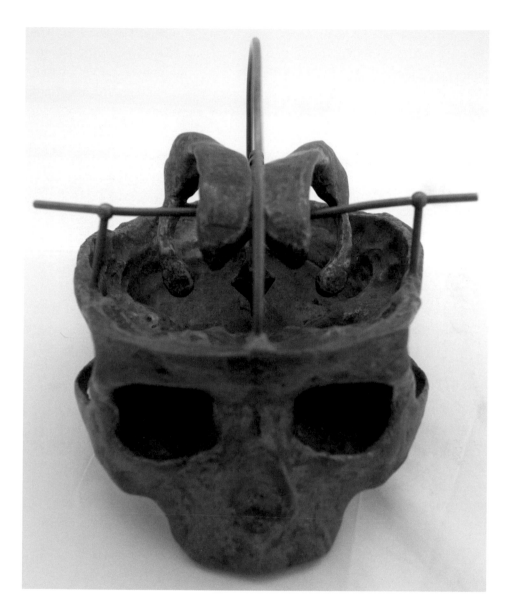

Norman Petersen and Arthur Elvidge represented McGill in the 1930 contingent of new residents and fellows. They would later play an inestimable role in the life of the Montreal Neurological Institute.[48]

Thomas I. Hoen

Thomas I. Hoen succeeded Arthur Elvidge as house surgeon in 1931.[49] Hoen is of great importance in the history of neurosurgery in Quebec and Canada. He graduated from Johns Hopkins School of Medicine and trained there with Halstead, the father of modern surgery. From Baltimore, Hoen went to Boston, where he was one of Cushing's last residents. He arrived in Montreal in 1931 to complete his neurosurgical residency and stayed at the end of his training to practise neurosurgery at Hôpital Saint Luc, becoming the first neurosurgeon to practise his specialty in a francophone hospital in Canada.[50] Hoen left Montreal in 1939 for the New York Medical College and, eventually, for New York University, where he chaired the Department of Neurosurgery from 1951 to 1961.[51]

George W. Stavraky

George W. Stavraky also came to the MNI in 1931, on a Rockefeller Fellowship. Stavraky studied the effects of the occlusion of the posterior inferior cerebellar artery with Colin Russel during his stay in Montreal[52] and later joined Charles G. Drake – who gained international fame for his skill in operating on aneurysms of the posterior circulation of the brain – at the University of Western Ontario, where he had a distinguished career as a prolific neurophysiologist and author.[53]

Fellows Come and Fellows Go

The year 1932 saw Norman Petersen leave for study abroad, his return uncertain. Arthur Elvidge did the same, but he was expected to return to take up the position of neurosurgeon at the Montreal General Hospital.[54] But there were newcomers: Jack Kershman, who would join the staff of the MNI, first came to study the cytogenesis of the nervous system; William Grant, of Ottawa, worked with Wilder Penfield on hyperpyrexia and with Cone on compression of the spinal cord; and Haddow M. Keith, already well established as a pediatric neurologist at the Mayo Clinic, came to study experimental epilepsy. They were joined by the ill-fated Wilbur Sprong.[55]

Wilbur Sprong

Wilbur Sprong decided early on a career in neurosurgery, having been influenced by Carl Rand from Los Angeles, one of Cushing's trainees. Sprong began his neurosurgical training at Johns Hopkins and came to Montreal to finish his residency and to work towards a PhD with Wilder Penfield.[56] Penfield selected Sprong to write the biographical sketch on Ramón y Cajal, to be published in *Neurological Biographies and Addresses* commemorating the opening of the MNI.[57] Penfield called upon Sprong because of "his power of expression ... and quick insight" and because, as Penfield wrote, "like Cajal ... he had the muscles of a giant and an unusual capacity for overwhelming enthusiasm in the pursuit of investigation."[58] Wilbur Sprong accomplished the task assigned to him but never saw the fruits of his labours in print: he died tragically in 1934 at the age of thirty-two. As Penfield noted of Sprong's passing, "With his rare gifts and high courage, Wilbur Sprong was ready to throw himself into that crusade against neurological disease and suffering which we as neurologists are bound to wage. 'Strange cancellings must ink th' eternal books' when he is called back to leave in the field many who are weary or half-hearted, many who have turned aside to follow 'wandering fires.'"[59]

Table 4.2
Residents and fellows, Sub-Department of Neurosurgery,
Royal Victoria Hospital, 1928–32

Year of arrival	Name	Origin
1928	Ottiwell Jones	University of California at San Francisco
1929	Dorothy Russell	London Hospital Medical College, UK
	Joseph P. Evans	Harvard University (Ottman scholar)
	Arthur Elvidge	McGill University
1930	Jerzy Chorobski	University of Warsaw (Ottman scholar)
	Lyle Gage	University of Pennsylvania
	J. Norman Petersen	McGill University (Ottman scholar)
	Isadore Tarlov	Johns Hopkins Hospital
	Arne Torkildsen	University of Oslo
	Earle Brewer	New York (research fellow)
1931	Thomas Hoen	Peter Bent Brigham Hospital
	George Stavraky	McGill (Rockefeller Scholar)
1932	Harold Elliott	Ontario
	William Grant	Ottawa
	Haddow M. Keith	Mayo Clinic travelling fellow
	John Kershman	McGill University
	Wilbur Sprong	Johns Hopkins Hospital

THE MONTREAL NEUROLOGICAL INSTITUTE OF THE
ROYAL VICTORIA HOSPITAL

The MNI was created at the RVH in 1933, before it moved to its new building under construction across University Street.[60] As the cornerstone was being laid for the MNI in 1933, Norman Petersen, back from London, Amsterdam, and Paris, his position secured by the Ottman Fellowship, took on responsibility for neuroanatomy and clinical neurology at the institute. Arthur Elvidge was appointed to the staff of the RVH in addition to that of the Montreal General Hospital. Joseph Evans was appointed registrar of Neurology and Neurosurgery and was in charge of the outpatient clinics. Theodore Charles Erickson arrived at the RVH in 1933, having interned in Philadelphia with one of the great figures of early twentieth-century neurosurgery, Charles H. Frazier.[61] Erickson was the first chief resident at the MNI when it moved to University Street. Others also came: Allan MacKay, a recipient of the Holmes Gold Medal from McGill

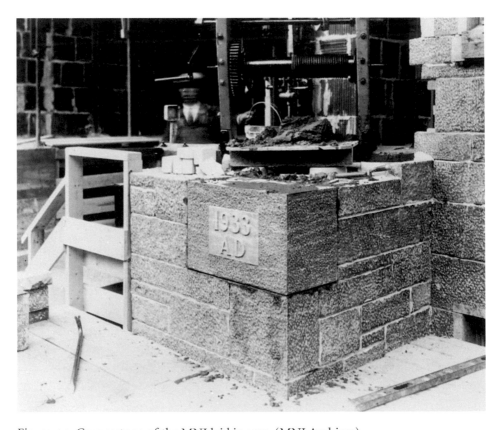

Figure 4.9: Cornerstone of the MNI laid in 1933. (MNI Archives)

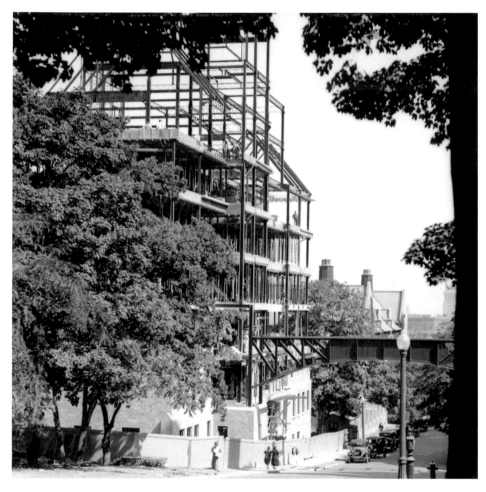

Figure 4.10: The MNI under construction. The ironwork of the bridge linking the institute to the RVH is visible at right. (MNI Archives)

University Medical School, would provide a lifetime of service to the Department of Neurology at the Montreal General Hospital; Robert W. Graves would later be head of the Department of Neurology at Albany Medical College; Robert Unwin Harwood, who worked on lead poisoning and its relationship to multiple sclerosis with Drs Russel and Cone; and Olan R. Hyndman, a Rocke-feller Fellow, who published a paper on agenesis of the corpus callosum – a subject that would be of great interest at the MNI four decades later.[62] J. Masson, a neurologist from Strasbourg, came to take on a temporary position as an extern.[63] Arthur Young joined the Neurological staff of the MNI upon its move across the street from the RVH and would render great service to the institute.

Table 4.3
The Montreal Neurological Institute, Royal Victoria Hospital, 1933*

Director	Wilder G. Penfield
Neuropathologist	William V. Cone
Biochemist	Donald McEachern
Registrar	Joseph P. Evans
Neurophysiological fellow	George W. Stavraky
Neuropathology fellow	Wilbur Sprong
Research fellow	Theodore Erickson
Research fellow	Robert Harwood
Research fellow	Haddow M. Keith
Research fellow	John Kershman
Voluntary fellow	Jerzy Chorobski
Voluntary fellow	Robert W. Graves
Voluntary fellow	Arne Torkildsen
Extern	Olan R. Hyndman (Rockefeller Fellow)
Extern	J. Masson (Strasbourg)
Consulting neurologist	F.H. MacKay
Associated consulting neurologist	Roma Amyot
Associated consulting neurologist	Émile Legrand
Associated consulting neurologist	Jean Saucier

*Also listed as members of the Department of Neurology and Neurosurgery of the RVH but not as members of MNI in 1933 are Lyle Gage, William Grant, and Ralph Stuck; and as associates in neurology: J.N. Petersen, Arthur Young, and A.G. Morphy. (RVH, *Annual Report, 1933*, 13–14, 17)

ACADEMIA

In their five years at RVH, Penfield, Cone, and their residents and fellows, produced noteworthy publications. Penfield was especially prolific and catholic in his interests, which ranged from the invention of surgical forceps to modifications of Río-Hortega's histological techniques.[64] He described the surgical treatment of intracranial hemorrhage by reporting two operative cases with excellent outcome, which was unusual at the time.[65] He also developed a method of treating infants with a myelocele or a meningomyelocele.[66] He brought order to the lesions associated with von Recklinghausen's disease and made significant, authoritative contributions to the classification of brain tumours.[67] Of note, Penfield's description of the oligodendroglioma in his "Classification of

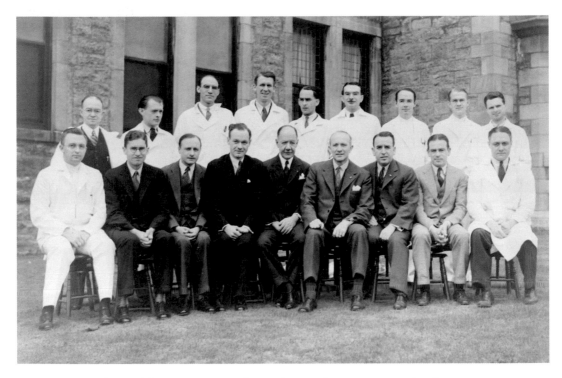

Figure 4.11: Members of the Department of Neurology and Neurosurgery, Royal Victoria Hospital, McGill University, spring 1934, before the opening of the Montreal Neurological Institute: (*seated*) Lyle Gage, Arthur Elvidge, Norman Petersen, Arthur Young, Colin Russel, Wilder Penfield, William Cone, Joseph Evans, Wilbur Sprong; (*standing*) Olan Hyndman, Jerzy Chorobski, Robert Harwood, Theodore Erickson, Arne Torkildsen, John Kershman, William Grant, Ralph Stuck, and George Stravrasky. (MNI Archives)

Gliomas and Neuroglia Cell Types" is clear, concise, and definitive, and would not be surpassed until the advent of molecular neurobiology.[68] Similarly, Penfield's stress on the hyper-vascularity of glioblastomas is prescient, as it has become a major area of research in contemporary neuro-oncology. Keasley Welch and Henry Garretson would further investigate this aspect of malignant gliomas in their MSc theses.[69] Most noteworthy of Penfield's academic efforts during this period was his editorship of the authoritative, multiple-volume *Cytology and Cellular Pathology of the Nervous System*, to which he, Elvidge, and Cone contributed.[70] Being entrusted with a project of such magnitude, involving so many well-regarded contributors, largely consolidated Penfield's reputation on the world stage.

Penfield was drawn to the physiology of the diencephalon in relationship to epilepsy, as revealed in a case that he encountered and published under the title "Diencephalic Autonomic Epilepsy," which he recognized, somewhat tentatively, as "a new conception in neurology."[71] The diencephalon would play a major

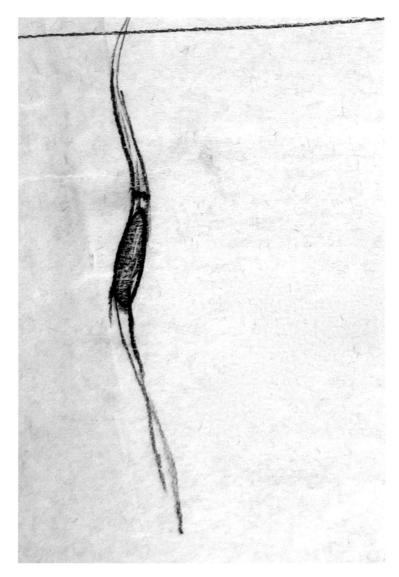

Figure 4.12: The neuropathology department under William Cone was decades ahead of contemporary laboratories in the diagnosis of tumours associated with Von Recklinghausen's disease, as illustrated in Cone's sketch and concise description of the microscopic appearance of a subcutaneous tumour: "In the silver stain for neurofibrils the tumour cells are seen to have long tails. Frequently the nuclei of cells lie along nerve fibres seen to pass through the cell … The long wormlike appearance of the nuclei … in the tumour place it in the group of tumours associated with Von Recklinghausen neurofibromatosis." (W. Cone, 28 October 1929, MNI Archives)

role in Penfield's later concept of the centrencephalic integrating system. Cushing expressed his regard for "Diencephalic Autonomic Epilepsy" in a letter to Penfield dated 13 October 1931, although not all agreed with him:

> Dear Wilder:
>
> On my return from abroad, I found your excellent bundle of the year's reprints – for which many thanks. Your diencephalic-autonomic epilepsy paper, which I of course saw when it came out, excited me greatly. It's a fine study. I made reference to it, as you will see, in my Welch Lectures a copy of which I am sending to you – not that I believe it's all true. [John Jacob] Abel, in fact, tells me that the most important part of it is wrong, which shows how foolish it is for one to trespass too far onto other people's provinces.
>
> Always yours
> Harvey Cushing[72]

Penfield's publications on epilepsy at this time were mostly derivative and owe much to Foerster's generous spirit in accepting Penfield as a co-author. Penfield, however, does raise the concept of the meningocerebral cicatrix as a cause of focal epilepsy in these publications. The investigation of this concept would occupy MNI fellows – most notably Chorobski, Erickson, and Evans – for the next few years. This would lead to new knowledge on the innervation of cerebral blood vessels and on cerebral ischemia. As such, the concept of the meningocerebral cicatrix represented a testable hypothesis that was a major step forward in the investigation of epilepsy and of neurophysiology.

5

The First Research Program at the Royal Victoria Hospital: A Vasomotor Mechanism of Focal Epilepsy

I was led to undertake the study of the cerebral blood vessels.
– Penfield

Penfield left Breslau and Foerster with a new treatment for post-traumatic epilepsy and an ambitious research program.

It would take many years for the new treatment to prove its worth. All that one could do at the time was to select patients with a focal component to their epileptic seizure, identify the area of the brain where the seizure originated as precisely as possible by history and physical examination, inducing a seizure by hyperventilation if necessary, and perform a PEG for corroboration. If all was concordant, an operation under local anaesthesia was performed to remove a scar, if one was found, while avoiding damage to functionally important structures. The results on the patient's seizure frequency and severity were observed over time. For how long? Fedor Krause, who had pioneered in the surgical treatment of epilepsy, suggested at least five years.[1] Penfield presented the results of surgery in his first series of seventy-five patients at the International Neurologic Congress in London on 30 July 1935, and published his results the following year.[2] A little less than a third of the patients were "cured." The cured included patients who had an exploratory craniotomy only, without resection of any cerebral tissue, or who had the ligation of one or more cerebral arteries, results for which an explanation was not forthcoming.[3] Nonetheless, the highest success rates were in patients in whom an MCC or other focal abnormality was resected.[4]

The research program that suggested itself to Penfield – the investigation of a localized, cerebrovascular cause for focal epilepsy, a concept that he inherited from Hughlings Jackson[5] – could readily be investigated in the laboratory and was quickly implemented upon his return from Breslau. There was some empirical support for this hypothesis, as Foerster had observed an area of cortical

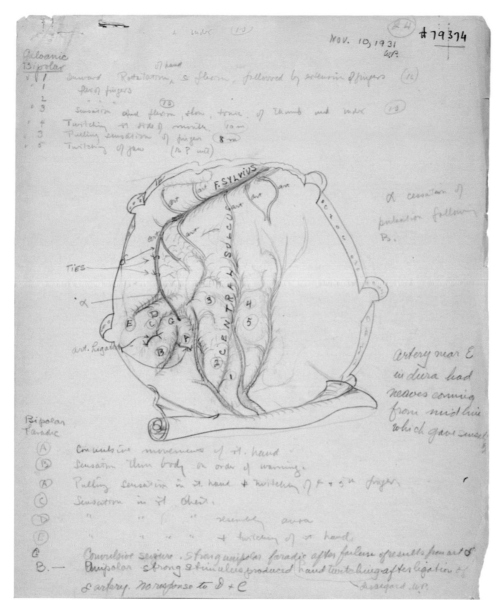

Figure 5.1: Operative sketch of a patient operated upon for the treatment of focal epileptic seizures. No gross abnormality was found, but some arteries appeared more prominent and appeared to become hyperemic in conjunction with seizures induced by cortical stimulation. These were ligated (∝). The drawing reflects the position of the left brain as the surgeon saw it from the head of the operating table: The dura is rolled over towards the midline of the brain at 6 o'clock. The patient's feet would be at 12 o'clock, his nose at 3 o'clock, and the occiput at 9 o'clock. Numbers indicate the sensory and motor responses to simulation. The letters indicate the sites where stimulation produced epileptic responses. The drawings resembling the "alpha" sign represent a knot where an artery was ligated. Although Penfield had high hopes for the beneficial effects of this procedure, it was performed in only half a dozen patients before it was abandoned. (MNI Archives)

anemia spreading outward along the cortex from the epileptic focus during an intra-operative seizure.[6] Further, Penfield had noted that disorganized blood vessels were a component of the MCC. They anastomosed freely with normal arteries and arterioles on the surface of the cortex about the scar. Penfield hypothesized that slow, progressive traction on these vessels by the contracting scar stimulated a reflex vasoconstriction that produced an area of focal ischemia, which, in turn, set off an epileptic seizure.[7] As he expressed it in 1930, "This pull, and the plexus of newly formed vessels caught in it, provide in our opinion a mechanism very important in the aetiology of the focal epilepsy which results from a penetrating wound of the brain."[8] Such an epileptogenic focus could be removed, Penfield asserted, with the same effect on focal seizures as if they has been caused by a tumour, because, as he had demonstrated with del Río-Hortega, a clean surgical incision did not produce a jagged, disorganized epileptogenic scar.[9] This was a testable hypothesis that suggests at least three areas of investigation: the demonstration that cerebral blood vessels are innervated; that focal cerebral ischemia produces epileptic seizures; and, as a corollary, that reflex vasodilation occurs as the seizure abates. One of Penfield's first laboratory projects in Montreal was thus the investigation of intracerebral vascular nerves.[10]

INTRACEREBRAL VASCULAR NERVES

Penfield took issue with the prevailing opinion that cerebral blood flow responds passively to changes in blood pressure, without an intervening neural mechanism. Rather, he believed that intracerebral blood vessels are innervated and capable of reflex vasoconstriction that he thought might even be a trigger for epileptic seizures. Thus he "was led to undertake the study of the cerebral blood vessels," which was facilitated by modifications to histological techniques developed by his technician Edward Dockrill.[11] Using these new techniques, Penfield was able to identify the presence of nerve fibres on intracerebral arteries and arterioles.[12] This finding was compatible with his theory of epileptogenesis, as he highlighted in the conclusion of his paper: "From a purely morphologic point of view, intracerebral vasomotor reflexes are possible."[13]

Penfield's interest in a neural component in the control of the cerebral circulation was shared by his colleagues Stanley Cobb at the Boston City Hospital and Henry S. Forbes. Forbes had developed the "Forbes window," a circular, transparent Lucite prosthesis the size of a trephine. This Lucite window was affixed to the skull of experimental animals, allowing one to observe the effects of extracranial neural stimulation on the cortical vessels.[14] Cobb and Forbes, and Cobb's research fellow, Jacob Finesinger, joined Penfield and his research fellow, Jerzy Chorobski, in one of the earliest exchanges between the MNI and Harvard, the study of cerebrovascular innervation.[15]

Five Monkeys

Penfield and Cobb had designed a collaborative project to study the influence of sympathetic innervation on the cerebral circulation. In Montreal, Penfield and Jerzy Chorobski performed sympathectomies in monkeys that, once recovered from surgery, were transported from Montreal to Boston. There the animals were fitted with a Forbes window, and the effects of neural stimulation on the diameter of the cortical vessels were measured using callipers and a standard scale.[16] Penfield's 6 March 1931 letter to Cobb reveals the simplicity of early twentieth-century cross-border research.[17]

> Dear Stanley,
>
> Dr Jerzy Chorobski will reach Boston on Wednesday morning the 11th. He will be bringing five monkeys. The monkeys will be sent directly to the Neurological Laboratory, City Hospital. I hope that is all right ... On Thursday I am having Edward Dockrill, the technician who is working on the staining of nerve fibers on the vessels of the brain, come down also. He will reach the Laboratory more or less the same time that I do. I wonder if a bench could be given him for histological work. For the sake of the best results we have to do the staining immediately and get immediate fixation of the head. He will bring along all of his own materials and instruments as nearly as possible. Perhaps you could let him have some alcohol and distilled water ...
>
> I am bringing some instruments along in order to be able to dissect the cranial nerves for stimulation. I hope to be able to bring a monkey along for control, but that depends on whether or not one of our present monkeys improves in health.
>
> I shall see you Thursday morning at the Hospital.
> WGP

As a result of this work, Cobb and Finesinger's "Vagal Pathway of the Vasodilator Impulses" and Penfield and Chorobski's "Cerebral Vasodilator Nerves" were published back-to-back in the *Archives of Neurology and Psychiatry* in 1932, and a reprint of Cobb and Finesigner's paper is included in Penfield's bound collected reprints.[18] Penfield and Chorobski's paper caught the eye of Harvey Cushing, who praised it highly in his letter to Penfield of 21 December 1932.

Dear Wilder:

I have just been reading with a great thrill your paper with Chorobski (to whom my compliments) in the last number of the *Archives*. It's simply a magnificent piece of work, and in combination with Stanley Cobb's paper sets a standard for a combined neuro-physiological study that will be hard to beat. I wish I might have been in Atlantic City last June to hear it and to add to the applause you must deservedly have received. You can well understand how stirred I am by your demonstration of a special parasympathetic bundle coming off from the brainstem in view of my long-arm lucubrations about a cerebral parasympathetic system, reprinted in a book I am sending you. I can scarcely wait to have you pursue this path-way headward, for I anticipate that it will have its central station in the interbrain …

With much power to your elbow, I am,

Always yours.[19]

"AT THIS TIME A STRANGE PHENOMENON WAS NOTED": PENFIELD, 1933

Chorobski, in his master's thesis "Vasodilator Nervous Pathway,"[20] and the combined experiments of Penfield, Cobb, and their co-workers had demonstrated that intracranial arteries are richly innervated, that vasoconstriction is mediated by the sympathetic system, and that vasodilatation is a parasympathetic function. These observations had been made on a small area of the cortex seen through a Lucite window in laboratory animals. Penfield was now set to make a bold statement on the cause of epilepsy, based on observations of patients in whom a larger portion of a cerebral hemisphere had been exposed in the operating room.[21] He reported that a focal seizure had been generated in twenty patients upon whom he had performed cortical stimulation. The seizure had been accompanied by the constriction of a superficial artery with arrest of blood flow in the cortex normally supplied by the constricted vessel. This constriction had persisted for the length of the seizure and for a variable period after it had stopped: "At this time a strange phenomenon was noted. The artery … showed a definite constriction. This was so sharp that it could not be doubted. The lumen was practically closed at this point. Proximal to this constriction the artery was pulsating. Distal to it no pulsation could be seen with the naked eye … Over a period of about ten minutes this constriction gradually passed off. At one time there persisted at the site of the previous constriction a little pallor but this eventually disappeared also." Penfield continued,

"The vasomotor spasms and changes seen so characteristically in the cerebral cortex of epileptics are due to vasomotor reflexes ... subserved by ... nerve cells upon the blood vessels of the brain ... Where such a lesion exists, excision of a focal scar with its vascular plexus is at present the most effective way of abolishing these malignant local reflexes." Penfield then concluded, unequivocally, that "the one constant, visible phenomenon in the brain during an epileptic seizure is cessation of arterial pulsation. Pallor may be present during a seizure but more often follows it."[22] In some cases, Penfield also observed that "the reddening of the veins after the seizure was so marked that they approached in colour the bright red of the arteries." Red cerebral veins would be the focus of much interest at the MNI over the ensuing years, and even into the twenty-first century. But for now, Penfield assigned a fellow, Francis Echlin, to investigate the epileptogenic effects of vasoconstriction on the cortex.

CEREBRAL VASOSPASM

Francis Echlin and Cerebral Vasospasm

Sherrington's student Howard Florey[23] relates that Sherrington had often observed that responses to electrical stimulation of the motor cortex of monkeys could be obtained if the cortex had a reddish hue. If, however, the cortex had a yellowish tinge, reflecting a state of hypoxemia, the cortex was non-responsive. Intrigued, Sherrington set Florey to investigate the vasoreactivity of the cerebral cortex through an enlarged trephine hole using a binocular microscope and a gentle probe. Florey observed that cortical arteries react to "mechanical, thermal, electrical, and chemical stimuli by contraction and dilatation." The most clinically relevant observation made by Florey was that "in cases where the artery is ruptured it can be seen, after bleeding is stopped, that it has contracted at the point of rupture and for a considerable distance on either side of it."[24] The importance of this observation, that cerebral arteries constrict when in contact with extravasated blood, would not be appreciated for another thirty years, when the occurrence of cerebral vasospasm following the rupture of a cerebral aneurysm was well documented and universally accepted by the neurosurgical community. But cerebral vasospasm following subarachnoid hemorrhage was the furthest thing from Wilder Penfield's mind when he asked Francis Echlin to study the role that cortical vasoreactivity might have on the genesis and propagation of epileptic seizures.

Francis Asbury Echlin, an American, graduated from McGill Medical School in 1931, then studied neurology, neurosurgery, and neurophysiology in the United States, France, and England.[25] Echlin served on the house staff and as a

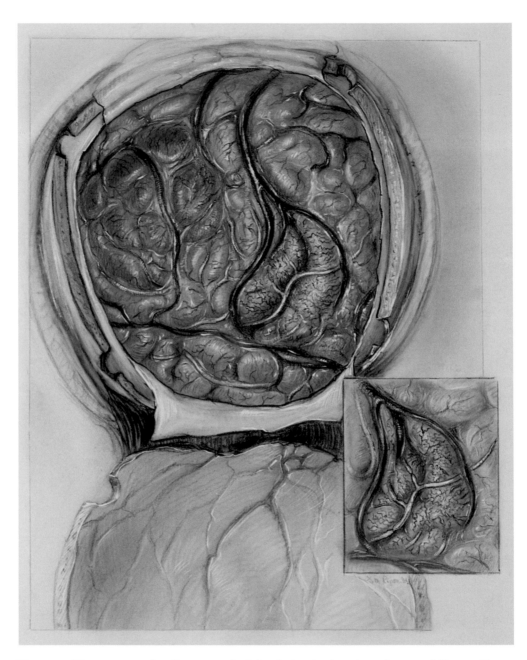

Figure 5.2: Vasospasm and epileptogenesis. Stimulation in the triangular area delineated by two large veins joining to form the Rolandic vein and the roughly horizontal Sylvia fissure (*inset*) produced a convulsion beginning with flexion of the wrist and arm. The convulsion was preceded by focal vasoconstriction of the cortical arteries supplying the area from which the convulsion was generated. (H. Blackcock, MNI Archives)

research fellow at the MNI from 1937 to 1939. His task as a research fellow was to determine if the constriction of cortical arteries could be induced in animals. Echlin took to the laboratory, where he performed large craniotomies and produced focal vasoconstriction much as Florey had in Sherrington's laboratory, by mechanically stimulating cortical arteries with a glass probe, by stretching a vessel with a small thread looped around it, or by applying an electrical current to the side of the artery. Unlike Florey, however, Echlin was able to record his results photographically, as Riser, Mériel, and Planques had done in France.[26] Echlin was able to confirm Florey's and Riser's observations on the vasomotor responses of cortical arteries. He further observed that prolonged, focal vasoconstriction resulted in histologically verified cortical ischemia – a phenomenon that he termed "vasospasm."[27] While Echlin stimulated the arteries along a gyrus, an assistant injected gentian violet intravenously, and they observed that "the brain rapidly turned a deep blue except in the area where the blood vessels had been constricted. This area remained white ... Coronal sections of the brain showed that ischemia had been almost complete through the entire depth of the cortex in a large portion of the area stimulated."[28] There were no immediate consequences to these observations, which were appreciated only a quarter of a century later, again largely through Echlin's efforts.

Francis Echlin left the institute in 1939 to join the faculty at New York University at Bellevue and Lenox Hill Hospitals, where he worked with MNI fellow Thomas Hoen.[29] Upon America's entry into the Second World War he joined the United States Army Medical Corps, then in 1951 Echlin became director of the neurosurgical service at Lenox Hill. While there, he developed a model for the study of acute cerebral vasospasm produced by whole blood, blood plasma, and serotonin applied to the exposed vertebral and basilar arteries.[30] In these experiments, Echlin also demonstrated that cerebral vasospasm could follow head trauma, with and without subarachnoid hemorrhage, a topic that is of great interest to those currently studying the effects of head injury. A few years later, Echlin also developed a model for the study of chronic vasospasm by injecting blood into the subarachnoid space of the monkey and observing the effects on arterial diameter by serial angiography performed over a period of days.[31] Echlin's seminal work on cerebral vasospasm was honoured by the First International Workshop on Cerebral Vasospasm, which reproduced key elements of his McGill thesis in the workshop's proceedings.[32]

Richard Lende and Manipulation Hemiplegia

At first Echlin's findings were met with resounding silence, an eloquent example of prematurity in science. However, Penfield's interest in this topic was rekindled by the occurrence of unexpected hemiplegia in patients upon whom he had operated. Careful analysis of these cases led Penfield to conclude that "interference with the blood supply of the internal capsule and thalamic radiation was the most likely cause," and that this was "probably related to manipulation of arteries."[33] The arteries felt to be responsible were the lateral lenticulostriate arteries, the branches of the middle cerebral artery that supply the internal capsule and thalamus.

As vasospasm was felt to be responsible, Richard Lende was given the task of studying vasospasm in animals in order to find an agent that could be applied topically to these arteries for relief or prevention of spasm. This project became his MSc thesis, "Local Spasm in Cerebral Arteries."[34]

Richard Allen Lende obtained his medical degree from the University of Oregon in 1951. During his studies, he came under the influence of Clinton Woolsey, the distinguished neurophysiologist who would later credit Penfield with the discovery of the supplementary motor area. Through Woolsey, Lende developed a life-long interest in cerebral localization and, after an interlude at Queen Square, he found his way to Wilder Penfield's laboratory at the MNI. Lende used Echlin's technique to expose the hemisphere of a variety of animals and to produce vasospasm. Spasm having been induced, Lende then applied a gelatine sponge soaked with a variety of putative vasodilating substances to the constricted artery and photographed the results for analysis. In this way Lende found that adrenergic blocking agent could reverse the induced vasospasm.[35] One of the substances that Lende tested, papaverine, came to be routinely used to relieve intraoperative vasoconstriction.

Richard Lende was destined for a brilliant career and a tragic fate. After he left the MNI in 1959, he practised neurosurgery at the University of Colorado, which he left in 1965 to become chair of neurosurgery at Albany Medical College.[36] Throughout his career, Lende remained true to the interest in cerebral localization that had brought him to the MNI, and he became an authority on the subject in a variety of animals, most notably the spiny porcupine and other woodland creatures.[37]

Richard Lende died unexpectedly at the age of forty-nine following a skiing accident. Wilder Penfield had a great fondness for Lende, as Phanor Perot recalled: "Dick … was charming, debonair, bright, and imperturbable. He ran the service just the way the Chief wanted it – an extraordinary accomplishment!"[38] The Richard Lende Winter Neurosurgery Conference commemorates Richard Lende's life, and at this writing, the conference is in its fortieth year.[39]

Continuum

The investigation of cerebral vasospasm runs as a rich vein through the first fifty years of the MNI. After a brief interlude following Lende's 1960 paper, Echlin, then at Lenox Hill, reinvigorated the field in 1965 with his investigation of vasospasm of the vertebro-basilar system. That paper stands as a landmark in vasospasm research and inspired other MNI fellows, most notably Guy Odom at Duke University and Eric Peterson at the University of Ottawa, to enter the field.

Guy Leary Odom, having obtained his medical degree from Tulane University in 1933, spent 1937 to 1943 training in neurology, neuropathology, and neurosurgery at the MNI. His time at the institute coincided with that of Francis Echlin, whose work on vasospasm Odom would remember after he left Montreal for Durham, North Carolina, and Duke University. Odom spent the remainder of his career at Duke where Blaine Nashold, another MNI trainee, later joined him.[40] During this time Odom published a series of influential papers on the response of cerebral arteries to various agents using Echlin's 1965 model.[41] A few years later, Eric Peterson and Richard Leblanc used the same model in their investigation of cerebral vasospasm.

Eric Weston Peterson

Eric Weston Peterson, a native Montrealer, graduated from McGill Medical School in 1942 and was the Holmes Gold Medalist of his graduating class. Peterson then joined the Royal Canadian Air Force on active service with the rank of captain. Peterson was later assigned to the Royal Canadian Army Medical Corps, and he was stationed at the First Canadian Neurological Hospital at Hackwood Park, Basingstoke, England. Peterson did landmark research during the war with William Cone and others. Upon his discharge from the Army in 1945 he resumed his training at the MNI under Penfield and Cone.[42] William Feindel, who would become the third director of the MNI, was Peterson's junior resident for a time.

His training at the MNI having come to an end, Peterson took an appointment at the Illinois Neuropsychiatric Institute of the University of Illinois, where he collaborated, most notably, with Horace Magoun on the role of the midbrain and pons in postural tremor. While in Chicago, Peterson also collaborated with Elwood Henneman on the cortico-collicular connections of the visual system. Henneman, also a McGill graduate, trained in neurosurgery at the MNI and became a noted neurophysiologist.[43] He held the Walter B. Cannon Chair of Physiology at Harvard University, where he created the first department of neurobiology.

Peterson befriended other prominent neurosurgeons then in Chicago, such as Loyal Davis; Paul Bucy, of the Kluver-Bucy syndrome and founder of the journal *Surgical Neurology*; Ralph Cloward, with whom he remained friends throughout Cloward's life; and Theodore Brown Rasmussen, also a MNI fellow, who had left the MNI in 1947 to become professor of neurosurgery at the University of Chicago. Peterson eventually left the Windy City for the University of Southern California to begin his clinical practice as an associate of Rupert Rainey, the inventor of the hemostatic clip that bears his name.

Scientific Contributions
Eric Peterson returned to Canada in 1954 to become the first head of Neurosurgery at the University of Ottawa. There he gained a formidable reputation as a rigorous scientist and a meticulous surgeon who had great respect for the cortex. It was also in Ottawa that Richard Leblanc first met him and became his collaborator, colleague, and life-long friend. Peterson's major academic interest was in cerebrovascular disease. Ever imaginative, he was the first to use the superior ophthalmic artery to induce electro-thrombosis of a carotid cavernous fistula.[44] However, his major research interest was in the investigation of the etiology of cerebral vasospasm and its reversal: Peterson and Richard Leblanc used Echlin's model for the investigation of acute vasospasm of the basilar artery and developed the first chronic model of experimental cerebral vasospasm.[45] Using these models, Peterson and his collaborators were the first to discover the role of cyclic adenosine monophosphate in the reversal of acute and chronic vasospasm.[46] These experiments led Leblanc to elaborate a theory of the antagonistic role of calcium and of cyclic-AMP in the cause of cerebral vasospasm and in its reversal.[47] Peterson retired from the practice of neurosurgery only when his health began to fail. He maintained a keen interest in the progress of his trainees until he quietly passed away at home, in the company of his family and in the thoughts of many.

Richard Leblanc left Ottawa for the MNI after graduating from medical school, to train in neurosurgery with Theodore Rasmussen, William Feindel, Gilles Bertrand, and André Olivier. As his neurosurgical training ended, Leblanc joined the Cone Laboratory for Neurosurgical Research, where he obtained his MSc under William Feindel and Lucas Yamamoto.[48] While in the Cone Laboratory, Leblanc and his co-workers established that platelet products are potent vasoconstrictors of the large arteries at the base of the brain and of the smaller cortical arteries and arterioles, and that their effect could be countered by calcium antagonism.[49]

MNI fellow Bryce Weir and his collaborators at the University of Alberta also developed a highly successful model for the study of chronic vasospasm in primates.[50] Weir had done his residency at the MNI, where he was greatly influenced by Theodore Rasmussen. Weir left the MNI for the University of Alberta at the end of his training, where he was eventually appointed chair of the Department of Neurosurgery. While in Alberta, Weir wrote a very well-received, encyclopedic textbook on cerebral aneurysms.[51] Like three MNI fellows before him – Theodore Rasmussen, Joseph P. Evans, and Sean Mullan – Weir was appointed chairman of the Department of Neurosurgery at the University of Chicago.

THE MNI AND THE UNIVERSITY OF CHICAGO

Theodore Rasmussen was the first of four successive chairmen of the Department of Neurosurgery at the University of Chicago to have trained at the MNI. Percival Bailey had established the neurosurgery program at Chicago in 1928, and Ted Rasmussen followed as professor and head of the department in 1947.[52] After seven years in Chicago, Theodore Rasmussen returned to the MNI and McGill University, to become professor and chairman of Neurology and Neurosurgery. He was replaced at the University of Chicago by MNI alumnus Joseph P. Evans, who had the distinction of delivering the MNI's first Fellows Lecture in 1957, in honour of William Cone. Then Sean Mullan replaced Evans as head of the Department of Neurosurgery at Chicago in 1967. Mullan, a native of County Derry, Northern Ireland, met Wilder Penfield in Oxford in the summer of 1953. Mullan began his training in neurosurgery in Belfast and completed it at the MNI. He wrote an important paper with Penfield on emotional reactions elicited by stimulation of the temporal lobe.[53] Mullan left the MNI In 1955 for the University of Chicago, where he was instrumental in the creation of the Brain Research Institute and the Brain Research Foundation.[54] Bryce Weir was recruited from the University of Alberta to replace Mullan upon his retirement.

MCGILL RED, MNI BLUE

These events occurred in the Windy City over a few decades. But in Montreal, on a warm autumn day in 1934, when the trees on Mount Royal display their splendour in red, yellow, and orange, the newly constructed MNI was holding its Foundation ceremonies.

PART TWO

The First Director
1934–1959

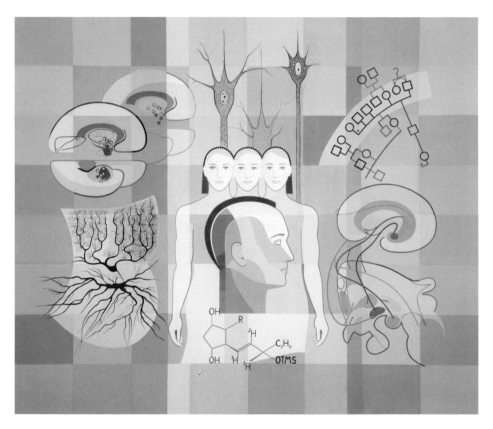

Luba Genush, *The World of Neurology* (*left panel*), "shows the points in and around the amygdala where stimulation produced epileptic automatism and memory changes; below is a giant nerve cell and astrocyte from the cerebellum; then we see brain cells, a map of sensory areas on the head and the formula for a compound used to analyze the brain's chemistry; followed by a family tree for neurogenetics and complex connections of the hypothalamus." (W. Feindel, *Images of the Neuro* [Montreal: Montreal Neurological Institute and the Osler Library of the History of Medicine, 2013)

6

The Founding of the Montreal Neurological Institute

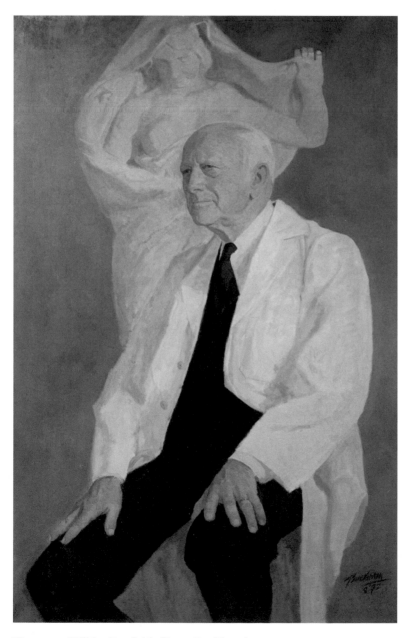

Figure 6.1: Wilder Penfield. (Lynn Buckham)

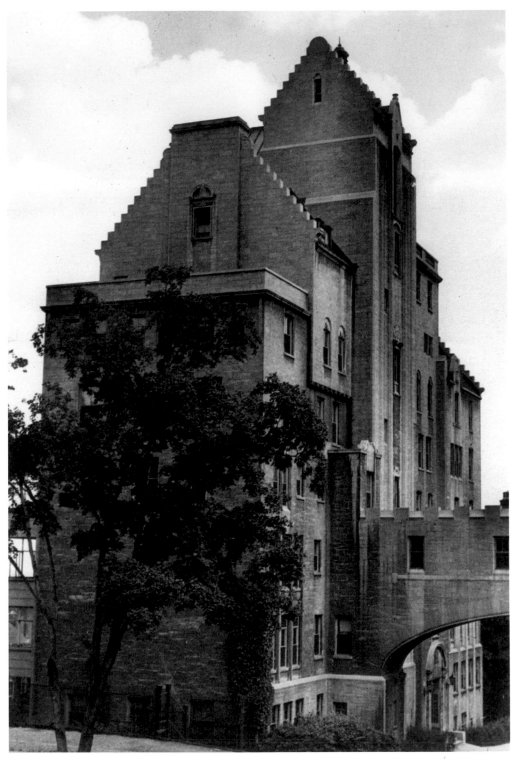

Figures 6.2 and 6.3: North (*above*) and east (*opposite*) aspects of Montreal Neurological Institute, 1934. (Penfield, *No Man Alone* [Boston: Little, Brown, 1977], 315; W. Penfield, "The Significance of the Montreal Neurological Institute," *Neurological Biographies and Addresses Foundation Volume* [London: Oxford University Press, 1936]

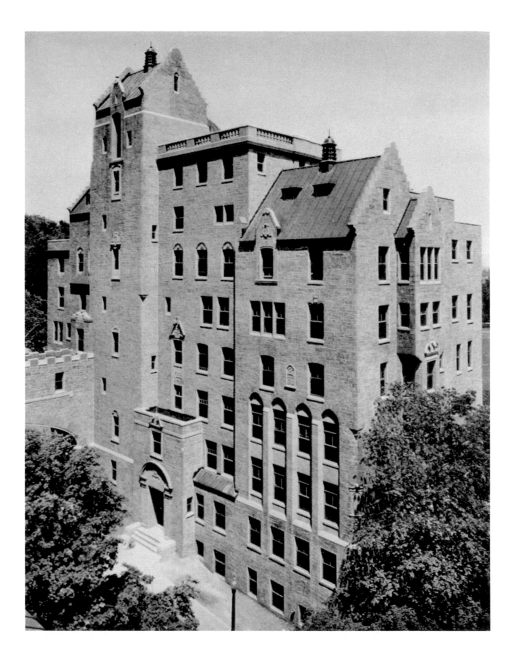

Vere Brabazon Ponsonby, ninth earl of Bessborough and fourteenth governor-general of Canada, laid the cornerstone of the MNI on 6 October 1933. On 27 September 1934 Sir Edward Beatty, chancellor of McGill University, declared the institute formally opened.

The Rockefeller Foundation provided funds to build and equip the laboratories of the institute and created an endowment fund of one million dollars in support of the scientific work of the Department of Neurology and Neurosurgery. The clinical, or hospital, part of the institute was built through

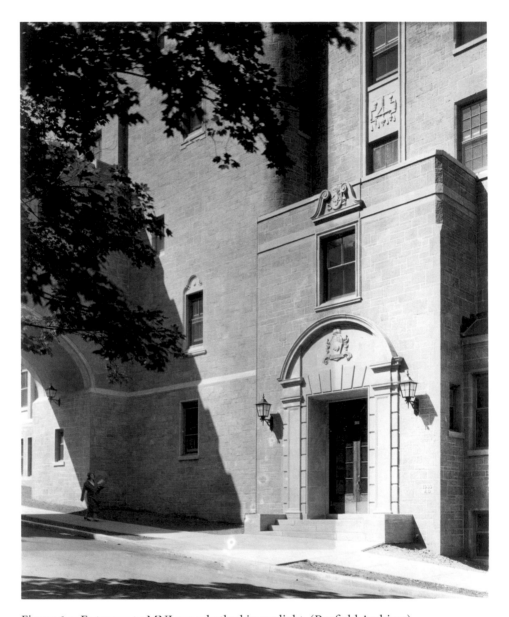

Figure 6.4: Entrance to MNI, 1934, bathed in sunlight. (Penfield Archives)

donations from private individuals. Quebec Premier Louis Alexandre Taschereau and Mayor Camillien Houde of Montreal agreed that the province and the city would be responsible for the hospital's yearly operation.[1]

The MNI is situated on the southern slope of Mount Royal along the east side of University Street. The doors to 3801 University lead up a few steps to a vestibule inlaid with the donor plaques. From the vestibule is a reception hall,

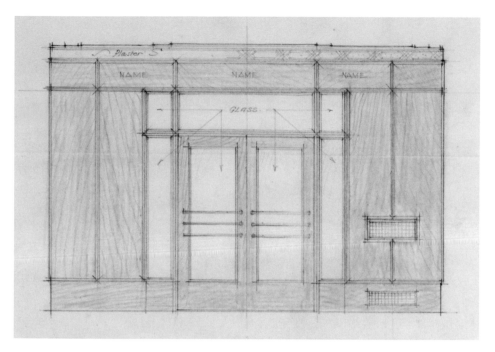

Figure 6.5: West wall, inner view of the entrance portico (*detail*). (Ross & Macdonald, Montreal Neurological Institute, interior elevations and plan for entrance hall, 1933, ARCH33404, Ross & Macdonald fonds, Collection Centre Canadien d'Architecture / Canadian Centre for Architecture, Montreal)

the centrepiece of the MNI. Decorations of the hall, recently renamed the Feindel Foyer, celebrate the rich history of neurology from its floor to its ceiling. A table of bird's-eye maple inlaid with an image that alludes to a cross-section of the human brain is in the centre of the small room. The lampstands and the floor tiles suggest the anatomy of the spine, and the radiator screens in the alcove represent modules of nerve fibres and Schmidt-Lanterman clefts.

NATURE UNVEILING HERSELF BEFORE SCIENCE

The Feindel Foyer's main feature is the elegant marble statue of a woman identified by the legend *La Nature se dévoilant devant la Science* (Nature unveiling herself before science). Penfield explained the statue's significance in *Neurological Biography and Addresses* commemorating the institute's Foundation ceremonies: "This figure embodies all the mysteries of nature, mysteries which only a scientist may hope to discover."[2] Penfield wrote to his mother on 17 July 1932, "I have always longed for a copy. The other day in Cleveland it occurred to me

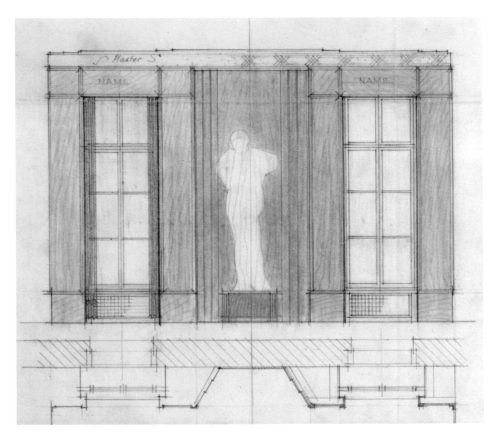

Figure 6.6: East wall of MNI lobby illustrating recesses for *La Nature* (*detail*).
(Ross & Macdonald, Montreal Neurological Institute, interior elevations and plan
for entrance hall, 1933, ARCH33404, Ross & Macdonald fonds, Collection Centre
Canadien d'Architecture / Canadian Centre for Architecture, Montreal)

as I was walking down the street, that we might have a copy made and placed
in such a position in the entrance that it would suggest to one entering the ideal
I have in mind for the whole Institute."[3] *Nature* has remained there to be con-
templated by all who cross the threshold of the institute.

High on the walls of the foyer are depictions of the ventricular cavities of
the brain and a frieze listing the names of famous neurologists, whose
biographies are included in the Foundation Volume: John Hughlings Jackson,
who had such a formative influence on Penfield's thinking; Sir Victor Horsley,
the first neurosurgeon; and Nobel laureate Sir Charles Sherrington, Penfield's
Oxford mentor, represent the British Isles. Sherrington is joined by two other
Nobel laureates, the histologists Santiago Ramón y Cajal and Camillo Golgi.

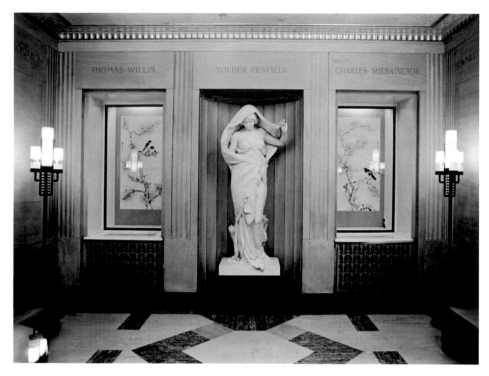

Figure 6.7: MNI lobby after Penfield's death. His name now appears above *La Nature*. Paintings on either side by Faith Feindel. (MNI Archives)

The French school is represented by Jean-Martin Charcot, for whom the first chair of neurology was created, and by Claude Bernard, the first proponent of experimental medicine. Wilhelm Erb, Franz Nissl, and Alois Alzheimer represent the German contribution to neuroscience, while Constantin von Monakow and Ivan Pavlov represent Russia, and Silas Weir Mitchell and Harvey Cushing represent the United States.[4] Wilder Penfield joined them, his name at the centre of the frieze, over *La Nature*, when the lobby was renovated after his death. Thomas Willis, the Oxford physician who coined the word *neurologist*, was also added, next to Penfield's name. Surprisingly the name of Broca, who proved the concept of cerebral localization of discrete neurological function, is not cited.

The foyer ceiling is decorated with frescoes depicting neuroglial cells within the cerebellum, as they appear under gold and silver stain and as they lie within a background of neurons and blood vessels. It is on this realistic background that the ram appears, as a metaphorical reminder of the goal of the MNI.

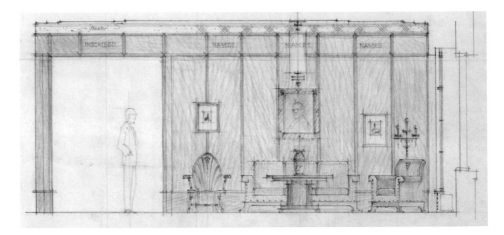

Figure 6.8: North wall of MNI lobby (*detail*). (Ross & Macdonald, Montreal
Neurological Institute, interior elevations and plan for entrance hall, 1933, ARCH33404,
Ross & Macdonald fonds, Collection Centre Canadien d'Architecture / Canadian
Centre for Architecture, Montreal)

THE INSTITUTE AND HOSPITAL

The floor space in the Rockefeller Pavilion, the central part of the building,
follows Penfield's original design, drafted on New York's Biltmore Hotel stationery. Private consultation offices on the first floor allowed neurologists and
neurosurgeons to conduct clinical research and teach within the same building. The studio for gross and microscopic photography was also originally on
the first floor, then moved to the sixth floor, where it currently resides. The
auditorium, later named in honour of John Hughlings Jackson, also situated
on the first floor, was a steep, semicircular amphitheatre as one might find in
ancient European universities where public dissections took place. At the MNI,
the amphitheatre served for student lectures, clinical case presentations during Grand Rounds, and venue for visiting speakers.[5]

Patient wards were on three clinical floors. The first two – the J.W. Mc-
Connell Ward on the second floor and the Sir Herbert Holt Ward on the third
floor – each accommodated fourteen public patients. The third floor was meant
to communicate with the Royal Victoria Hospital via a bridge spanning University Street. But, as William Feindel recalled,

> The bridge led into the children's ward of the [Royal Victoria] hospital.
> The hospital staff, headed by the Physician in Chief Jonathan Meakins
> and supported by Holt, was unwilling to allow such a thoroughfare.

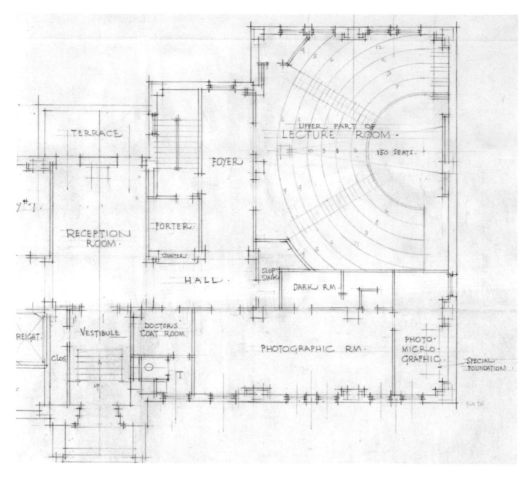

Figure 6.9: First floor of MNI (*detail*). The amphitheatre, named in honour of Hughlings Jackson in 1974, centre of MNI academic activities (*upper right*), was later converted into office space and replaced by the Jeanne Timmins auditorium. The photography laboratory (*lower right*), relocated to the sixth floor, where it remains today. (Ross & Macdonald, Montreal Neurological Institute, first floor plan, 1932, ARCH33375, Ross & Macdonald fonds, Collection Centre Canadien d'Architecture / Canadian Centre for Architecture, Montreal)

The bridge was not functional until 1942, eight years after the opening of the Institute. Meanwhile, patients had to be transported by a circuitous route from the RVH through a grungy service tunnel under University Street and a lugubrious passage past the pathology morgue to the Institute.

Eventually, in 1941 a patient in the RVH, who had to be moved by stretcher through this subterranean passageway for EEG tests in the Institute, offered to fund the bridge's functional completion. As a silent historical foot-note to the end of all this commotion, a plaque on the bridge records the donation in 1942 from the Aaron and Bronfman families.[6]

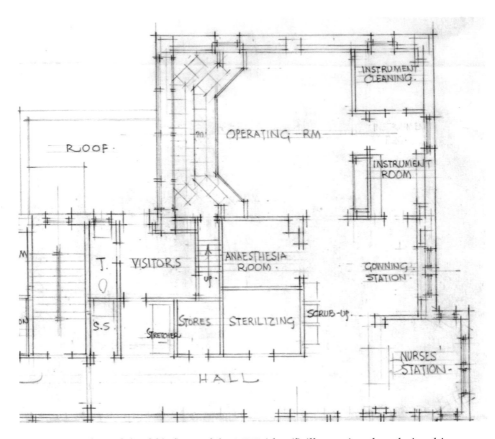

Figure 6.10: Plan of the fifth floor of the MNI (*detail*) illustrating the relationship of the operating room to the adjoining anesthesia induction room and the visitor's gallery. (Ross & Macdonald, Montreal Neurological Institute, fifth floor plan, 1932, ARCH33372, Ross & Macdonald fonds, Collection Centre Canadien d'Architecture / Canadian Centre for Architecture, Montreal)

The fourth floor was reserved for fifteen private and semi-private patients.[7] The lighting of the wards was "entirely from windows at the end of each ward, and, with reflection from the cream coloured ceiling, the light [fell] evenly on every patient. Nursing control [was] facilitated by placing a desk in a bay of glass which [projected] into the ward, so that every bed [might] be seen by the nurse. A common dressing room [was] so arranged that patients [might] easily be moved into it for surgical dressings, examinations or therapy."[8]

On the fifth floor, which separated the patient wards from the laboratories on the floor above, there were two operating rooms and smaller induction and service rooms. The main operating room was of unique, novel, and practical design. As described by Norman Petersen, the institute's registrar, the room is provided with a viewing gallery which is entered by a narrow pair of stairs from the

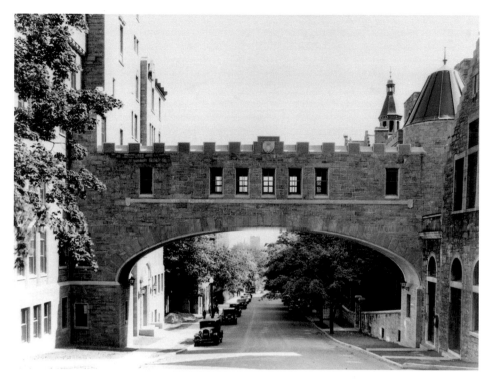

Figure 6.11: The Bronfman Bridge looking south down University Street. Built through the generosity of the Bronfman Family and Mr B. Aaron, the bridge made life more tolerable for patients who required transportation between the MNI and the RVH. (MNI Archives)

visiting physicians' room. This obviates the necessity of visitors or research fellows, who come in to watch operations, passing through the operating room at all. Beneath the viewing gallery is a small photographic cellar with a window. The photographer enters this cellar from the viewing gallery and sets up his camera behind the window. A photographic mirror adjustable from the cellar is maintained over the operating field and above the operator's head. In this mirror the photographer can see the field and can take photographs routinely at every operation without fear of contamination and without confusion. The temperature and moisture of the air in the operating room are automatically controlled and the ventilation is carried out with thoroughly washed air, so that windows will never be open and danger of wound contamination from the air is thereby reduced to a minimum.[9]

This arrangement was essential to expose large photographic plates of the brain and of the sterile numbered tickets marking the points of positive response to stimulation of the cortex. These photographs were life-sized and, with

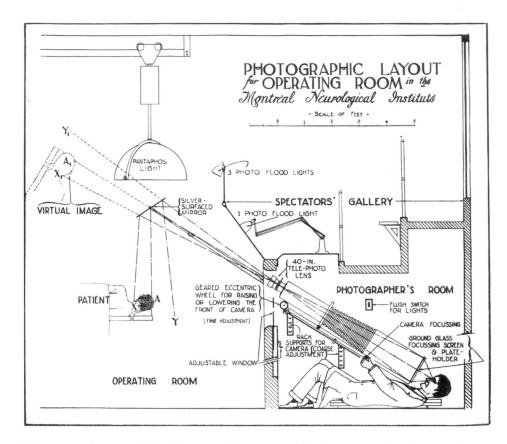

Figure 6.12: Cartoon of the photographic apparatus for intra-operative photography, main operating room, 1936. The photographer and his camera are outside the operating room in a cubby below the viewing gallery. The camera points through a window in the wall of the operating room towards a mirror above the operative field, angled to reflect the operating site and not interfere with the surgeon nor cast a shadow on the field. (H.S. Hayden, "A New Technique for Surgical Photography in the Operating Room," *Photographic Journal* 76 [1936]: 205–9) (See figure 29.4)

the surgeon's operative drawing, they remain within the MNI Archives as an unmatched database for the study of human brain function. A smaller operating room, used mainly for ventriculography and pneumography, was connected to the Radiology Department. After these procedures, the patients could be brought directly into the main operating room, if necessary.

The sixth floor housed the director's office at one end and the Fellows Library at the other, the two joined by a long corridor smelling of pyridine and xylol, reagents used in the silver staining method, as the walls of the corridor were lined with doors, each opening into a research laboratory.[10] These included

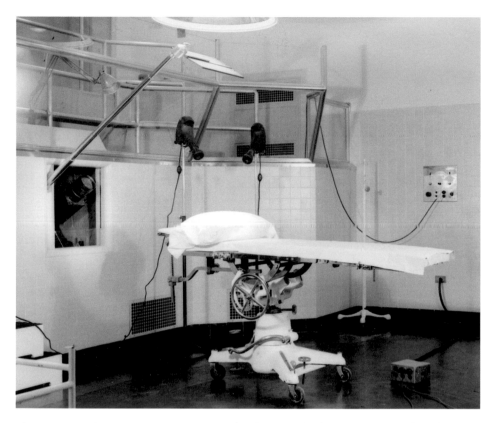

Figure 6.13: Main operating room, 1936. The photographer's camera lens (*left*) is focused on the mirror on the end of the boom. (MNI Archives, photographer H. Hayden)

laboratories for pathology, chemistry, and physiology. The seventh floor had operating rooms for animal experimentation and carefully planned animals quarters with an outdoor runway for the dogs. Finally, the eighth floor provided rooms and living space – and a squash court – for half a dozen residents and fellows. Unfortunately, the animal runway was immediately below the eighth-floor bedroom windows that had to be kept open during Montreal's hot summer nights as the dogs were let out; many a resident lay awake serenaded by the sounds of dogs out for their run above the city.

Every afternoon at four o'clock, as the neurological clinics closed, the experiments ended, and the post-operative patients were safely in the recovery room, the neurologists, neurosurgeons, residents, and fellows gathered, a few at a time, and then a few more, until the corridor from the director's office to the library door was filled with chatter and shop talk, as bracing hot tea was had from a giant samovar and butter cookies disappeared from colourful tin boxes.

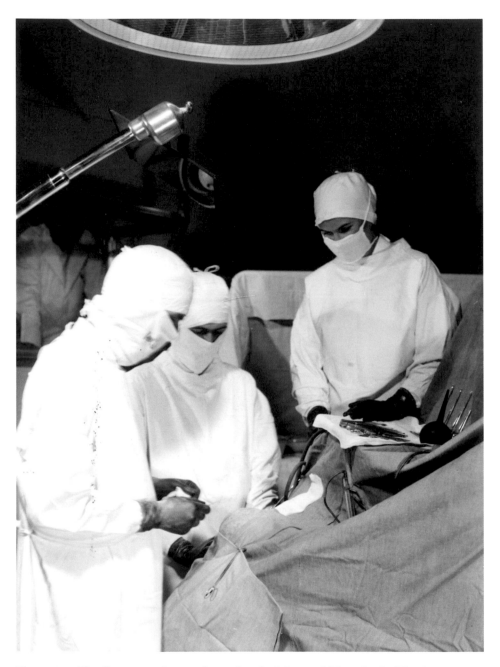

Figure 6.14: The first operation performed at the Montreal Neurological Institute, 1934. In the usual order are Theodore Erickson, Donald Coburn, and Cora McLeod, assistant operating room nurse. David Reeves, a research fellow, is in the gallery. Notice the boom holding the overhead mirror. Donald F. Coburn was one of the first members of the house staff after the institute opened in 1934. He later relocated to the University of Kansas Medical Center. David L. Reeves became president of the American Association of Neurological Surgeons in 1962–63. (MNI Archives, photographer H.S. Hayden)

NEUROLOGICAL BIOGRAPHIES AND ADDRESSES

Undoubtedly the most important publication of the first year of the institute was *Neurological Biographies and Addresses* gathered within a Foundation Volume, commemorating the opening of the institute and published for the staff by the Oxford University Press.[11]

This small, handsome volume contains a hidden pearl. In it, Penfield describes his motivation for the creation of the institute. As he relates, General Sir Arthur Currie had just recently died from a stroke at the age of fifty-seven, "as we stood by his bedside helpless." Penfield continues, determinedly, "The task to which this Institute is dedicated in all humbleness of spirit is the achievement of greater understanding of the neurological ills to which man is heir so that physicians may come to such a bedside with healing in their hands."[12] This sentiment was expressed more succinctly and most earnestly, carved in stone at the entrance of the building: "Dedicated to relief of sickness and pain and to the study of Neurology.[13]

Penfield continues his Foundation Address by welcoming some of the distinguished visitors: Harvey Cushing from Boston, Allen Whipple from New York, Gordon Holmes and Godwin Greenfield from Queen Square, and "from London … our most distinguished pupil, if it shall not be thought vainglorious of Dr Cone and me that she should be named thus, Dr Dorothy Russell."[14]

Gordon Holmes, the dean of British neurology, gave one of three Foundation Lectures, on, appropriately, neurology. Harvey Cushing's lengthy piece, titled "Psychiatrists, Neurologists and the Neurosurgeon," followed. Cushing's lecture is notable for the frustration that he expresses at his own unsuccessful efforts to create an institution similar to the MNI in Boston.[15] Penfield followed Cushing with "The Significance of the Montreal Neurological Institute." A handsome photograph of the entrance's ceiling illustrates Penfield's address.

Not part of the addresses, but undoubtedly more precious to Penfield than the words spoken that day, is a telegram found deep in the Penfield Archives stamped "Via Marconi" in vivid red and "Sept 27 1934" in royal blue, which reads, "BEST WISHES AND CORDIAL GREETINGS OTFRID FOERSTER." Henceforth, these two colours, McGill red and MNI blue, would govern Penfield's life.

The keynote addresses were followed by biographical sketches of the individuals whose names appear in the foyer.

◆◆◆

FRANCOPHONE CONSULTANTS

Penfield addressed the linguistic duality of the city of Montreal and the French School of Neurology. Penfield had promoted close ties with French-speaking colleagues from the two great teaching hospitals of the Université de Montréal, by naming three young neurologists, Roma Amyot and Jean Saucier from Hôpital Notre-Dame and Émile Legrand from Hôpital Hôtel-Dieu, as neurological consultants to the institute. They were, Penfield said, "distinguished leaders in the field of neurology," who brought with them "the high tradition of the French school of neurology."[17]

Roma Amyot

Roma Amyot obtained his medical degree from the Université de Montréal in 1924, then studied neurology at the Université de Paris for four years, most notably with André Thomas, who had been a student of Jules Dejerine. He obtained a doctoral degree from the Université de Paris, and a bronze medal from its Faculty of Medicine for his dissertation on convulsions in amputees.[18] "The first francophone neurologist in Québec,"[19] Amyot became a neurological consultant to the Montreal Neurological Institute in 1934.

A true academic, Amyot published an early paper on spinal epidural abscess that underscored the high mortality of this condition in the pre-antibiotic era, despite surgical drainage.[20] Although Amyot published in English, he saw the need for a didactic and research publication that would speak to francophone physicians and medical scientists in their own language, and that would serve as an outlet for their publications. He became the editor of the major francophone medical journal *L'Union Médicale du Canada*, where he, Saucier, and others could publish their works in French. Amyot's and Saucier's interests were wide-ranging, and they published extensively on brain tumours, on tuberculosis and syphilis as they affected the brain and spinal cord, on poliomyelitis, on multiple sclerosis, and on other degenerative diseases of the nervous system.[21]

Jean Saucier

Jean Saucier obtained his medical degree from the Université de Montréal in 1922. Like Amyot, he was awarded a doctorate in medicine from the Université de Paris, in 1927, for a thesis on hypertrophic neuritis. While in Paris, he studied neuroanatomy with Augusta Dejerine-Klumpke, neurology with André Thomas, and neuropsychiatry with Joseph Babinbski.[22] With Amyot and

Legrand he became a neurological consultant to the Montreal Neurological Institute in 1934. Saucier was the first francophone member of the Canadian Neurological Society and its first francophone president. Saucier, like Amyot, was a prolific writer on a variety of neurological subjects.[23]

Émile Legrand

Émile Legrand, age thirty-eight at the opening of the MNI, was the eldest of its three francophone consultants. Under the pressure of work, he largely left the practice of neurology to Amyot and Saucier, devoting himself to psychiatry. His career was short lived, as his life ended prematurely in an airplane accident in 1949.[24]

Antonio Barbeau

The three original francophone neurologists were joined by a fourth, Antonio Barbeau, shortly after the institute opened its doors. Barbeau graduated from the Université de Montréal in 1924, the same year as Roma Amyot, but instead of making his way directly to Paris for postgraduate training, he attended the Université de Montpellier, in the south of France, then spent a year in Paris, also with Dejerine-Klumpke, Thomas, and Babinski. Unlike his French-Canadian colleagues, Barbeau did not feel the need to return directly to Montreal, but rather chose to go to Harvard, where he worked with Stanley Cobb and Henry Forbes, Penfield's friends and colleagues. Barbeau became a consultant in neurology at the Montreal Neurological Institute in 1936 and was appointed as the first chair of the Department of Neurology at the Université de Montréal in 1939.[25]

A CANADIAN SCHOOL OF NEUROLOGY

Penfield ends his Foundation address with the hope that the institute would act as a catalyst for Canadian neurology: "And yet this inauguration is not of a colonial branch of London's National Hospital, not a lesser Salpêtrière springing up in the new world, not an upshoot from an aberrant American root which has tunneled its devious way across the unguarded border. We dare to hope that this is the inauguration of an institute of medicine that is characteristically Canadian, the birth of a Canadian School of Neurology. In my own case," Penfield underscores, "it means a change of national allegiance."[26]

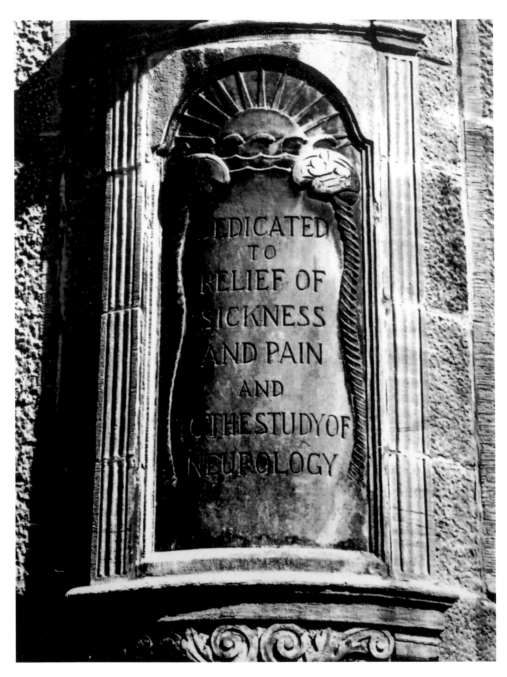

Figure 6.15: The original stone plaque now on the exterior facade at the right of the main entrance shows a carving of the brain and spinal cord and the phrase selected by Penfield, "Dedicated to relief of sickness and pain and to the study of neurology." (MNI Archives)

7

The First Year and the Second

The newly opened institute provided neurologists and neurosurgeons with private consultation offices, allowing them to carry on clinical research and teaching in the same building, while public outpatient clinics were conducted at the RVH.

André Cipriani was an early recruit who had an immediate impact on the clinical and scientific activities of the institute. Born in Trinidad, Cipriani first studied mathematics and physics at McGill University before studying medicine, also at McGill. He joined the staff of the institute in 1936 and quickly became a vital member of the Department of Electrophysiology. His first task was the construction of a cathode ray oscillograph to improve the accuracy of cortical stimulation. Cipriani later became director of the Biology Division at Atomic Energy of Canada at Chalk River, Ontario, where he pioneered the use of Cobalt-60 for the treatment of cancer.[1]

THE NEUROSURGICAL TRAINING PROGRAM

The creation of a residency training program was a first priority of the MNI. The neurosurgical training program consisted of an internship that included six months of neurosurgery, six months of neurology, and six months as senior intern in the Outpatient Department. A two-year residency was offered to candidates who had previous clinical and laboratory experience at the institute, which could be achieved through fellowships in neuropathology, neuro-anatomy, neurophysiology, or biological chemistry. There were also voluntary fellowships and externships that allowed participation in the clinical services. Clinical teaching was supplemented by weekly sessions in pathology, medical

Table 7.1
Clinical staff, Montreal Neurological Institute, 27 September 1934
to 31 December 1935

Director	Wilder G. Penfield
Registrar	J. Norman Petersen
Neurologist	Colin Russel
Consulting neurologist	F.H. MacKay
Associate neurologist	Donald McEachern
Associate neurologist	A.G. Morphy
Associate neurologist	J. Norman Petersen
Associate neurologist	Arthur Young
Associate consulting neurologist	Roma Amyot
Associate consulting neurologist	Emile Legrand
Associate consulting neurologist	Jean Saucier
Associate consulting neurologist	Norman Viner
Assistant neurologist	Haddow Keith
Neurosurgeon	William V. Cone
Associate neurosurgeon	Arthur Elvidge
Roentgenologist	E.C. Brooks
Associate roentgenologist	A.E. Childe

Table 7.2
Laboratory services, Montreal Neurological Institute, 27 September
to 31 December 1935

Neuroanatomist	Colin Russel
Biochemist	Donald McEachern
Neurophysiologist	Arthur Elvidge
Neurophysiological fellow	Donald Coburn
Neurophysiological fellow	William Grant
Fellow in roentgenology	Arthur E. Childe
Neuropathologist	William V. Cone

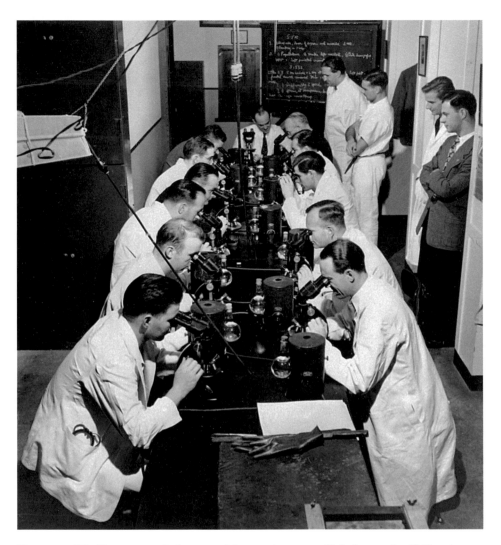

Figure 7.1: Weekly neuropathology teaching session, 1947: (*left, front to back*) Fleming, Daly, Fisher, McRea, Steelman, Elvidge, with Welch at the top of the table; (*right, front to back*) Rasmussen, Dooglever-Fortuyn, Peterson, Jackson, Penfield; (*standing, front to back*) Rosen, Meyer, Hunter, Pavrovsky. (MNI Archives)

conferences, and weekly and monthly didactic lectures. Regular meetings of the Montreal Neurological Society – the neurology section of the Montreal Medico-Chirurgical Society – were later included as a part of the curriculum. Meetings of the Montreal Neurological Society were held alternately at the MNI and at the Montreal General Hospital, and, on occasions, at Hôpital Notre-Dame. The Neurological Society meetings allowed attending staff and fellows to present interesting clinical cases and research findings. The reports were given in French

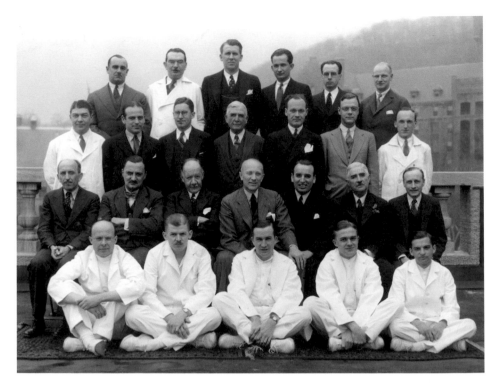

Figure 7.2: Attending physicians, house staff, and fellows of the Montreal Neurological Institute, 1936, after its opening on University Street. (*Front row, left to right*) W.M. Witherspoon, E.B. Boldrey, D.L. Reeves, R. Pudenz, I.M. Tarlov. (*Second row*) R. Amyot, J. Saucier, C. Russel, W.G. Penfield, W.V. Cone, F.H. MacKay, J.N. Petersen. (*Third row*) E. Walker, J.P. Evans, A.R. Elvidge, A.G. Morphy, A.W. Young, A.E. Childe, F.L. McNaughton. (*Top row*) W.L. Reid, J. Kershman, T.C. Erickson, A.J. Cipriani, K. von Santha, J.S.M. Robertson. (H.M. Keith, E. Legrand, D. McEachern, and N. Viner are absent.) (MNI Archives)

if the speaker was from the Université de Montréal or in English if from McGill University. Most importantly, the meetings provided a forum for invited speakers of the highest calibre from the United States, the United Kingdom, and other European universities.

Notable in figure 7.2 is Edwin Barkley Boldrey, who obtained his MD from Indiana University in 1932. He began his postgraduate training at the Montreal General Hospital and became one of the first research fellows at the MNI in 1935. He began service on the house staff in July 1936 and rose to resident house officer in 1938. During this time Boldrey carried out a critical review of operations for epilepsy performed by Penfield and Cone from 1928 to 1936. Boldrey earned an MSc for his thesis, "Architectonic Subdivision of the Mammalian Cerebral Cortex Including a Report of the Electrical Stimulation on One Hundred and Five Human Cerebral Cortices," one of the most important theses produced at the institute (figure 3.5).[2] Part of Boldrey's thesis was published in *Brain* in 1937, in which the sensorymotor "homunculus" makes his first appearance.[3]

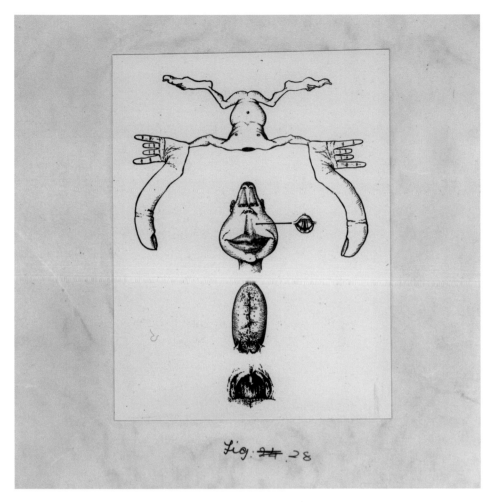

Figure 7.3: Original sketch of the homunculus by Mrs H.P. Cantlie. The thumbs are more exaggerated in size, the head more pear-shaped, and the tongue fatter than in the version published by Penfield and Boldrey in *Brain*, 1937. (Penfield Archives)

Table 7.3
House staff and fellows, Montreal Neurological Institute, 1934–1935

E.M. Atkinson	F.L. McNaughton
E.B. Boldrey	N.C. Norcross
D.F. Coburn	D.L. Reeves
T.C. Erickson	W.L. Reid
W. Gibson	J. Sanchez-Perez
W.T. Grant	G. Stavraky
W. Haymaker	R. Struck
J. Kershman*	I.M. Tarlov
L. McConnell	E. Walker

* John Kershman was the first resident in neurology at the MNI. Adapted from P. Robb, *The Development of Neurology at McGill* (Montreal: Montreal Neurological Institute, 1989).

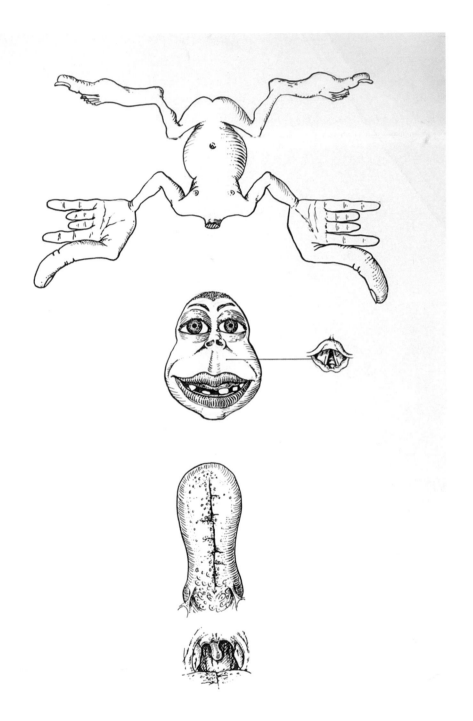

Figure 7.4: Sketch of the homunculus Mrs H.P. Cantiles for publication. (MNI Archives. W. Penfield and E.B. Boldrey, "Somatic Motor and Sensory Representation in the Cerebral Cortex of Man as Studied by Electrical Stimulation," *Brain* 60 [1937]: 389–443)

NURSING

Provisions were made for nursing on the private and public wards. A head nurse and three or four duty nurses staffed the fifteen-bed private wards during the day, and two duty nurses replaced them at night. The two public nursing wards were similarly staffed. A six-month postgraduate course, which met the special needs for nursing neurological and neurosurgical patients, was created, and could be extended to two years if training in operating room procedures was desired. The course included lectures in neuroanatomy, neurophysiology, neurology or neurosurgery, as well as nursing classes. Postgraduate trainees were assigned to the public wards, where they were "given a considerable amount of supervision and teaching while on duty."[4]

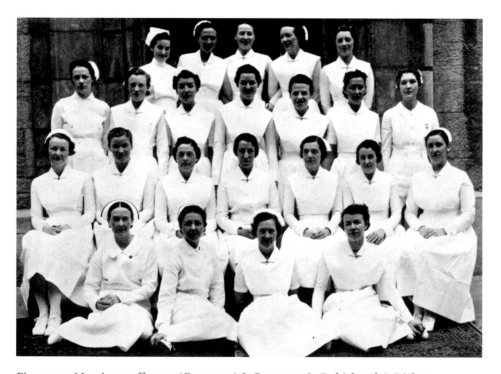

Figure 7.5: Nursing staff, 1936. (*Front row*) J. Cameron, L. Robichaud, I. Dickson, I. Gillispie. (*Second row*) C. Lambertus, C. MacLeod, B. Cameron, F. Flanagan, H. Eberle, L. MacNichol, M. Collins. (*Third row*) J. Young, G. Gordon, D. Fischer, M. Fenwick, C. Colpitts, L. Millette, M. McDonald. (*Top row*) C.T. LeBlanc, M. Howlett, A. Hudson, M. Reid, E. Scott. (MNI Archives)

Table 7.4
Nursing staff,* Montreal Neurological Institute, 1934–35

Supervisor	E. Flanagan
Assistant supervisor and ward teacher	H.M. Eberle
Night supervisor	B. Cameron
Operating room supervisor	K. Swicker
Ward nurse	M. Currie
Ward nurse	M. Goldie
Ward nurse	L. McNichol
Assistant operating room nurse	C. McLeod
General operating room duty	E. Kelly
General ward duty	M. Casselman
General ward duty	K. Kidd
General ward duty	C. Lambertus
General ward duty	E. Scott

* Mary Roach served as nurse-anaesthetist

ACADEMIA

The exuberance of the opening of the research laboratories at the institute was followed by the realization that the cost of proposed research programs exceeded income projections, as was made painfully obvious in Norman Petersen's 1936 report: "Because of decreased income from securities, the funds derived from the endowment given by the Rockefeller Foundation are ten thousand dollars less annually than the minimum which was estimated as necessary for the proper maintenance of the laboratory and research activities. Consequently the laboratory work has been handicapped and has fallen short of its full possible realization. Increased income is needed particularly for the endowment of research fellowships."[5] Nonetheless, a large number of publications came from the MNI in its first two years on University Street, many with observations obtained at surgery.

Insights from Surgery

Brain Tumours
Arthur Elvidge, Wilder Penfield, and William Cone read a paper at the annual meeting of the American Association for Research in Nervous and Mental Diseases on cerebral gliomas, based on the study of over 200 pathologically

verified cases[6] – a startlingly large number accumulated over a short time, which reflected Elvidge's interest in brain tumours. The reading of this paper generated a few irksome comments from Israel Strauss and Joseph Globus, of New York, who had coined the term *spongioblastoma multiforme*, which Penfield had favoured until this presentation. Penfield now preferred *glioblastoma multiforme*, which he felt required an explanation:

> I do still feel that spongioblastoma was a happier name. I do agree that it was better chosen in some ways. I do agree that his [Strauss] and Dr Joseph H. Globus was the first adequate description of this tumor type. On the other hand, when I found that Roussy and the French school had adopted glioblastoma, that Dr Dorothy Russell and others adopted that term, it seemed best not to claim to personal preference in names … Glioblastoma is the term which now appears in the nomenclature that was adopted by the National Organization on Nomenclature and was approved by the American Neurological Association. It seems to me that we would do well to have done with worrying about the names, to accept the national nomenclature and to carry on.[7]

Penfield had maintained his interest in tumours of the cranial nerves and, with his colleague Tremble, an otolaryngologist, published a beautifully illustrated paper of the exposure of tumours within the facial canal.[8] Penfield also pursued his interest in intracranial innervation to the dura as a cause of head pain, which was a vexing problem during awake craniotomies when certain areas of the dura were stimulated.[9]

Epilepsy and Surgical Therapy

A most important paper published in the first two years of the institute was Penfield's "Epilepsy and Surgical Therapy,"[10] which was first read at the International Neurologic Congress in London in July 1935, but was submitted late to the symposium organizer, Professor Otto Marburg, Penfield's opposite number at the Neurological Institute of the University of Vienna. Penfield felt that a personal note might mitigate his tardiness. In his note Penfield expresses his sadness at the death of Walther Spielmeyer, who had visited the institute and had provided advice on the treatment of one of the patients discussed in the submitted paper. Spielmeyer had succeeded Alzheimer in Munich and had worked with Franz Nissl. Both their names appear on the frieze in the MNI lobby.

26 April 1935.

Dear Professor Marburg,

Enclosed you will find the paper which I propose to read in London this summer. I shall not, of course, read all of it but shall abbreviate it so that I can present the important features of it in the time allotted to me. I hope that my delay has not made your management too difficult.

It was a great sorrow to me to learn of Spielmeyer's death. He will be very much missed. There are so few sincere and well trained workers in the field of neuropathology.

Yours sincerely

WGP[11]

Later published in the *Archives of Neurology and Psychiatry*, the paper is wonderfully written and comprehensive: it reviews epilepsy as a surgically treatable condition and discusses interventions from sympathectomy to subtemporal decompression, and from arterial ligation to cortical excision. For the first time, Penfield reports his surgical results in the treatment of focal epilepsy and stresses the importance of finding a resectable scar at surgery in order to achieve satisfactory seizure control. These included meningocerebral scars, which involved the meninges, and cerebral scars, which did not. Many patients had an explorative craniotomy with no other procedure performed, since a scar was not found on the surface of the exposed cortex. Some of these untreated patients were nonetheless inexplicably cured or improved. More than half of the patients (forty of seventy-seven) were improved by surgery, including some who had no curative procedure at all! It would take many years and the discovery of the role of incisural sclerosis in temporal lobe epilepsy by Penfield and Baldwin before these numbers would be improved upon.

Joseph Evans, in a very well-illustrated and innovative paper, reviews Penfield's patients in whom resections in the parietal lobe had produced loss of one or more sensory modalities.[12] A more complete assessment of the sensory localization would come thirty-five years later from the systematic observations of Penfield and Rasmussen in their monograph *The Cerebral Cortex of Man*.[13]

Basic Research

Financial shortfalls notwithstanding, basic research was inaugurated in the laboratories of the new institute. Evelyn Anderson and Webb Haymaker reported their study of hormones produced by pituitary cells grown in vitro, and on the in vitro growth of pituitary grafts.[14] They later wed. Evelyn Anderson would go on to a distinguished career at the University of California's Institute of Experimental Biology. Webb Haymaker would have a unique career, first as the head of neuropathology at the Armed Forces Institute of Pathology, and later as the head of Life-Sciences Research at the National Aeronautic and Space Administration's Ames Research Center. While still at the MNI, Haymaker and Jesus Sanchez-Perez, who, like Penfield, had worked with del Río-Hortega, described a new staining technique for tissue cultures, which appeared in *Science*.[15] Maude Abbott of McGill University rendered a great service to the history of neuroscience when she invited Sanchez-Perez to demonstrate del Río-Hortega's staining technique at the the International Association of Medical Museums in New York, in April 1935, as del Río-Hortega's technique had never before been fully described in English.[16] This was the technique that Rio-Hortega and Penfield had used to discover the oligodendro cyte and to study the glial reaction to brain wounds. George Stavraky, from Hungary, worked on the interaction of the thalamus and hypothalamus, an area that would later be a major focus of the Department of Neurophysiology at the MNI. He and Haddow Keith used thujone, a component of absinthe long used in France to induce experimental convulsions, to study the effects of seizures on the endocrine and autonomic nervous systems.[17]

Events

The American Neurological Association met in Montreal in June 1935, under the presidency of Colin Russel. Jason Mixter of Boston presented one of the earliest reports on the successful removal of a ruptured cervical intervertebral disc. William Cone was present and, in future years, he would become one of the most expert neurosurgeons operating upon this type of lesion. Wilder Penfield was president of the American Association of Neuropathologists, which also met in Montreal that year. It is a reflection of the high regard in which Russel and Penfield were held that this was the first time these two associations had their annual meeting outside of the United States.

As was often the case, the institute hosted a famous visitor during the academic year: "On two occasions during 1936, His Excellency, the Right Honorable Lord Tweedsmuir, governor-general of Canada, visited the Institute and following the second visit both he and Lady Tweedsmuir sent autographed photographs to us."[18] Lord Tweedsmuir would return to the institute later, not as a visitor, but as a patient, when he suffered a brain injury from a fall at Rideau Hall, the governor general's residence in Ottawa. Despite emergency surgery by Penfield and Cone in Ottawa, and then reoperation at the Montreal Neurological Institute, Tweedsmuir never recovered from his accident and died in February 1940.[19]

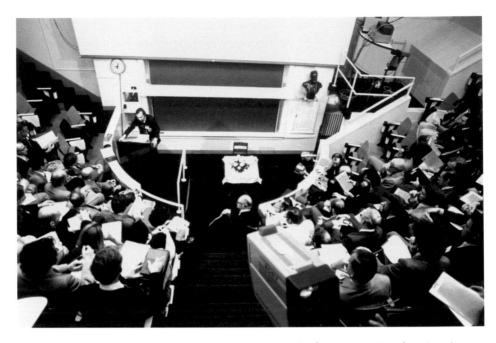

Figure 7.6: Hughlings Jackson amphitheatre during the first international symposium on computed tomography scanning, 1973. Roméo Ethier is at the podium, introducing William Feindel, sitting on a step, waiting to speak. (MNI Archives.)

THE FIRST HUGHLINGS JACKSON MEMORIAL LECTURE

The annual Hughlings Jackson Memorial Lecture is the MNI's oldest tradition, originally held in the institute's multi-tiered auditorium, later named the Hughlings Jackson amphitheatre. The amphitheatre was split by steep, narrow steps that challenged everyone's surefootedness. The stairway led to a small semi-circular area. Patients whose case was to be discussed gained access, in wheelchair or on a gurney, stage left, through a recessed side door. A bronze of Hughling's Jackson looked down on the patient as he or she entered. Stage right held the podium, where the lecturer addressed an audience that often had standing-room only. The Hughlings Jackson lecture remains the most prestigious event of the MNI's academic year and has been given by Nobel laureates, Gairdner Foundation award-winners, and other notable neuroscientists. Penfield gave the inaugural lecture, and although he never published his address, his very rough draft is reproduced here, as it sheds light upon Penfield's great admiration for Jackson, which guided his career. Noteworthy is Penfield's mention of Jackson's concept of a vasomotor etiology of epileptic seizures.

4 April 1935

To-day is the one hundredth anniversary of the birth of John Hughlings Jackson, the greatest leader of neurological thought. The event is being celebrated in many academic centres and the International Neurological Congress is held this summer in London in honor of Jackson. Otfried Foerster will there give the quinquennial Jackson Lecture which was inaugurated by Jackson himself. We in Montreal will be represented in that celebration by Dr. Colin Russel who is Vice-President of the Congress.

It is true of a number of great religious leaders that the influence of their teaching continues to be a guiding power long after they are dead. The same is true of some philosophers – Rousseau and Marx for example. But the number of physicians is few indeed of whom this may be said. It is true of Hughlings Jackson.

He was not a laboratory man like Pasteur. He was never an exhaustive recorder of clinical cases like his associate Sir William Gowers. He was a student of the neurological mechanisms which he surmised must lie behind the complaints and disabilities of sufferers from disease of the nervous system. His true interest lay, not in the nature of the lesion, he was not a pathologist; not in the remedy for the condition, he was not a therapeutist; and not primarily even in the alleviation of the suffering. He was a physiologist who never conducted an experiment, a philosopher who interested himself in the principle behind the manifestation.

At one time early in his career Jackson determined to forsake medicine for philosophy. Jonathan Hutchinson is credited with dissuading him, but I believe it was the challenge which epilepsy offered the philosophical mind that held him. "Epilepsy," he said, "is an experiment which disease carried out upon the brain."

One half of his writings, as collected by James Taylor, deal with epilepsy …

Jackson gave many definitions to the subject of his favourite preoccupation. "A convulsion," he said, "is but a clotted mess of innumerable movements." "Convulsion is the mobile counterpart of hemiplegia." Finally he defined epilepsy carefully as "the name for occasional, sudden, excessive, rapid and local discharges of grey matter."

The essential feature of his conception was that all epileptic fits result from local discharges of grey matter. His great French contemporary, Charcot, realizing the significance of this concept was the first to call localized motor fits "Jacksonian epilepsy" in his honor. Passing logically from the conception of local discharge he conceived the idea that convolutions represented specific movements and taught this ten years before the motor gyrus was demonstrated experimentally by Hitzig and by Ferrier.

In discussing representation Jackson, who knew nothing of chromosomes and less of genes said "A very small part of the body (the germ cell) represents the whole of the man it is detached from, even the tone of his voice and the tricks of his manner." This illustrates his way of using whimsical similes. He seems to have accepted the current view that blood vessel change was somehow the cause of these seizures but he expanded the conception characteristically. "It is, I speculate," he said, "through the arteries that sequence of movements is developed, whether these movements be spasm passing up the arm and down the leg, or whether they be orderly sequences of movements in health."

This involved a startling hypothetical attempt to explain the mechanism of control of voluntary movement, as well as the sequence of convulsive movement, by vascular control.

He saw no basic difference between essential (or idiopathic epilepsy) and focal epileptiform seizures, or between a sensory aura and a motor fit. It was all a matter of difference in localization of the discharge. Genuine epilepsy, for him, was highest level epilepsy. Epileptiform fits he considered middle level or motor province fits, and lowest level fits he called ponto-bulbar. Hence there were (1) epileptic fits, (2) epileptiform fits and (3) ponto-bulbar fits.

He saw immediately that in the lowest level of the brain stem and spinal cord the body and its parts are represented; in the cortex of the hemispheres there is a higher re-representation of a middle level which includes complicated movements and different aspects of sensation such as touch, vision and smell. He did not know until others discovered it that these movements were represented accurately in the precentral gyrus or vision in the calcarine cortex but long before these details were worked out he knew in a general way that it must be so. Observation of epileptic patterns had told him this and much more. Hemianopsia, he said, is the sensory homolog of the paralysis of the conjugate deviation.

But not stopping there and as usual limited only by the vaguest consideration for anatomy he reasoned that there must be on a still higher level centres which re-re-represent all the lower nervous arrangements and thus the whole body. Consciousness, he argued, is evolved out of and potentially contains all the lower sensori-motor series, and he quoted Herbert Spencer: "The seat of consciousness is that nervous centre to which mediately or immediately, the most heterogeneous impressions are brought."

And yet he did not consider himself a materialist for he said: "to give a materialistic explanation is not to give an anatomical one." He believed in a parallelism between mind and matter but did not concern himself as to what the actual connection might be.

A seizure initiated by primary loss of consciousness "begins," he said, "in the very highest nervous arrangements." In such cases there is "pallor, flow of saliva and universal movement." He observed further that when an aura preceded loss of consciousness it was most often a sensation in the epigastrium, that essential epilepsy had its discharge in this highest level and that petit mal seemed to be associated with the anterior cerebral arteries, but no Hitzig has yet come forward to follow Jackson's pointing finger and to delimit this highest level in terms of anatomy.

Curiously enough it has been stated, by those who should know better, that Jackson considered a convulsion to be a manifestation of release from control. This is quite untrue. He considered it to be due to a *discharge* of grey matter. The concept of release he applied to the automatic states which follow confusion. In this case the seizure, he believed, usually took place on the highest level and was followed by paralysis of the same sensori-motor substratum. Such a paralysis in the middle level might produce post-convulsive monoplegia but the paralysis occurring in the highest level served only to paralyze the substratum of consciousness thus releasing temporarily a completely irresponsible "automatic" individual. Recurring epileptic insanity due to this cause interested him much.

In these efficient and highly mechanized times we record exhaustively, experiment enthusiastically and publish data interminably. To the study of much evidence we often bring little insight. What a contrast is the picture of Hughlings Jackson observing a patient in the National Hospital in Queen Square and retiring to his carriage to spin constructive hypotheses behind a team of trotting horses. He did not subject these hypotheses to laboratory tests, but he tested them just the same. He returned again to the wards of the hospital to see how disease had carried out her multiform experiments for him upon the nervous systems of suffering human beings. Observing and musing thus he conceived logical principles and he became the founder of modern neurology and his conjecture still runs before our laboured thought.[20] [The following seventeen pages are missing. The last six pages contain a description of seizure patterns.]

JACKSON IN HEAVEN

The inaugural Hughlings Jackson lecture and celebrations required some preparation, on which Penfield elaborated to his friend at the time, Sir Francis Walshe, imminent editor of *Brain*, 22 March 1935:

> We are having a small celebration here in Montreal on the fourth of April with a Jackson Memorial Lecture in the afternoon and short papers by some of the fellows in the evening on different aspects of Jackson's contributions. The latter meeting will be softened or somewhat liquefied with beer and even a short skit by some of the younger members of the clinic. I believe that in the skit Jackson returns from the neurological heaven where he is said to live entirely alone …
> Yours sincerely,
> WGP[21]

Penfield may have gotten more than he bargained for: William Gibson had suggested to Penfield that the MNI celebrate the centenary of Hughlings Jackson's birthday. William Graham, a resident in neuropathology, wrote a "take-off on the faculty and staff" to mark the occasion. As Gibson recalled, "Webb Haymaker was Sir Victor Borsley and I was Jughlings Hackson. The quips which Grant had incorporated in the play were pretty close to the bone, as we hung up our respective haloes on a hat stand supposedly in heaven. No one escaped and the 'humor' was savage."[22] Fortunately, as Penfield mentioned, the affair was well lubricated, and everyone's budding career was saved. But a tradition was born: the Annual Hughlings Jackson Lecture and Dinner.

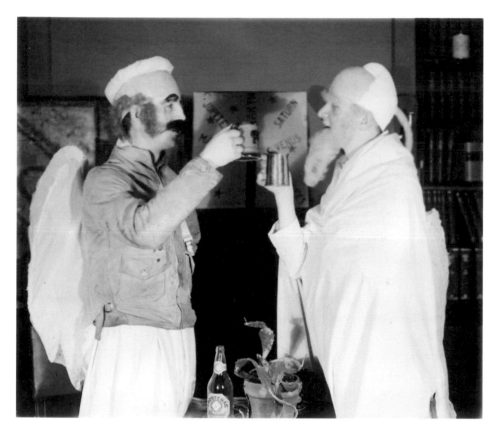

Figure 7.7: First Hughlings Jackson Day celebrations by the Fellows Society of the Montreal Neurological Institute, 1 April 1935. Webb Haymaker appears at the left as Sir Victor Horsley. William Gibson is at right, as John Hughlings Jackson come down from Heaven – it is not stated where Horsley resided at the time. (Haymaker had a distinguished career as director of the Armed Forces Institute of Pathology. He later contributed greatly to the American space program and was awarded the NASA Exceptional Scientific Achievement Medal. Gibson became one of the most influential academics of his day, and was instrumental in the founding of two colleges, one at Oxford University and the other at the University of British Columbia. Penfield Archives.)

8

Elvidge, McNaughton, and Jasper

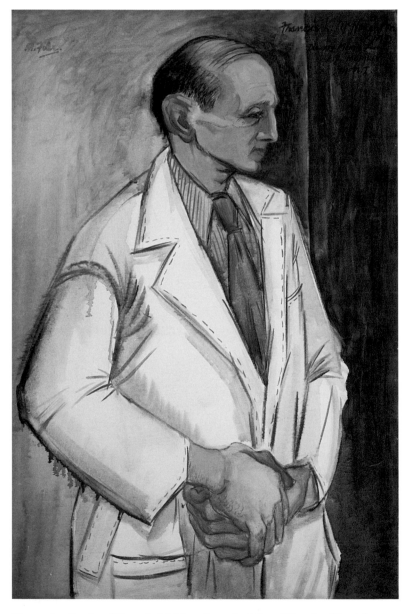

Figure 8.1: Study of Francis McNaughton by Mary Filer, for *The Advance of Neurology*. (Courtesy Dr Fred Andermann)

ARTHUR ELVIDGE AND THE INTRODUCTION OF
CEREBRAL ANGIOGRAPHY IN NORTH AMERICA

Arthur Roland Elvidge, born in London, England, in 1899,[1] immigrated to Canada with his family when he was twelve and eventually settled in Montreal. Elvidge enlisted in the Royal Canadian Army at seventeen and fought at Passchendaele. He obtained his MD, CM (Doctor of Medicine, Master of Surgery) from McGill University in 1924, and postgraduate degrees for research on the reticulo-endothelial system from the same institution. Penfield held Elvidge in high esteem and his words, to his life-long friend Stanley Cobb, express his feelings candidly: Arthur Elvidge, Penfield wrote,

> emerged from the laboratory and put in two years as surgical intern. At that tme Dr Archibald was willing to offer him a permanent position in the lung clinic. We managed to get him away from there and he spent three years as Resident and Neuropathologist … He is the neurosurgeon in charge at the Montreal General Hospital and is more or less in charge of the neurophysiological work here at the Institute. He does practically all of his operating at the Institute, bringing his cases up from the General. He has a good mind and I think will have a future of continued service to the cause of neurology.[2]

Elvidge completed his training in neurosurgery with Penfield and Cone in 1932. He then took the familiar road to Queen Square, but his most productive time abroad was spent in Lisbon with António Egas Moniz, the neurologist who introduced angiography of the brain in 1927.[3] Elvidge headed his own neurosurgical service when the MNI opened in 1934. There, he developed an interest in the treatment of malignant gliomas, and Cone often referred such cases to him. As Preston Robb noted, "He was a remarkably skilled neurosurgeon and had a great interest in brain tumours. His skill in removing them was extraordinary."[4]

Perhaps the most noteworthy contribution to clinical neurology at the nascent MNI was Arthur Elvidge's introduction of cerebral angiography to North America.[5] Elvidge performed this examination on three patients in 1934 and six in 1935. By 1938 his experience was broad enough for Elvidge to publish his methodology and to assess the usefulness of this technique in the diagnosis of cerebral lesions.[6]

Prior to angiography, radiological diagnosis of intracranial lesions relied on skull X-rays, PEG, and ventriculograms.[7] Radiography of the skull was of limited value unless the pineal gland was calcified and shifted to one side,

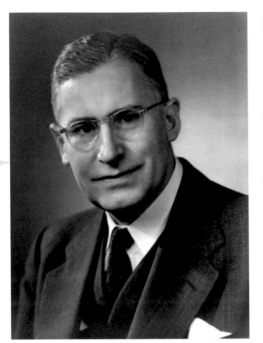
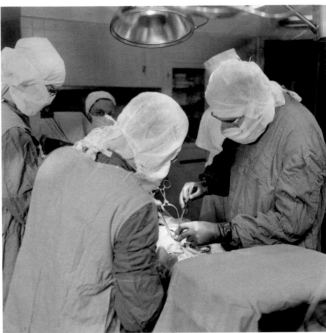

Figures 8.2 and 8.3: Arthur Elvidge (*left*) operating on a spinal lesion (*right*).
(MNI Archives)

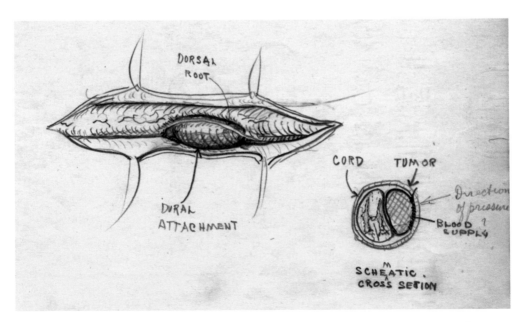

Figure 8.4: Operative drawing of one of Elvidge's cases, illustrating the relationship of
an intradural, extramedullary tumour to the spinal cord and nerve. (MNI Archives)

indicating the presence of a mass lesion. Hyperostosis could signify the presence of a meningioma, especially if accompanied by a widening of the groove of the middle meningeal artery, which supplied the lesion. Stippled areas of calcifications could suggest the presence of a tumour, such as an oligodendroglioma, the type of tumour that affected Penfield's sister. One or many partially calcified angiomas could also be seen on plain skull X-ray. Nonetheless, astute observation and a prepared mind could still exploit skull X-rays to advantage and even make novel observations. This was the case for two landmark papers published by Penfield and his collaborators. The first was published with Rawle Geyelin, a physician at the Presbyterian Hospital, New York, describing the familial occurrence of what Penfield referred to as *endarteritis calcificans cerebri*, consisting of calcified arteries at the junction of the white and grey matter and associated with cerebral induration resembling "pink coral with a shade of tan," as colourfully reported by William Cone in his description of the histopathology.[8] The second paper was published with Arthur Ward, then a fellow at the MNI, and is an early report of a calcified cavernous angioma, which Penfield and Ward termed *hemangioma calcificans*.[9] A genetic contribution to the ethology of cavernous angiomas and other cerebrovascular hamartomas is currently a very active area of investigation.[10]

Pneumoencephalography required a lumbar puncture, the injection of air into the subarachnoid space, and placement of the patient in a series of positions to allow the air to fill every part of the ventricular system. It most often resulted in severe headache, nausea, and vomiting, sometimes lasting for days. Ventriculography added the possible complications attendant to puncturing the brain with a blunt needle. All that could be achieved with these studies was observation of either the distorted shape of the ventricular system by a mass lesion; focal enlargement, most frequently of the temporal horn, indicating atrophy of the mesial temporal lobe structures in patients with temporal lobe epilepsy; or diffuse ventriculomegaly. Neither of these examinations could reveal a vascular malformation or an aneurysm, the blush of a vascularized tumour nor its displacement of the vascular tree. Cerebral angiography was thus a major advance in the diagnosis of intracranial vascular lesions and of brain tumours.

Angiography, as Arthur Elvidge described it, was a major undertaking. It began in the operating room with the patient under general anaesthesia and the common carotid artery exposed low in the neck. The patient, still covered with surgical drapes, was then transported to the Neuroradiology Department. There, the common carotid artery was punctured with a needle whose tip was advanced into the internal carotid artery. Two or three radiological plates were

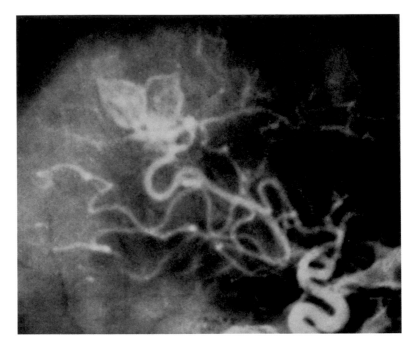

Figures 8.5 and 8.6: Case M.G. Angiogram obtained by Elvidge of an arteriovenous malformation of the right central cortex, and photograph taken during the excision of the AVM by Wilder Penfield, showing the location of the lesion just behind the motor strip (*opposite*). Note the numbered tickets that mark the locations of motor responses obtained by electrical stimulation. This is the first example published of the use of angiography together with intraoperative cortical mapping. (A.R. Elvidge, "The Cerebral Vessels Studied by Angiography," *Proceedings of the Association for Research in Nervous and Mental Disease* 18 [1938]: 110–49. Copyright Wolters Kluver)

exposed to obtain the angiogram, after which the patient was returned to the operating room for surgery upon the newly revealed lesion. Visualization of the vertebro-basilar circulation was even more complicated. After the common carotid artery was punctured, the tip of the needle was directed proximally toward the aorta or subclavian artery. The surgeon compressed the distal carotid artery to allow the contrast material to flow in a retrograde fashion. At the same time an assistant compressed the axillary artery so that the contrast material could make its way up the vertebral artery into the basilar artery and reveal the posterior circulation of the brain. Since a mechanized system for the rapid exposure of a series of X-ray films had not yet been invented, the angiographer had to expose the X-ray plates at the proper time after the injection of the contrast material to show the arterial and venous phases of the cerebral circula-

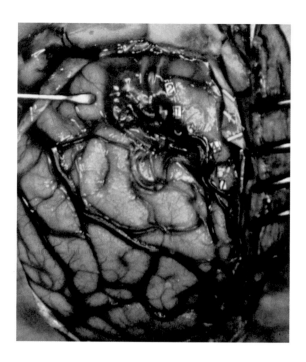

tion. As Elvidge described it, "For ordinary purposes in angiography two plates may suffice – one to show the arterial tree and a second, taken some three to four seconds later, to demonstrate the venous channels. One may, of course, vary the time interval to obtain the desired results, with some success, but obviously, the best way is to produce a succession of plates, one second apart if this is possible."[11] During the mid-1930s, Elvidge and research fellow Jesus Sanchez-Perez "fashioned a mechanical changer from castoff materials, including a bicycle chain and pedal … this machine was one of only three semiautomatic film changers in existence at the time."[12]

Using these techniques, Elvidge was able to demonstrate arteriovenous malformations, aneurysms, and mass lesions. Angiograms were obtained in stereotactic mode by exposing successive films with a separation of seven degrees. This had a distinct advantage in demonstrating the arteries that supplied an arteriovenous malformation (AVM) and the veins draining it, and in demonstrating small vascular lesions. The technique of stereoscopic angiography remained in everyday use at the MNI into the twenty-first century.

The iconic images from Elvidge's 1938 paper are of an arteriovenous malformation revealed by arteriography and by operative photography, the latter demonstrating the relationship of the AVM to the motor strip as identified by cortical mapping under local anaesthesia. This case was retrieved for this publication and Penfield's operative drawing is reproduced here for the first time.

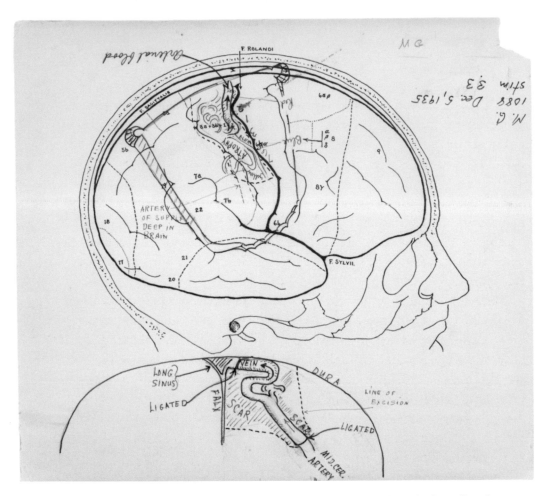

Figure 8.7: Penfield's operative drawing of case M.G., initially drawn "upside down," as the surgeon views the brain from the vertex during surgery. Here it is reproduced in the more conventional orientation. The numbers represent motor responses. Note the *U*-shaped artery that also appears at the centre of the angiogram and operating photograph, which represents a superficial branch of a deeper artery supplying the AVM. The draining vein and the direction of blood flow are indicated by the arrow. The vein is noted to drain "arterial blood," indicating shunting of arterial blood directly into the veins draining the lesion. This is also illustrated at the lower aspect of Penfield's drawing, showing the AVM in frontal view. (MNI Archives)

Of this case, Penfield commented in his operative note, "The arteriogram which had been made by Dr Elvidge had demonstrated the structure as it was found very beautifully."[13] Cortical mapping in the treatment of arteriovenous malformations within eloquent brain regions remained a routine procedure at the MNI for many years thereafter.

By the mid-1940s angiography had become commonplace, but the treatment of cerebral aneurysms lagged behind. When Elvidge and Feindel reported a case of direct, intracranial obliteration of an anterior circulation aneurysm in 1947, only nine similar cases had been previously reported.[14] In the same report they also discussed the insightful use of electroencephalography, which had been introduced at the MNI by Herbert Jasper in 1938, to monitor a patient's progress post-operatively. They observed that sub-arachnoid hemorrhage could result in "changes in the normal circulatory equilibrium with a resulting ischemia of the cerebral tissue lying beyond the aneurysm," presumably from cerebral vasospasm.[15]

Cerebral angiography, with improved methodology and equipment, remained within the purview of neurosurgery at the MNI until Roméo Ethier became head of the Department of Neuroradiology and introduced the transfemoral approach for the selective catheterization of the carotid and vertebral arteries.

Residents and nurses who held Penfield in awe and were exhausted by Cone's work schedule, had a great fondness for Elvidge and found him more approachable.[16] He was "extraordinarily good-natured, relaxed, and friendly," and he always seemed to find the right words to relax the atmosphere in the operating room, especially when the unexpected occurred.[17] One of his residents tells of the time when he had suggested to Elvidge that an aneurysm that both thought had been satisfactorily clipped should be excised, as was often done at the time. Elvidge hesitated for a moment and began to dissect the aneurysm further with a view to following this suggestion, when suddenly a gush of arterial blood filled the operative field. Elvidge, with some difficulty, arrested the bleeding and, when all was under control, turned to the resident, deadpan, and said, "Thank you, Bill," without further comment.[18]

Unlike Cone, who regularly made rounds promptly at 7:45 every evening and expected to be met by the residents, Elvidge arrived unnoticed at irregular hours, sometimes as late as 11:00 p.m. The nurses then quietly called the residents down from their quarters on the eighth floor. They joined Elvidge for ward rounds, and the next day's operating list was finalized.

Arthur Elvidge retired in 1962, but his later years were marred by the onset of Parkinson's disease. Despite Elvidge's severe disability, Richard Leblanc recalls seeing him in his wheelchair at the back of the Hughlings Jackson amphitheatre, his eyes beaming with pride, as he listened to David Hubel, former resident and fellow, give his first lecture after being awarded the Nobel Prize.

FRANCIS LOTHIAN MCNAUGHTON

Francis McNaughton, like Arthur Elvidge, appears in Mary Filer's evocative mural *The Advance of Neurology*. It is striking that the central figure of this mural is not Penfield but Francis McNaughton, universally known as Saint Francis, warmly, lovingly, respectfully, and never in his presence.

McNaughton was physician to, and a close personal friend of, Stanley Knowles, the parliamentarian and promoter of universal health care in Canada. McNaughton attended Knowles through a dozen political campaigns over four decades, encouraging him to participate in political life despite his multiple sclerosis. Knowles wrote of his friend Francis, "He gave many hundreds of other people a similar chance to live and to have a better life. He was a fine gentleman, a kindly person, and a remarkable physician."[19]

First and foremost, McNaughton was a physician. To William Feindel, McNaughton's "success as a neurologist can be attributed not only to his skill and knowledge of the anatomy of the brain and nerves but as well to the honesty and warmth of his character."[20] McNaughton began his career at the MNI in 1934 as an experienced clinical researcher, having investigated the use of ergotamine in the treatment of migraine. He later wrote his MSc thesis on the distribution of pain fibres of the dura and cerebral vessels.[21] He remained true to *migraineux* and others suffering from head pain, trigeminal neuralgia, and post-traumatic headache throughout his career.[22]

Francis McNaughton became neurologist-in-chief at the MNI in 1951, and in 1959 he became the first professor of neurology to be appointed at McGill University. McNaughton elevated teaching and research at McGill to new levels.[23] He recruited wisely and attracted the likes of Miller Fisher, Bernard Graham, Donald Lloyd-Smith, Roy Swank, Reuben Rabinovitch, and Donald Tower to McGill and the institute. As Preston Robb wrote of McNaughton, "In his kindly and forceful way, he was able to get things done where others had failed. Perhaps most importantly, he ran a happy ship and was beloved by all."[24] McNaughton held many administrative posts in learned societies during his tenure at the MNI, including the vice-presidency of the American Neurological Association, and the presidencies of the Canadian Neurological Society and of the American Epilepsy Society.

Although headache and migraine were major interests, McNaughton was equally preoccupied with the care of epileptic patients. He was one of the earliest investigators to use mysoline and other medications in the treatment of epileptic seizures.[25] He also recognized the role of surgery in the treatment of medically intractable epilepsy and was especially expert in the selection of patients who would benefit from surgery. Penfield held McNaughton in such high regard as an epileptologist that he invited him to write the chapter on the medical management of epileptic seizures in *Epilepsy and the Functional Anatomy of the Human Brain*.[26]

McNaughton remained true to his friends – he was a member of the Norman Bethune Foundation to the end of his days.[27] He was often seen on the

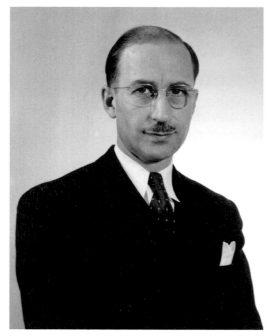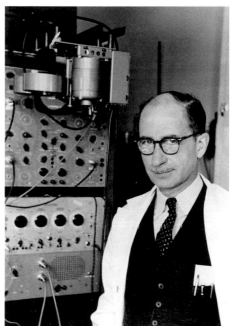

Figures 8.8 and 8.9: Herbert Jasper. (MNI Archives)

wards of the MNI well into retirement, looking in on an old patient whose care he had transferred to a younger colleague, or consulting at the request of a colleague on a patient whose condition was difficult to diagnose. McNaughton provided these services as long as his health permitted, and when he was in decline, his first students at the institute cared for him as one would an elderly parent. He died in 1986.

HERBERT JASPER AND THE ELECTRICAL ACTIVITY OF THE BRAIN

In 1937, the year that Elvidge presented his paper on angiography, Herbert Jasper crossed the Canadian border heading north carrying a primitive EEG machine in the back seat of his car. Jasper was on his way from Brown University, in Providence, Rhode Island, to the MNI, to help Wilder Penfield come to a more precise localization of epileptic seizures. Jasper would have an enormous impact on the diagnosis and treatment of epilepsy, the development of neurophysiological research, and the international recognition of EEG as a clinical and scientific tool.[28]

Herbert Henri Jasper was born in La Grande, Oregon, in 1906. A keen student of psychology and philosophy, he earned a BA in 1927 and an MSc in 1929. Jasper then left Oregon for the University of Iowa, where he obtained his first PhD. Jasper had the good fortune of attending a conference where he met Alexandre and Andrée Monnier, who were working with Herbert Spencer Gasser then at Washington State University. Gasser won the Nobel Prize in 1944 for his studies on axonal transmission and gave the Hughlings Jasckson Memorial Lecture at the MNI in 1957. The Monniers invited Jasper to join them in Paris, at La Sorbonne, where he worked with them and Louis Lapicque on chronaxie – a measure of neuronal excitability.[29] As Jasper recalls his first crossing of the Atlantic, "We sailed from Oregon on a passenger freighter through the Panama Canal in the summer of 1931. It was a long and delightful trip and we arrived in Paris in time to start the year at the Sorbonne in the fall of 1931. It was a most important turning point in my career."[30]

Jasper returned to the United States in 1932 and took a position at Brown University, where he developed an EEG laboratory. Then in 1935 he and Leonard Carmichael published the first report in the United States on the human EEG, in which they cautiously predicted, "It may well be that the electroencephalograms … may prove significant in psychology and clinical neurology. It is even possible that this technique may provide information in regard to brain action which will be comparable in significance to the information in regard to heart function which is provided by the electrocardiograph."[31]

Jasper returned to Paris in 1935 to defend his *Doctorat ès Science* thesis, which included a supplement entitled "Electroencéphalographie chez l'homme" (Electroencephalography in man) based on his work at Brown. In the same year Foerster and the physiologist Altenburger reported the first use of EEG for recording directly from the cerebral cortex during surgery.[32]

A CHANCE ENCOUNTER

Herbert Jasper first met Wilder Penfield in 1937, when Penfield was invited to Brown University to give a seminar on the electrical stimulation of the cortex, and after the seminar Penfield visited Jasper's laboratory. It was isolated from electrical interference by chicken wire. As Penfield recalled, "Inside the maze was a young man, moving about like a bird in an aviary. This was a rare bird, a *rara avis*, Herbert Jasper, a young man driven by one creative idea after another. He could, he said, localize the focus of an epileptic seizure by the disturbance of brain rhythms outside the skull. I doubted that but hoped it might be true."[33]

As a result of this encounter Jasper sent two patients to the MNI, in whom he claimed to have localized an epileptogenic focus by EEG. Penfield operated upon the two, and in each case he confirmed Jasper's localization. Penfield immediately recognized the potential value of Jasper's EEG methods and suggested that he spend more time at the institute. Clearly, Jasper also recognized the value of such a partnership, as he wrote to Penfield on 5 February 1938.

My Dear Dr Penfield:

The more I think about your proposal that we should join forces in our respective fields of research, the more I believe that such collaboration should result in some very important progress in the interpretation of electroencephalograms, and I should hope that also it would make some significant contributions to our general understanding of epilepsy … I am also very much interested in following up the operated cases to obtain a good record of the change in the electrical activity of the brain.

This should yield important information in regard to some general questions of brain physiology as well as test the efficiency of the operation in removing a discharging focus and possibly result in the discovery of new foci in some cases.

I feel that this is such an excellent opportunity that you have suggested, that I would like very much to spend the next three months in Montreal, but I do not see how that can be arranged in the immediate future … Do you think that our collaboration might be satisfactory if I could plan on being in Montreal Thursday, Friday, and Saturday of each week? This would necessitate considerable expense for travel, but in view of the importance of the work I believe that it would be worth the expense.

In regard to equipment, I have a very good portable set-up which could be very easily transported to Montreal in my car. It is now being used for some of our own work in the hospitals, but I will be glad to remove it temporarily in case you wish to have some cases run before your equipment is completed.

Very sincerely yours,
Herbert H. Jasper[34]

Penfield agreed, and the results were gratifying for both men. Penfield invited Jasper to relocate to the MNI permanently, and an annex "dedicated to clinical electroencephalography for the study of epilepsy and mental illness" was added in the basement of the institute in the fall of 1938.[35] Of his career at the institute, Herbert Jasper later wrote, "My time with Wilder Penfield and his family, in which I became an adopted member, working with his splendid enthusiastic staff and hundreds of colleagues and students from all over the world who worked with us, was certainly a most pleasant and productive 27 years of my life."[36]

The work of the Department of Electroencephalography began on 15 September 1938, its activities concerned mainly with localization of epileptogenic foci as an aid to the clinical investigation of potential surgical candidates. The MNI held a symposium on EEG on 24 February 1939, and as an indication of the interest in this subject at the time, participants came from elite New England colleges, including Brown, Harvard, the University of Pennsylvania, and Yale. The MNI was well represented as well: John Kershman spoke on focal epilepsy and the results of surgery, Theodore Erickson discussed the spread of epileptic discharge and excitation across the cortex and the corpus callosum in monkeys, and Penfield addressed the propagation of epileptic seizures in man.[37]

Very rapidly after his arrival, the Department of Neurophysiology, under Jasper's direction, published a number of significant papers.[38] A few years later, Jasper was able to contribute the first comprehensive description of the essential role of EEG and electrocorticography in the diagnosis and treatment of epilepsy in Penfield and Erickson's *Epilepsy and Cerebral Localization*.[39] Jasper had an even greater role in the magnum opus *Epilepsy and the Functional Anatomy of the Human Brain*, which he co-authored with Penfield, and which remains unique in its genre.[40]

Feeling the need for more medical training, Herbert Jasper enrolled as a medical student, taking his MDCM at McGill in 1943. Much to his surprise and consternation, he received a failing grade on his final examination because he defined death as a cessation of electrical activity in the brain, when his professors had a more mechanical conception based on the inactivity of the heart. After some petitioning, Jasper was granted a passing grade and added a medical degree to his PhD and DSc. When the time came, Jasper dedicated his department to the war effort, as did others at the MNI. He served as a captain in the Royal Canadian Army, although, like Cone, he had not taken Canadian citizenship, but would do so later.[41] With the end of the war, Jasper found a new focus for his research, delving into the deep grey nuclei of the brain and exploring their relationship to the cortex.[42] With the assistance of the brilliant and insightful Pierre Gloor, the department also investigated the physiology and connections of the limbic system, for which Gloor was awarded a PhD for his dissertation "Electrophysiological Studies of the Amygdala in the Cat."[43] The international success of the Department of Neurophysiology attracted a great number of trainees over the years, many of whom achieved prominence in the clinical and basic neurosciences.

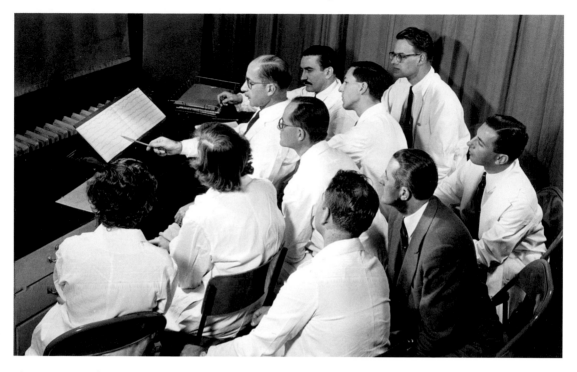

Figure 8.10: Herbert Jasper teaching. Cosimo Ajmone-Marsan is the mustachioed gentleman at Jasper's right, while Gilles Bertrand is directly behind Jasper, straining to see the EEG recording to which Jasper is pointing. (W. Feindel, "Brain Physiology at the Montreal Neurological Institute: Some Historical Highlights," *Journal of Clinical Neurophysiology* 9 [1992]: 176–94)

JOURNAL OF ELECTROENCEPHALOGRAPHY AND CLINICAL NEUROPHYSIOLOGY AND THE INTERNATIONAL BRAIN RESEARCH ORGANIZATION

In 1947, the International Federation of Electroencephalography was inaugurated in London, England, and the *Journal of Electroencephalography and Clinical Neurophysiology* was launched, with Herbert Jasper as editor-in-chief. Jasper's wife, Goldie, who had been head nurse on the Children's Ward at the MNI, took on the organization of this new journal, which quickly grew to international stature.

Jasper attended a meeting of the International Federation of EEG and Clinical Neurophysiology in Moscow in 1958. As a result of this meeting – and more importantly, of Jasper's influence – the International Brain Research Organization (IBRO) was created. As Jasper retells it, "After the close of the Moscow Colloquium in 1958 I had a private conference with the president of the Soviet

Academy of Science which resulted in his agreement to collaborate with our international efforts in this direction."[44] Jasper took a sabbatical year and moved to Paris as IBRO's first executive secretary.

Herbert Jasper left the MNI in 1964 to join Jean-Pierre Cordeau, a former MNI fellow, at the Université de Montréal. Jasper remained a consultant in neurophysiology at the institute and collaborated with Gilles Bertrand in the exploration of the deep nuclei during the treatment of patients with Parkinson's disease.[45] Jasper also worked with K.A.C. Elliott and others from the MNI in elaborating the functions of gamma amino butyric acid – GABA – and of acetylcholine in the cerebral cortex.[46] Jasper was called upon to develop the first workshop on research into the epilepsies, which published its deliberations as the classic *Basic Mechanisms of the Epilepsies*.[47] *Basic Mechanisms* has been rejuvenated every decade since and serves as Dr Jasper's enduring legacy.

9

Rumours of War

Herbert Jasper was not the only new arrival at the institute in 1937. Antonio Barbeau, from the Université de Montréal, joined Amyot, Saucier, and Legrand as an associate consulting neurologist at the MNI, further strengthening the ties of the institute with the French-speaking population of Montreal. Barbeau's son André later trained in neurology at the MNI and gained international recognition for his work on Parkinson's disease. Roy Swank came to the institute in 1939 and achieved international recognition for his work in multiple sclerosis, while others came as clinical and research fellows. Notable among these was Y.-c. Chao, who became the first neurosurgeon in China and cemented a relationship between that country and the MNI that still thrives.

Others came to the institute as the political situation of Europe deteriorated. One was Karl Stern, who had studied neuropathology with Walther Spielmeyer in Munich and J. Godwin Greenfield at Queen Square before coming to the MNI in 1939. Stern's interests at the MNI were many, a reflection of the quality of his training and the quickness of his mind. He worked on the thalamico-cortical connections with Francis McNaughton, on tumour invasion with Guy Odom, and on intracellular neurofibrils in Alzheimer's disease with K.A.C. Elliott. Stern also provided clinical service to the institute, working in neuropathology with Cone.[1] Karl Stern is known to the general public for his very successful *Pillar of Fire*, about a man's spiritual quest in troubled times.[2] Miguel Prados, a student of Cajal, left Franco's Spain for the MNI and joined the staff as a research fellow and clinical assistant in neuropsychiatry. Like Stern, Prados later relocated to the Allan Memorial Institute and became one of Canada's earliest psychoanalysts.

The MNI received a portentous visit in 1937, from Propper Graschenko. Graschenko was destined for an influential career in the Soviet medical hierarchy and was instrumental in fostering future interaction between the institute and the Soviet Union. Graschenko, as director of the Institute for Investigation of the Nervous System, proposed that Penfield visit the Soviet Union during the Second World War to assess their medical services and invited him to the Soviet Union again two decades later, to attend to the physicist Lev Davidovich Landau (see below).[3]

EPILEPTOGENIC LESIONS AND SEIZURE PROPAGATION

Cortical Microgyria

The immediate pre-war period was especially fertile for research at the MNI. One of the most important contributions to the broad field of epilepsy was the discovery of focal polymicrogyria and its role in epileptogenesis. Penfield and Cone's contribution to our understanding of one of the important causes of epilepsy has been largely forgotten and is revived here. Interest in this condition was renewed with the advent of magnetic resonance imaging, and focal polymicrogyria and other cortical malformations are now major areas of epilepsy research.

Penfield and his collaborators first used the term *microgyria* in print in 1939.[4] It is now commonly referred to as *focal polymicrogyria*, a term used to describe a section of the cerebral cortex with multiple malformed convolutions resulting in an irregular "bumpy" cortical surface. The first patient in whom "microgyria" was described was a thirteen-year-old girl whose mother had a difficult pregnancy and a prolonged labour, and who was cyanotic at birth. She developed seizures characterized by numbness of the fingers of the right hand, with occasional Jacksonian march and generalization, starting at the age of twelve years. Radiological investigation revealed that the left cranial fossa was smaller than the right, the left lateral ventricle was larger than its opposite number, and the septum pelucidum was deviated to the left, all attesting to longstanding atrophy of the left cerebral hemisphere. An epileptic focus was recorded over the left parietal area. Wilder Penfield and William Lister Reid operated upon the patient on 16 December 1938. Penfield's operative report states,

> Just posterior to what seemed to be the post-central gyrus, there was a white crusty patch where the pia arachnoid was very much thickened and there was obvious connective tissue. This surmounted an atrophied gyrus. In a narrow line or in a zone about one cm. in width, passing downwards as far as the fissure of Sylvius there was an area of obvious

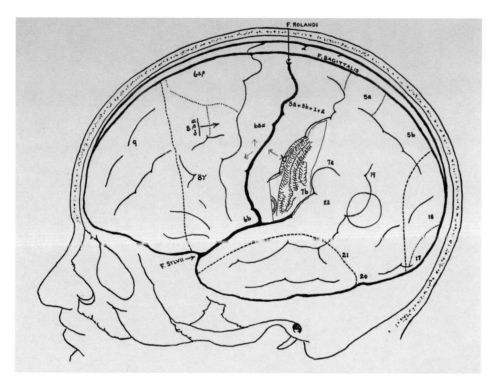

Figure 9.1: Penfield's operative drawing of case LB. The area of focal microgyria is enclosed within the red line, outlining the area of resection. "Sensation in palm & fingers. Almost Like Aura" were rerecorded at point X. (MNI Archives)

focal microgyria. During the removal it became evident that there were at least three gyri within the zone. At some places the width of each gyrus was only 1–2 mms. These passed inwards to the bottom of the fissure, at a depth of about 2 cms where it was continuous with rather dense resistant white matter.[5]

Penfield's operative sketch is seen here (figure 9.1) for the first time since it was drawn.

The lesion was resected and examined microscopically by William Cone and Robert Pudenz, who observed that the

specimen is seen to be comprised of two small bits of cortex. In the grey matter there has been a striking diminution of ganglion cells. Those remaining have been isolated into groups by projections of tissue upward from the white matter. These projections consist of a close feltwork of

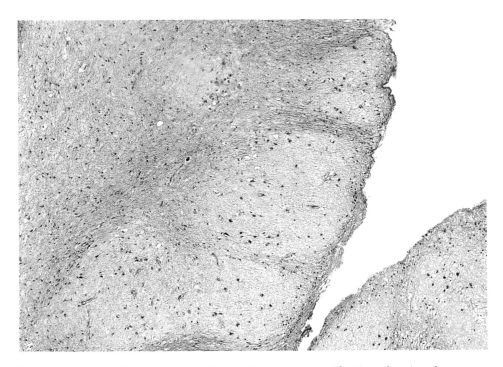

Figure 9.2: Histopathological slide of case LB at 100x magnification, showing the markedly thinned cortex with an overly convoluted, nodular appearance. The darker material arranged in bands extending towards the cortical surface are "upward projections" of white matter. (Courtesy Jason Karamchandani, MNI)

delicate fibrils staining bluish. This is especially dense in the white matter ... there is no architectonic pattern whatever. The majority of the remaining cells stain poorly and are seen in various stages of chromatolysis. Many of the nuclei are pyknotic ... Ganglion cells stain poorly ... There is disorganization of the entire structure.[6]

Penfield did not publish an illustration of the histopathology of this important case, but the original blocks were retrieved from the Department of Neuropathology at the MNI in 2014 and examined by Jason Karamchandani, neuropathologist at the institute.[7] He observed that the specimen shows markedly thinned cortex with an overly convoluted, nodular appearance. Bands of material extending towards the cortical surface are also present, constituting the "upward projections" of white matter that William Cone noted in his original report. Thus, Penfield and Cone had "unequivocally and accurately identified his patient's lesion as what is now recognized as focal polymicrogyria."[8]

Penfield's exuberance on encountering microgyria is displayed in an operative note: "On coming to the bank over which point 18 lay we suddenly and quite unexpectedly came upon a small, buried, yellowish, tough microgyrus."[9] His interest in this pathology persisted well into the 1950s and a very informative section on this topic is to be found in "Epilepsy and the Functional Anatomy of the Human Brain."

Penfield correctly surmised that microgyria can result from anoxia-ischemia, stating,

> Focal Microgyria … is produced by localized ischemia during birth … It seems evident that the combination of cranial compression and molding and defective fetal circulation results in ischemia of one gyrus or a group of gyri. In such gyri there is destruction of the nerve cells, which can survive complete anoxemia for only a few minutes. There results rapid convolutional shrinkage during the first year of life, the period of maximum growth of the brain. The normal convolutions are forced to move toward the area in question, and the cranial chamber, which enlarges only in response to the thrust of the brain, remains smaller on the affected side, while the underlying ventricle is moulded into a normal general outline.[10]

This results in a small, shrivelled gyrus: "Histological examination of these small gyri shows non-ganglionic areas bordered by islands of grey matter and thinned out grey layers."[11]

Penfield would later invoke a similar mechanism – compression of the brain in the birth canal – to explain the occurrence of what he referred to as *incisural sclerosis*, a major cause of temporal lobe epilepsy (see below).

Although Penfield was correct in invoking a vascular cause for polymicrogyria, most authors would agree that the vascular insult occurs in utero, after cortical migration has occurred, and not during labour, as Penfield surmised.[12] Further, the causes of polymicrogyria are varied. In addition to intrauterine ischemia, intrauterine infection with viral and bacterial organisms, parasitic infection, metabolic disorders, and genetic alterations are also recognized as causative agents.[13]

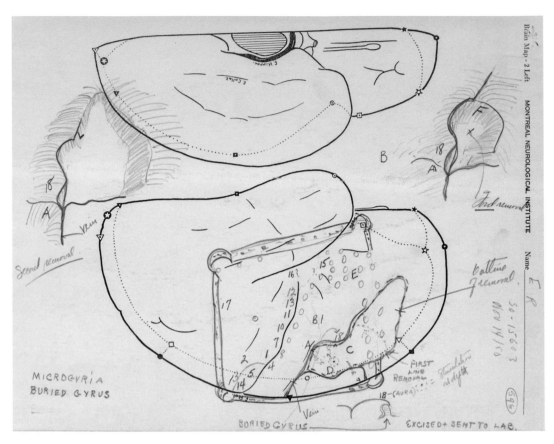

Figure 9.3: Penfield's operative drawing of a case of focal microgyria discovered at surgery, surgeon's view. The numbers indicate areas where electrical stimulation elicited sensory and motor responses, and the letters encircled in the red (*C, D*) area where epileptic activity was recorded. As the area encircled in red was resected, a "buried" microgyrus became apparent (insert, right of center at the inferior border of the illustration) under number 18. The inserts labeled *A* and *B* at the left and right borders, respectively, indicate the first stage of the resection (*B*) and the completed resection (*A*). (MNI Archives)

CEREBRAL BLOOD FLOW AND METABOLISM

The mechanism that Penfield proposed for the process of microgyration was in keeping with his broader theory of a dynamic role for the cortical circulation in the aetiology of focal epilepsy, and his early work was directed at exploring this theory. Penfield published a wonderfully illustrated paper in 1937 entitled "The Circulation of the Epileptic Brain" and showed a particular interest in the phenomenon of oxygenated – red – cerebral veins in association with epileptic seizures.[14]

In "The Circulation of the Epileptic Brain," Penfield elaborated on his conception of the interplay of vasomotor reactivity and focal epileptic discharges.

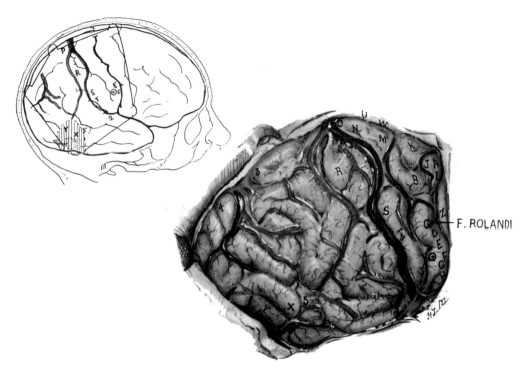

Figure 9.4: Cerebral hyperemia demonstrated by arterialized veins following a seizure induced by electrical stimulation at a point indicated by the letter *X*. The presence of red veins, reflecting the presence of arterialized blood, is an indication of increased blood low to match increased metabolic demand. (W. Penfield, "The Circulation of the Epileptic Brain," *Proceedings of the Association for Research in Nervous and Mental Disease* 28 [1937]: 605–37)

He proposed that localized vasoconstriction decreased the oxygen supplied to the cortex, triggering the onset of a seizure. Excessively discharging neurons then increased the metabolic activity in the epileptic area, which in turn stimulated a reflex increase in local cerebral blood flow. As the seizure abated, the blood flow exceeded the metabolic needs of the epileptic area, and oxygenated blood entered the veins draining the epileptic focus.[15] The phenomenology of red cerebral veins was later fully explored in the Cone Laboratory for Neurosurgical Research by Feindel, Yamamoto, and their co-workers, and by Leblanc and colleagues.

As a result of Penfield's clinical observations, a talented group of fellows were set to work on the effects of cortical, thalamic, and hypothalamic stimulation on cortical and subcortical blood flow, which resulted in a significant number of graduate degrees. The fellows included Francis Echlin, Theodore Erickson, Storer Humphreys, Martin Nichols, Nathan Norcross, and Kalman

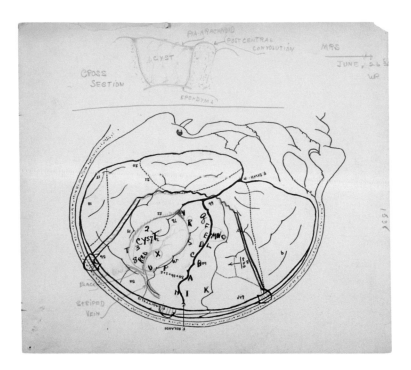

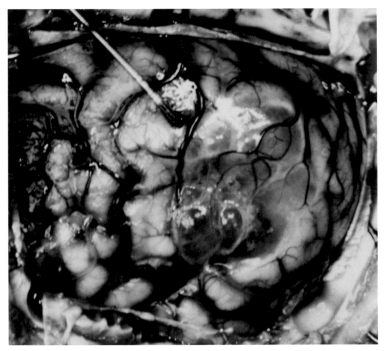

Figures 9.5 and 9.6: Operative images of case 21. (*Top*) Penfield's operative drawing, surgeon's upside-down view, of his findings at operation, delineating the cyst and the red vein emanating from it. The relationship of the cystic cavity to the pia-arachnoid and to the ependyma are also illustrated in the usual orientation. (*Bottom*) operative photograph of the same case in the usual orientation, demonstrating the hourglass shape of the red draining veins drawn in the previous illustration.[16]

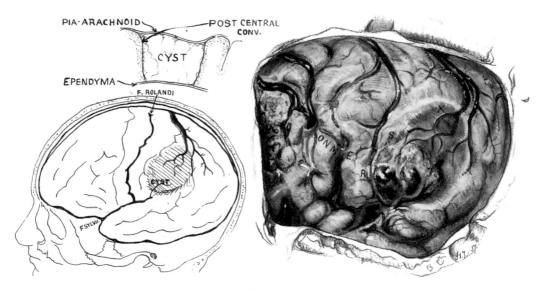

Figure 9.7. Post-convulsive hyperhemia following a spontaneous seizure in a patient (case 21) with a post-embolic cyst. The letter *X* indicates a vein filled with arterialized blood draining the cyst. The red cerebral vein eventually meets another draining vein to enter the superior sagittal sinus. (W. Penfield, "The Circulation of the Epileptic Brain," *Proceedings of the Association for Research in Nervous and Mental Disease* 28 [1937]: 605–37)

von Santhe.[17] Norcross's thesis was especially influential for his use of the newly described thermocouple method to measure cerebral blood flow, and a review of the MNI library loan card reveals that his thesis was consulted by von Shanta, Erickson, and Nichols in pursuit of their own investigations.

Penfield's opinion on the role of vascular mechanisms in the onset, propagation, and attenuation of epileptic seizures evolved with time. One major instrument of change was the introduction of the thermocouple method to measure subcortical blood flow. Using this device, Kalman von Santha and André Cipriani showed that local cerebral blood flow increases to meet the metabolic demands of functioning cortex.[18] Similarly, Penfield, von Santha, and Cipriani published a few anecdotal case reports in which increased subcortical blood flow accompanied increased metabolic activity during an epileptic seizure.[19] The coupling of cerebral blood flow and metabolic activity as demonstrated by von Santha and Cipriani is now exploited by functional brain imaging, which has become one of the most active and productive fields in neuroscience.

EPILEPTIC PROPAGATION

The discovery of polymicrogyria and of the close coupling of cerebral blood flow and electrical activity of the brain were not the only discoveries that were premature for their time. Such was the case also for Theodore Erickson and the role of the corpus callosum in the propagation of epileptic seizures.

Table 9.1

Graduate theses investigating a putative vascular mechanism in epilepsy

Investigator	Thesis
Lyle Gage (1931)	The Effects of Vasomotor Nerve Section on Experimental Epilepsy.
Jerzi Chorobski (1932)	Part 1: A Vasodilator Nervous Pathway to the Vessels from the Central Nervous System Part 2: On the Occurrence of Afferent Nerve Fibers in the Internal Carotid Plexus
Nathan Norcross (1936)	Studies in Cerebral Circulation
Joseph Evans (1937)	Study of Cerebral Cicatrix
Martin Nichols (1938)	Changes in the Circulation of the Brain and Spinal Cord Associated with Nervous Activity
Francis Echlin (1939)	Cerebral Ischemia
Storer Humphreys (1939)	Study of the Vascular and Cytological Changes in the Cerebral Cicatrix
Theodore Erickson (1940)	The Nature and the Spread of the Epileptic Discharge
Francis McNaughton (1941)	The Distribution of Sensory Nerves to the Dura Mater and Cerebral Vessels

Theodore Erickson obtained a PhD in 1939 for his highly imaginative and prescient, two-part dissertation, "The Nature and the Spread of the Epileptic Discharge."[20] In the first part of his dissertation, Erickson was unable to create epileptogenic scars by a variety of methods. This led him to conclude that neurovascular mechanisms, contrary to Penfield's hypothesis, do not contribute to the development of epileptic seizures.[21] Erickson was forceful in stating "that neither focal nor general decrease in the blood flow in the cerebral cortex is responsible for precipitating an epileptiform fit," and that "the theory that cerebral cicatrices may induce epileptiform fits by causing abnormal local variability in blood flow … has not received any support from the results of the present series of experiments."[22]

SECTIONING THE CORPUS CALLOSUM

The second part of Erickson's dissertation was on the spread of epileptic discharges from an experimental epileptic focus, using a device built by André Cipriani. Once a pattern of spread was established from the experimental epileptic focus to the opposite side, the corpus callosum was sectioned, and the effects of callosotomy on the spread of electrical activity were recorded. Electrographic recordings demonstrated that the epileptic activity, which had been bilateral before sectioning of the corpus callosum, was now limited to one hemisphere. Erickson was unequivocal: "My observations on the spread of the epileptic discharge from one cerebral hemisphere to the other prove definitely that this spread occurs largely or entirely via the corpus callosum."[23] Sectioning of the corpus callosum would later become a staple in the surgical treatment of certain types of medically refractory generalized epilepsy, and Roger Sperry would win the Nobel Prize in 1981 for his study on callosotomised patients.[24] Interestingly, in this same period Oland Hyndman and Wilder Penfield demonstrated agenesis of the corpus callosum using PEG.[25] Agenesis of the corpus callosum is a defining feature of some familial syndromes that were later described at the MNI (see below).

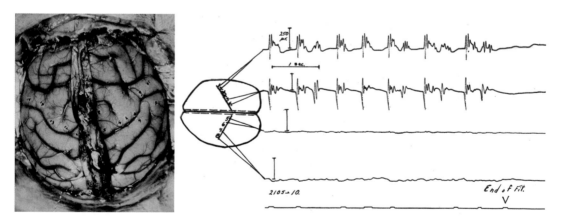

Figure 9.8: EEG after callosotomy. The seizure activity spreads along the hemisphere where an epileptogenic focus has been created (*left hemisphere, top two tracings*), but the opposite hemisphere is electrographically silent. (T. Erickson, "The Nature and the Spread of the Epileptic Discharge" [PhD diss., McGill University, 1939])

KINDLING

Like Erickson, Penfield and Boldrey also addressed the question of propagation of epileptic seizures and proposed a novel mechanism wherein "acquired … neuronal connections [are] established by the conditioning influence of previous individual experience. In this sense habitual epileptic seizures should be considered true conditioned reflexes in the cortex of any patient."[26] This idea is heavy with meaning and pits the Pavlovian conditioned reflex against the Hebbian concept of the *engram* in the facilitation of synaptic transmission, and anticipates the discovery of the phenomenon of kindling in the spread of epileptic activity.[27]

DIAGNOSIS

Most importantly for the future activities of the institute, Arthur Childe and Wilder Penfield studied the radiological appearance of the temporal horns of the lateral ventricles.[28] Focal enlargement of a temporal horn would be recognized in the 1950s as a surrogate marker for mesial temporal sclerosis, and its demonstration by PEG became a determining factor in the decision to operate upon patients with temporal lobe epilepsy. The informative value of the PEG in temporal lobe epilepsy was surpassed only when mesial temporal sclerosis could be visualized directly by magnetic resonance imaging almost half a century later.

BRAIN TUMORS

John Kershman, a fellow in neurology who would play a vital role at the institute for the remainder of his career, undertook a taxing and exacting project in the study of the cytogenesis of the human central nervous system, with the goal of identifying the cells of origin of common glial tumours.[29] His most noteworthy efforts were directed at the medulloblast, felt to be the cell of origin of the highly malignant medulloblastoma, a common tumour of the cerebellum. Kershman was able to identify undifferentiated cells originating from the roof of the fourth ventricle that migrated to the intermediate, external granular zone of the cerebellum. "These cells of the external granular zone," Kershman felt, "may justifiably be called medulloblasts," a hypothesis that is still valid.[30]

Penfield's own interest in brain tumours had not abated. He wrote an informative paper on the symptoms produced by brain tumours with Theodore Erickson and Isadore Tarlov.[31] But the high point of Penfield's writings on brain

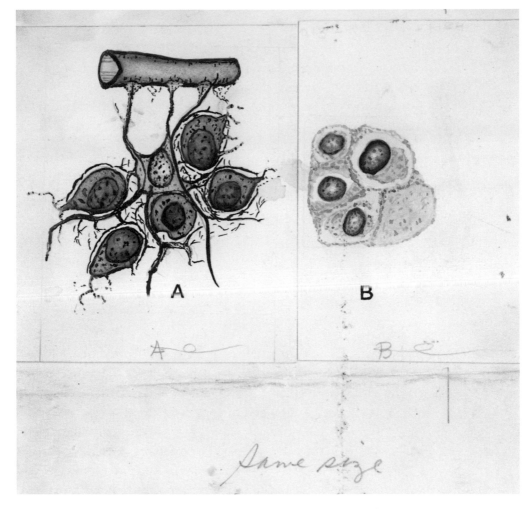

Figure 9.9: Sketches of an oligodendroglioma. The illustrations are from case R.I., Penfield's sister. (Penfield Archives. Final illustration appeared in W. Penfield and D. McEachern, "Intracranial Tumours," *Oxford Medicine* 6 [1938]: 137–224)

tumours is the authoritative "Intracranial Tumours," published in 1938. The text is clear, comprehensive, and insightful. It is especially masterful in its description of the histology of brain tumours. It must also have been of great personal significance for Penfield, as the illustrations that he chose for the histopathological features of oligodendrogliomas are from his sister Ruth's case.[32]

THE HUGHLINGS JACKSON LECTURES

Wilder Penfield had delivered the first Hughlings Jackson Lecture at the MNI in 1935 and set the tone for future lectures. The staff of the Neurological Institute gave the second Hughlings Jackson lecture, on Hughlings Jackson's teachings. Karl Lashley, professor of psychology at Harvard University and Donald

Hebb's mentor and collaborator, delivered the third lecture, "Factors Limiting Improvement after Central Nervous Injuries." Detlev W. Bronk, then at the University of Pennsylvania and later president of Rockefeller University and of the National Academy of Sciences, gave the 1938 Hughlings Jackson Lecture, "Nerve Cells and Synapses in the Regulation of Organic Function."

THE TANGIBLE AND THE IMMATERIAL

Wilder Penfield's most significant publication of 1937 was undoubtedly "Somatic Motor and Sensory Representation in the Cerebral Cortex of Man," on the structure–function relationship of the brain, written with Edwin Boldrey and based largely on Boldrey's thesis.[33] Penfield also published another seminal paper the following year, "The Cerebral Cortex and Consciousness."[34] These two papers in many ways symbolize Penfield's life's work: the localization of cortical function and the search for the intangible source of human consciousness. In "Cortex and Consciousness," Penfield states his firm belief that there is a "level of integration within the central nervous system that is higher than that to be found in the cerebral cortex," which would lead him to the concept of the centrencephalic integrating system, and ultimately to *The Mystery of the Mind*.[35] The advent of war, however, interrupted Penfield's research as the MNI geared up for the war effort.

WE'LL MEET AGAIN

The first years of the MNI must have exceeded Penfield's expectations. An institute had been built to his specification and was associated with a major university. Neurology, neurosurgery, and psychology were represented. New diagnostic methods were developed and helped in the diagnosis of many neurological conditions that were previously diagnosed solely by clinical acumen. Novel treatments were established. Scientific hypotheses were formulated and rigorously investigated by dedicated, imaginative clinician-scientists working in well-equipped laboratories. The institute achieved international stature and attracted fellows from all over the world, who came for instruction, insight, and experience, and most would become leaders in their chosen field. Sadly, this antebellum state was not to last. The clouds of war were gathering at the horizon and cast long, dark shadows. Most of the MNI class of 1938 would be caught up in the coming storm.

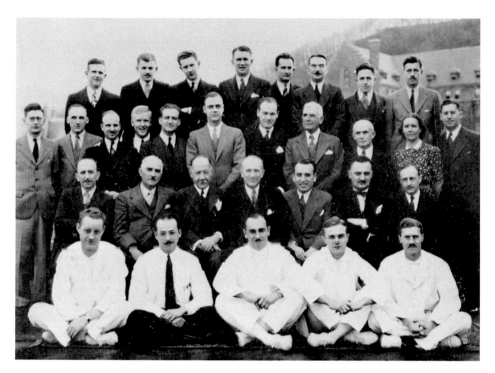

Figure 9.10: Staff photograph 1937. (*Front row, left to right*) F.H. Hanson, R.H. Stevens, W.L. Reid, R.H. Pudenz, O.W. Stewart. (*Second row*) R. Amyot, F.H. Mackay, C.K. Russel, W.G. Penfield, W.V. Cone, J. Saucier, J.N. Petersen. (*Third row*) W.M. Nichols, F.L. McNaughton, H.M. Keith, D.O. Hebb, D. McEachern, A.E. Childe, A.W. Young, A.G. Morphy, N. Viner, M. Harrower, A.R. Elvidge. (*Back row*) G. Odom, E.B. Boldrey, G.Y. McClure, T.C. Erickson, A. Cipriani, J. Kershman, S. Humphreys, F. Echlin. (MNI Archives)

10

"Cry 'Havoc' and let slip the dogs of war"

The 1939 annual report of the MNI opens with group photographs of the medical and nursing staff. Unlike in previous years, however, the photographs are of interest not for those present, but for the six physicians and thirteen nurses who are absent: Colin Russel, Arthur Childe, and William Vernon Cone had been given ranks in the Royal Canadian Army Medial Corps and posted overseas, near the hamlet of Basingstoke, in Hampshire, England, on the estate of Lord Camrose, publisher of the *Daily Telegraph*. There, under the directorship of Lieutenant-Colonels Russel and Cone the Number One Canadian Neurological Hospital was organized and staffed.[1]

Although America had not yet entered the war, three American MNI fellows, Storer Humphreys, Oscar Wilhelm Stewart, and Fred Hanson accompanied Cone, Russel, and Childe to Basingstoke. Fred Hanson transferred to the United States Army in May 1942 but was permitted to accompany the Canadian troops on the Dieppe Raid, to know first-hand the mental toll of combat and to better treat neuropsychiatric casualties. Hanson would later be influential in organizing the care of neuropsychiatric patients in the US Army, "based on the lessons learned at Basingstoke."[2] Stewart came to the Neurological Institute in 1938, after having trained at Harvard and Johns Hopkins. He was first stationed at Basingstoke and later sent to Queen Elizabeth Hospital in Birmingham, later to return to Basingstoke as neurosurgeon-in-chief until the unit was disbanded.[3] W. Martin Nichols is also absent from the 1939 photograph. A graduate of Edinburgh University, Nichols had been at the MNI in 1936 and 1937,[4] joined the British Army as a medical officer, was captured at Dunkirk in 1940, and was transferred to a prisoner of war camp, where he attended to ill and wounded prisoners.

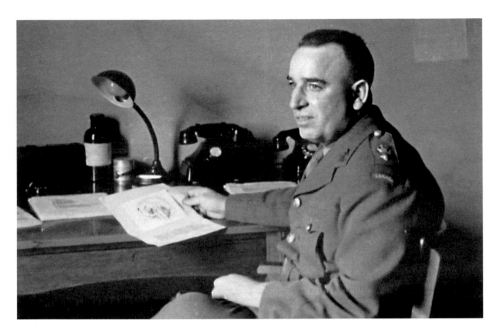

Figure 10.1: William Cone, on active duty in England. (Penfield Archives)

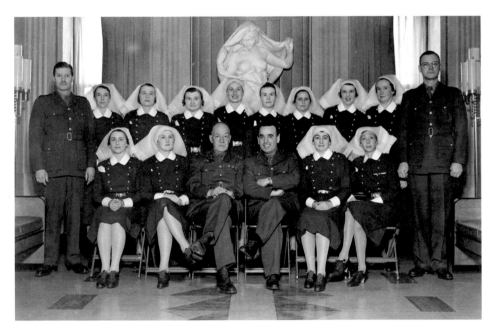

Figure 10.2: The MNI contingent of Number 1 Canadian Neurological Hospital prior to departure for England. (*Sitting*) E. Scott, M. Roach, C. Russel, W. Cone, J. Mackay, H. Kendal. (*Standing*) O. Stewart, E. Jones, C. Winter, F. Bossy, A. Hudson, I. Gillispie, M. Swartz, E. Grimes, H. Shanks, A. Childe. Fred Hanson appears in the 1938–39 annual photograph (figure 9.10). (MNI Archives)

COLIN K. RUSSEL

It is a measure of Colin Russel's stature that he had been summoned to Ottawa at the outbreak of war to advise the Royal Canadian Army on the organization of overseas medical services, which led to the creation of the Number 1 Canadian Neurological Hospital. The task was not an easy one: with fewer than fifty medical officers and not even a dozen nursing sisters, "the Royal Canadian Army Medical Corps … was magnificently unprepared for the Second World War."[5]

Colin Russel was born in Montreal in 1877, graduated from McGill University Medical School in 1901, and interned at the Royal Victoria Hospital, where he studied internal medicine for two years. He then had the good fortune of studying neurology and psychiatry at Johns Hopkins University with William Osler, who had not yet moved from Baltimore to become the Regius Professor of Medicine at Oxford University. Russel then did his own Grand Tour of Continental Europe, stopping first in Zurich to study with Constantin von Monakow, on to Berlin to work with Hermann Oppenheim, then to Paris and the clinics of Jules Dejerine, Pierre Marie, and Joseph Babinski. By 1905 Russel was at the National Hospital, Queen Square, London, where Hughlings Jackson still attended patients and David Ferrier, Sir William Gowers, Sir Charles Beevor, Sir Gordon Holmes, and especially Sir Victor Horsley were in their prime. Russel and Horsley established the somatotopic arrangement of the post-central gyrus in man, which was later more precisely elaborated upon by Penfield and Rasmussen.[6] Colin Russel held the rank of captain in the Royal Canadian Army Medical Corps during the Great War and went overseas with the McGill General Hospital Unit, based in England. Once there, he took charge of neuropsychiatric patients suffering from conversion hysteria, referred to in the colourful yet descriptive trench short-hand as "shell shock."

Colin Russel returned to Montreal in 1906 and became a clinical assistant in medicine and neurology at the RVH. He was appointed neurologist to the hospital in 1910, and by 1922 he was promoted to clinical professor of neurology at McGill University. Aware of Hughlings Jackson's writing on the subject, and perhaps with an element of foresight, Russel wrote one of his first papers on a patient with a tumour of the antero-mesial temporal lobe who had experienced episodes of a "dreamy state," in many ways identical to Jackson's own description of uncinate fits.[7] The role of the mesial temporal structures in temporal lobe epilepsy would later be firmly established by Penfield, Jasper, and Feindel (see below). Undoubtedly as a result of his work with Victor Horsley, Colin Russel realized the need to develop the specialized field of neurosurgery in Montreal and he worked closely with Archibald in this endeavour. Russel was instrumental in Archibald's efforts to recruit Penfield and Cone, and he became the MNI's first neurologist-in-chief when it opened in 1934.

Russel was reactivated in the Royal Canadian Army at the outbreak of the Second World War and summoned to Ottawa to advise the Royal Canadian Army Medical Corps on how best to organize a medical unit to accompany the Canadian Forces overseas. Russel proposed the creation of a hospital, much like the MNI, staffed by neurologists, neurosurgeons, and specialized nurses who would receive troops with injury to the nervous system. Thus, the Number One Neurological Hospital was created, with Russel as overall commander and William Cone as the neurosurgeon-in-chief, seconded by Harry Botterell from the University of Toronto. After the war it was reported that "under the spell of Lt-Col. W.V. Cone's persuasiveness the hospital came overseas with more luxurious and expensive hospital furniture than surely ever went to war since Hannibal crossed the Alps."[8]

Penfield kept the MNI faculty and staff apprised of the developments at "No. 1," as the Number 1 Canadian Neurological Hospital was referred to, in his annual report: "Late in June 1940 the unit reached England and in September the Nursing Sisters followed[9] … In September 1940 the admission of patients began. From the middle of December 1940 the unit was enrolled in the Emergency Medical Service as a surgical center for the treatment of head injuries among the troops as well as among the civilians. Huts are being built to enlarge the accommodation of the hospital. On several occasion during the year the Canadian Broadcasting Corporation broadcast greetings from the unit to relatives in Canada and the United States."[10]

A report received from Lt-Col. Russel provided a front-line account of the creation of No. 1 and of its early activities at Basingstoke: "We have built up a hospital which will shortly have 250 to 300 beds, with operating rooms, x-ray department, laboratories, pathological and chemical, where the estimation of total protein can be done in ten minutes, or the sulfonamide content of the blood and cerebrospinal fluid can be carried out, and sections made of autopsy material … Dr Cone and I are called in consultation two or three times a week to other hospitals, and, seriously, he is making a great reputation among the English hospitals, and it is well deserved. He has had some splendid results."[11]

The casualties in the first year of operation at No. 1 were mainly head injuries. Cone's treatment of complex depressed cranio-facial fractures – an injury very common in Canadian motorcycle dispatch riders unaccustomed to driving on the left side of the road – was noteworthy, as reported in the *British Medical Journal*:

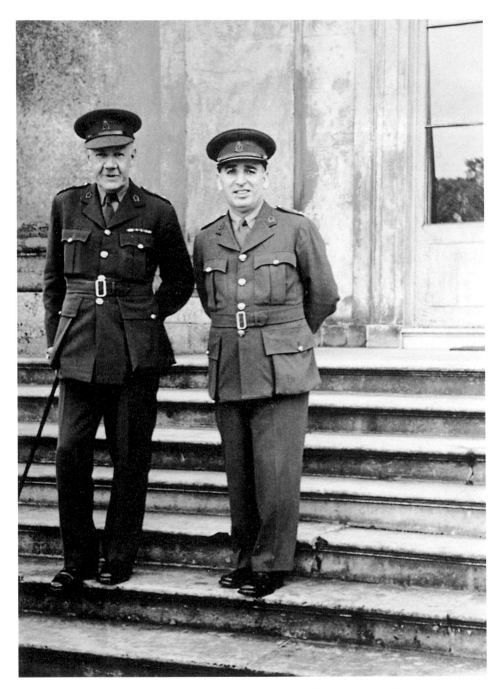

Figure 10.3: Colin Russel and William Cone at Basingstoke. (MNI Archives)

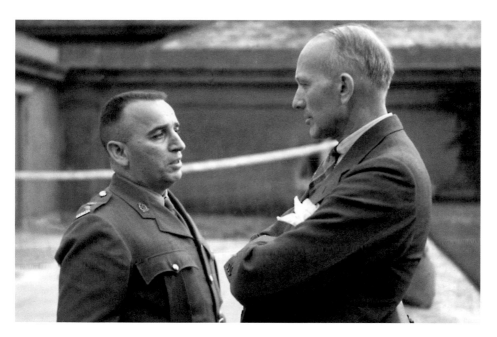

Figure 10.4: Cone and Penfield confer during the latter's visit to Basingstoke. (Penfield Archives)

> Lt-Col. Cone showed particular enterprise in the management of compound fractures of the skull involving the frontal sinuses. Those with a lacerated wound across the forehead, severe bleeding from one or both nostrils, and X-ray evidence of fracture line involving both walls of the frontal sinuses were his special field … The amount of anterior basal damage usually greatly exceeds that seen on the skull films, with great comminution not only of the frontal sinuses but of the ethmoids as well, with tears in the dura and pulped brain tissue plugging the holes and even protruding into the remains of the sinuses. Lt-Col Cone attacked these, exenterating the sinuses, sucking out damaged brain, and patching the dura with fascia.[12]

Cone's technique for the management of cranio-facial injuries was included in *Military Neurosurgery*, a field manual prepared by Penfield for the Canadian Medical Corps.[13]

Beside his clinical load, Cone took every opportunity to advance the care of neurosurgical patients, but his publications were few. Nonetheless, while at Basingstoke, he, Stewart, and Russel published an interesting paper on the pathophysiology of avian blast injury. The publication is a single case report of a pheasant that had the misfortune of perching near an exploding shell during a bombing run on London. He had the double misfortune of being observed in a dazed condition by three neuroscientists who felt it their duty to submit the unfortunate fowl to necropsy.[14] (Inspiration favours the prepared mind.) More prosaically, and undoubtedly of greater utility, Botterell, Carmichael, and Cone reported on the use of sulfa drugs in head-injured patients.[15] Harry Botterell replaced Cone as head of the neurosurgical division of the hospital when Cone returned to the institute in the autumn of 1941.[16] Botterell was later replaced by William Stewart.

Russel left for Montreal after a stint as special consultant in London in 1942. Although his return was a joyous occasion for his many friends and colleagues at the MNI, it became obvious that his service in two world wars had taken its toll: "On his return to Canada, Dr Russel resumed his duties at the Neurological Institute and only gradually retired from its activities in the post-war years. Even when ill health and the burdens of age interfered with his life, he usually managed to attend Monday ward rounds, and executive meetings, and contributed vigorously and emphatically (sometimes with mild profanity) to the discussion of important issues. He resented every inroad that ill health made on his activities. Frequently the spirit protested against the limitations of the body."[17]

Russel died on 5 March 1956. He is immortalized in Mary Filer's *Advance of Neurology*, in which Russel sits at the patient's bedside, his head as if gently cradled by Bill Cone's powerful hands.

SISTERS OF MERCY

Thirteen MNI nurses also answered the call to colours: Freda Bossy, Isabel Gillespie, Evelyn Grimes, Anna Hudson, Etta Jones, Helen Kendall, Janet C. Mackay, Evelyn Scott, Helen Shanks, Margaret Stewart, Myrtle Swartz, Mary Roach (head matron), and Constance Winter.[18] For Helen Kendall it was a second tour of duty overseas, since she had been a sister with the Canadian Expeditionary Force in France, in 1917, as close to the front as one could be without carrying a rifle. She was awarded the Royal Red Cross Class II medal, the ARRC, a British Commonwealth decoration awarded to a military nurse "who has performed some very exceptional act of bravery and devotion at her post of duty."[19]

Lucie Millette Stewart recounts the preparation of the nursing staff for service overseas:

On January 6, 1940, chest x-rays were taken of the Neuro personnel that had enlisted, then measurements for uniforms, followed by two evenings of drill and instruction at the Royal Canadian Grenadier Armory. On

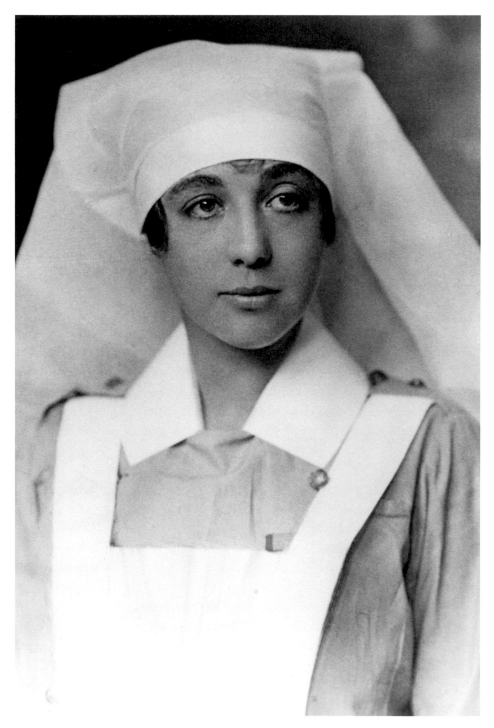

Figure 10.5: Helen Kendall, age seventeen, with the Canadian Expeditionary Force in France, 1917. (Photographer unknown, 97-550-28398 B, Beaton Institute, Cape Breton University)

February 2nd inoculations against typhoid and smallpox were given. On February 15th Dr Cone went home to Iowa to visit his mother. He was back on the 19th to cover the wards for three weeks to give Dr Penfield a respite. On Feb. 16th the last inoculation of the nurses was given and they were in uniform by February 17th. Departure took place on June 6, 1940 from Windsor station, Montreal and on to Basingstoke and the residence of Lord Camrose in Hampshire.[20]

THE ESTATE

The estate of Lord Camrose, some sixty miles from London, was reached by

> a quarter mile driveway, framed by stately elms. The front of the manor had a wide, crescent-shaped courtyard, in the center of which stood a life-sized statue of Edward the Seventh on his magnificent horse … The three storied manor house was sufficiently large to accommodate nurses in its left wing, and doctors in its right. The main floor was unique with dining hall, kitchen, music and games' room, and a very large living or entertainment room. This room featured eight-foot high doors opening onto a large patio. From the patio, steps led down to the lawn from which the psychiatric unit could be observed in the distance. The main hospital complex was to the left, made up of quickly-erected Nissen Huts.[21]

Number 1 Canadian Neurological Hospital rapidly outgrew the confines of Lord Camrose's home and, now joined by a plastic surgery division, expanded behind the very large house and grew to a 750-bed facility that eventually cared for some 16,000 patients.[22]

BEYOND THE CALL

Freda Bossy was from New Carlyle, Quebec, and went to Basingstoke with the original contingent of nursing sisters. She was in charge of a ward in a Nissen hut that "was connected to the admitting room, operating theatres, physio and occupational therapy, kitchen and supply rooms." By all accounts, her ward was an oasis of sanity in the hubbub as patients, nursing sisters, and orderlies came to and fro, from the Admitting Department to operating theatres and rehabilitation rooms. Despite the traffic, Bossy ran a tight ship: "She had her convalescent, wheelchair and mobile patients at the far end of the ward where there were two tables used for meals, card games, correspondence, and anything

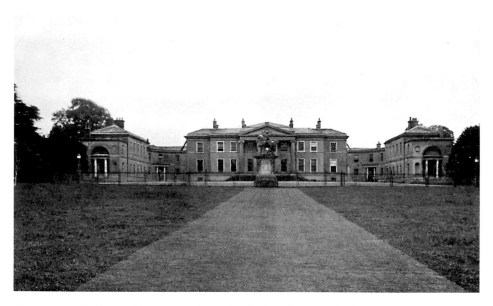

Figure 10.6: Hackwood House, Basingstoke, before the arrival of No. 1 Canadian Neurological Hospital. Nissen huts were attached to the back of the house, where 16,000 patients were treated. (Penfield Archives)

else. The sickest men were placed near the front of the ward close to the nursing station," as they were at the MNI, "and where they were under her constant supervision."[23]

What is remembered of Freda Bossy, however, is not the grit and determination needed to run a ward full of sick and dying servicemen, but her kind heart and gentle nature. The story is told of a French boy, found unconscious in a ditch in France, who was evacuated to Basingstoke with other casualties. He was admitted, unconscious and alone, to Freda's ward, where, under her care, he recovered consciousness, recuperated, and acted like any typical boy – save for a head bandage and a walking cast. He soon found a place in the routine of the hospital. When the colonel in charge of the unit found that the boy was well enough to be transferred out, Miss Bossy asked, "Where will he go?" His village in France, she had been told, was still under German occupation, and it had been planned that the boy would be sent to a refugee camp in England. Bossy would have none of it: "Surely he could stay here where he is loved," she insisted. The boy stayed on Miss Bossy's ward, happy and well cared for, until he was reunited with his mother after the Liberation of France.[24] A MNI nurse can stare down a full-bird colonel anytime.

Freda Bossy's devotion to the men under her care did not escape Penfield's attention, and he wrote to her after the Allied landing at Normandy: "You are in our thoughts and now that D-Day has arrived I fear the flow of wounded is reaching your hospital. We wonder how long before they will begin to reach us. It is a lucky man who is nursed by you for you have something that is granted to very few. Nursing is sometimes a gift which has something to do with the best type of love. You will not misunderstand me. I hope you will come back to the MNI sometime."[25]

Freda Bossy did return to the MNI, but under the worst of circumstances, not as a nurse but as a patient. Stewart tells her story in a letter to Penfield, dated 23 April 1945. In it, he reveals not only Miss Bossy's heroic struggle but also poignantly reveals his own character and dedication to duty.

> Dear Doctor Penfield,
> ... About three weeks ago we had a call from Headquarters announcing that six of our Sisters were to be returned to Canada and among this six were four of the head Sisters on my seven surgical wards. This was quite a blow, particularly because it included Freda Bossy and Myrtle Schwartz, two of our trusted stand-bys. Freda and Myrtle were both very disappointed for they wanted to stay on here until the finish. Freda took a few days' leave prior to her departure date, which was to have been yesterday. That night, on the 18th [of] April, she waked from her sleep and tried to get out of bed to go to the bathroom when she found that she was paralyzed in her right arm and leg. She was brought by ambulance here, arriving the following evening. You can imagine the thoughts that were racing through her mind and also sympathise with me in my task of talking with her and examining her ... X-ray films taken the next morning revealed an area of calcification in the Rolandic region on the left side, rather near the falx ... and I felt that it was most probably calcification in either an astrocytoma or an oligodendroglioma ... Because of my very close association and deep regard for her, I did not want to operate and felt, in view of the absence of increased pressure ... that she could be returned to Canada by hospital ship with safety and that there either you or Doctor Cone could take charge of her and operate ... She insisted that she be operated on here and I did not feel justified, under the circumstances, in insisting that she return to Canada without operation.
> Her decision having been made, I operated the next morning for I did not want her to have any more time to brood over it than could be helped and also, I wanted to do it before I myself was more tired from cases which might have continued to pile up from the European Theater

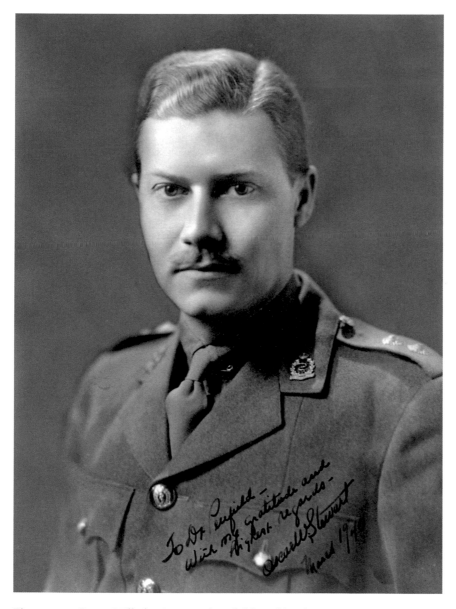

Figure 10.7: Oscar Wilhelm Stewart. (Penfield Archives)

… Since operation she has done very well. She is alert and cheerful and has as much movement as she had before and movement is increasing each day. She, of course, knows that the tumour is a relatively malignant one and that my removal was only a sub-total one. She knows this, simply by reason of the fact that I did not tell her otherwise. It has been very hard on me to talk with her and to help her over this period and only her grand personality and bearing has enabled me to think clearly and act in a way that I have felt best. We have reserved a bed for her on the next hospital ship and I told her that she will be going directly to Montreal where she will be under you and Doctor Cone ...

Bill [Stewart][26]

Miss Bossy's convalescence was long and arduous, but she met it as she met every challenge in life, with courage and determination. She eventually recovered well enough to nurse some of her former patients from Basingstoke at the Queen Mary Veterans Hospital in Montreal.[27]

Oscar Wilhelm Stewart survived the war but not its aftermath. He died in 1950 of complications of pulmonary tuberculosis contracted during his service overseas, and for which he had delayed treatment to stay with the wounded. He was forty-four years old.

11

Home Front

The outbreak of the Second World War drastically changed the nature of the MNI's activities: the war increased its clinical workload to barely tolerable levels, caused a reorientation in its research priorities, and had an almost disastrous effect on its finances.

The institute's dedication to the war effort at home and abroad is reflected in Penfield's comment on the MNI's research priorities, in his 5 May 1941 address to the staff: "In regard to research, some of it should now be considered secret, as it may aid the enemy. The result of such work may not be published, but if of value may be communicated through the Canadian Research Council to the British Research Council. Other research which might also conceivably help the beleaguered people of England is best published in whole or in part."[1] This type of secretive, directed research required a shift in the prevailing attitude of openness and academic freedom among the institute staff. Penfield addressed this point head-on: "But now, when the existence of academic freedom is threatencd, when survival of the culture of the English-speaking people is at stake, the members of the University faculty may legitimately forsake abstract study. They may introduce a previously unknown element of secrecy into their work."[2] The times justified the secrecy, as Penfield reflected the dark period when Britain and the Commonwealth stood alone in the struggle against Fascism, and his tone is Churchillian, as he sounds a clarion call of determination and duty: "The gaps left in our ranks by those gone overseas have been closed until we can welcome them back. If others of us go, these new gaps will be closed again, and the work of the institute will go on."[3]

Secret or open, the intimate relationship fostered in the five years of the MNI's existence by the proximity of clinicians and researchers had created a unique atmosphere in which, as Penfield observed, "much of the work has been carried out by co-operation between different activities in laboratory departments of the Institute, so as to utilize to the full all the possible research tools which are available. Fortunately there are no rigid departmental lines to ob-struct research."[4] The same spirit of cooperation prevailed during the war, as different departments and individuals with specific expertise combined their ef-forts to the common cause.

WARTIME RESEARCH

Early in the war, the MNI was host to high-echelon guests from Great Britain who gave talks on medicine and the war. Rear Admiral Gordon-Taylor pre-sented "Surgical Aspects of Modern Warfare"; Wing-Commander R.D. Gilles-pie, psychiatrist to the Royal Air Force, read his "Psychological Aspects of the War in Great Britain"; and Sir Harold Gillies, consultant in plastic surgery to the Royal Navy, Army, and Air Force, gave an address, "Treatment of Burns."[5] These and other related topics would form the core of the MNI's war-related research.[6]

Aviation Medicine

A giant apparatus exerting centrifugal force was constructed in the EEG Labo-ratory, which allowed investigation of the effects of gravity and acceleration on fighter pilots. As casualties were to be transported from the field to Basingstoke by air, the transport of head-injured patients at high altitudes required special attention. Thus a decompression chamber equipped for measuring vital signs up to a simulated altitude of 30,000 feet was built by André Cipriani and in-stalled at the MNI. Night vision, important in pilots as nighttime bombing was introduced, was also investigated at the institute. Murray Bornstein, a MNI re-search fellow who would gain great prominence in multiple sclerosis research, participated in many of these projects, especially with Eric Peterson and Her-bert Jasper.[7] Molly Harrower-Erickson studied fatigue in bomber pilots, and Herbert Jasper approached muscle fatigue in other combatants as a "biochem-ical problem with neurological aspects."[8] Jasper and Harold Vineberg, who was later to become a pioneering cardiac surgeon, investigated skin burns, a fre-quent occurrence in pilots.[9]

Seasickness

The prevention and treatment of seasickness was a special problem for troops and merchant seamen who were crossing the Atlantic in convoys in increasing numbers, to supply Britain with men and materiel. Research at the MNI tar-geted "the role of the vestibular system, the movement of heavy abdominal or-gans, and certain psychological elements" in this condition. To further study this phenomenon, Herbert Jasper suggested that experimental seasickness could be produced "by apparatus constructed in the laboratory with man as the un-happy subject." This device was a giant seasickness cradle built in what had been the squash court at the MNI and christened HMS *Mal de Mer*. An effective rem-edy was found to protect military personnel against motion sickness from the studies performed on the good ship *Mal de Mer*, in cooperation with a research group at the Banting Institute in Toronto.[10]

Boris Petrovitch Babkin, Ivan Pavlov's former assistant, collaborated with the staff of the MNI, quite appropriately, on the effects of repeated swinging motions on the stomach of the dog.[11] Babkin was born in Koursk, Russia, in 1877. He began work with Pavlov in 1902 after graduating from medical school and performed the first experiments on conditioned reflex with him at the In-stitute of Experimental Medicine in St Petersburg. Babkin was appointed pro-fessor of physiology at the University of Odessa in 1915, but in 1922, his revolutionary fervour deemed lacking, he was sentenced to a term in prison be-fore being exiled from the Union of Soviet Socialist Republics. Babkin took refuge in Starling's laboratory at University College, London, where he stayed for two years, then was appointed chair of Physiology at Dalhousie University, Halifax, in 1924. He subsequently relocated to Montreal as professor in the De-partment of Physiology at McGill University, where he was chair of the de-partment in 1940 and 1941 and stayed on as professor, post-retirement, until 1947. It was then that Penfield invited him to continue his work as a research fel-low at the MNI, where he remained until the end of his life. His principal in-terest at the institute was investigating the role of the cerebral cortex and subcortical centers in the regulation of gastro-intestinal function, joining Pavlov and the Montreal school.[12]

Head Injuries and Cerebral Edema

Head injuries and their sequelae in combat troops and motorcycle dispatch riders were of obvious concern. Much of the MNI's research in this area fo-cused on the acute effects of head injuries; post-traumatic headache and post-traumatic epilepsy; and the biochemical and electrophysiological effects of head trauma.[13] Robert Pudenz made a significant contribution to the field, studying the use of tantalum to repair large cranial defects,[14] the same mate-rial that was widely used in military and civilian practice well into the last half of the twentieth century. In addition, Guy Odom, Yi-cheng Chao, and Storer Humphreys investigated several materials to repair dural defects in compli-cated head wounds.[15]

The role of cerebral edema in head trauma and the possible deleterious ef-fects of prolonged exposure of the cortex during surgery or on the battlefield were poorly understood at the time. The importance of cerebral edema is reflected by the calibre of the researchers – Elliott, Jasper, and Prados – who dedicated their time to its study. They were aided by especially gifted assistants in William Feindel and John Stirling Meyer, both from McGill, and in Berk Strowger, from Stanford. It was in these circumstances that Elliott began his work on fluids for cortical irrigation during surgery, which led to the development of Elliott's solution.[16]

Infection was also an ever-present concern in patients with open head wounds, for which the newly discovered sulfa drugs held much promise. Their use when applied topically to open wounds or injected intravenously and intrathecally was studied by a number of investigators at the MNI.[17]

Spine and Peripheral Nerve Injuries

Other parts of the nervous system were not forgotten. William Cone published important papers on intervertebral discs, spinal fusion after discoidectomy, and the avoidance of complications from spinal cord injury.[18] Herbert Jasper and his collaborators studied the pathophysiology of peripheral nerve injuries.[19] Claude Bertrand and Mr Hurtz investigated different methods of suturing nerves, and Peter Lehmann studied the reaction of nerves to different suture material.[20]

Although not strictly related to the war effort, Harold Elliott, who had trained in neurosurgery at the MNI before the war, devised the Swiss Army knife of neurology, the McGill hammer, "a compact instrument for testing reflexes, light touch, pain sensation and two-point discrimination."[21] Elliott would eventually serve at Basingstoke, after serving at No. 1 Canadian General Hospital. He was later neurosurgeon-in-chief at the Montreal General Hospital, where he was succeeded by Joseph Stratford.

The Montreal Neurological Institute's contribution to the Canadian war effort is unique in Canadian history. From the creation on the Number One Neurosurgical Hospital at Basingstoke, to war-related research in Montreal, the MNI staff dedicated themselves to the care of military and civilian casualties and to the safety and well-being of our troops, whether they served on land, sea, or air (figure 11.3).

ACADEMIA

Visiting speakers addressed mainly the subjects in which the MNI was involved with wartime research. Two addresses, however, dealt with shock, a subject that was not studied at the MNI, but was of obvious interest to neurosurgeons dealing with patients suffering major trauma to other parts of the body as well as

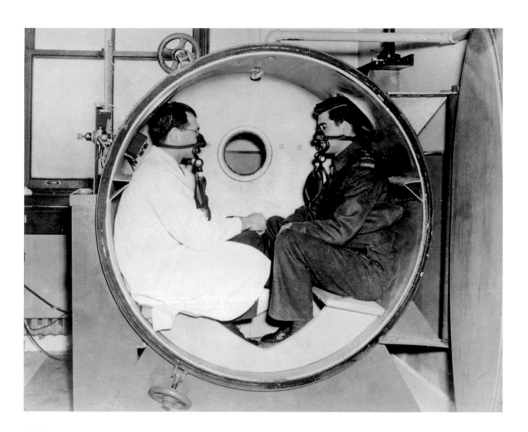

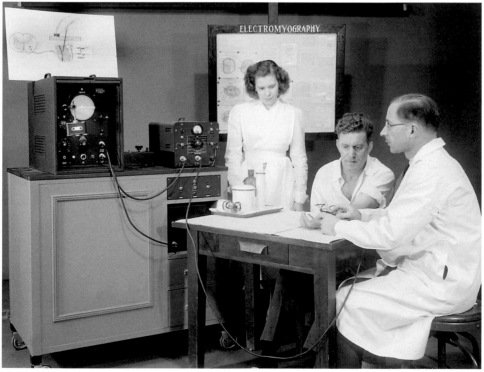

Figures 11.1 and 11.2: (*Above*) Murray Bornstein and Eric Peterson (*in uniform*) in the MNI decompression chamber. (*Below*) Herbert Jasper performing an electromyogram on a patient with recovering nerve damage, assisted by Marjorie Matthews. (MNI Archives)

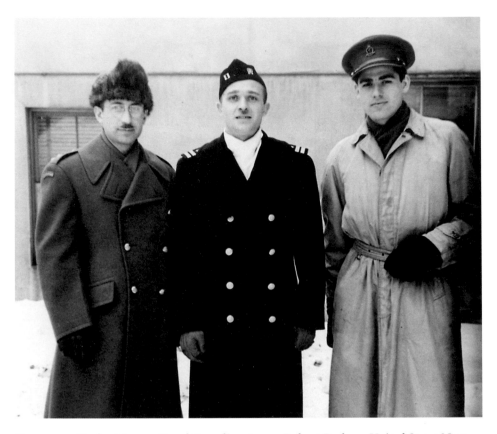

Figure 11.3: Herbert Jasper, Royal Canadian Army; Robert Pudenz, United States Navy; Eric Peterson, Royal Canadian Air Force. (MNI Archives)

to the head. The institute therefore invited international authorities on the subject to bring the staff, fellows, and residents up to date on this important topic. Virgil Moon, of the Jefferson Medical College in Philadelphia, was invited to address the topic of surgical shock. Moon was an authority on the subject and his studies and writings had "profoundly influenced the way battle casualties were managed in World War II."[22] John Scudder, an expert on blood transfusion from Columbia-Presbyterian Hospital in New York, was invited to speak on shock and blood studies as a guide to therapy. Scudder was very influential at the time and promoted the use of dried, reconstituted blood plasma on the battlefield.[23] Before the United States entered the war, Scudder was instrumental in the promotion and organization of the Blood Plasma for Great Britain Project, credited with saving many a Tommy's life.[24]

Two other addresses stand out: Robert Pudenz's "Lucite Calvarium: A New Method for the Observation of Intracranial Phenomena," and John Fulton's

"Blast Injuries."[25] Fulton was the distinguished physiologist from Yale University and Harvey Cushing's biographer. It is not known if Fulton referred to game fowl in his talk.[26]

Other topics discussed were not related directly to the war, but, in anticipation of psychological sequelae in combat troops – what is now referred to as post-traumatic stress disorder – treatment of mental conditions came to the fore: Zygmunt Pietrowski of the New York State Psychiatric Institute presented "Psychological Investigations of Insulin Treated Schizophrenics" – so-called insulin shock – and the controversial Walter Freeman spoke on the radical therapy of psychoses and neuroses – more widely to be known as frontal lobotomy. In opposition, Wilder Penfield, Ewen Cameron, and Miguel Prados reported their observations in "The Treatment of Certain Chronic Behaviour Disorders by Convolectomy [the resection of a cortical convolution] as a Substitute for Lobotomy" and discussed the neuroanatomical and neurophysiological implications of frontal removals.[27] These two addresses were published after the war as part of a symposium held by the Association for Research in Nervous and Mental Disease.[28]

Theodore Erickson discussed some problems of the scalenus anticus syndrome. It is unknown if he related this condition to the second topic that he addressed at the institute, "Erotomania as an Expression of Cortical Epileptiform Discharge."

THEODORE CHARLES ERICKSON

It would be difficult to surpass Theodore Charles Erickson's career at the Montreal Neurological Institute. He obtained an MSc in anatomy in 1929 from the University of Minnesota under A.T. Rasmussen, the father of Theodore Rasmussen, the second director of the MNI. Erickson obtained his MD from Minnesota in 1931. He then came to the institute while it was still at the RVH and was its first resident when it crossed University Street. He was a resident and fellow until 1939 and stayed at the institute for two years thereafter as assistant surgeon and lecturer in neurosurgery in charge of the Laboratories of Neurophysiology. During his time at the MNI, Erickson obtained a second MSc in 1934 for his thesis "Neurogenic Hyperthermia," and a PhD in 1939 for his dissertation "The Nature and the Spread of the Epileptic Discharge."[29] Erickson's crowning achievement at the institute was co-authoring *Epilepsy and Cerebral Localization* with Penfield in 1941.[30] Their book contains a chapter by Molly Harrower, the MNI's first psychologist, on the application of psychometric methods for assessing patients with epilepsy. She and Erickson married

Table 11.1
War-related addresses at the MNI

Speaker	Topic
Head injuries	
H. Botterell (Toronto)	Management of Acute Head Injuries in Royal Canadian Army Medical Corps Overseas
J.P. Evans (Chicago)	Pathological and Clinical Observations of Brain Injury
W.O. Gliddon (Ottawa)	Gunshot Wounds of the Head: A Review of the After-effects in 500 Pensioners from the Great War 1914–18
R. Pudenz (Passedena)	The Lucite Calvarium: A New Method for the Observation of Intracranial Phenomena
Earl Walker (Chicago) & D. Denny-Brown (Harvard)	The Pathogenesis and Experimental Studies of Concussion
A.A. Ward (MNI)	Effect of Cholinergic Drugs on Recovery of Function following Experimental Lesions of the Central Nervous System
Spine and peripheral nerves	
J.B. Camp (Mayo Clinic)	The Roentgenologic Diagnosis of Lesions Affecting the Spinal Cord
L.J. Pollock (Northwestern)	Injury and Repair of Peripheral Nerves
J.E. Samson (Cartierville)	Experiences with Low-Back Pain
B. Stookey (Columbia)	Surgery of Peripheral Nerves in War
I. Tarlov (New York)	Plasma Clot Suture of Nerves
F. Turnbull	Management of Nerve Injuries in the Late Stages
Other topics	
B.A. Campbell (MNI)	The Medical Officer at Sea
J. Fulton (Yale)	Blast Injuries
G. Horrax (Lahey Clinic)	Neurosurgery in Wartime
F. Kennedy (Cornell)	Functional Disorders Associated with Warfare
V.H. Moon (Jefferson)	Surgical Shock
C.P. Rhoads (Rockefeller)	Deficiency Disease and the Nervous System
J. Scudder (Columbia)	Shock and Blood Studies as a Guide to Therapy
S.B. Wolbach (Harvard)	Avitaminosis and Diseases of the Nervous System

while both where at the institute, one of many matrimonial matchings at the MNI. Erickson and Harrower-Erickson left the institute in 1942 when Erickson established the Department of Neurosurgery at the University of Wisconsin Medical School, in Madison. This was a highly successful venture for which he created a residency training program, an EEG laboratory, and a vigorous neuro-physiological research program headed by the renowned Clinton Woolsey.[31]

Table 11.2
Other addresses

Speaker	Topic
T. Erickson (Wisconsin)	Scalenus Anticus Syndrome
	Erotomania as an Expression of Cortical Epileptiform Discharge
F. Ingraham and O. Bailey (Harvard)	Subdural Hematoma in Infancy
H. Howe (Hopkins)	Neurobiological Aspects of Poliomyelitis
T.I. Hoen (NYU)	Herniation of the Intervertebral Discs
M.E. Knapp (Minneapolis)	The Kenny Treatment
W. McCulloch (Illinois)	The Functional Organisation of the Primate Cortex
I. McQuarrie (Mayo Clinic)	Physicochemical Studies on the Mechanism of Convulsive Phenomena
H.H. Merritt (Harvard)	The Medical Treatment of the Convulsive Disorders
A. Morris (MNI fellow)	Herniation of Cervical Intervertebral Discs
B.M. Patten (Michigan)	Development Defects of the Nervous System
T. Putnam (Harvard)	The Treatment of the Dyskinesias
A.T. Rasmussen (Minnesota)	Organization of the Trigeminal Nerve
E. Walker (Hopkins)	The Thalamus and Some of Its Connections
A.O. Whipple (Columbia)	Evaluation of Penicillin in Its Relation to Surgery

THE HUGHLINGS JACKSON MEMORIAL LECTURES

The Hughlings Jackson Lectures continued without interruption, seeming to be a reminder of better times past and of better times to come, when science could be pursued for its own sake, and not directed at men and women damaged by war.

Detlev Wulf Bronk had given the fourth Hughlings Jackson lecture on 6 April 1938. The lectures for 1939 and 1940 were given by Walter B. Cannon – of the fight-or-flight reaction, and Charles H. Best, co-discoverer of insulin. Professor Cannon discussed "A Law of Denervation," and Professor Best presented "Factors Affecting the Liberation of Insulin from the Pancreas." Stephen Walter Ranson of Northwestern University, Chicago, member of the National Academy of Science, and frequent collaborator with Horace Magoun, delivered the 1941 lecture, "Experimental Studies on the Corpus Striatum," in what was the last named lecture he gave, as he died in 1942. Lord Edgar Douglas Adrian was the first Nobel laureate to give the Hughlings Jackson Lecture, in 1942, "Sensory Areas of the Brain." Lord Adrian had been awarded the Nobel Prize with Sherrington in 1932, and it is an eloquent testimony to the high regard in which Penfield and the MNI were held that Adrian chanced the crossing of the Atlantic in wartime to deliver his lecture. Subsequent Jackson lecturers would only need to cross the forty-ninth parallel to come to Montreal, at least until the cessation of hostilities. Thus, Philip Bard, professor of physiology at Johns Hopkins University, who had obtained his doctorate from Harvard under Cannon, gave the 1943 lecture, "Re-representation as a Principle of Central Nervous Organization." The singular Percival Bailey, whose autobiography *Up from Little Egypt* inspired many a budding neurosurgeon, gave the 1944 Hughlings Jackson Lecture, "The Cortical Organization of the Chimpanzee Brain." Finally, Penfield's lifelong friend Stanley Cobb gave the 1945 lecture, "Some Problems on Neurocirculatory Asthenia."

THE DEATH OF HARVEY CUSHING

Penfield received a telegram from Louise Eisenhart, Cushing's long-time collaborator on 7 October 1939, stating simply, "Chief died quietly this morning."

Cushing had an unprecedented understanding of Canadian medicine, particularly of McGill Medical School, because of his strong personal and professional relationship with Sir William Osler, and the research that he carried out for his monumental biography of Osler, which appeared in 1925.[32] His surgical

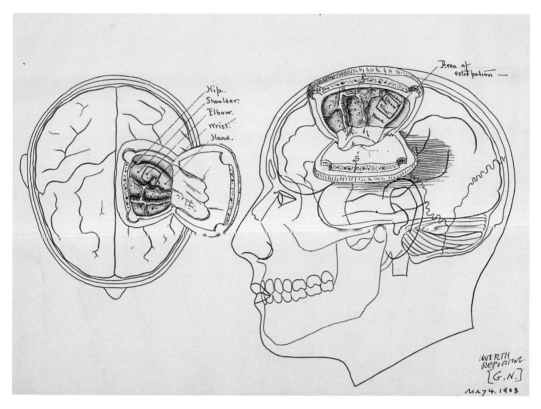

Figure 11.4: Drawing by Harvey Cushing, one of a set of four he sent to Wilder Penfield in 1932. Cushing performed the operation in 1903, while he was at Johns Hopkins. It depicts the result of stimulation in the hip, shoulder, elbow, wrist, and hand regions of the cerebral cortex. (MNI Archives)

ritual influenced Penfield and Kenneth Mackenzie, who established the two major Canadian schools for neurosurgical teaching and treatment in Montreal and Toronto.

The death of Cushing was deeply felt at the MNI. A memorial meeting was held in his memory on 15 November 1939, presided by Dean Charles Martin, in the presence of Gerald Birks; William Francis of the Osler Library; Wilder Penfield; and William Cone.[33] For Penfield, Cushing was "technician, operator, artist, physiologist, he set up a new standard in his surgical clinic … and now it may be said that neurosurgeons throughout the world belong to the Cushing school."[34] Penfield had good reason to pay a warm tribute to Cushing. He had been a surgical intern on Cushing's service at the Peter Bent Brigham Hospital at Harvard in 1919, and while he was at the Columbia Presbyterian Hospital in

New York, Penfield made frequent visits to Cushing in Boston. As Penfield noted later, "I was very greatly influenced in the development of my own particular technique by the Cushing ritual. I made drawings of every instrument and listed the routine steps of every operation. It seems fair to say, therefore, that throughout my surgical career I have used Cushing's method as a sort of classic and have constantly referred to the general principles which he laid down in neurosurgical operating."[35]

Harvey Cushing, knowing of his interest in cerebral localization, sent Wilder Penfield four operative sketches drawn by his own hand of cases in which Cushing had performed electrocortical stimulation. One is reproduced here for the first time (figure 11.4).

12

Life at the Institute

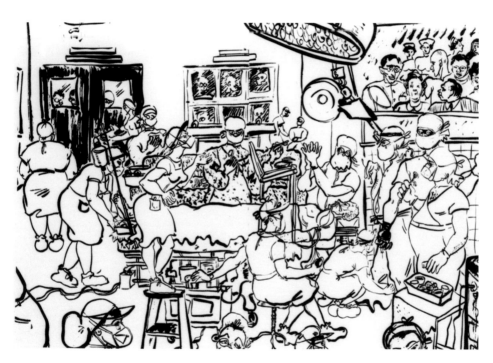

Figure 12.1: Life in the operating room at the MNI. (Drawing by Mary Filer)

Clinical services at the MNI met the challenge of an increasing patient population augmented by the repatriation of casualties from Basingstoke, but they were pressed to the limit of their capacities. Donald McEachern sounded an alarming note on behalf of the Department of Neurology:

> The most serious problem facing the service is that of survival. For several years the Institute has been filled to capacity and it has frequently been impossible to admit all patients for whom admission has been recommended. In the past year the shortage of beds has become acute and

a large waiting list has developed. Surgical "emergencies" are perforce admitted ahead of cases from the waiting list and the number of beds available for neurological cases has steadily dwindled … The lack of beds is a serious threat to our service, which bears the responsibility of training nurses, students and interns in the principles of neurology. It also means that we are unable to serve the needs of the neurologically ill of the City and Province.[1]

Indeed, the only patients admitted to the hospital at the time were neurosurgical emergencies and servicemen, while the waiting list for elective patients could be well over a year.[2] As a result of the high occupancy rate, the hospital, which, unlike the institute, did not have an endowment fund, had seen almost a quadrupling of its annual deficit.[3] Yet patients needed to be cared for, as John Kershman emphasized:

A serious problem which merits consideration is what can be done for the indigent patient who arrives penniless at the door of the Institute from outside the Province of Quebec. Many on them came hundreds of miles, using their last resources for railroad fare, arrive here and place themselves at our mercy. At the present time the institute has five such patients under its care … Three of these patients have brain tumours and two suffer from a neurological illness as yet undiagnosed. It is impossible to turn these patients away, nor do we wish to. They are sick people who rightfully come to us for help.[4]

The need for space did not spare the neurosurgeons, who had to adjust their practice to meet the ever-increasing demand on their services. Most surgical patients admitted were so seriously ill when they arrived at the MNI that they required priority over others. Dressing rooms on the wards served as "treatment rooms" for some surgical procedures that would otherwise have been performed in the operating rooms. These included twist-drill craniectomies for ventriculography, tumour biopsy, and aspiration of abscesses. The dressing rooms were also used to apply skull tongs to reduce and stabilize neck fractures and to apply plaster body casts. The use of the large, well-equipped, and brightly lit dressing rooms for such procedures continued for another five decades.

Although the clinical services were coping with an increase in patients, they were doing so in the face of a dwindling number of residents and fellows who entered the military as they finished their training.[5] Clearly, something needed to be done. The obvious solution was to repatriate William Cone, as Penfield re-

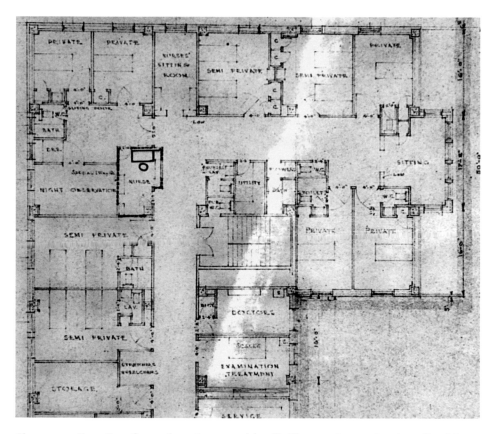

Figure 12.2: Four East floor plan, circa 1934 (*detail*). The nursing station is outlined in bold. The treatment room, where ventriculograms, biopsies, cyst aspirations, and the application of Cone-Barton tongs for spinal stabilization were performed, is visible inferiorly at centre. Single private rooms and double semi-private rooms are indicated. (MNI Archives)

lated to the staff: "When I addressed the annual meeting twelve months ago, I was expecting myself to leave the Institute for service overseas to No. 1 Neurological Hospital to relieve Dr Cone. Owing to factors over which I had no control, this was prevented.[6] However, as the result of our urgent request, the Director General of Medical Services allowed Lt Col. William Cone and Major Arthur Childe to return to take up their essential work here."[7]

WILLIAM CONE'S RETURN

William Cone returned from Basingstoke in the autumn of 1941. In his first report to the institute in two years, he first addressed the situation of No. 1 Neurological and acknowledged Colin Russel's role in its creation.

The organization we left is a going concern. It is very well staffed and well equipped to handle the neurological and neurosurgical casualties of our active service force. They are doing excellent work at No. 1 Neurological and are making a name for Canadian neurology and neurosurgery in England. We from the Montreal Neurological Institute and the Royal Victoria Hospital claim a big stake in the unit. Dr Colin Russel, as a result of his experience in the last war, felt such a unit was essential and dreamed the dreams of its organization. Then he implemented the dreams until the Unit took form. All of us here had a part in helping him plan it.[8]

Russel's organizational talents were also recognized outside of the MNI: he was promoted to the rank of full colonel and attached to the Canadian Headquarters of the Royal Canadian Army Medical Corps (RCAMC) in London, England, as neurological consultant. Having acknowledged Russel's essential contributions, Cone then recognized the nurses who elected to stay at No. 1 and those who returned: "Miss Bossy, Miss Hudson, Miss Winter, Miss Swartz, Miss Gillespie, Miss Roach, Miss Jones and Miss Sharpe are there now and where in this wide world could a better group of specially trained nurses be found? The Unit will miss Miss MacKay and Miss Kendall who were such balance wheels for all of us over there. We are pleased to have them back in Canada."[9]

With Cone's return to clinical practice, new records for the number of patients operated upon were reached. Meeting the needs of these patients, Cone stated, rested entirely with the superlative dedication of the nurses: "The nursing staff in the operating room and on the wards has been untiring, efficient and kindly, in spite of the added responsibilities and added load. The nurses have recognized the importance of fear, anxiety and uncertainty as a factor in illness and have shown sympathy, understanding, dignity and courage in managing patients who have lacked faith and confidence. I mention this because with the rapid turnover and increased work, it might seem that there would be no time to consider the patient as a person. Somehow, however, they have made time to do so."[10]

The daily activities in the operating room in wartime are recounted in a letter from Elizabeth McRea-Welch:[11]

Nurse's Training at the Royal Victoria Hospital began for me the day after World War II was declared. In that first year of training I was sent to the M.N.I. to get a student's experience in Neurological and Nerosurgical

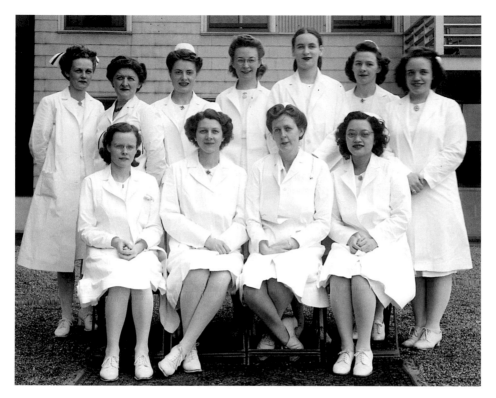

Figure 12.3: Operating room nurses, assistants, and technicians, 1946, in front of the Military Annex. (*Seated*) Marieleurrie Lachrité, Elizabeth McRae, Helene Calender, and Eva Chong Wong. (*Standing*) Margaret Haggart, Mary Roach, Mabel Darville, Irene Bloomer, Mary Filer, Margaret McNichol, and Isabelle Miller. (MNI Archives)

Nursing … After graduation I applied for work as a floor duty nurse at the "Neuro" … I was sent … to the Operating Room where a nurse was needed. Training me in Operating Room technique was done on the job by the nurses who were already there. I was touched and grateful for their generous kindness – for I was assigned to the Operating Room as assistant head nurse … Rita Edwards, the Operating Room Supervisor, was also Dr Penfield's scrub nurse. She handled the dual responsibility with grace. I have never seen another operating room nurse work with the smooth speed which Rita displayed. When Rita Edwards resigned in 1944 to marry Dr Peter Lehmann, I became head nurse …

Mary Filer worked "part time" as a nurse on our staff, while she studied art. Her talents were enjoyed by all when, during the Christmas Seasons, she decorated the windows of the Institute with her painting. She used her art to poke fun at the scenes of confusion that accompany Operating Room preparations … One used to hang in the Operating Room's coffee nook (figure 12.1).[12]

Besides his duties as a surgeon, Cone was also head of the Department of Neuropathology, where medical students had been called upon to fill the breach created by the departure of the junior medical staff for military service. One of them, William Feindel, had transferred from Dalhousie Medical School in September 1942 to continue his medical studies at McGill. He was assigned to neuropathology as a research fellow on 1 January 1944.[13]

William Cone inspired many in their neurosurgical career. He also stimu lated creativity in other areas, as witnessed by a poem by Stanley Ellis, Cone's orderly, whose job it was to maintain illumination on the operative field:[14]

Dear Lord please send me from thy throne
A perfect light for Willie Cone.
Make it so strong that he will see
Right-through the whole anatomy,
and more.
Lord as it is my arms are sore
Twisting light from left to right,
From early morn till late at night.
Oftimes I pray while thus I fight
If only thou would shout aloud,
For Cone, let there be light.
Stanley
June 25, 1946

DEPARTURES

Despite the return of Cone, Childe, and Russel, wartime demands continued to thin the institute's roster. Captain Donald McEachern and Lieutenant André Cipriani joined the RCAMC to direct research at a "special branch" in Ottawa, and McEachern was later called to London. John Kershman joined the Royal Canadian Air Force as consulting neuropsychiatrist, while Herbert Jasper and junior staff members Claude Bertrand, Peter Lehmann, and Donald Ross also joined the RCAMC.[15]

After 7 December 1941, American fellows also left the institute to answer the call to duty, while others took up academic practice in the United States. One was Theodore Erickson, Penfield's collaborator on *Epilepsy and Cerebral Local- ization*. Erickson's departure struck a double blow to the academic activities of the institute, as Molly Harrower, who had built up a new Department of Clin- ical Psychology at the institute, accompanied him as his wife.[16] Erickson and Harrower's was not the only wedding celebrated at the institute. Captain Peter

Lehmann married Rita Edwards, operating room supervisor and Penfield's surgical nurse. Cone fared no better, when *his* operating room nurse, Faith Lyman, married William Feindel.[1]

◆ ◆ ◆

Although a small lung nodule prevented Penfield from wearing the colours, he contributed greatly to the war effort as the leader of the British-American-Canadian Surgical Mission to England, Russia, and China, whose primary focus was to assess the organization of wartime medical services in the Union of Soviet Socialist Republics.[18] The mission arrived in Moscow in May 1943, a few months after the Battle of Stalingrad.

The mission to Moscow was the brainchild of Propper Graschenko, director of the Institute for Investigation of the Nervous System, who had visited the MNI in 1937, and who had suggested to his political superiors that Penfield should lead the delegation.[19] Penfield seems to have been most impressed with the Soviets' success in returning "70% of the injured" to active service.[20] One can't help but wonder at the veracity of this staggeringly high percentage of injured troops returning to the firing line. Penfield was also struck by the remarkably low incidence of psychoneurosis – shell shock – reported by the Soviet authorities. This Penfield ascribed to "an enormous supply of its specific antidote, i.e., high morale manufactured in Russia."[21] How morale was "manufactured" is left unsaid. Penfield contrasted the attitudes prevailing in American theatres of operation and on the Russian front. The Americans, he felt, were going down the wrong path in not creating specialized hospitals like the one at Basingstoke. Not so in Russia, he found: "Specialization has been pushed farther forward towards the front than ever before, even in the Sorting and Evacuation hospitals of the front line. The next level of reception is made up of special hospitals, in which head cases, wounds of the chest and abdomen, and wounds of the extremities are segregated."[22]

The surgical mission to China was largely restricted to Chungking, a limitation dictated by the situation in the field, but Penfield was given the opportunity of a private audience with Chiang Kai-shek, an encounter that left him convinced that "no one in China doubts the integrity and ability of the Generalissimo," whose role in the struggle against the Japanese Penfield equated with "that of George Washington during the long years of the American revolution."[23] Penfield made the same analogy after meeting Mao Zedong during a second visit to China in 1962.[24]

◆ ◆ ◆

The institute suffered a great loss with the death of Norman Petersen on 18 July 1944,[25] and Surgeon Lieutenant-Commander J. Preston Robb of the Naval Medical Service, a former resident in neurology, was seconded to the institute as acting registrar to help with the overwhelming burden of clinical administration after Petersen's death. The numbers were truly staggering: "The increase in the number of patients cared for in 1944 over those cared for in 1935, the first full year of operation of the institute, was 97%. The increase in hospital days over 1935 was 104%. The increase in operations was 148%." At times, Robb added, while the original forty-seven beds had not increased, there had been as many as 100 patients in the institute,[26] so the "treatment rooms" were often used to accommodate the overflow of patients. The end of the war would only add to the numbers of those cared for at the MNI, as troops with head injuries and spinal cord lesions were repatriated.

VE DAY

Wilder Penfield addressed the changes that he foresaw with the coming end of the war in an address to the MNI on 9 May 1945: "On the day before yesterday, victory was delivered in Europe; the full threat of military casualties is now reaching Canada; crowding of civilian patients is at a maximum; the teaching of medical students on an accelerated plan is soon to be terminated, and refresher courses for the returning medical officers are prepared; wartime research is now to be oriented toward the Pacific and peacetime research re-established." Penfield then listed three broad concerns for the coming years: "the care of Canadian military casualties, the care of civilians, [and] scientific and academic needs."[27]

For military casualties, Penfield was able to announce that a military annex was almost completed that would add twenty-seven beds to the MNI. However, it did not alleviate the lack of beds for the civilian population, which Penfield estimated would require the building of a new wing. Further, Penfield proposed that the MNI create additional space to accommodate six or eight graduate fellows to pursue post-war research. Penfield's concerns were echoed by John Kershman, who put it succinctly: "The most striking feature of the past year was the very marked increase in our expenses." He feared, specifically, that "scientific laboratories might be starved at the expense of maintaining the hospital wards." In this context, he recalled that the laboratories "were specifically endowed by separate funds from the Rockefeller Foundation, and if the cost of hospitalization threatens to drain these limited resources then the roots of our work become stagnant and devitalized." Referring to the annual grants from the city and province, Kershman noted that it might soon be necessary to test their generosity further.[28]

As if in answer to Kershman's plea, generous donations continued to benefit the institute, as George Savoy[29] made generous contributions for epilepsy research. Two other donations were quite poignant: $18.00 from In His Name Society for the purchase of dentures for a patient, and $93.60 from the Montreal Lions Club for the purchase of an accordion for a crippled patient – small but most thoughtful comforts.[30]

ACADEMIC ACTIVITIES

A six-week refresher course in neurology for newly discharged officers was instituted. It was comprehensive, intense, and rigorous, encompassing a review of neuroanatomy by Francis McNaughton, didactic lectures on the interpretation of X-rays by Arthur Childe, tutorials on EEGs by Herbert Jasper, and lessons on the interpretation of the cerebrospinal fluid by K.A.C. Elliott.[31] Participants also attended neurosurgical and neurological ward rounds and assisted at outpatient clinics. Evenings were "kept free to provide time for reading and study," and it was suggested that "the Fellows Library, and the McGill Medical Library may be used for this purpose."[32]

NEWS FROM ABROAD

There was mixed news from abroad. Arne Torkildsen had survived the German occupation of Norway and was working in Oslo. To everyone's relief, and contrary to previous reports, it was learned in August 1944 that Jerzy Chorobsky was alive. But the war was far from over in the summer of 1944, and the razing of Warsaw by the Nazis, one of the bloodiest actions of the war, was underway. It took a year to confirm the well-being of Chorobski and of his wife Victoria. In a letter dated 13 August 1945, three months after VE Day, Chorobsky wrote to Penfield from a devastated Warsaw: "I take the first opportunity to get in touch with you. We both are safe and sound, although we passed through some rather terrible times … I hope I will be able some day to come over to America and see what interesting things you have done in the field of neurosurgery during these six black years."[33]

13

Valour

To paraphrase Penfield on the MNI, the significance of the building lies in the people it houses.[1] Four fellows – Martin Nichols, Jerzy Chorobski, C. Miller Fisher, and Reuben Rabinovitch – tempered by war, resistance, and incarceration, exemplify the character, singularity of purpose, and devotion to duty of those who had been at the institute and those who would come later.

DUNKIRK

The reality of war was brought home early to the MNI. Martin Nichols was a former fellow and a handsome, bespectacled young neurosurgeon who came to Montreal from Edinburgh in 1937 and worked with Wilder Penfield and André Cipriani on the coupling of cerebral blood flow and electrical activity of the cortex and basal ganglia.[2]

Nichols joined the Royal Army Medical Corps at the start of hostilities and was initially posted at Edinburgh Castle. He wrote to Penfield on 12 December 1939, before deployment:

> I heard some very exciting news from Mr Jefferson [Sir Geoffrey Jefferson] that I was to be appointed second surgeon to … the experimental mobile neurosurgical unit of the B.E.F. [British Expeditionary Force] … From what I have been able to find out, it is designed to work either at casualty clearing stations or at advanced bases and consists of several fitted trucks. In one of them the motor will drive the generator for lights and electrosurgical unit and also the suction pump. Mr Dott [Norman McComish Dott, Scottish neurosurgeon] carried out some experiments on electrocautery sets and found that an ordinary spark gap set was quite impossible for the battlefield … as a result … a very powerful electro-magnet has been designed to run off automobile batteries. I sincerely hope I get a chance to use these things.[3]

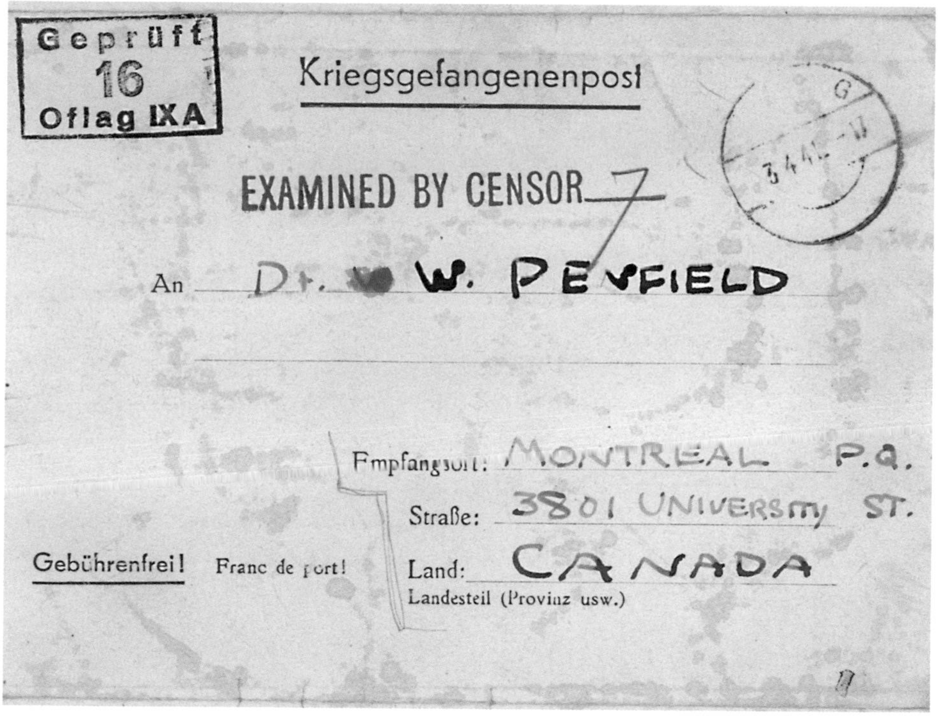

Kriegsgefangenenpost

EXAMINED BY CENSOR 7

An Dr. W. PENFIELD

Empfangsort: MONTREAL P.Q.

Straße: 3801 UNIVERSITY ST.

Gebührenfrei! Franc de port! Land: CANADA

Landesteil (Provinz usw.)

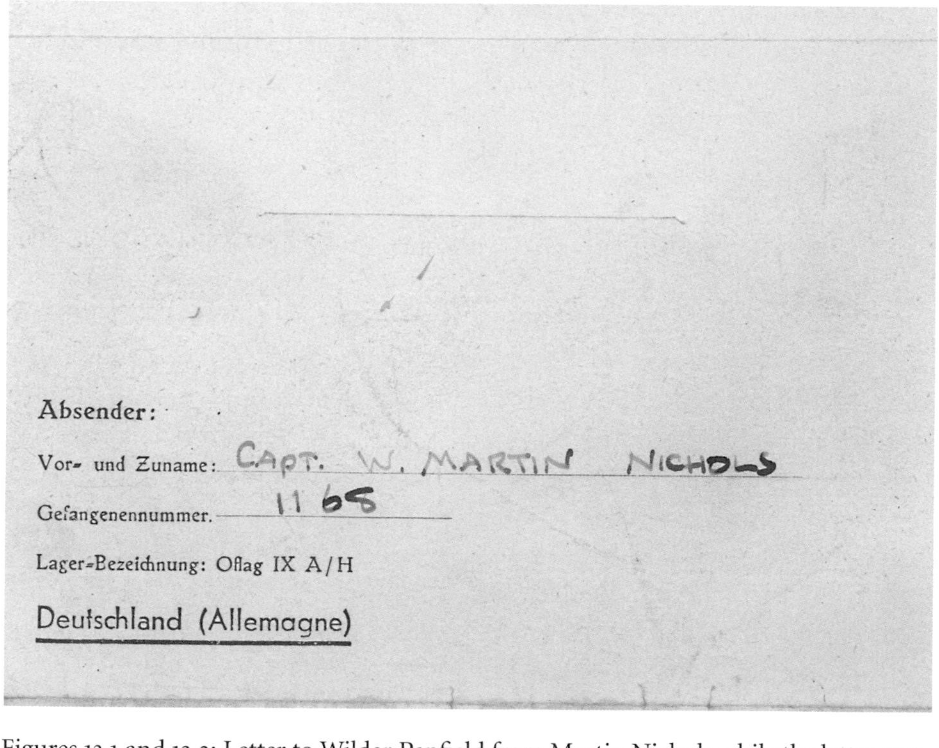

Absender:

Vor- und Zuname: CAPT. W. MARTIN NICHOLS

Gefangenennummer. 1165

Lager-Bezeichnung: Oflag IX A/H

Deutschland (Allemagne)

Figures 13.1 and 13.2: Letter to Wilder Penfield from Martin Nichols while the latter was a prisoner of war in Stalag Luft I. (Penfield Archives)

Nichols crossed the Channel into France with the BEF. But the combined British and French Forces were no match for the German Blitzkrieg, and what remained of the BEF was evacuated, with great effort and sacrifice, from the beaches of Dunkirk, between 26 May and 4 June 1940. On the afternoon of 6 June, William Cone wrote to Wilder Penfield, "Nichols … took over a head team and special truck and though they have not returned are probably staying with their wounded. It is said they did a splendid job."[4] Nichols had indeed stayed with his wounded and was taken prisoner but remained active as a surgeon in a prisoner of war camp, Stalag Luft I.[5] Nichols wrote Penfield on 28 March 1941 from the camp, asking about old friends, enquiring of family members, reminiscing about better times, the small things that help us through difficult times: "I am here in a small hospital – part of a state mental home – with one general surgeon and a Jesuit priest. We let out pus and remove sequestra and even remove the odd appendix. Our patients are our own British wounded and French and Poles from nearby working camps, my rounds are in three languages for I have to speak German to the Poles as well as my limited vocabulary of Polish phrases. These Poles are very gallant & friendly. Wonder where Chorobski is." Penfield responded on 9 May 1941: "George Chorobski is at home and alive, but we do not hear anything from him."[6]

Nichols survived the war and his internment and had a distinguished career in the United Kingdom. He returned to the MNI in October 1959 and spoke at the twenty-fifth anniversary of the founding of the institute.[7]

THE RAZING OF WARSAW

Jerzy Ludwik Chorobski was born in 1902 in what is now Pidhaitsi, then in western Poland, now in eastern Ukraine. His father was a physician, as was his brother, who died in the First World War. Chorobski obtained his medical degree from the University of Krakow in 1926, and while there, Chorobski worked in a psychiatric clinic, which perhaps stimulated his interest in neurology.[8] True to his interest in psychiatry, however, Chorobski travelled to Zurich after graduation to work with Eugen Bleuler, an authority on schizophrenia. From Zurich, Chorobski went to Paris to study with George Guillain, of the Guillain-Barré syndrome, and with Joseph Babinski, for whom he had a life-long admiration. While in Paris, Chorobski observed operations performed by Thierry de Martel, founder of French neurosurgery, and by Clovis Vincent, who had studied with Cushing and would succeed de Martel upon his death.[9]

Still feeling the need for further instruction, Chorobski obtained a Madeleine Ottman Fellowship in 1930 and travelled to Montreal to study with Penfield,

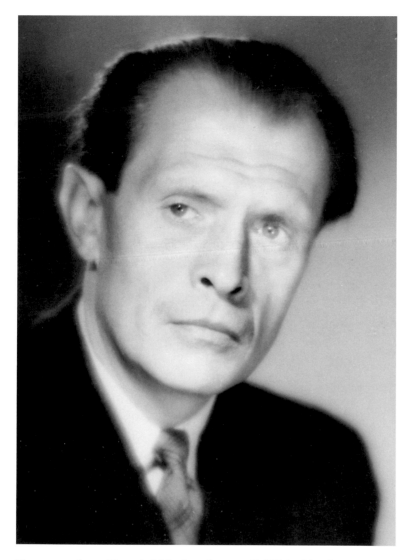

Figure 13.3: Jerzy Chorobski, before the war. (MNI Archives)

then still at the RVH. There he did ground-breaking work on the innervation of cerebral blood vessels.[10] From Montreal, Chorobski travelled to Chicago where he met and worked with the influential neurosurgeon Loyal Davis and observed Percival Bailey operate.[11] Chorobski also visited Hugh Cairns at Oxford and Foerster in Breslau. He returned to Montreal the following year, before returning to the University of Warsaw in 1935. Chorobski's return to Poland was not as happy as his stays in Paris, Montreal, and Chicago. He became the head of neurosurgery at the Academy of Medicine in Warsaw, where he spent most of his career, in the words of a colleague, "in the shadow of Satan," first under Nazi occupation and later under Soviet rule.[12]

With the invasion of Poland in September 1939 and the subsequent siege of Warsaw, Jerzy Chorobski was called upon to operate in a number of military hospitals, "close to the front, most frequently under artillery fire and during continuous air raids."[13] The Polish Cavalry was no match for German mechanized units and dive-bombers, and, after the fall of Poland, Chorobski led a double life: director of neurosurgery at the university by day, and partisan by night. "Chorobski, aware of his patriotic traditions, was able to participate in actions undertaken by the Underground Army. He used his knowledge of foreign languages to work in radio monitoring and to prepare news for underground bulletins. He treated the wounded soldiers of the Underground Army. These activities were forbidden under penalty of death."[14] Paul Bucy, who had met him in Chicago, remembers Chorobski as "a tough character" and tells of his visit to Warsaw after the war, when Chorobski showed him "the radio set camouflaged in a toaster, which was still buried under the floorboards of his kitchen and on which he had listened to the broadcasts of the BBC throughout the war."[15] Discovery of a clandestine radio meant summary execution. Jerzy Chorobski was awarded the Virtuti Militari Cross, "the highest Polish military order, for his activities during the war."[16]

The Underground Polish Army had risen against the Germans in 1944 as the Russians approached Warsaw. Seeing the magnitude of the fighting, the Soviets stopped short of the city, to let the battle play out. Thus, for over two months, Warsaw was the scene of some of the most vicious fighting of the war. Chorobski continued to operate in unspeakable circumstances until the university hospital itself was destroyed in October 1944. Chorobski and his staff left the city, taking with them whatever serviceable equipment they could.[17]

PENFIELD IN WARSAW

The war over, Jerzy Chorobski returned to Warsaw and set upon the task of rebuilding his department. His efforts were rewarded in 1949 by promotion to professor of neurosurgery at the University of Warsaw and by the opening of a new seventy-eight-bed neurosurgical clinic in 1951. The new professorship, however, and the clinic were not sufficient to compensate for life under Stalinism.

Chorobski's plight had come to the attention of Edward Arnold Carmichael, an honorary physician to the National Hospital, Queen Square, and director of the Medical Research Council's Neurological Research Unit.[18] Carmichael wrote Penfield about Chorobski on 19 November 1951.

Dear Penfield,

You probably know that I was over in Poland a matter of three or four years ago and met Chorobski. At that time I was a little bit worried at his attitude to the regime, feeling that he might by verbal indiscretions get himself into an unavoidable position. I have in the last 24 hours heard that it is possible he might lose his position and be transferred to a colder climate further east. I have also heard through a definite source that he sent a message to me that he was not happy. I took this as an indication that he would like us if possible to take some steps to bring him across the Iron Curtain into more civilized regions, … and wonder if one might approach the Rockefeller people giving them this information. If you think anything might come of this or can think of another way to help Chorobski I would indeed be glad to hear. I will certainly do all I can.

With kindest regards,

Yours sincerely,

E. Arnold Carmichael[19]

Penfield did not delay in forwarding Carmichael's letter to the Rockefeller Foundation and to Howard Naffziger, who, it will be recalled, had arranged for Ottiwel Jones to study with Penfield and Cone when they were still at the Royal Victoria Hospital.[20]

Dear Howard:

I am enclosing a copy of a letter from Arnold Carmichael which you will treat as completely confidential. I suppose you know very well the danger that he [Chorobski] has been in and probably can size up the situation very much better than I can … The matter of getting anyone moved from East to West is something that I know nothing about. I would be delighted to do anything for George that I can if he gets out, and I know that you have a similar feeling.

Yours sincerely,

WGP[21]

However, as the affair progressed, Carmichael injected a note of caution and tradecraft in his response to Penfield on 27 November 1951:

Dear Penfield,

I am indeed very grateful to you for being so quick in handling this matter I wrote to you about … My information is that it is inadvisable for any of his friends such as yourself or myself to write to him or get in touch with him – it might be as well for you to know this. I have a way open to me by which I can get in touch with him, so if you want anything passed through to him do let me know.[22]

Penfield replied to Carmichael on 8 December 1951:

Dear Carmichael:
   … You have spoken of getting a message to the man in question. I think it would be all right to say that I would be glad to provide money for travel, if necessary, with a view to this being used for any useful purpose in his getting out. We would also be glad to welcome him at the Montreal Neurological Institute until other arrangements can be made.
   As ever yours,
   WGP[23]

Penfield reiterated his willingness to help Chorobski in any way that he could in a follow-up letter four days later but underlines the gravity of Chorobski's situation should their efforts come to light.

   … We will be glad to have George work here until some permanent arrangement can be made for his future, but I am much concerned for fear that he will end in Siberia rather than here.[24]

Chorobski invited Penfield to attend the Congress of Polish Neurologists, which was to be held in Warsaw in October 1952. Although Penfield's initial response had been positive, he later declined the invitation. Penfield received correspondence on this issue and on its implications in a letter 24 September 1952, received from Leolyn Dana Wilgress, McGill alumnus and Canadian diplomat. Wilgress had been the Canadian ambassador to the USSR and Canadian high commissioner to London. At the time of his writing to Penfield, Wilgress was Canadian undersecretary of state for external affairs and deputy minister of foreign affairs, and later the Canadian permanent representative to NATO.[25]

Dear Dr Penfield:
   … Our Chargé d'Affaires in Warsaw has learned from the British Embassy that Dr George Chorobski is regarded with suspicion by the authorities and is endeavouring to defend western theories in his field against those propounded by the Soviet authorities … it is hard for us at

this distance to get a clear picture of the issue involved and the sort of risks that Dr Chorobski might run by associating closely with western scientists whose views would be in conflict with those held by Soviet scientists …

Yours sincerely,

[*Signed*] Mr Dana Wilgress[26]

Three days later, Dr Penfield received a telegram from Chorobski: "Wic died suddenly Chorobski." Penfield later learned that Victoria, Chorobski's wife, had committed suicide.

Honoris Causa

Chorobski eventually left Poland for Montreal, but only temporarily. In 1959, at the twenty-fifth anniversary celebration of the founding of the institute, Wilder Penfield presented Jerzy Chorobski with the degree of Doctor of Science *honoris causa*, on behalf of McGill University. In his presentation, Penfield said,

Mr Chancellor:

I have the honour to present to you, that you may confer upon him the degree of Doctor of Science, *honoris causa*, Jerzy Chorobski, Doctor of Medicine of the University of Krakow …

He came to Montreal in 1930, already well trained in Neurology and Psychiatry. He turned his eager mind to neurosurgery and to research in the physiology of the brain and its circulation.

Three years we worked together, and I can say that few men in any university have a broader knowledge and none a more unquenchable enthusiasm than George Chorobski. Returning in 1934 from his wander-years of graduate study in Montreal, Chicago, London and Paris, he introduced the specialty of neurosurgery in Poland in the face of many obstacles and trained a school of loyal neurosurgeons.

In the face of danger and uncertainty he carried on his surgery and his pursuit of truth with incredible keenness, contributing to our knowledge of the nerve control of cerebral blood vessels, and to many varied neurosurgical problems …

Through the years that followed 1939, the years of Poland's agony, he stood steadfast with that heroic race, his countrymen. In the story of that nation, Chorobski's contribution will rank high indeed. I am proud and happy to present this friend, distinguished scientist, outstanding surgeon … [*sic*] this stalwart son of Poland.[27]

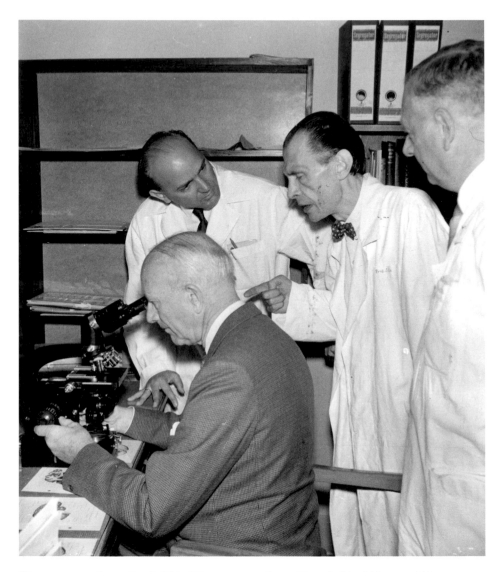

Figures 13.4 and 13.5: Penfield in Warsaw, 1960. Jerzy Chorobski, old beyond his years, standing behind Penfield at the microscope. (*Opposite*) Jerzy Chorobski (*extreme left*) reads the proclamation conferring the title of Doctor of Medicine *honoris causa* from the University of Warsaw upon Penfield (*centre*). Sitting at Penfield's left is presumed to be Marcin Kacprzak, rector of the Academy of Medicine. Partially hidden by Chorobski is Roszkowski, dean of the academy. (MNI Archives)

The following year Penfield finally made his way to Warsaw and in turn received the title of Doctor of Medicine *honoris causa* from the University of Warsaw, conferred upon him by Jerzy Chorobski.

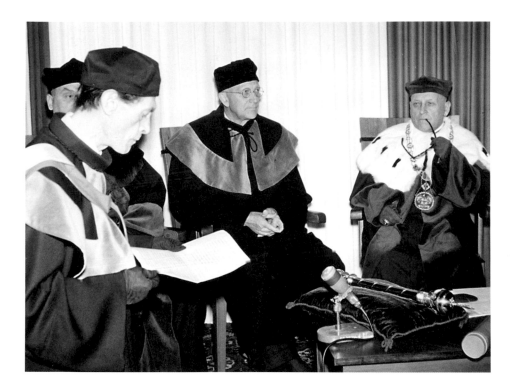

STALAG X B

Charles Miller Fisher's medical residency at the RVH was cut short when he joined the Royal Canadian Navy as surgeon lieutenant commander in 1940.[28] A German raider, the *Kriegsmarine* auxiliary cruiser *Thor*, sank his ship, the convoy escort HMS *Voltaire*, in 1941. Fisher survived the blast and spent many hours in the South Atlantic while the *Thor* machine-gunned gathering sharks. Fisher was eventually taken aboard the *Thor*, where he aided the German medical officers in treating the wounded. Fisher spent ten days on the *Thor* as it continued its mission, before being transferred to a prison ship headed for La Rochelle, a major French seaport and site of the North Atlantic U-boat pens.[29] From La Rochelle Fisher and the other prisoners of war were transported, under heavy guard, to Stalag Xb Sandhostel in northern Germany, between Hamburg and Bremen.[30] At Stalag Xb the POWs were showered, deloused, and vaccinated against typhoid. Fisher was assigned to the infirmary, where the "entire medical supply consisted of paper bandages, liquorice tablets for gargling with, and a one piece scalpel somewhat corroded with ¼ inch of the tip of the blade missing."[31] Fisher was transferred to a new camp, Marlag und Milag Nord, fifteen miles from Bremen, in the summer of 1942.[32] There he "had sterilizers, a few needles and suture material. Medicines provided included sulfapyridine, calcium, antacids, cough tablets and aspirin."[33] Fisher occupied his time with learning German so that he could keep up with the medical literature. Recreation at Stalag Xb included poker, bridge, ersatz cabaret reviews, and watching German searchlights play off Royal Air Force Wellington bombers heading for a night raid on Hamburg.

In 1944 Fisher was moved to a camp in Annaburg to accompany prisoners sick or injured enough to be allowed repatriation to England, when a fellow physician generously offered his place to Fisher, a husband and a father.[34] While waiting for transport that would take the prisoners from Annaburg to England, those who were able enough played sports – mostly soccer, softball, and rounders, a primitive form of baseball popular with British schoolgirls. From Annaburgh, the British sick and injured and their medical escorts boarded a Red Cross ship bound for Sweden and eventual repatriation to England. Then Fisher and some other Canadians set sail for New York and freedom. From there Fisher boarded a Canadian Pacific train to Toronto, where he saw his daughter for the first time.

Still on active service, Fisher was assigned to the RVH, where he encountered Reuben Rabinovitch for the *second* time:

> On occasion, I ate at the same table as Dr Reuben Rabinovitch, a young neurosurgeon in training. He eventually gave up the profession for neurology. Regularly he would say in his gravelly voice, "I know you, we have met before." I was embarrassed not to be able to recall the occasion, although his voice sounded somewhat familiar … One day he explained. At the beginning of World War II he had been studying neurosurgery in Paris [at La Pitié, with Clovis Vincent] and was arrested when the Germans overran France … At some point, he developed paraplegia, a paralysis of both legs due to spinal cord disease. He was moved from hospital to hospital and finally was repatriated via Annaburg in the same group as I. I was the officer who certified that he had to travel to Sweden by stretcher. During the softball games I played second base for the Canadians, and a familiar sound at every game was the loud booming voice of a heckler lying on a stretcher at an open window. It had been "Rab." For three years he had feigned paraplegia and was successfully rescued from the Germans.[35]

STALAG XVII B

Stalag 17 is the title of a movie about life in a German prisoner-of-war camp, directed by Otto Preminger, whose plot revolves around suspicion by fellow POWs that one of them is a German spy posing as an American. Although the story may be fictional, Stalag XVII b did exist, and there was someone among the prisoners, Harry Vosic, who was not what he made himself out to be. Vosic, who posed as an American airman, was in fact a Canadian doctor who had come to France to train in neurosurgery with Clovis Vincent. His real name was Reuben Rabinovitch, from La Macaza, Quebec.[36] Rabinovitch attended high school in Montreal and university in New York City,[37] then studied medicine at the University of Paris and graduated in 1940. Rabinovitch chose to stay in Paris after graduation to train in neurology and neurosurgery with Clovis Vincent, at La Pitié hospital. Vincent at that time had been shouldering the brunt of neurosurgical practice in Paris since Thierry de Martel's death.[38] Rabinovitch, as a foreigner and a Jew, was interned by the Gemans for seven months but was released, at Vincent's urging, to meet the needs of La Pitié in caring for neurosurgical cases. Rabinovitch himself recounts, with great emotion and abounding respect, the work of Clovis Vincent under Nazi occupation.[39]

Like Chorobski, Rabinovitch did not limit himself to caring for the sick and the wounded. He was active in the French Underground, aiding US airmen shot down over occupied France. Rabinovitch was arrested in the company of two American airmen and identified himself as Harry Vosic, gunnery sergeant, using a fictitious serial number that he had memorized for such an eventuality.[40] Harry Vosic – the first name was that of a cousin and the surname that of another – eventually found himself in Stalag 17 b near Krems, Austria. Milton Seldin, a fellow POW, tells of his first encounter with Sergeant Vosic, which gives the true measure of the man:

> It was October 12, 1943, Columbus Day, but the 1300 or so American GIs who had that day arrived in Krems, Austria, had little to celebrate. The first group of prisoners moved up to the delousing station where they were to take hot showers and have their hair clipped to the scalp … Suddenly … one of the boys writhed on the cement floor, clutching at his middle. A comrade [Vosic] … came forth and with practiced fingers explored the affected area of the sick lad's body. Quickly, and with evident authority, he spoke in French to the prisoner-bath attendant and in

German to the officer who came in response to the summons. The American had suffered an attack of appendicitis, he told them, and should be operated on immediately. The officer, in turn, called in a German doctor who confirmed the diagnosis.[41]

Questioning why a gunnery sergeant had such medical knowledge, the Germans apparently believed Vosic's story of a love affair gone bad that had caused him to abandon medicine and join the Air Force. Rabinovitch was then put in charge of an infirmary of sorts, in a filthy, louse-infested barracks previously occupied by Russian prisoners. After overseeing the clean-up and delousing, Rabinovitch was assisted by other POWs who had no medical knowledge whatever. Rabinovitch performed his duty despite suffering from excruciating back pain, to the point of needing a cane to see to his rounds. Seldin recounts how Rabinovitch trained and used his newly acquired medical assistants for the good of their fellow prisoners: "Once he discovered a case of diphtheria. He taught us how to recognize the white spots in the throat and in the next twenty-four hours our makeshift medical corps examined every throat in the camp while he argued with the German officials into providing us with serum. It would be impossible to estimate how many boys might have perished had an epidemic gotten under way."[42]

Showing uncommon courage in the face of certain death should he be discovered, Rabinovitch "used everything he could lay his hands on, to get as many boys as possible out of the camp. He faked x-rays, mixed up case histories, and with … medical double talk 'bamboozled' German medical officers into approving the release of many GI's, some of whose scars came from football games and accidents back on the farm."[43]

Rabinovitch's subterfuge could only go on for a certain time before the beleaguered Germans acted upon their growing suspicions. Fearing discovery, Rabinovitch converted his back pain into paraplegia and found himself on a stretcher in Annaberg, fooling even Miller Fisher but cheering him on at second base from a stretcher he didn't need. As Fisher recounted, they next saw each other in the cafeteria of the Royal Victoria Hospital.

THE WATCH THAT ENDS THE NIGHT

A letter to the editor of the now defunct *Montreal Star* was reproduced in a small, privately published collection of addresses in memory of Reuben Rabinovitch.

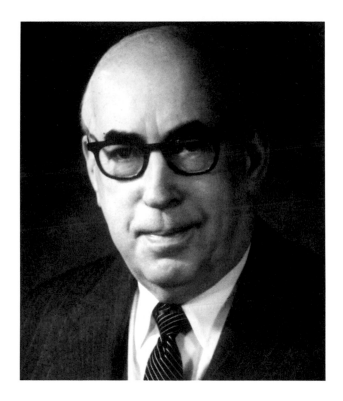

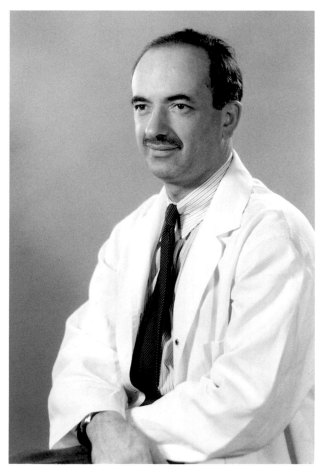

Figures 13.6 and 13.7: C. Miller Fisher (*above*) and Reuben Rabinovitch (*below*) in better times. (MNI Archives)

Sir,

On September 16 Dr Reuben Rabinovitch, neurologist of this city, died at the age of only 56 at the height of his powers … Dr Rab was a very great, a very rare healer. Whether from his concentration camp experience or from his native sensitivity, he had acquired what seemed to me to be a Shakespearean knowledge of men. Like many of his patients I often had the feeling that he was literally inside my own mind – not out of curiosity but merely because he was there. And being there, he took my fears away, and when he got out again, I found that some of his own courage had been left behind inside of me. He loved life. Few men more subtly and accurately understood its fragility; he was also indignant at it, as most of us are without daring to admit it.

When my novel, "The Watch That Ends The Night" appeared, it was widely believed that its doctor protagonist, Dr Jerome Martell, was modelled on the famous Dr Norman Bethune. He wasn't, for I never knew Bethune. But Martell's way of dealing with his patients was Dr Rab's way. This is not to suggest that Martell was modelled off him; he wasn't. But if I had not known Dr Rab, I could never have understood Dr Martell.

I went to Dr Rab because I had been troubled for years by back trouble – nothing serious as the Neurological Institute considers a case to be serious – but bad enough to paralyze my movements pretty often. Dr Rab taught me how to deal with that, but he also taught me much more. He helped me to deal with myself; he enabled me to become a better writer. In saying this, I know that hundreds of his patients would say the same of their own experience with this very rare doctor who, when we visited him, seemed rather to be visiting us; to know us better than we knew ourselves, and then with a mysterious luminous smile, a blend of irony and kindliness, to return again to himself.

Hugh MacLennan.[44]

14

The Postwar Period

The immediate post–World War II period was a golden era
at the Montreal Neurological Institute.
– Donald Tower

The end of the war was a period of rejoicing and reunion at the MNI. The annual photograph shows the house staff in their starched white uniforms, lined up and ready to meet the challenges of neurosurgical training (figure 14.1). Eric Peterson is present, recently discharged from the RCAF. Reuben Rabinovitch is seen for the first time in a staff photograph, to be decorated in the coming year by the American and French governments for the aid and comfort he gave to downed American airmen and for his clandestine work in the Resistance. Standing erect, almost at attention, Miller Fisher is also present for the first time. William Feindel is there, at the extreme left of the top row, as is Theodore Rasmussen, back from Burma, at the extreme right. It is the first time that the first three directors of the institute, Penfield, Rasmussen, and Feindel, are photographed together. Their mandates would see the MNI through its first half-century. Preston Robb, one of the most distinguished neurologists at the MNI and at McGill University, is absent, although his influence at the institute was already being felt.

PRESTON ROBB

J. Preston Robb acquired his distinguished broken nose on the gridiron of Percival Molson Stadium playing in the 1938 Canadian Intercollegiate Football Championship, one year before he graduated from McGill Medical School.[1] Robb joined the Royal Canadian Navy upon his graduation, and, like Miller Fisher, served in the Atlantic. However, Penfield had been so impressed with Robb as a medical student that he personally arranged for him to be seconded to the MNI, where his services were urgently needed, since other members of the staff were serving in England. Robb thus returned to the MNI as assistant neurologist and registrar in 1944 and 1945. Upon his discharge from

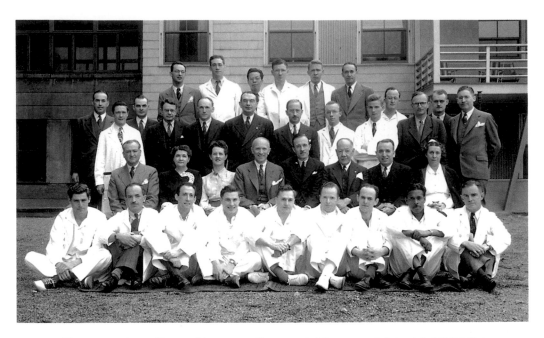

Figure 14.1: Attending and house staff, 1945–46. (*Front row, left to right*) E.W. Peterson, R. Rabinovitch, I. Schiffer, G.W. Thomas, C. Bertrand, W. Gibson, W.K. Welch, J. Chandy, W.F. Caveness. (*Second row*) D. McEachern, E. Davidson, F. Richardson, W. Penfield, C. James, C.K. Russel, W.V. Cone, E.C. Flanagan. (*Third row*) C.M. Fisher, J.M. Thompson, D. McRae, K.A.C. Elliott, F.L. McNaughton, J. Kershman, H.H. Jasper, A. Pope, J.S. Meyer, G.E. Joron, J. Fortuyn, A.A. Bailey, A.R. Elvidge. (*Top row*) W.H. Feindel, H.F. Steelman, C.J. Chen, A.A. Morris, C.W. Cure, T.B. Rasmussen. (MNI Archives)

the Navy, Robb trained in his first love, pediatric neurology, at Johns Hopkins and at Harvard.[2] It was a cold heart that was not warmed at the sight of this tall, imposing man with a crooked nose playing with hospitalized toddlers at Christmastime.

Robb succeeded Francis McNaughton as professor of neurology at McGill University in 1968, a position he held until 1976.[3] During his tenure Robb improved undergraduate teaching and the neurology training program, and strived to protect the neurology staff from administrative duties so that they could devote more time to research. Significantly, Robb recruited the likes of Eva and Fred Andermann, Stirling Carpenter, Andrew Eisen, George Karpati, Allan Sherwin, and Ivan Woods to the MNI.

Preston Robb was a great advocate for the care of epileptic patients. His expertise in this area was recognized by the National Institutes of Health, Bethesda, which commissioned him to survey and report on the basic and clinical research in epilepsy being performed in major institutions across the United States.[4] He was also a great champion for the surgical treatment of epilepsy refractory to medical management. Robb was especially concerned with the lack of adequate medical care in deprived areas: he travelled to the Canadian far north during the summer months to bring neurological care to the Inuit, and during a sabbatical Robb was a consultant to the Kenyatta General Hospital, Nairobi, where he devised a manual for epilepsy care in the field for the Kenyan government.[5] He was also instrumental in creating treatment facilities for patients living with epilepsy and other neurological conditions in Asia and South America. Robb was a founding member and president of the Canadian Neurological Society and president of the American Epilepsy Society, from which he received the William Lennox Award. Preston Robb went to his reward at the fine old age of ninety, a short time after he was awarded the MNI's lifetime achievement award and was celebrated by his friends and colleagues.

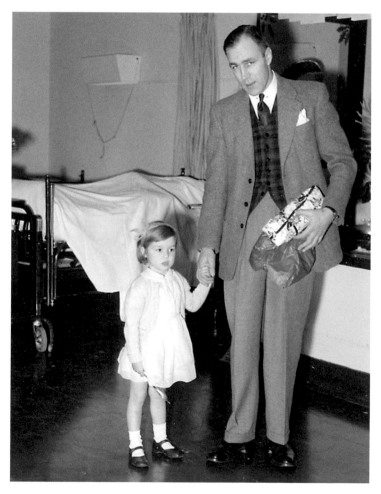

Figure 14.2: Preston Robb at Montreal Children's Memorial Hospital, Christmas 1955. (MNI Archives)

BIRTH OF NEUROSURGERY IN INDIA

Jacob Jaya Chandy, who sits in the front row of the 1945–46 annual photograph, would become India's first neurosurgeon and one of his country's leading medical educators. Chandy arrived at the MNI after the Second World War and trained as a neurosurgeon for three years with Penfield and Cone, then in 1948 he became chief resident in neurosurgery at the University of Chicago under Theodore Rasmussen, who later succeeded Penfield as director of the MNI. Chandy returned home in 1949 and established India's first Department of Neurological Sciences at the Christian Medical College and Hospital in Vellore, in the state of Madras (now Tamil Nadu) in southern India, where he promoted the MNI model of an integrated clinical-research facility for the next twenty years. Chandy arranged for key members of his department to train at the MNI, including J.C. Jacob and G.M. Taori in neurology, Sushil Chandi in neuro-pathology, and Elizabeth Mammen and S. Sarojini in neurosurgical nursing. Jacob later headed the Department of Neurology at Memorial University in St Johns, Newfoundland. Ramchandra Gindé from Bombay, B. Ramamurthi from Madras, and Jacob Chandy's son, Mathew, also came to train in neurosurgery at the MNI. Mathew Chandy later became head of neurosurgery in the department that his father had founded. Compelled by India's laws to retire in 1970, Jacob Chandy continued to contribute to his country's medical education. His numerous students and colleagues recall him as a powerful influence on several generations who went on to work in major academic centres in India and elsewhere.

FREEDMEN'S HOSPITAL: THE MNI
AND HOWARD UNIVERSITY

"Visitors tell us," Penfield reported in 1948, "that they consider the unique feature of our organization to be the close integration of research and teaching with clinical work. This is, of course, no more than should be expected in a clinical institute." As if to prove his point, Penfield noted that twenty-five fellows were occupied in various laboratories, nine of whom were pursuing graduate degrees. They came, Penfield went on, "with varied training and abilities from the fighting forces around the world, from the French and English Universities of Canada, coast to coast in the United States, Mexico, Uruguay, Brazil, Norway, Holland, France, Switzerland and Czechoslovakia, from India, China and Australia."[6] Clarence Greene was one who had come from the United States.

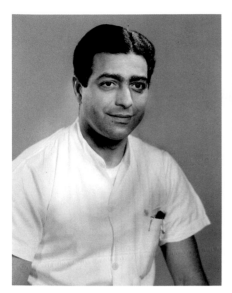 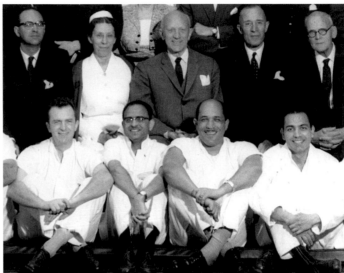

Figures 14.3 and 14.4: (*Left*) Clarence Greene, house staff, Montreal Neurological Hospital, 1947. (*Right*) Jesse Barber sits third from the left, in front of Wilder Penfield. To Penfield's right are Eileen Flanagan and William Feindel. (MNI Archives)

The winds of change were gathering for African-Americans after the Second World War, and they were blowing northward, to Montreal as promising young men, thwarted in their ambition of becoming neurosurgeons in the United Sates, looked to the MNI. So it was that Clarence Greene Sr, who would become the first African-American neurosurgeon in the United States, found himself climbing the steep southern slope of Mount Royal to 3801 University Street in the summer of 1947.

Clarence Sumner Greene Sr had studied pre-medicine at Harvard College and eventually entered Howard University College of Medicine, where he earned his medical degree in 1936. He practised surgery and taught at Howard University for eleven years before arriving at the MNI for neurosurgical training. Greene also participated in research during his stay at the institute, on new methods for staining nerves in the meninges with Francis McNaughton, and on the histopathology of gliomas with William Cone.[7]

Clarence Greene left Montreal in 1949 to return to Washington, DC, where, based at Freedmen's Hospital, he was appointed chair of neurosurgery at Howard University. Greene earned the distinction in 1953 of becoming the first African-American to be certified by the American Board of Neurological Surgery and was also the first African-American to be named to the Harvey

Cushing Society, predecessor of the American Association of Neurological Surgeons. Greene was very active at Freedmen's, performing diagnostic angiography and PEG, and operating on cerebral aneurysms, brain tumours, and other conditions affecting the nervous system. He practised there until his untimely death in 1957. But in his short career he became a model for other African-Americans seeking careers in medicine and other professions. Jesse Barber Jr was one of them.[8]

Jesse Barber Jr received his undergraduate degree from Lincoln University in Oxford, Pennsylvania, and then undertook medical studies at Howard University Medical College, graduating in 1948. Barber was Clarence Greene's resident at Freedmen's Hospital and came to the MNI in 1958, after Greene's passing, to complete his residency in neurosurgery. In 1995 Barber recounted how he came to the institute: Clarence Greene "died in 1957 and I had been encouraged and supported in trying to secure a Neurosurgical Residency and to become his replacement. My application for residency was accepted by MNI although turned down by ten other programs."[9] Jesse Barber trained with the same neurosurgeons with whom Clarence Greene had studied – Penfield, Cone, and Elvidge – and with the new generation, Theodore Rasmussen, William Feindel, and Gilles Bertrand. Barber recounts that Cone, during one of his habitual 1 a.m. rounds, engaged him in conversation and remarked, "I guess Dr Greene could be called the father of neurosurgery at Howard. If that's so I guess I could be called the grand-father because I sent Charley Drew to Presbyterian, I trained Clarence Greene and now I am training you."[10]

Jesse Barber left the MNI in 1961 to become chief of neurosurgery at Howard University, where he remained for the next twenty-two years. Under Barber's direction, Freemen's Hospital introduced new diagnostic procedures such as EEG and radioactive isotope brain scanning, and new operations. The Division of Neurosurgery, from a poorly financed and meagerly equipped one-man operation under Greene, now expanded with the addition of a neuropathologist, neuroradiologists, and allied specialties. Barber also reached out to neurosurgeons at other institutions in and around Washington and Georgetown, an initiative to which many responded, most notably MNI alumnus Maitland Baldwin. Barber also prioritized the teaching of undergraduate students with formal lectures, small group presentations, and taught members of other divisions within the Department of Surgery. But despite these measures and Barber's recognition by his peers, neurosurgery at Freedmen remained poorly staffed, with Barber being the only full-time neurosurgeon. Nonetheless, he inspired many students to follow him into the profession. Among them was Clarence Greene Jr.

Returning to Montreal for the 1995 MNI reunion, Jesse Barber reflected on the institute, stating that the "MNI has played an integral role in my neurosurgical training and a major role in African American neurosurgery."[11] Barber stressed the point by adding, of his own role, "I have been reasonably successful in promulgating the memory of Clarence Greene and the MNI in the development of AA NRS [African-American neurosurgery]."[12] This self-assessment is all the more poignant as Barber added it to his typewritten text in his own hand.

The reputation of the MNI as a place where talent and self-motivation were all that were required to learn the science and craft of neurosurgery extended beyond Washington DC and reached the African-American community as far as the West Coast of the United States. And so it was that Lloyd Dayes came from Loma Linda University in balmy San Bernardino County, Califiornia, to cold Montreal. Dayes came to the MNI at an earlier stage in his career than Greene and Barber, having interned at the Montreal General Hospital before travelling the quarter mile down Pine Avenue to the institute. Dayes arrived at the MNI in 1961, the year Jesse Barber left for Howard University. Dayes stayed at the institute until 1965, before returning to Loma Linda as a newly minted, MNI-trained neurosurgeon. While at the MNI, Dayes worked with Hanna Pappius on the effects of urea on the fluid and electrolyte distribution in the brain.[13] Dayes became the fourth African-American neurosurgeon certified by the American Board of Neurosurgery, in 1967.[14] Lloyd Dayes had a remarkable career at Loma Linda where, in 1987, he became the first African-American to chair a board-certified neurosurgical program in the United-States, and the second MNI fellow, after George Austin, to hold that position at Loma Linda.[15]

A NEW DIRECTOR WOULD HAVE TO BE FOUND

Many changes had occurred to the MNI during the last two years of the war. The X-ray Department had been expanded, and a third operating room had been added to the fifth floor. Sadly the squash court was no more, sacrificed for K.A.C. Elliott's neurochemistry laboratory. The Department of National Defence had built a two-story wooden military annex, accommodating twenty-seven patients, behind the institute.[16] Although very useful at the time of its construction, the annex proved problematic in the following years, as it doubled the number of active beds but without an increase in the operating budget, and the MNI faced "the menacing specter of a rapidly mounting clinical deficit."[17] Penfield, whose responsibility it was to assure adequate funding for the hospital function of the MNI, expressed his frustration unequivocally: "Ten years of active directorship remain to me (God willing) under the university statutes and I would ask no better fate, provided this Institute is to fulfill a reasonable destiny. But for the purposes of retrenchment, should that become necessary, *a new Director would have to be found.*[18] The problems were easily identified: the military annex must be torn down and replaced by a new wing, and an adequate budget must be provided for the care of patients. Penfield had a surprising solution: "Either the public must support voluntary hospitals voluntarily or *medicine must be socialized.*"[19]

William Cone, above the financial fray, was more upbeat and looked to Wilder Penfield for a model of how the MNI could meet its clinical and academic responsibilities, and did so with a wink in Penfield's direction:

No better example of how productive the scientific approach to clinical medicine and the scientific results obtained from clinical studies controlled in the laboratory can be cited than the work Dr Penfield has done on epilepsy. Out of it has come new facts on localization of function in the cerebral cortex applicable to all neurological problems; new facts on the pathological lesions causing epilepsy; new facts on treatment; *he may yet find the seat of the soul!* This approach needs to be applied as intently to so many other problems if progress is to be steady and not fortuitous.[20]

Herbert Jasper also remained optimistic and, looking ahead, defined the major direction that the Department of Neurophysiology would follow in the coming years and that Penfield would emphasize for the remainder of his career: the study of the diencephalon, "which seems to exert a control on cortical activity with special reference to consciousness."[21]

◆ ◆ ◆

Jasper's interest in the interrelationship of the cortex and diencephalon was reflected in his work with Jan Droogleever-Fortuyn, from Amsterdam, and John Hunter, from Sydney, Australia.[22] At a more basic level, Kristian Kristiansen worked with Wilder Penfield and Guy Courtois on epileptic discharges in isolated cerebral cortex.[23] Birger Kaada, a pioneer neurophysiologist from Oslo, studied the effects of stimulation of the mesial temporal and limbic structures, work that he had started with Karl Pribram at Yale and continued with Herbert Jasper at the institute.[24]

On the clinical side, Wilder Penfield, Harry Steelman, and Herman Fanigin described the results of cortical excision in the last series of patients operated upon at the MNI that did not include the resection of the mesial temporal structures.[25]

Of great clinical interest, Herbert Jasper and John Hunter developed a system "for cinematography of epileptic patients simultaneous with their E.E.G. tracing."[26] The method consisted of photographing the patient and the EEG tracing on the same 16 mm frame, thus eliminating the possibility of errors in synchronization of two separate recordings. This system would be greatly improved upon in the coming years and serve as the model for epilepsy centres throughout the world.

Despite the financial challenges of the institute's hospital function, the MNI added a Pleiades of research fellows to help with its work, many of whom would achieve distinction in their chosen fields. Perhaps the most notable were Igor Klatzo and Jerzy Olszewski, both of whom had come from Oskar and Cécile Vogt's laboratory.

Table 14.1
Notable research fellows, 1945–49

Name	University	Name	University
C. Ajemone-Marsan	Turin	C.-l. Li	Shanghai
George Austin	Pennsylvania	D. Lloyd-Smith	McGill
Maitland Baldwin	Queen's	William Magnus	Utrecht
Jacob Chandy	Madras	Gabriel Mazars	Paris
Guy Courtois	Montreal	Jerzy Olszewsky	Freiburg
Jan D-Fortuyn	Amsterdam	Jean Panet-Raymond	Montreal
William Feindel	McGill	Bernard Pertuiset	Paris
Miller Fisher	Toronto	Reuben Rabinovitch	Paris
Herman Flanigin	Oklahoma	Lamar Roberts	Duke
Clarence Green	Howard	Harry Steelman	Duke
John Hanbery	Stanford	Joseph Stratford	McGill
John Hunter	Sydney	Donald Tower	Harvard
Igor Klatzo	Freiburg	John Van Buren	Columbia
Kristian Kristiansen	Oslo	Keasley Welch	Yale

ACADEMIA

William Gibson

A special meeting in honour of the late Pio del Río-Hortega was held at the institute in the academic year 1945–46, where Pierre Masson, Wilder Penfield, Miguel Prados, and MNI fellow William Gibson spoke.[27]

William Carleton Gibson was one of the most distinguished Canadian academics of the last century. Born in Ottawa and raised in Victoria, Gibson obtained his MSc from McGill University in 1936 and was then awarded a research fellowship to work with Penfield, who, immediately recognizing his brilliance, arranged for Gibson to study with Sherrington in Oxford. After obtaining his doctorate in 1938, Gibson returned to McGill, where he obtained his medical degree. He moved again for his internship, to the University of Texas. While in Texas, Gibson befriended fellow UBC graduate Cecil Howard Green, founder of Texas Instruments. Green thereafter referred to Gibson as "my most expensive friend." Among other philanthropic gifts directed to medical education, Gibson encouraged Green in the founding of Green College, Oxford, in 1979, and of Green College at the University of British Columbia.

Gibson did war-related research while in the RCAF during the Second World War, then trained in neurology at the MNI and graduated in 1947. During his residency he modified the silver impregnation method and applied it to the study of *boutons terminaux* in the cerebral cortex.[28] William Gibson's most notable contribution in clinical care while at the institute was singled out by the MNI's neurologist-in-chief, Donald McEachern: "Last summer [1946], Montreal was again visited by a considerable epidemic of Infantile Paralysis. Through the energy and foresight of Dr William C. Gibson, and with the backing of Dr G.F. Stephens, a diagnostic clinic for Poliomyelitis was organized. This provided free diagnostic facilities to all physicians in Montreal and surrounding areas. One hundred and thirty-six patients were examined at this clinic, which was equipped to carry out all the specialized procedures. Dr Gibson's account of this experience has been awarded the annual prize of the Montreal Medico-Chirurgical Society, and will be published in due course."[29]

William Gibson had a remarkable career after leaving the institute: he held positions at the University of Sydney, Australia, and at the University of California at San Francisco. He returned to British Columbia and the new medical school at UBC, where he became professor of neurological research, research professor of psychiatry, and professor (and head of the department) of the history of medicine and science.[30] Gibson was also chancellor of the University of Victoria, from 1985 to 1990.

The Hughlings Jackson Lectures

A coup for the postwar MNI was to have two Nobel laureates give succeeding Hughlings Jackson lectures: Otto Loewi presented "Problems Connected with the Effects of Nervous Impulses" in 1946, and Sir Henry Dale read "Chemical Transmission and Central Synapses" in 1947. Loewi and Dale had been awarded the 1936 Nobel Prize in Medicine or Physiology jointly for their studies on acetylcholine. The 1948 Hughlings Jackson Lecture was given by Derek Denny-Brown, titled "Disorganization of Motor Function Resulting from Cerebral Lesions," and H. Cuthbert Bazett of Oxford delivered the 1949 lecture, "Blood Temperature in Man and Its Control."

This last lecture was an apt topic, as Penfield's blood remained decidedly up over the unresolved financial shortfall in the MNI's finances. These preoccupations must have been mitigated by the increasing recognition of his work, as he was invited to give prestigious, named lectures in the United Kingdom and in the United states. Two stand out: the Ferrier Lecture of the Royal Society, London, "Some Observations on the Cerebral Cortex of Man" on 20 June 1946,[31] and the Lane Medical Lectures of Stanford University, delivered in San Francisco, November 1947. These lectures were later incorporated in Penfield and Rasmussen's *Cerebral Cortex of Man*.[32] Penfield's achievements were also recognized by his peers in Canada, as he was elected the first president of the newly created Canadian Neurological Society and gave its inaugural address on 22 May 1949.[33]

The Organ of the Mind

A significant event of 1949 was the beginning of publication of the journal *Electroencephalography and Clinical Neurophysiology* under Herbert Jasper's editorship, and papers from the Montreal Neurological Institute were prominent in the inaugural issue. Indeed Penfield had the honour of publishing the first paper in the journal, "Epileptic Manifestations of Cortical and Supracortical Discharge."[34] The unusual appellation of *supracortical* discharge indicated Penfield's hypothesis, the basis of his conceptualization of the centrencephalic system, that the diencephalon and mesencephalon, although anatomically subcortical, may "represent a level higher in the scale of functional representation than the cortex,"[35] This was a singular view that was not shared by all and was challenged by many, and most notably by Boris Babkin in a symposium held at the MNI.[36] Babkin had been Pavlov's assistant in the very early days of Pavlov's research on the conditioned reflex, and his "Origin of the Theory of Conditioned Reflexes: Sechenov, Hughlings Jackson, Pavlov" is a brilliant summation of the evolution of the concept of the conditioned reflex. A reading of Babkin's informative paper makes it obvious that Pavlov's conception of the higher mental function is at odds with Penfield's emphasis on the diencephalon. As Babkin relates, "The conditioned response requires the participation of the central nervous system, especially that of the cerebral cortex, which may be considered the chief organ of conditioned reflexes. After the removal of the cerebral cortex in animals, only crude conditioned reflexes can be established, for which certain, as yet unknown, subcortical parts are responsible."[37] Babkin then asks the fundamental question: "How is one to reconcile these two concepts – the mechanistic and the psychologic, the reflex action and the free expression of will in … man?"[38] For Babkin, the answer was obvious: "It is most probable that the highest manifestations of the human spirit also require preliminary reflex activity of the cerebral cortex."[39] Penfield would spend half his life pondering this question (figure 30.4).[40]

Two other influential speakers addressed the institute during the immediate post-war period: J.M. Nielsen and Clinton Woolsey. Neilsen was a highly regarded aphasiologist, who presented "The Application of Aphasia to Cerebral Localization." Clinton Wolsey, the neurophysiologist from Johns Hopkins University who shared Penfield's interest in sensory-motor localization, spoke on the second sensory area. In many ways Woolsey's and Neilsen's addresses foreshadowed the institute's future scientific endeavours in the localization of sensory-motor function and of language.

15

The Cerebral Cortex of Man

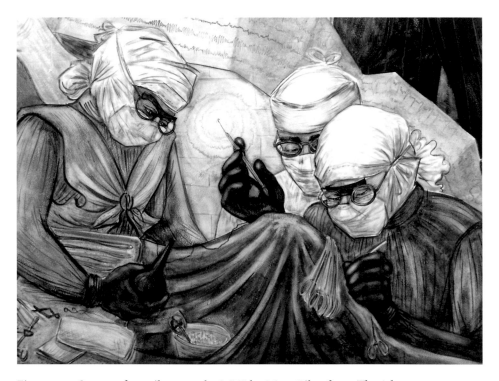

Figure 15.1: Surgery for epilepsy at the MNI by Mary Filer, from *The Advance of Neurology*.

THE CEREBRAL CORTEX OF MAN

The Cerebral Cortex of Man was long in germinating.[1] It began in 1936 with Boldrey's thesis, followed in 1937 by Penfield and Boldrey's "Somatic Motor and Sensory Representations in the Cerebral Cortex of Man." Penfield and Erickson's *Epilepsy and Cortical Localization*, which marked the end of the pre-EEG era in epilepsy research, followed in 1941. With the return of Theodore Rasmussen to the MNI, an ever-increasing number of patients underwent stimulation of the cortical motor and sensory areas during surgery. Finally, with the results of some four hundred cortical stimulations in hand, Penfield previewed *The Cerebral Cortex of Man* in the fall of 1947, with the Lane Lectures at Leland Stanford University.[2] Penfield's introduction was genuine and touching: "I am the first Lane lecturer who was from a family of pioneer parents in this west country of yours … My father entered Spokane, Washington, on horseback. He came to hunt but he remained there and became the first physician to that city, and my mother joined him on the first passenger train to cross the Rocky Mountains."[3] On the data that he was to present, the results of cortical stimulation, Penfield was quick to point out, "these surgical procedures are not experiments, for we are dealing with human beings. But from time to time conditions present themselves which would satisfy the most exacting requirements of a critical investigator."[4] Three years later a book appeared with the same title as Penfield's Lane lectures, this time by Penfield and Rasmussen.

The Cerebral Cortex of Man is, to some, Penfield's greatest publication, not the least because of the rigorous analyses of his co-author Theodore Rasmussen. It is concise and detailed and speaks with the authority of a mature clinician-scientist secure in his observations, which are novel, detailed, and exhaustive. Hortense Douglas-Cantlie illustrated the book with line drawings that are striking in their clarity. The whimsical full-frontal homunculus as originally drawn by Cantile for the 1937 paper, upside down save for the face, reappears one last time, to be replaced by sensory and motor homunculi in profile, laid upon cross-sections of the hemispheres. There were other attempts at illustrating the homunculus, some more successful than others, but these images have reached iconic status and are indelibly imprinted in the mind of all neuroscientists.[5]

Donald Tower, a contemporary observer, described Penfield and Rasmussen's method of cortical stimulation under local anaesthesia:

> The crux of my residency year was the exposure to Penfield's surgical treatment of cortical epileptogenic foci. These were long operations, largely because of the observational studies carried out by Penfield on the exposed cerebral cortex. Because the patients were awake, Penfield could examine by gentle electrical stimulation the extent of the focus, often reproducing aura or seizure patterns as described by the patient and observers, together with the EEG recordings from the surface of the cortex as interpreted in the operating room gallery by Herbert Jasper. Localizations of sensory and motor responses were also elicited by Penfield's stimulation. It was customary to mark the points of stimulation and of EEG abnormalities by sterile tickets (of letters or numbers) placed

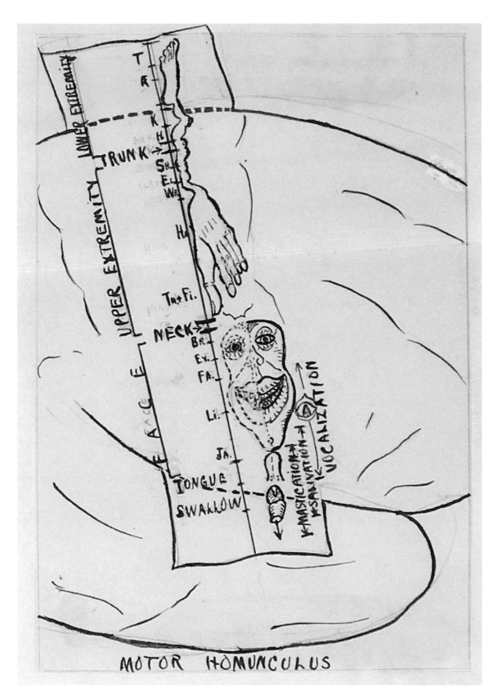

Figure 15.2: Sketch of the motor homunculus, never published. (Penfield Archives)

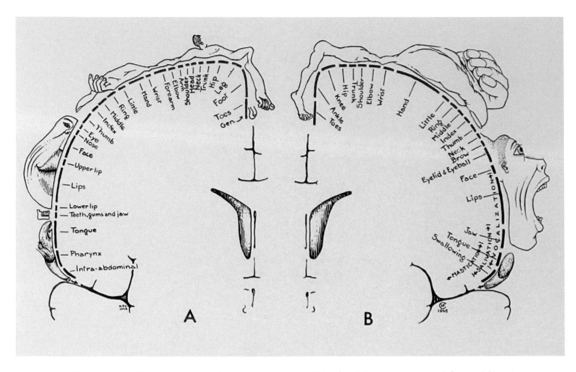

Figure 15.3: The sensory and motor homunculi in final form, mounted for publication (Penfield Archives). Final versions of the homunculi were published as separate illustrations in W. Penfield and T. Rasmussen, *The Cerebral Cortex of Man: A Clinical Study of Localization of Function* (New York: Macmillan, 1950).

on the exposed cortex together with a white thread delineating the focal area to be excised. These findings were photographed with the gallery camera by Charles Hodge, the MNI's master photographer. In addition, Penfield made sketches and annotated diagrams of the observations. Surely this was history in the making. I personally think that Penfield was frustrated by some skeptical critics or nonbelievers in localization. *He never got the full recognition or the surely deserved Nobel Prize*, but for us participants it was a tremendous experience … We who scrubbed in on these cases saw and heard very clearly and without uncertainties. They stick with you unforgettably.[6]

Penfield and Rasmussen's most detailed observations were of the sensory and motor "strips," within the pre- and post-central gyri. It was from these responses that the homunculus came to be. But Penfield and Rasmussen were careful to point out that the results obtained with stimulation, especially of the motor strip, were crude and lacked dexterity: "It is a far cry from the gross movements produced by cortical stimulation to the skilled voluntary perform-

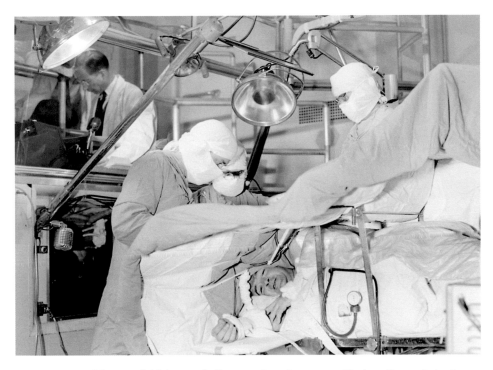

Figure 15.4: Wilder Penfield (*centre left*) operating circa 1950s. Herbert Jasper is in the gallery studying the electrocorticogram. The window at left allows the photographer to photograph the operative exposure through a mirror held by a boom rising at forty-five degrees from the side of the window. (MNI Archives)

ance of the hand of man and monkey. Our problem is to discover, if we can, how this cortical mechanism is utilized in the composition of such performance."[7] Further, Penfield realized that the cartoon of the homunculus could lead to an unwanted, concrete interpretation of the somatotopic relationship that it symbolized: "The relative length of the central cortex devoted to any one structure *varies from individual to individual* so that it is impossible to locate the arm area, for example, by measuring from the Sylvian or medial longitudinal fissure." To ensure that the reader understood, he reiterated, stating that the homunculus is but an "illustration of the order and comparative extent of elements in the sensory and motor sequence," that "it is a cartoon of the representation in which scientific accuracy is impossible."[8] The best way to think of the homunculus, therefore, is as a probabilistic map. *The Cerebral Cortex of Man* also summarized work that Penfield and Rasmussen had performed since the Lane Lectures, delineating the second sensory area and detailing the areas of the cortex responsible for vocalization.[9] The book was more tentative on the localization of functions where only a few stimulation points had been obtained, such as the classical language areas and the supplementary motor area.

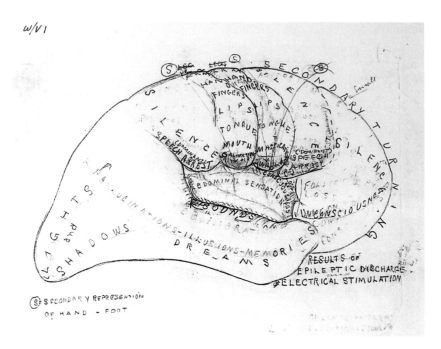

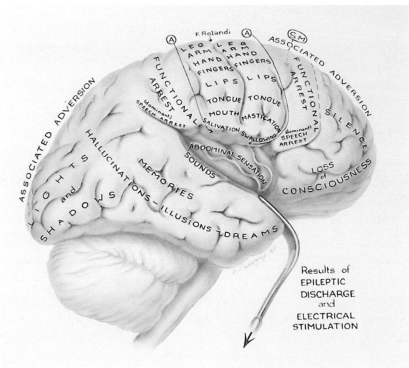

Figures 15.5: (*Top*) Original sketch of the cortical functional areas of the non-dominant hemisphere, 1950. The supplementary motor area is not illustrated. (Penfield Archives)

Figure 15.6: (*Bottom*) Final drawing of the cortical functional areas of the non-dominant hemisphere, 1950. The supplementary motor area is not illustrated. (Penfield Archives)

DECEPTIVE MONSTROSITY

Francis Walshe was the author of the well-regarded *Diseases of the Nervous System*, and the editor of *Brain* from 1937 to 1953.[10] Despite these literary accomplishments, "Walshe's happiest literary medium lay in his letters. Whether published in the Press or in medical journals, or whether transmitted for private perusal, they proved to be consummate accomplishments in the sphere of mordant invective."[11] Walshe was a vocal critic of the representation of sensory-motor responses as a homunculus, to which he had referred as "a deceptive monstrosity" in a letter to Penfield in 1943.[12] Walshe was no gentler on 6 August 1946, as Penfield was preparing the Ferrier Lecture of the Royal Society, "Some Observations on the Cerebral Cortex of Man":[13]

> I feel that your "homunculus" does indicate graphically your observations, but that it does not indicate any plan of organization in the motor cortex. It represents a partial aspect of the truth, an aspect so fragmentary that no inferences can be drawn from it. I surmise that you will be heartily tired of its horrific appearance – copied uncritically from text to text – before you see the last of it. You may even have to slay it yourself – an infanticide that might find attenuation.[14]

This call to infanticide was met with a cordial response from Penfield, who answered on 20 August 1946:

> As far as the homunculus is concerned, it was one of a number of illustrations which we used to try to illustrate the truth. Of course, there is nothing like the homunculus as far as cortical representation is concerned, but it seems to be the only sort of thing that people in general understand. I would kill the damn thing if I could, but that is never possible. It does call attention to certain facts, such as the reversal of the order of representation in the face and neck, as compared with the rest of the body.[15]

The matter did not end there, and was revived after the publication of *The Cerebral Cortex of Man*, when Penfield and Walshe met in Banff, Canada, in 1952, as reported by Donald Tower:

> Penfield tried to summarize much of his cerebral localization results by diagramming them in the form of an homunculus, e.g., of localizations

in the primary motor and sensory strips of the cerebral cortex. Critics unmercifully ridiculed these homunculi. I vividly remember sitting through a lecture at University College, London, at which F.M.R. Walshe engaged in such ridicule. Walshe was an able speaker and had the audience rolling in the aisles with laughter. I was embarrassed and angry. However, Penfield had his revenge. At a 1952 meeting of the Canadian Neurological Society in Banff, Alberta, Canada, both Penfield and Walshe were featured speakers. Walshe gave his usual sarcastic critique. Penfield was not a good speaker, tending to read a carefully crafted exposition. However, Walshe angered him. He literally tore up his talk and launched into a spontaneous defense of his findings and concepts that utterly demolished Walshe and led us MNI staffers to literally stand up and cheer for Penfield.[16]

Penfield and Walshe would cross swords again after the publication of Penfield and Jasper's *Epilepsy and the Functional Anatomy of the Human Brain* in 1954, on the concept of the centrencephalic integrating system (see below).

Language and the Supplementary Motor Area

Although a great achievement, the *Cerebral Cortex of Man* has deficiencies: the role of the dominant supplementary motor area is only alluded to, Broca's area is limited to Brodmann's area 44, the boundaries of the temporal language zone are indefinite, and the language function of the inferior parietal lobule – the supramarginal and angular gyri – is not mentioned.[17] But the MNI would address these deficiencies in the early 1950s.

THE SUPPLEMENTARY MOTOR AREA

Area X

Boldrey's 1936 thesis and the paper that Penfield and he published *Brain* in 1937 both illustrate, among other responses, the result of stimulation producing vocalization.[18] In one instance, referred to as "point 22" in both publications, "arrest of speech" was obtained during stimulation in front of the precentral sulcus towards the midline, in area 6a *beta* of Vogt and Vogt.[19] Boldrey finds case 22 worthy of note: "Inability to speak was, of course, subjective in most instances. Case 22, however, was told to count aloud, and while doing so, appropriate stimulation caused a definite hesitation though it did not stop her. Afterwards she volunteered that it had been difficult to speak."[20] Case 22 is the first demonstration that language function resides in what is now referred to as the supplementary motor area (SMA).

Richard Brickner was the next to foray into the mesial aspect of the frontal lobe. Brickner was a neurologist at the Neurological Institute of New York. In 1940, he prevailed upon neurosurgical colleagues to apply a stimulating electrode to the left frontal lobe of a patient upon whom they were operating in an attempt to cure her of epileptic seizures.[21] During the stimulation of the superior and medial aspect of the left precentral region, "low down in area 6, probably just above its junction with the posterior tip of area 32," a locus that Brickner referred to as "area X," an unexpected response was elicited: the patient perseverated in repeating the letter *H* while reciting the letters of the alphabet, and continued to recite correctly, starting at the letter *I*, when the stimulating electrode was removed. Richard Brickner had chanced upon what Penfield, a decade later, would refer to as the SMA, and characterized the interruption of its function by electrical stimulation as "perseveration of speech," an element of dysphasia. The postwar era saw the MNI focus much of its attention on the characterization of "area X," and on the localization of language. Keasley Welch, Preston Robb, and Lamar Roberts were the three fellows principally involved in these endeavours.

Penfield and Welsh 1949

Penfield first refers to the SMA in June 1949, in "The Supplementary Motor Area in the Cerebral Cortex of Man," co-authored with Keasley Welch.[22] Penfield and Welch outline some of the effects produced by stimulation of the SMA in Jacksonian terms, as positive or negative responses. The positive responses, obtainable by stimulation of either hemisphere, were vocalization, movements of the face and the jaw, and synergic movements of the trunk, the extremities, the head, and the eyes. Pupillary dilatation and tachycardia were also observed. Negative effects of stimulation consisted in "inhibition of voluntary activity," which some have referred to as bradykinesia. With regard to language, Penfield and Welch state that "a few examples of true aphasia [were] elicited by stimulation of the supplementary area on the dominant side … Our impression is that a small *posterior part* of this area is more important in speech function than is the remainder."[23] Penfield next referred to the SMA in a lecture delivered at the Congrès Neurologique International in Paris, in September 1949. Almost in passing, Penfield summarized his thinking on language localization as a result of his observations on the SMA: "It is now evident that speech has three and perhaps four separate areas of representation in the cortex of man."[24]

SPEECH AND BRAIN MECHANISMS

Although the localization of the anterior and posterior speech regions was broadly known when Penfield and his fellows applied themselves to this topic, the evidence was crude and indirect, based as it was on the post-mortem analysis of patients whose lesion often extended beyond what we now recognize as the language areas. Thus, there was a need for a more systematic research program directed at setting the localization of the language on firmer ground. Preston Robb was Penfield's first fellow to address this question.

Robb, 1946

Preston Robb's research towards his MSc was "The Effects of Cortical Excision on Speech."[25] Robb analyzed fifty-one cases operated upon by Penfield for the resection of an epileptogenic focus in or near the two major speech areas known at the time. Robb illustrated his observations with composite diagrams of the resected areas and indicated the degree of aphasia that the original injury and/or the resection produced. As expected, aphasia was present when the left posterior temporal lobe and the inferior parietal lobule were affected. There were no cases in which the superior-most aspect of the frontal lobe was involved, and thus Robb remained silent on the language function of the SMA. Robb's case studies were complex and too few for one to arrive at general conclusions, as he himself recognized. Nonetheless, very practical information came out of his study, of great importance to neurosurgeons venturing into the dominant temporal lobe, as he states, "When 4 cm from the tip [of the temporal lobe] posteriorly were excised the postoperative aphasia was only very transient. When 7 cm were excised the postoperative aphasia was more persistent."

Roberts, 1949, 1952

Lamar Roberts first took up the stimulating electrode for his MSc thesis, "A Study of Certain Alterations in Speech during Stimulation of Specific Cortical Regions," published in 1949,[26] in which he analyzed a series of eighty-eight patients in whom cortical stimulation had produced an aphasic response.[27] As he undoubtedly expected, positive responses were obtained from the posterior third of the third left frontal convolution (Broca's area), from the posterior aspect of the first and second temporal convolutions (Wernicke's area), and from the inferior parietal lobule, whose language competency was first described by Jules Dejerine.[28] Surprisingly, aphasic responses were also obtained from "the intermediate precentral region at the midline." Cautious at first, Roberts commented that these responses were "too few in number to be conclusive."[29] By the time he published his doctoral dissertation, "Alterations in Speech Produced

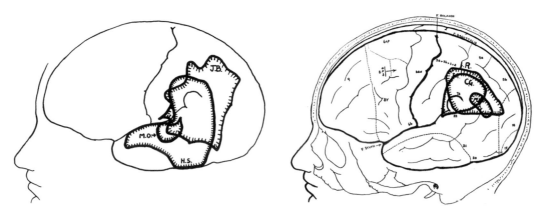

Figure 15.7: Figure 6 (*left*) from Robb's thesis outlining the lesions in three patients whose initial injury had rendered them aphasic. Figure 7 (*right*) from Robb's thesis outlining the lesion in two patients whose initial injury had rendered them dysphasic. (P. Robb, "A Study of The Effects of Cortical Excision on Speech in Patients with Previous Cerebral Injuries" [master's thesis, McGill University, 1946])

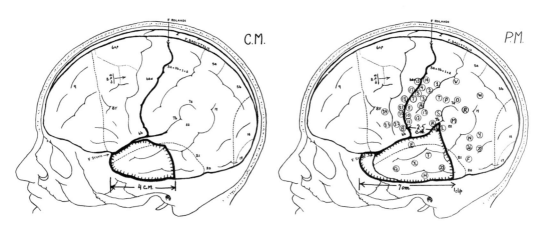

Figure 15.8: The excision of the dominant temporal neocortex extending to 4 cm from the temporal tip did not produce aphasia (*left*), while resection extending to 7 cm did (*right*). (P. Robb, "A Study of The Effects of Cortical Excision on Speech in Patients with Previous Cerebral Injuries" [master's thesis, McGill University, 1946])

by Cerebral Stimulation and Excision," in 1952, he was unequivocal: "Electric interference has produced alterations in speech similar to the disordered speech of aphasic patients. The areas involved are Broca's, inferior parietal, posterior temporal and supplementary motor of the left hemisphere."[30]

Roberts also made a prescient observation: "The left hemisphere is dominant in practically all individuals regardless of handedness except those who have gross lesions of the left hemisphere within the first few years of life."[31] These assertions would be confirmed a decade later through the work of Milner, Rasmussen, and their collaborators.

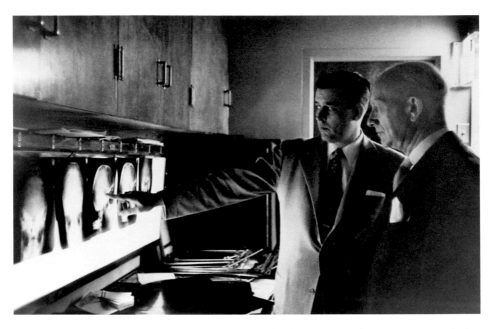

Figure 15.9: Lamar Roberts (*left*) and Wilder Penfield examining the pneumoencephalo-gram of a patient to be operated upon the following day, 1950. (MNI Archives)

Penfield and Roberts, 1959

Penfield and Roberts published their final statement on the cortical localiza-tion of language in *Speech and Brain Mechanisms*.[32] Based largely on Roberts's thesis and dissertation, it could not have achieved its status without the dis-covery of the language function of the SMA, which rendered incomplete all previous treatises on the subject of language. Unlike other important works on the subject – those of Dejerine, Marie and Foix, and Luria – *Speech and Brain Mechanisms* is not based on lesion analysis alone, with its inherent tentativeness, but relies also on direct evidence obtained through cortical stimulation.[33] Al-though elaborated upon by others since its publication, *Speech and Brain Mech-anisms* remains authoritative to this day.[34]

Penfield, Roberts, and Dejerine

Penfield and Roberts's map of the speech areas demonstrated by cortical stimulation, with the exception of the SMA, can be superimposed on Jules Dejerine's map published in his monumental treatise *Anatomie des centres nerveux* (Anatomy of neural centres) in 1901.[35] Indeed, it is unfortunate that neither Penfield nor Roberts appears to have read Dejerine, as they echo many of his points.

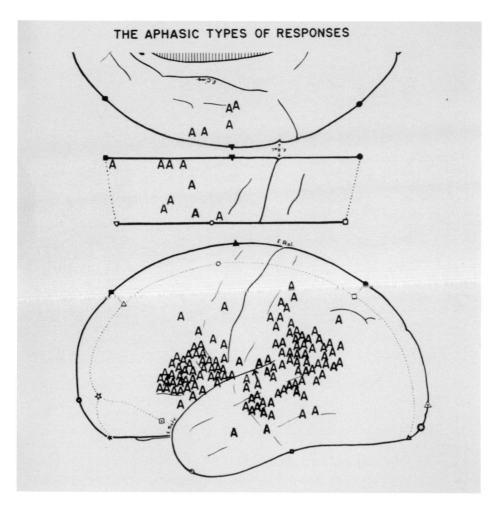

THE APHASIC TYPES OF RESPONSES

Figure 15.10: Figure 10 from Roberts's dissertation (*detail*). Each letter *A* illustrates a point where an aphasic response was obtained on the lateral, superior, and medial aspects of the hemisphere. The illustration was later reproduced in W. Penfield and L. Roberts, *Speech and Brain Mechanisms* (Princeton: Princeton University Press, 1959). (L. Roberts, "Alterations in Speech Produced by Cerebral Stimulation and Excision" [PhD diss., McGill University, 1952], 50)

For Dejerine, language is derived from the coordinated action of three primary centres – Broca's area, Wernicke's area, and the angular gyrus – which are joined by connecting fibres into a *zone du langage* (language zone) about the Sylvian fissure.[36] For Dejerine, "*any alteration of the language zone at any point in the surface that it occupies does not result in difficulties limited to this or that modality of language, but an alteration in* ALL *modalities of language, with predominance of those difficulties corresponding to the … centre directly affected by the lesion.*"[37]

Penfield and Roberts held a similar view: "So far as can be determined, there is no difference between the effects of the electrical current when applied to the

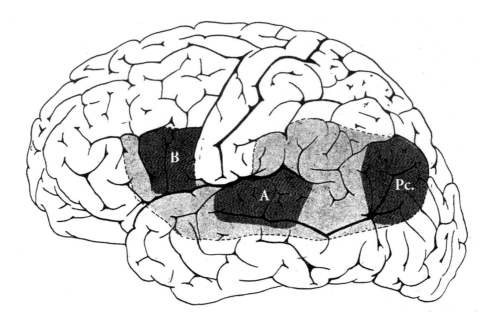

Figures 15.11 and 15.12: Dejrine's "language zone": *B*, Broca's area; *A*, Wernicke's area; *Pc*, *pli courbe*, the angular gyrus. The intensity of the shading reflects the probability of finding a speech deficit, articulate, interpretive, or written, particular to each area. A lesion in any part of the whole shaded area, or of the subcortical fibres joining them, can affect all aspects of language, but the aspect most affected will be determined by the proximity of the lesion to area *A, B,* or *Pc*. (*Opposite*) Penfield and Roberts's three language areas delineated by cortical stimulation. (MNI Archives) The yellow colouration is in the original. (J. Dejerine, *Anatomie des centres nerveux* [Paris: Ruff, 1901]. See also W. Penfield and L. Roberts, *Speech and Brain Mechanisms* [Princeton: Princeton University Press, 1959].)

dominant Broca's area, supplementary motor area, or parieto-temporal region as regards the various alterations of speech. The reason for this lack of difference could be that these three areas are connected by transcortical and subcortical pathways in a single system. An electrical disturbance set up in any part of the system might disrupt the function of the whole system."[38]

There is another striking similarity between Dejerine and Penfield and Roberts: they both recognized a hierarchy in the language centres. Dejerine's hierarchy was psychological and based on education, while that of Penfield and Roberts was based on functionality. Dejerine first: "It should not be believed … that a lesion anywhere within the language zone produces equal alterations of the different modalities of language: there exists a veritable hierarchy of the centers presiding over the different modalities of language arising from education and the organization of [language]."[39] Thus, for Dejerine, Wernicke's area is most important because, as children, we first learn the meaning of words. Then comes Broca's area, because we learn to speak words after we have learned

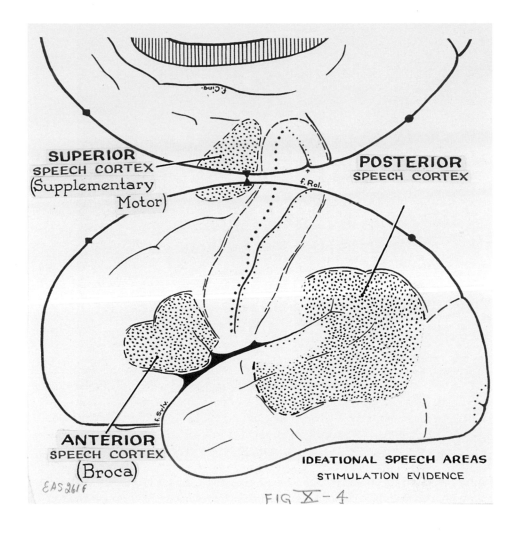

SUPERIOR
SPEECH CORTEX
(Supplementary
Motor)

POSTERIOR
SPEECH CORTEX

ANTERIOR
SPEECH CORTEX
(Broca)

IDEATIONAL SPEECH AREAS
STIMULATION EVIDENCE

FIG X-4

their meaning and how to link them into a meaningful sentence. Dejerine's area – the angular gyrus – is third in the hierarchy, because we learn to read and to write only after we have mastered spoken language.[40]

Penfield and Roberts also recognized a hierarchy: "We believe that the most important area for speech is the posterior temporo-parietal region ... The next important area for speech is that of Broca ... The supplementary motor area ... is dispensable; nonetheless, lesions here can produce prolonged dysphasia, and it probably is very important if the other areas for speech are destroyed."[41]

Rasmussen and Milner elaborated upon the findings of Penfield and Roberts in their 1975 paper "Clinical and Surgical Studies of the Cerebral Speech Areas in Man," especially on the delineation of the two major speech regions, the anterior (Broca's) and the posterior (Wernicke's and Dejerine's).[42] They and their co-workers would also add to our understanding of the functional organization of language by establishing its hemispheric *lateralization* with the use of the Wada test (see below).

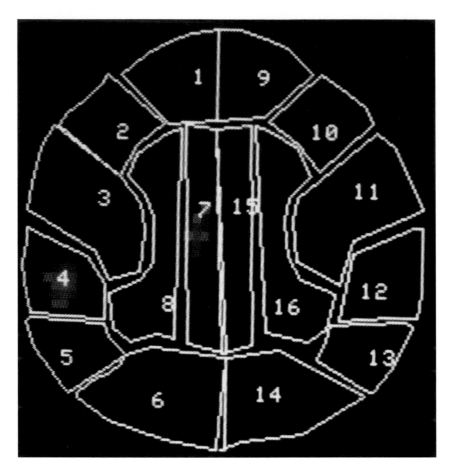

Figure 15.13: Early functional positron emission tomography scan superimposed on a region of interest template from a matched magnetic resonance image scan. The PET scan shows increased blood flow in the left post central gyrus (template area 4) and supplementary motor area (template area 7) in response to vibrotactile stimulation of the right hand. Ernst Meyer and Richard Leblanc later used this technique to identify the central area and language competent regions in patients with structural brain lesions. (R. Leblanc and E. Meyer, "Functional PET Scanning in the Treatment of AVMs," *Journal of Neurosurgery* 73 [1990]: 615–19; R. Leblanc, E. Meyer, R. Zatorre, D. Bub, and A. Evans, "Language Localization with Activation-PET Scanning," *Neurosurgery* 31 [1992]: 369–73.)

BROCA'S BIOGRAPHER

Francis Schiller came to the MNI in 1948 as a special assistant to Wilder Penfield. He had graduated from the University of Prague medical school in 1933, then, perhaps as a sign of those troubled times, he served as a medical officer in the Czechoslovakian army. He subsequently moved to La Pitié hospital, Paris, where he assisted Clovis Vincent.[43] Schiller was thus one of three MNI fellows to assist this greatest of French neurosurgeons, the other two being Jerzy Chorobski and Reuben Rabinovitch. Schiller found himself at the Radcliffe Infirmary, Oxford, after the Fall of France. There he worked with Sir Hugh Cairns and the influential neurologist and aphasiologist William Ritchie Russell. While in Oxford, Schiller wrote an interesting paper on aphasia produced by missile wounds to the head.[44]

Lamar Roberts benefitted greatly from Schiller's presence at the MNI, receiving support and advice throughout his years of study on language localization. Roberts acknowledged Schiller "for his excellent criticism," and refers to his paper "Aphasia Studied in Patients with Missile Wounds" in his MSc and PhD theses, in the same sentence in which he mentions Milton Shy and Donald Hebb![45] Roberts even favours Schiller's classification of aphasia over that of others.[46] One can't help but think that Roberts's work on language might have inspired Schiller to write his excellent biography of Pierre Paul Broca, for which he is justly famous.[47]

CONSCIOUSNESS RECONSIDERED

Wilder Penfield was able to reciprocate Francis Schiller's kindness to Roberts when Schiller asked for his assistance with "Consciousness Reconsidered,"[48] a paper that was to appear in a special Symposium on Brain and Mind published by the *Archives of Neurology and Psychiatry* in 1952.[49] Stanley Cobb, a participant in the symposium, was unapologetically materialistic and succinct: "Everyone is interested to find out how the brain works and what it does. Mind is … what it does."[50] Schiller's position was more nuanced and stressed a role for a semantic approach in the discussion of brain, consciousness, and mind.[51] The major interest of the symposium rests in a discussion between Penfield and Karl Lashley. Penfield unabashedly defended the role of the centrencephalic integrating system, stating that without it "there can be no conscious processes of the mind." Lashley, dubious, negated any cognitive or mindful role of the brainstem and thalamic reticular formation – the heart of Penfield's system – and bluntly concluded, "That system is anatomically very simple, and if it fulfills its function as a dynamic center [for arousal] … I think it will probably have exhausted all of its possibilities."[52] Francis Walshe would later use this amicable exchange between Penfield and Lashley less amicably, in a frontal assault on Penfield's centrencephalic system.

16

Incisural Sclerosis

Speech and Brain Mechanisms did much to clarify the localization of language and is one of the singular achievements of the MNI. The surgical treatment of epilepsy was also a major concern of the institute and made great strides in the 1950s with the discovery by Wilder Penfield, Maitland Baldwin, and Kenneth Earle of the cause of temporal lobe epilepsy, and by William Feindel and Wilder Penfield on the role of the amygdala in its symptomatology.

MESIAL TEMPORAL LOBE EPILEPSY

Penfield and Erickson had analysed the results of the surgical treatment of focal epilepsy in 1941, largely on patients operated upon before the EEG was in common use at the MNI.[1] They noted, "The best results from … surgical therapy occur in those cases in which a removable localized lesion is found in an otherwise comparatively normal brain."[2] Despite rigorous pre-operative selection, therefore, if a cortical lesion was not found at surgery, the procedure was terminated and the case was classified as a "negative exploration." The number of negative explorations was significant. Clearly, a better method of selecting patients for craniotomy was required. Would the routine use of EEG help to meet this challenge? Herbert Jasper and John Kershman thought so: "A single, well restricted focus of random spikes or sharp waves, with normal activity from all other regions of the head, usually leads to the site of onset of an epileptic seizure … the electrogram [EEG] therefore provides a reliable guide to further study of the possibility of successful surgical therapy."[3] Wilder Penfield was not convinced.

To elucidate the role of EEG in the treatment of focal epilepsy, Wilder Penfield and Harry Steelman undertook a review of all cases operated upon since the advent of EEG at the MNI and reported their results in 1947.[4] The first striking observation was that during this period the incidence of negative

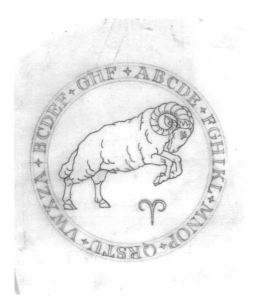

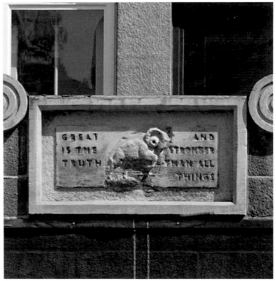

Figure 16.1: Sketch for an architectural device for the McConnell Wing. The ram is the astrological symbol of the brain. Early anatomists referred to the hippocampus as Ammon's horn, and early pathologists referred to scarring of this region in epileptic patients as Ammon's horn sclerosis. (Penfield Archives)

Figure 16.2: The ram, battered and weather-beaten, but still surging. (Photographer Richard Leblanc)

explorations had been greatly decreased. The proportion of successfully treated temporal epilepsy cases, however, was barely better than chance. With regard to the EEG, Penfield and Steelman were of two minds and lukewarm at best: "The simpler the electrographic record is and the better it is localized, the better the prognosis of a successful excision … However, the electrogram *without objective change in the cortex … is not yet to be trusted as the final guide to excision.*"[5] But, unknown to Penfield at the time, the pathology in temporal lobe epilepsy most often resides within the mesial structures, unseen within the operative exposure; and, although the epileptic activity may have been reflected from these structures to the lateral neocortex, if no structural pathology was evident, excision was not carried out. Penfield stressed this point in the discussion that followed the reading of his paper: "So far as electroencephalographic records from the exposed brain are concerned, we have been doing this for six or seven years *but are not ready to make final judgment as to its value.* It does help, but it is possible also, that it may misdirect the surgeon because of the altered condition of the cortex after exposure."[6]

Thus, for Penfield, further progress on the treatment of focal epilepsy still required the demonstration of a structural lesion visible to the surgeon's eye at the time of operation. This opinion was undoubtedly reinforced by the great success that he and Arthur Ward reported the following year in a small series of patients with temporal lobe epilepsy in whom a calcified cavernous angioma was seen on skull X-ray.[7] Could similar results be brought to light if a large series of temporal resection were reviewed?

Wilder Penfield and Herman Flanigin set themselves the task of analyzing all cases of patients operated upon for temporal lobe epilepsy at the MNI from January 1939 to April 1949.[8] The results, again, were hardly better than chance: the proportion of successfully treated cases stood at an unimpressive 53 per cent. One case, however, stood out, of a patient, previously reported by Penfield and Steelman, whose first operation had been unsuccessful and who was re-operated upon: "One patient has been operated on a second time since the termination of this analysis. It was found that there was *induration of the cortex* in the remaining uncus and hippocampal gyrus. This was excised, and he has had no further seizures during the few months that have followed operation."[9] From this single case arose the modern surgical treatment of temporal lobe epilepsy.[10]

MESIAL TEMPORAL SCLEROSIS

"He has shown us where the lesion lies"

The pathology responsible for temporal lobe epilepsy – scaring of the mesial temporal structures contained within the uncus and hippocampus – was characterized by Penfield and Jasper and two fellows, Maitland Baldwin and William Feindel.

Figures 16.3 and 16.4: (*opposite*) Brain maps originally drawn by Penfield in blue in 1945, and completed by Rasmussen in red in 1950. The patient first underwent a right lateral temporal resection in 1945. Electrocorticography revealed epileptic activities at letters *A, B, D,* and *E* in blue, and he underwent the resection of the first and second temporal convolutions. His seizures remained problematic and he was operated upon for further lateral neo-cortical resection in 1950. The electrocorticogran demonstrated epileptic activity at letters *B, C,* and *D* in red, in the now exposed mesial temporal structures. These, and the third temporal convolution, were resected. The patient remained seizure-free after his second operation. This case, and similar cases where the mesial structures were removed after lateral neocortiocal resection proved ineffective, resulted in a change in the surgical treatment of temporal lobe epilepsy, to include the mesial temporal structures, most notably the amygdala and varying lengths of the hippocampus. (MNI Archives)

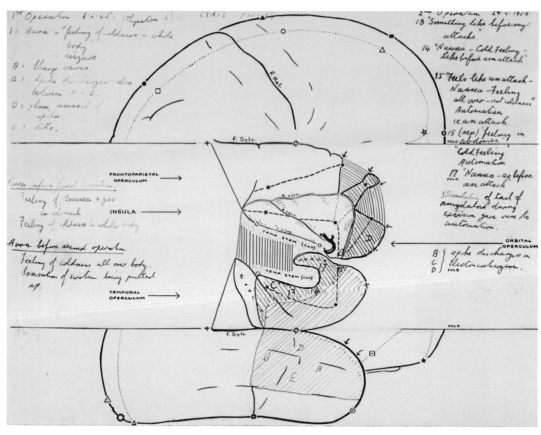

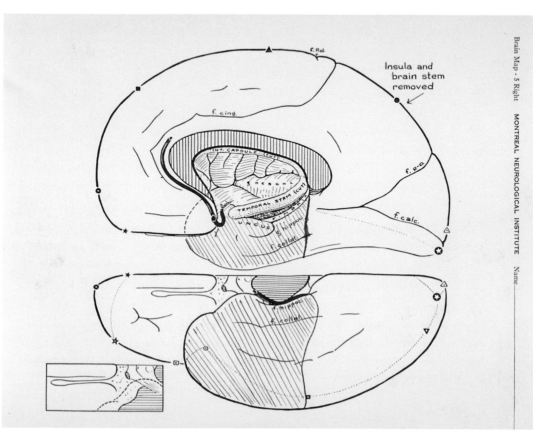

Insula and brain stem removed

Brain Map - 5 Right   MONTREAL NEUROLOGICAL INSTITUTE   Name

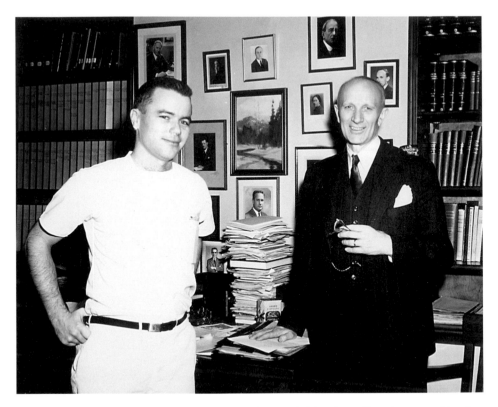

Figure 16.5: Maitland Baldwin (*left*) with Wilder Penfield in his office. (MNI Archives)

Maitland Baldwin was one of the most influential fellows to have trained at the MNI. With Wilder Penfield he brought order and clarity to temporal lobe epilepsy and its treatment. Baldwin analyzed the results of stimulation of the temporal lobe on the production of such psychical phenomena of temporal lobe epilepsy as "involuntary recollection," "illusions," "psychical hallucinations," and "emotion," most notably fear, in the first part of his MSc thesis, "Functional Representation in the Temporal Lobe of Man."[11] Although observing that these psychical responses often resulted from stimulation of the mesial structures, Baldwin was unable to determine the exact position of his depth electrode and recognized the "need for more accurate estimation of point localization in this type of stimulation."[12] Ever resourceful, Baldwin devoted the second part of his thesis to determining a set of Cartesian coordinates of the amygdala and anterior hippocampus that could be referred to during craniotomy, and to designing an "electrode holder" by which a set of depth electrodes could accurately reach these structures.[13]

The resultant technique for recording in clinical cases was described by Penfield and Baldwin in a landmark paper, "Temporal Lobe Seizures and the Technique of Subtotal Temporal Lobectomy," read before the American Surgical Association in April 1952: "It is possible to pass an electrode, coated except at the tip, into the temporal lobe and stimulate the uncus, amygdaloid nucleus or various portions of the superior temporal surface before deciding on excision. The electrode is introduced and then the current is switched on and off. An electrode, for example, passed directly inward in a plane 4 cm from the temporal tip will enter the amygdaloid nucleus at a depth of 4 to 5 cm."[14] This approach would be of great significance in the work of Feindel and Penfield in establishing the importance of the amygdala in psychomotor epilepsy.[15]

But Baldwin and Penfield's paper went further as they highlighted the case of a patient with temporal lobe epilepsy in whom it was found at operation that "the anterior part of the first temporal convolution appeared small and atrophic. The whole right temporal lobe seemed small, but the most marked objective abnormality lay in the uncus, hippocampus and hippocampal gyrus. Here the tissue was yellowish, tough and avascular. The electrocorticographic localization coincided with the objective abnormality."[16] With this last sentence, Penfield and Baldwin reconcile the electro-physiological findings of Jasper and Kershman to a physical, abnormal substrate, unifying the field of temporal lobe epilepsy in a clinical and patho-physiological whole.

Penfield, Baldwin, and Kenneth Earle, a neuropathology fellow at the MNI, referred to this pathology as incisural sclerosis, implying that they believed that the lesion resulted from a pathological event occurring in the region of the tentorial incisura.[17] This lesion, now referred to as mesial temporal sclerosis, is universally recognized as the most common cause of temporal lobe epilepsy, although its etiology is still debated. Penfield and Baldwin believed that incisural sclerosis resulted from ischemia produced as the mesial temporal lobe herniated through the incisura, compressing the anterior choroidal and branches of the posterior cerebral arteries as the result of undue pressure on the head during childbirth. Etiology aside, the importance of Penfield's work in this area was recognized by the editor of the *Annals of Surgery*, in which Penfield and Baldwin's paper appeared like a beacon. In response, William Jason Mixter, the first head of neurosurgery at the Massachusetts General Hospital and a man of few words, stated, "He has shown us where the lesion lies."[18]

THE AMYGDALA AND TEMPORAL LOBE EPILEPSY

The crucial role played by the mesial temporal structures, especially the peri-amygdaloid region encompassing the amygdala itself and the anterior part of the hippocampus overlying it, was firmly established by Feindel, Penfield, and Jasper in "Localization of Epileptic Discharge in Temporal Lobe Automatism," a paper that was read before the American Neurological Association in 1952, and in a greatly expanded paper by Feindel and Penfield published in 1954.[19] Feindel and his co-authors observed that the habitual aura and other typical features of epileptic attacks could be reproduced by electrical stimulation within and around the amygdala, and less frequently in the ventral claustrum and the anterior insula. The responses obtained by stimulation of these structures were a sensation of fear, a poorly described epigastric sensation, loss of contact with the environment, and amnesia, all features of temporal lobe – or psychomotor – epilepsy. Significantly, no new memories could be laid down during the amnesic period, but older memories were retained, suggesting that mesial temporal structures might be involved in recall. The resulting seizure discharges spread rapidly from the mesial structures to the lateral temporal cortex, as Jasper and Kershman had surmised.[20] Stimulation of the body of the hippocampus did not produce similar results. Jasper and Rasmussen later reproduced the results of Feindel, Penfield, and Jasper in a much larger series of patients.[21] Similarly, Gloor and his colleagues at the MNI observed similar findings in patients with percutaneously placed depth electrodes.[22]

TOWARDS A NEW WING

The discovery of the SMA, the cortical localization of language, the discovery of incisural sclerosis, and the demonstration of the role of the amygdala in the semiology of temporal lobe epilepsy, achieved through the mid-1950s, were made possible by renewed funding that came early in the beginning of the decade. Indeed, by 1950, Penfield was no longer speaking of resigning or of closing the hospital and was almost elated as he announced new funding from the university, and from public and private sectors:

> Last year, at this time, I pointed out that, following five years of financial deterioration, hospitalization had reached an economic impasse. We were forced to paint a gloomy picture; the accumulated clinical deficit, the insuperable problem of balancing Hospital books, the crowding everywhere, the menace of a non-fireproof annex. I closed my report with

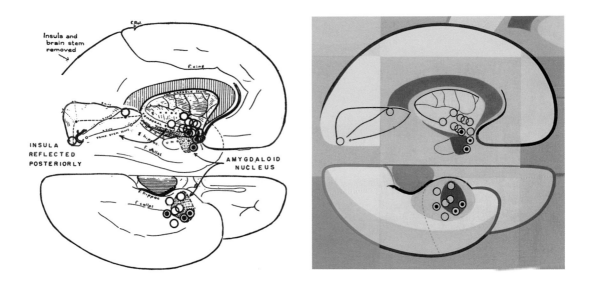

Figures 16.6 and 16.7: (*Left, right*) Points stimulated by Feindel and Penfield that produced psychical responses in patients with temporal lobe epilepsy and artistic rendering of the same, which appears in Luba Genush's triptych *The World of Neurology*, at the MNI. (W. Feindel and W. Penfield, "Localization of Discharge in Temporal Lobe Automatism," *Archives of Neurology and Psychiatry* 72 [1954]: 605–30; W. Feindel, R. Leblanc and A.N. de Almeida, "Epilepsy Surgery: Historical Highlights 1909–2009," supplement 3, *Epilepsia* 50 [2009]: 145)

these words of desperation: "If there is no Canadian, or group of Canadians ready to make permanent the Hospital organization of this Institute – then let the doors of the Hospital close." During the past year, a wonderful thing has happened. Support has come which makes possible the clinical reorganization so desperately needed. The Hospital doors do not need to close. The Montreal Neurological Institute may now fulfill its destiny as a provincial hospital and a national institute and its doors will never be closed.[23]

Thus, for the hospital function of the institute, the slate was clean. McGill had authorized the paying of its $1 million deficit, and Quebec Premier Maurice Duplessis, through an order-in-council, assured annual payment of $90,000 to meet future hospital needs. This Penfield considered to be of the highest significance: "*The interview with Mr Duplessis was crucial in the history of the Institute* … His words of encouragement … constitute for us an assurance that this Institute has served the people of Quebec well. It means that *our future is linked indissolubly with the future of this Province*."[24] Further, the federal finance minister, Paul Martin Sr, and his provincial counterpart, Albiny Paquette, agreed to provide moneys for the purchase of specialized equipment. There was more, and it came from the institute's most stalwart friend, J.W. McConnell, who "contributed a lump sum sufficient to construct the projected wing."[25]

This welcome news would help the institute with the coming of "new types of investigators who call for more space and larger budgets."[26] Neurophysiology was foremost among the most active laboratories in its study of the interplay between the cerebral cortex and the brainstem.[27] Neurochemistry was pushing forward with its work on the chemistry of the epileptogenic cortex.[28] Neuroanatomy had also expanded its sphere of interest with the arrival of Jerzy Olszewski, and neuropathology was now heavily committed to the study of multiple sclerosis with the arrival of Roy Swank.[29] Penfield estimated that another $1.5 million endowment was necessary to meet the demands of these "new types of investigators" and even conceived of higher goals for research in the advancement of neurology: "The laboratory work shows great promise of benefit to mankind. We must seek the truth. We must apply what we learn to the relief of sickness and suffering. We must orient our investigations wisely so that in distant perspective *we work toward an understanding of the physical basis of the mind.*"[30]

THE FELLOWS SOCIETY

The MNI's Fellows Society, created during the academic year 1938–39, was now entering its twelfth year.[31] The first president had been Theodore Erickson when there were seventeen fellows at the institute. Subsequent presidents were Guy Odom, Everett Hurteau, Theodore Rasmussen, Herbert Jasper, Edward Lotspeich, William Feindel, Arthur Morris, Keasley Welch, Harry Steelman, and Maitland Baldwin. The 1950 executive included Lamar Roberts, president; Revis Lewin, vice-president; and Choh-luh Li, secretary-treasurer; and there were a record number of forty-seven fellows. The Fellows Society and the Montreal Neurological Society, this year as before, hosted notable guests at the MNI, including Francis Schiller, then at the Nuffield Department of Surgery, Oxford, and later Paul Broca's biographer, who discussed aspects of amnesia. Two other eminent British visitors addressed the institute. Sir Henry Dale, Nobel laureate and chairman of the Wellcome Trust, who had given the 1947 Hughlings Jackson lecture, returned to the MNI to present "Chemical Transmission and Central Synapses." J. Godwin Greenfield, neuropathologist at Queen Square, gave the 1950 Hughlings Jackson Lecture, "The Pathology of the Cerebellum." Marthe Vogt, daughter of Oskar and Cécile Vogt, an honoured guest of the institute, read "Secretion of the Adrenal Cortex," and Jerzy Olszewksi, who had worked with the Vogts, spoke of her parents. Boris Babkin also reminisced about his old colleague on the centennial anniversary of Pavlov's birth in Babkin's last address at the institute.[32] He died in 1950 shortly after he had been elected to the Royal Society of London.[33] *Death comes before it is called.*

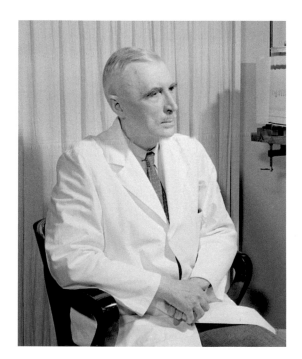 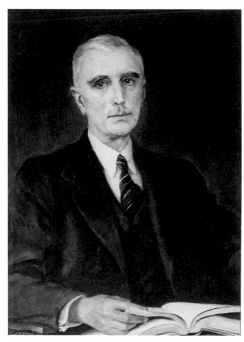

Figures 16.8 and 16.9: Boris Petrovitch Babkin in the laboratory (*left*). Watercolour on photographic print of Boris Babkin by Baroness Anna de Romer (*right*). (MNI Archives)

17

Bridging Two Solitudes

Penfield was in a reflective mood when he prepared his report for the academic year 1950–51, especially as he addressed the influence of the MNI on the medical and scientific landscape in Quebec. It is perhaps one of Penfield's most significant statements on his attempt to bridge the two solitudes in the practice of medicine in the province.

> The Montreal Neurological Institute occupies a unique position in the Canadian scene; first because of the nature of its scientific work in that field of medicine which is least understood.
>
> Secondly, the position of the Neurological Institute is unique in the field of clinical practice. During the first ten years of its existence here in Montreal it enlarged the special field of Neurology by addition to it of a new specialty, Neurosurgery, and both were made strong by new scientific methods.
>
> Once the new field of treatment was opened, some of the larger general hospitals that were not situated as close to the Institute as the Royal Victoria began to consider the need of having their own neurosurgeons.
>
> The University of Montreal and Laval University enlarged their academic departments correspondingly and appointed distinguished French-speaking neurologists and neurosurgeons to new posts.
>
> This is excellent. I think it is not vainglory for us to say that the Montreal Neurological Institute has opened up a new field of medical practice here in the Province of Quebec, and, to a certain extent in other parts of the world.
>
> But there is further work for the hospital to do, teaching, coordination, research, consultation. There are many new fields of treatment to be opened up. The clinical staff in neurology and neurosurgery of most of the hospitals of Montreal are also members of our staff, or are working

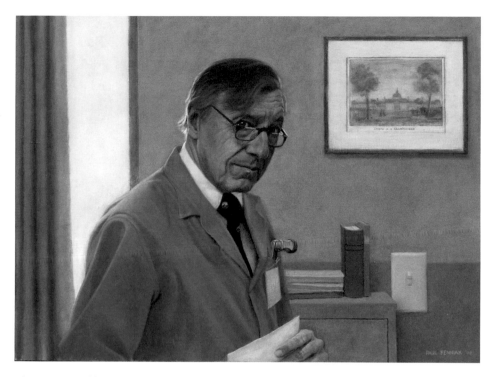

Figure 17.1: Gilles Bertrand. The painting within the painting is a study of La Salpêtrière, where Bertrand did postgraduate work on the venous circulation of the brain. (Paul Fenniak)

with us. Conferences back and forth on clinical problems are frequent and stimulating.

Thus the Institute is a meeting ground for the specialist in this area. This has been of great benefit to all of us. And now I am glad to be able to announce that this clinical alliance will unite Quebec City with Montreal in this field.[1]

The new alliance with Laval University in Quebec City was forged through two individuals: Sylvio Caron, professor of neurology and neurologist at Hôpital Hôtel-Dieu, and Jean Sirois, neurosurgeon at Hôpital de l'Enfant-Jésus. Penfield welcomed them in French as adjunct consultants: "Ces nominations ne font que rendre officielles les relations amicales que nous avons entretenues avec la Neurologie de Québec pendant de nombreuses années, et, plus récemment, avec sa Neuro-Chirurgie. Elles constituent un hommage à l'excellence du travail accompli par nos confrères dans la capitale de cette Province."[2] Caron and Sirois helped to fill the void created by the deaths of Antonio Barbeau – a man whose intellectual horizons knew no national boundaries – and of Émile Legrand, whom Penfield described as a "distinguished clinician, gay, debonair – a good friend."[3]

A DISSONANT NOTE

Distinguished French-Canadian neurologists had been listed as consultants since the very foundation of the MNI, and many able francophone fellows had trained at the institute. But the relationship with Montreal's French-Canadian medical community had not always been to everyone's satisfaction, as reflected in a letter from Francis McNaughton to Wilder Penfield on 10 November 1943.[4]

Dear Dr Penfield,

During the past year, I have been more convinced than ever of the urgent need for closer cooperation between the French- and English-speaking neuropsychiatric groups in Montreal. I have the impression that at the present time the French group feel very much outside of the active work of the M.N.I ... The M.N.I. is regarded by them as a purely English institution in spite of the fact that it is subsidized by the City and the Province, and serves both the French and English population. I realize of course that the fault is not all on our side, and there are many obstacles in the way of full cooperation which must be faced frankly, and overcome ... If the present trend continues, this ideal will become more difficult than ever to accomplish. It is quite possible that a few years will see the development of a rival French-Canadian Neurological Institute in Montreal, which would be unfortunate from many standpoints.

In the interest of a more positive policy of cooperation between our two groups, and as a basis for discussion, I would make the following proposals:

1. Immediate extension of teaching privileges in the Montreal Neurological Institute (neurological and neurosurgical) to the Neurological Department of the University of Montreal.

2. Appointment at an early date of a French-Canadian neurologist, and a neurosurgeon to the active teaching and visiting staff of the Montreal Neurological Institute and McGill University.

3. Encouragement of research at the Montreal Neurological Institute by younger graduates of the University of Montreal, with the idea of adding some of their number to the Montreal Neurological Institute staff in later years.

4. Extension of the research facilities in the Montreal Neurological Institute to the Department of Neurology of the University of Montreal.

5. Arrangement for regular exchange lectures and clinics in the undergraduate course, between the two University Departments of Neurology.

6. Provision of a regular course in the French language for all English-speaking interns, fellows and nurses on the Montreal Neurological Institute staff, and encouragement in the use of the French language on the wards.

7. Appointment of a French-Canadian representative on the Executive Committee.

Yours sincerely,

FLMcN

As it was, a French-Canadian neurologist would not be recruited to the attending staff of the MNI for another quarter century, until the appointment of Michel Aubé in 1974.[5] Aubé – able, intelligent, a polyglot with a quick wit – greatly admired and respected Francis McNaughton, and he carried on his tradition of care for patients suffering from migraine with compassion, dedication, and great insight into their condition. Serge Gauthier followed Aubé in 1977. Like Aubé, Gauthier fell under the spell of McNaughton and decided to devote his career to the care of patients with Alzheimer's disease.[6]

Gilles Bertrand was the first francophone neurosurgeon to be appointed to the MNI. Bertrand was the cousin of Claude Bertrand, the first French-Canadian neurosurgery resident trained at the MNI. Gilles Bertrand was born in Montreal and obtained his medical degree from the Université de Montreal in 1949, at the age of twenty. Following graduation he studied neurology with Raymond Garcin at La Salpêtrière, and while in Paris, he also studied the cerebral venous system with André Delmas, the noted neuroanatomist, under whose direction he obtained an MSc from the Faculty of Medicine of the Université de Paris.[7] After an internship in Toledo, Ohio, Bertrand began his residency in 1951 at the MNI and was Wilder Penfield's last resident. Bertrand came under the irresistible influence of William Cone during his residency and joined him as a junior partner in 1955. Bertrand was especially involved in the care of patients with spinal problems, concentrating his efforts, most notably, on lesions of the cranio-vertebral junction. In this regard, Bertrand produced the most complete theory of the etiology of syringomyelia and became expert in its treatment.[8] Bertrand also pioneered in the stereotactic treatment of movement disorders and carried out single-unit recordings of the human thalamus in awake patients being operated upon for Parkinson's disease.[9] Bertrand and Chris Thompson were the first to introduce computers into the operating room for the stereotactic surgery of movement disorders.[10] Bertrand was appointed a professor in the Department of Neurosurgery at McGill in 1971, was named William Cone Professor of Neurosurgery in 1988, and served as neurosurgeon-in-chief at the MNI from 1972 to 1991, when he was succeeded by André Olivier.

Francis LeBlanc was born in Nova Scotia. He obtained his medical degree at the University of Ottawa in 1959, and a doctorate in neurophysiology from the Université de Montreal in 1964. He then trained at the MNI from 1964 to 1968, whereupon he was appointed to the staff of the Department of Neurosurgery.[11]

André Olivier obtained his medical degree from the Université de Montreal in 1964. Following graduation he pursued a postgraduate degree with Professors Louis Poirier at Laval University and Rolf Hassler at the Max Planck Institute in Germany, then obtained his PhD from Université Laval in 1970, for his dissertation titled "Chemoarchitecture of the Primate Thalamus," and in that same year completed his neurosurgical training at the MNI. Olivier was then recruited to the Department of Neurosurgery at the institute, becoming a professor in 1984. Olivier was appointed the William Cone Professor and chairman of neurosurgery at McGill University in 1991, a position that he held for over twenty years. Olivier achieved international prominence for his treatment of epileptic patients, as an expert and innovator in stereotactic neurosurgery, and as a pioneer in image-guided neurosurgery.[12] Jean-Guy Villemure and Richard Leblanc, who both trained under them, later joined Bertrand and Olivier at the MNI.

IT TAKES A VILLAGE ...

Joan Thomas and Elabel Davidson, respectively assistant director and director of the Social Services Department, published *Social Problems of the Epileptic Patient / Problèmes sociaux de l'épileptique.* Their concerns about the medical care and social integration of epileptic patients were far-sighted, and their study is population based, rigorous, and comprehensive. Their book has the added virtue – rare in publications of the institute at the time – of being bilingual. Thomas and Davidson studied the social difficulties of 178 patients followed regularly at the epilepsy clinic at the MNI, and addressed their medical status with the collaboration of Francis McNaughton. They then evaluated the social status of the patients, their relationship with parents and family, their experience with schooling and employment, their interpersonal and intimate relationships, and child-rearing difficulties. Thomas and Davidson conclude, "No

Table 17.1
Graduate degrees awarded, Montreal Neurological Institute, 1950–51

Name	Degree	Thesis title
H. McLennan	PhD	Factors Effecting the Synthesis of Acetylcholine by Brain Tissue Preparation
J. Olszewski	PhD	An Atlas of the Thalamus of Macaca Mulatta
D.B. Tower	PhD	"Acetylcholine in the Cortex of Various Mammals and in the Human Epileptogenic Focus and Certain Factors Which Affect Its Activity"
J. Webb	PhD	Effects of Narcotics and Convulsants on Brain Tissue
G.M. Austin	MSc	An Investigation of the Facilitatory and Inhibitory Activity of the Suprabulbar Regions of the Cat
A.S. Dekaban	MSc	The Human Thalamus: Anatomical and Developmental Study
K.M. Earle	MSc	The Tract of Lissauer and Its Possible Relation to the Pain Pathway
R.M. Gibson	MSc	The Effects of Cortisone in the Healing of Incised Cerebral Wounds
I. Klatzo	MSc	A Study of the Tumors of the Nervous System by the Golgi Method
C-L. Li	MSc	Anatomical Study of Fiber Connections of the Temporal Pole in the Cat and the Monkey
H. Rosen	MSc	Influence of Massage on Rate and Down Growth of Regenerating Axons
J. Stratford	MSc	A Study of Certain Cortico-thalamic Relationships
J. Van Buren	MSc	The Cortical Representation of the Feeding Reflex

proposal can be a complete and final answer to the problems faced by the epileptic in our Province. Nor can a blueprint of needs be written for all time. The picture will inevitably change with shifting emphasis and development throughout our social structure … The magnitude of the problem requires that all forces in the community, both public and private, share the responsibility."[13]

ACADEMIA

Academic activities of the institute underwent a veritable British invasion during the academic year 1950–51. J. Godwin Greenfield had preceded that contingent when he gave the 1950 Hughlings Jackson Lecture, "The Pathology of the Cerebellum and Related Motor Pathways." The British visitors were no less distinguished: Sir Charles Symonds, from Queen Square, discussed "Migrainous Variants"; Sir Hugh Cairns, neurosurgeon at Oxford, presented "Consciousness and Memory"; and Sir Geoffrey Jefferson, from Manchester, read "Cerebral Aneurysms." Jefferson also provided "A Postscript to Descartes' Treatise on the Localization of the Mind." Jefferson's address at the institute was taken in part from his 1949 Lister Oration, "The Mind of Mechanical Man," delivered at the Royal College of Surgeons of England.[14] Bertram Collip, co-discoverer of insulin and past chair of biochemistry at McGill, gave the 1951 Hughlings Jackson Lecture, "The Endocrines in Relation to Neurology."

The academic year 1950–51 was perhaps unique in the history of the institute in the number of graduate degrees that it awarded to individuals who would make significant advances in the neurosciences.

18

The New Half-Century

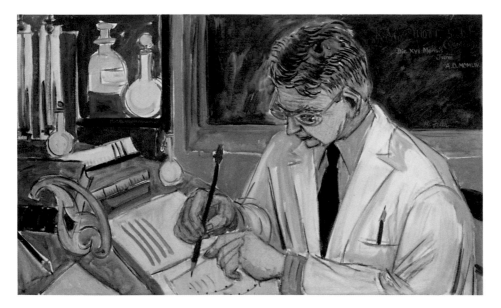

Figure 18.1: K.A.C. Elliott by Mary Filer. (Courtesy Hanna Pappius)

A NEW WING IN PROGRESS

"The boom of dynamite, the drone of cement mixers, and the staccato excitement of hammers" echoed in the summer of 1951, as the McConnell Wing, the latest addition to the MNI, was slowly rising along the north end of University Street, inching towards the slope of Mount Royal.[1] But the generosity of the patrons of the institute extended beyond grey brick and mortar: the Donner Canadian Foundation provided an annual grant in support of research in neurochemistry, and K.A.C. Elliott was appointed the first Donner Fellow and director of the newly named Donner Laboratory of Experimental Neurochemistry.[2] Experimental neurophysiology also benefited from a generous gift, from the Bronfman family, which endowed a fellowship that allowed Cosimo Ajmone-Marsan to join the staff.[3] He and Herbert Jasper mentored Davis Hubel during his fellowship in neurophysiology.

The MNI welcomed David Hubel, its Nobel laureate in the making, in 1952 (figure 18.2). Hubel was born of American parents in Windsor, Ontario, grew up in Outremont, in the francophone section of Montreal, and graduated from McGill University in 1947, with a degree in mathematics and physics. Almost on a whim he entered McGill's Medical School and arranged to meet with Wilder Penfield to discuss a burgeoning interest in research. Hubel recalled this first encounter with the MNI in a biographical sketch that he prepared for the Society for Neuroscience in 1996:

> By second year medical school I began to develop a strong interest in the brain. Luckily for me the MNI was part of McGill … [It] was perched high on the hill to the southeast of Mount Royal, a sort of ivory tower that medical students seldom climbed. I decided to grab the bull by the horns and made an appointment to see Penfield himself. Finally the day arrived. I borrowed the family car, parked it on University Street, and in a state of some terror climbed up to the fourth floor of the institute. Penfield was at his most charming, and when I told him of my physics background he immediately took me up to see Herbert Jasper, who in turn, immediately offered me a summer job doing electronics in his physiology group. When I got back to the car I found it running, with the keys locked inside. I took the streetcar home to get a spare key, and 90 minutes later was back. It was a stressful afternoon.[4]

Hubel worked with Jasper for the following two summers, and, after his internship at the Montreal General Hospital, he began a residency at the MNI, followed by a year of fellowship, again with Herbert Jasper. Hubel was greatly impressed with Jasper as a scientist, and wrote of him,

> His scientific outlook was wonderfully broad and he had a clarity of mind and scepticism that made him stand out among brain scientists. The first time we spoke, the day of the locked car, he asked me what I had read in the field. I told him I had just read *Cybernetics*, by Norbert Wiener. He gave me an odd look, and said, "Did you understand it?" I thought I had, even if through a glass, darkly, and when I said so, he grinned. It was clear that he thought that Wiener's brain science was off the wall, but he was nice enough not to want to put me down.[5]

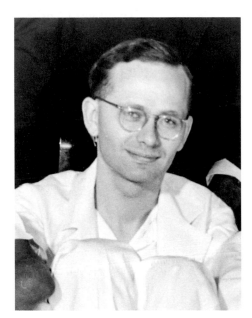 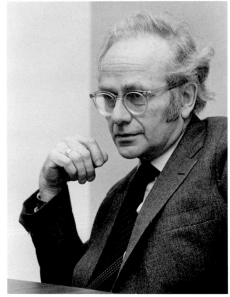

Figures 18.2 and 18.3: David Hubel, MNI resident in 1952 (*left*), and Nobel laureate and 1982 Hughlings Jackson lecturer (*right*). (MNI Archives)

Jasper was not Hubel's only mentor at the MNI: "I began learning EEG from Cosimo Ajmone-Marsan, who was then a teaching fellow at the MNI, and Jasper's main assistant. Ajmone-Marsan was a wonderful teacher, bright and witty, and I felt privileged to work with him. It didn't last: after three months he accepted a position at the National Institutes of Health (NIH) in Bethesda, Maryland, in clinical neurophysiology … Suddenly I found myself Jasper's main assistant, having to read most of the EEGs of the institute and attending all the Penfield temporal lobe excisions. It was a busy year."[6]

Jasper's influence on David Hubel would be far-reaching, as Hubel later recognized: "All the fellows at the institute took part in a seminar series that covered neurophysiology. By some lucky chance Jasper assigned me the visual system." Thus, Jasper set Hubel on a path that would lead him to Stockholm to receive the Nobel Prize.[7]

Hubel moved to Johns Hopkins University for further training in 1954, but was soon drafted into the US Army and sent to serve at the Walter Reed Army Institute of Research in Washington, DC. In 1958, Hubel moved to the Johns Hopkins Hospital, where he collaborated with Torsten Wiesel in Stephen Kuffler's laboratory. One year later Kuffler's laboratory moved to Harvard and, within five years, formed the nucleus of its new Department of Neurobiology. Hubel became professor of physiology at Harvard in 1965. David Hubel and

Torsten Wiesel were awarded the Nobel Prize in Physiology or Medicine in 1981, along with Roger Sperry. Hubel's first address as a Nobel laureate was the 1982 Hughlings Jackson lecture, "The Eye, the Brain, and Perception."

CORONATION

As was sometimes the case, Wilder Penfield deviated from purely clinical or academic – even metaphysical – issues in his annual report and touched on broader concerns, as in 1953, the year of Queen Elizabeth's coronation. First, he reflected on the role of the MNI in Canada:

> The Montreal Neurological Institute has a function which the casual observer would not suspect. It serves as a melting pot for Canadian citizenship. Herbert Jasper, Professor of Experimental Neurology, who was born in the United States and whose university education was carried out in Washington, Iowa, Paris and McGill, became a Canadian citizen during the past year. Allan Elliott, who was born in South Africa and who completed his education at Cambridge, England, has done the same. Jerzy Olszewski, born in Poland, is in the process of Canadian naturalization, and Choh Luh Li, born in China, likewise. Canadians may take reasonable pride in these acts, for these men are outstanding scientists. They have all of them refused flattering offers from universities elsewhere. But they have chosen to cast in their lot, once and for all, with us and to accept the full responsibilities of citizenship.[8]

Perhaps it was the pomp and grandeur of a young Queen's coronation or gratitude to the country that had received him and allowed him to create a great institute, but Wilder Penfield was moved to affirm himself Canadian: "We are proud of the heritage of this Province, which is now our heritage also; proud of the culture and sagacity that comes to us through our French ancestors, and the traditions of democracy and freedom that come to us from Great Britain. We are proud of the position of this Institute in the British Commonwealth of Nations. In this year of the Coronation, we are proud to own allegiance to our gracious Queen, Elizabeth the Second."[9]

ACADEMIA

Professor John C. Eccles addressed the MNI on the brain-mind liaison, which he published in *Nature* the following year.[10] His address contains the intriguing notion that "in brain-mind liaison the traffic is both ways, from brain to mind no less than from mind to brain." Penfield also had his opinion on the subject, which was less enigmatic: "We are beginning to surmise where and how memories are stored, where the nerve impulses originate that produce voluntary action. We cannot analyze the spirit, the mind, the soul. But we can analyze the mechanisms of the brain which make understanding and initiative possible and without which these things vanish."[11] Eccles also gave the 1952 Hughlings Jackson Lecture on a more tangible topic: "Electrophysiology of the Neuron." James C. White, chief of neurosurgery at the Massachusetts General Hospital, was even more down to earth in his 1953 Hughlings Jackson Lecture, "Pain Conduction in Man." Ragnar Granit, who would be honoured by the Nobel Foundation in 1968, also visited the MNI in 1975 and presented "Reflex Excitability of Motoneurones." Granit returned to the institute in 1975 to deliver the Hughlings Jackson Lecture, "Functional Roles of the Muscle Spindles." Other distinguished speakers included Brian McArdle from Guy's Hospital, London, who had just described the form of myopathy that bears his name.[12]

The most determined invited speaker was undoubtedly Charles M. Pomerat of the University of Texas, whose topic was "Tissue Cultures of the Human Brain." He flew up from Texas with a number of petri dishes containing astrocyte cultures strapped around his generous midriff to keep them warm.

EILEEN CONSTANCE FLANAGAN

The year 1952–53 saw the greatest addition of grey stone and mortar to the institute since its opening: "This year," Penfield wrote to the principal of McGill University, "the McConnell Wing, which is, in itself, a beautiful building of Montreal stone, stands complete."[13] The transfer of patients to the new wing was put in the hands of one of the most accomplished people to tread the halls of 3801 University Street, the MNI's first director of nursing, Eileen Flanagan: "During the coming summer, one after another of our activities will be transferred into the wing while essential supplementary alterations are made here in the main building. This will be carried out according to the dictates of Miss Eileen Flanagan. She has a genius for administration in the nursing field, but in other fields as well we know that, had she been a man, she would have made an able general. We are indebted to her for many things."[14]

Eileen Flanagan was born the daughter of a deacon of the Church of England in Pontiac County, western Quebec, in 1896, and her family moved to Montreal when she was two months old. As a child, she suffered from rheumatic heart disease and was confined to bed for a prolonged period of time, so she took the opportunity to study Greek from her father, who had himself studied it at Trinity College, Dublin.

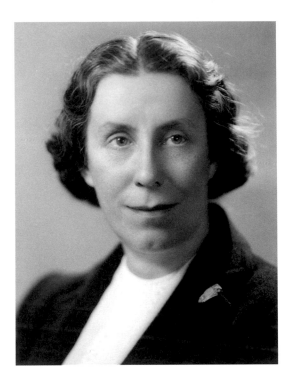

Figure 18.4: Eileen Flanagan.
(MNI Archives)

Young Eileen Flanagan entered the Faculty of Arts at McGill University in 1916, studying philosophy and the classics, most notably with Professor Stephen Leacock, the great Canadian wit. Like all true scholars, Flanagan "found Greek Literature much more enjoyable than Latin."[15] During weekends she served coffee to departing troops in Dominion Square, on their way to Windsor Station to board a train for Halifax, then on to a troop carrier bound for Southhampton. Hers was the last friendly face many of them would see.

Flanagan developed an interest in nursing after a bout of Spanish influenza, which followed the end of the Great War. Upon her recovery in 1920 she entered the School of Nursing at the RVH. A few years after graduation she was entrusted with the position of head nurse of the newly opened metabolism ward at the Vic. Her major interest then was the care of diabetic patients, a heavy burden before the discovery of insulin. Her devotion was such, and her intellect so keen, that she translated Joslin's *Diabetic Manual* into French, to better inform her francophone patients. Seeing a rising star, her superiors at the RVH gave Flanagan a leave of absence to study teaching and administration at the graduate School of Nursing at McGill, in 1928. The following year she took further instruction in England, at the Royal College of Nursing and at the London Hospital, where she assisted Sir Hugh Cairns and met Wilder Penfield and William Cone for the first time. "Little did I know," she later wrote, "that I would spend the next 27 years of my life with them."[16]

Eileen Flanagan returned to Montreal in 1933 and completed her baccalaureate at Royal Victoria College, then returned to full-time nursing at the RVH and was immediately told that she was to be the first director of nursing at the soon-to-be-opened MNI, "at a salary of $100 a month, living in residence."[17] Flanagan soon realized that the young men training in neurosurgery with Penfield and Cone would return to their home hospitals without the benefit of specialized nurses to look after their patients. "We therefore decided to organize a graduate course in Neurological and Neurosurgical Nursing, and to ask the hospitals sending doctors for training to send two nurses with them who could return and build up a nucleus of trained staff in their own hospitals. This had been a great success, the result being that there are now [1983] over one thousand graduates in all parts of the world with McGill University Montreal Neurological Certificates."[18]

Eileen Flanagan ran the Nursing Department at the institute with great ability and devotion. When she retired, in 1961, she was surprised to see the principal of McGill University, Cyril James, at her retirement dinner. James was there to announce that the governors of the university had awarded her a scholarship for the study of law![19]

The opportunity to study law arose from Eileen Flanagan's involvement with provincial, national, and international nursing organizations, which had been one of her preoccupations since 1940. Within these associations, she had worked with many distinguished jurists, some of whom were later elevated to the highest benches of the provincial and federal courts. In her capacity as president and chairperson of the Legislation and Labour Relations Committee of the Quebec Association of Nurses, Flanagan was instrumental in the passage of the Quebec Nursing Act, which elevated nursing to the same professional level as the College of Physicians and the Bar. This required the assent of the hard-nosed and reputed misogynist premier of Quebec, Maurice Duplessis. In this, Flanagan proved herself an able negotiator. When she met Duplessis to discuss the proposed Quebec Nursing Act, she told him that the federal authorities had said, "The Québec government would never give women such wide powers!" Duplessis, bolting back in his chair asked, "They told you this in Ottawa?" Flanagan replied innocently with the single word "Yes." Then, as she relates, Duplessis "straightened up, slapped his hand on his desk and said, 'You will be the first Provincial association to obtain such an act.'" And so it was; and not just in Canada, but in the whole of North America.[20]

Eileen Flanagan's talents extended beyond nursing and the law. She co-wrote the definitive history of nursing in Quebec, *Heritage: History of the Nursing Profession in Quebec from the Augustinians and Jeanne Mance to Medicare*.[21] She also collaborated on the more widely distributed *Miracle of the Empty Beds*, on the eradication of tuberculosis.[22] During her research for *Empty Beds*, she recalled her acquaintance with Norman Bethune: "I was surgical nurse supervisor while Bethune was at the R.V.H. He was working with Dr Archibald on lung surgery. I was impressed with his attention to his patients but also found him impatient, exacting and ingenious."[23] Undoubtedly, Flanagan had better luck working with Penfield, since she remained the director of nursing at the MNI for twenty-seven years.

CEREBRAL ISCHEMIA

Francis McNaughton was appointed professor of neurology at McGill University in 1951, upon Donald McEachren's death. Much was expected of McNaughton in his new position, but he was fortunate in having surrounded himself with exceptional young clinicians and researchers, as Penfield pointed out in announcing his new role at McGill and at the MNI: "Many years of leadership lie before Francis McNaughton, years in which to pursue his special interests, such as epilepsy and the cause and cure of headache. With the support of Robb, Young, Swank, Fisher, Lloyd-Smith, Tower, Rabinovitch, and others to come, the prospect for Neurology during the next twenty years is bright indeed."[24] C. Miller Fisher undoubtedly met Penfield's expectations in the field of cerebrovascular disease.

The MNI's interest in cerebrovascular physiology and pathology focused primarily on the cortical circulation until Miller Fisher's arrival, and attention changed to extracranial occlusion of the internal carotid artery. William Cone, however, had an early interest in cebebrovascular occlusion that straddled his time in New York at the Presbyterian Hospital and the beginning of his stay in Montreal at the RVH. At the time there were few diagnostic means to differentiate between ischemic and hemorrhagic stroke, and sterile emboli from septic ones. The former were especially common in the pre-antibiotic area when rheumatic fever was rife. Cone reasoned that if reactive ischemic changes were reflected in the cerebrospinal fluid, the cellular analysis of the CSF could become a powerful diagnostic tool to differentiate embolic strokes from other acute events affecting the brain. Thus, Cone undertook the study of the inflammatory changes produced by the injection of melted wax into the carotid artery of dogs. The emboli lodged in the middle cerebral artery and its branches and produced hemiplegia. Cerebrospinal fluid was obtained for analysis at different times prior to sacrifice. Cone and his co-worker concluded that "when a sudden or moderately sudden cerebral accident has occurred and polymorphonuclear leukocytes, but no organisms, are present in the cerebrospinal fluid, a cerebral infarction must be considered."[25] Not much came of these observations because of the unreliability of the experimental model, and interest in the effects of middle cerebral artery occlusion at the institute waned until Joseph Evans undertook his doctoral studies on the effects of ischemia on the brain by applying a silver clip to the main branches of the middle cerebral artery. The purpose of the experiment was to produce elements of Penfield's meningocerebral cicatrix.[26] But rather than supporting Penfield's hypothesis, Evans's results constituted a major challenge to it. Significant interest in cerebral ischemia was therefore not a priority at the institute until the early 1950s, with the work of Miller Fisher.

Charles Miller Fisher attended medical school at the University of Toronto, graduating in 1938, and interned at the Henry Ford Hospital in Detroit.[27] Fisher then came to the RVH for his residency and spent six weeks on the neurology service at the MNI before going off to war. After his discharge from the Navy, Fisher returned to the institute to continue his training in neurology. Although he has expressed great respect for Wilder Penfield and his accomplishments in his memoirs,[28] he was not beyond some gentle ribbing,[29] as in a story told to Richard Leblanc, perhaps apocryphal: Miller Fisher was rounding with Penfield early one morning when Penfield whipped off his glasses in that familiar gesture of frustration and irritation and said, "Fisher, the dressings haven't been done! Come and see me in my office after rounds!" and left in a huff. It was one of those steamy, hot, humid, mid-July mornings in Montreal, when there is not breeze enough to ruffle a feather. Penfield had left the door to his office open in a vain attempt to let in a bit of air. Finding this insufficient, he tried to open his window, but it was swollen shut by the humidity. Undeterred, Penfield put a chair under the windowsill and, propping himself on his bent right leg, struggled to open the window. Just then, Miller Fisher walked into the office and, seeing Penfield red-faced, teeth clenched, and determined, cried out, in mock alarm, "Wait Dr Penfield, don't jump! I'll do the dressings!"[30]

Despite his *rocambolesque* introduction to neurology at the MNI, Miller Fisher was nonetheless offered the position of acting registrar during Preston Robb's sabbatical. After a few years at the institute and as neurological consultant at the Queen Mary Veterans Hospital, Fisher went, on Roy Swank's advice, to the Boston City Hospital for a year of postgraduate training under Raymond D. Adams, to study the neuropathology of stroke. This would be the turning point of his career. Upon his return from Boston, Miller Fisher was appointed clinical assistant in neurology at the MNI, neuropathologist at the Montreal

General Hospital, and consultant in neurology at Queen Mary Veterans Hospital, which had a large population of stroke patients. It was there that he observed the cases that he later studied in the Pathology Department at the MGH, where "a methodical search for disease of the internal carotid artery at necropsy was … undertaken and [was] surprisingly rewarding."[31] However, all was not smooth sailing for this retired mariner: his technique required the removal of the carotid bifurcation at post-mortem examination. This made it impossible for the undertaker to perfuse the face, precluding an open casket. Complaints eventually reached the dean of medicine and a solution had to be found if Fisher was to continue his work. Thus, with the resourcefulness of an ex-POW, Fisher inserted one end of a red rubber catheter in the stump of the common carotid artery and the other into the external carotid artery, thus allowing perfusion of the face even if the carotid bifurcation was removed.[32] Through these studies, Miller Fisher forever changed our understanding of stroke.

Fisher observed that stenosis or occlusion of the internal carotid at its origin in the neck is a frequent cause of stroke, and he concluded that the underlying process affecting the carotid arteries is arteriosclerotic.[33] He also observed that many patients who later had a completed stroke had had transient premonitory symptoms, often a temporary hemiparesis or aphasia, but most commonly transient monocular blindness. This occurrence, Fisher surmised, was caused by a small embolus originating from the arteriosclerotic plaque. Fisher was able to confirm this when he chanced to observe a small platelet embolus in a retinal artery of a patient who had an episode of transient monocular blindness as he was being examined.[34] Miller Fisher ascribed the occurrence of asymptomatic carotid occlusions, and the variable clinical picture that can accompany a completed stroke, to "many factors, such as the patency of the opposite carotid artery, the efficacy of the collateral circulation, or the size of the component vessels of the circle of Willis." Thus, the whole of our current understanding of arteriosclerotic cerebrovascular disease and its manifestations were explained. But Miller Fisher went further and suggested a possible treatment of carotid disease in the neck, based on his improvised bypass, stating that "it is even conceivable that some day vascular surgery will find a way to by-pass the occluded portion of the artery during the period of ominous fleeting symptoms," and that "anastomosis of the external carotid artery, or one of its branches, with the internal carotid artery above the area of narrowing should be feasible."[35] Both suggestions were prescient, as surgeons rapidly focused their efforts at re-establishing carotid circulation by endarterectomy and, later, by extracranial to intracranial bypass. But Fisher recognized the underlying pathophysiological mechanism leading to carotid occlusion and in this he also foresaw our current therapeutic approach: "Since the pathological substrate of carotid disease is atherosclerosis, the fundamental approach to therapy must be directed at the prevention or cure of that disorder."[36]

While Fisher was revolutionizing the field of ischemic vascular disease, rumours were abuzz that Wilder Penfield was about to retire as director of the institute – as he indeed did in 1954. Contemporaneously, Raymond Adams had been awarded the Bullard Professorship at Harvard University, replacing Penfield's old friend and collaborator Stanley Cobb. Adams was quick to offer Miller Fisher the opportunity of joining him, and despite Penfield's best efforts to dissuade him, the talk of Penfield's retiring and the academic uncertainty that it entailed carried the day: Fisher went to Boston, where he continued on what can only be described as a stellar career.[37]

Miller Fisher's departure from the MNI was but a harbinger of what was to come, as some of the brightest and best residents and fellows left the institute for Bethesda, Maryland.

19

The MNI and the National Institutes of Health

It was the largest collection of MNI trainees anywhere except in Montreal.
– D. Tower

By far the most significant of the MNI's international influence was its role in the formation of a neurological institute within the National Institutes of Health in Bethesda, Maryland.

At the end of the Second World War, more than fifteen US states had no qualified neurologist. In August 1950, the US Congress authorized the creation of the National Institute of Neurological Diseases and Blindness as one of the National Institutes of Health, with Pearce Bailey as its first director. Shortly after his appointment of the newly created, but largely unstaffed NINDB, Bailey joined Milton Shy and Maitland Baldwin at a meeting of the American Medical Association, in Denver, where they had both relocated after leaving the MNI. As a result of the meeting, Shy and Baldwin agreed to join Bailey: Shy, thirty-three years old, as the director of the Clinical Research Program and head of Medical Neurology, and Baldwin, two years older than Shy, as chief of Surgical Neurology, effective 1 May 1953.[1] The NINDB eventually became the National Institute of Neurological Diseases and Stroke, the leading funder of neurological research in the world.[2]

Milton Shy obtained his medical degree from the University of Oregon in 1943 and interned there before coming to the RVH to begin a residency in internal medicine. Shy served the United States Army as a medical officer towards the end of the Second World War and was seriously wounded in action in Italy. After his recovery he completed his military service in the Army of Occupation in Germany.[3] Upon discharge from the Army in 1947, he entered the neurology program at the National Hospital for Neurology in Queen Square, London, then came to the MNI in 1949 as a neurology fellow, where he stayed until 1951. During that time the first seeds of his career in the field of neuromuscular disease were sown, in a paper entitled "The Effects of Cortisone in Certain Neuromuscular Disorders."[4] Three years later he and Glenn Drager described the condition that bears their name.[5] After a decade at the NINDB, Shy was

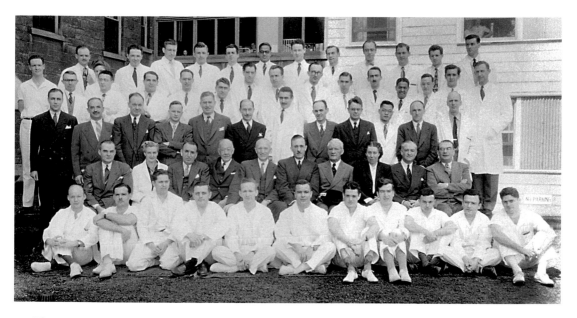

Figure 19.1: 1949–50 annual photograph of the staff of the Montreal Neurological Institute showing the nucleus of the soon-to-be-created National Institute of Neurological Diseases and Blindness. Maitland Baldwin and Milton Shy are seated in the front row, sixth and seventh from the left. Cosimo Ajmone-Marsan and Choh-luh Li are seventh and tenth in the third row. Igor Klatzo, Donald Tower, and John Lord are in the fourth row in the ninth, tenth, and eleventh position, and John Van Buren is tenth in the last row. Not shown are Shirley Lewis, an operating room nurse from the MNI who also relocated to Bethesda and later married Maitland Baldwin; Maureen Benson-DeLemos, who left the institute to become chief EEG technologist at the NINDB; and Anatole Dekaban, pediatric neurology consultant to the MNI. (MNI Archives)

appointed head of Neurology at the University of Pennsylvania and subsequently director of the Neurological Institute at Columbia-Presbyterian Hospital in New York, in 1967, but he suffered a fatal heart attack three weeks into his mandate. He was forty-eight.

Maitland Baldwin graduated from Harvard College in 1938. He obtained his medical degree from Queen's University, in Kingston, Ontario, in 1943 and interned at the Montreal General Hospital. Baldwin then joined the United States Navy and participated in the landing at Iwo Jima and in the preparations for the invasion of Japan at Okinawa. Following the end of hostilities, Baldwin served with the American Army of Occupation in Japan, as Shy was doing in Germany. After his release from service, Baldwin came to the MNI as resident and fellow from 1947 to 1952.[6] Baldwin joined Shy at the University of Colorado, in Denver, in 1952, where they had that fateful meeting with Pearce Bailey.

Maitland Baldwin's friend and fellow MNI alumnus, the candid Cosimo Ajmone-Marsan, recalls Penfield and Baldwin's relationship: "Baldwin, in the course of his residency at the MNI, had become one of the preferred pupils and a *protégé* of Wilder Penfield … Baldwin himself had the greatest admiration for his teacher and made no secret that he aimed to emulate him … in many endeavours."[7] Baldwin was named clinical director of the NINDB in 1960. Like Shy, Baldwin was not destined for long life, for he died in 1970 at the age of fifty-two.

◆◆◆

Pearce Bailey and Maitland Baldwin's interest in making the NINDB a referral centre for the surgical treatment of epilepsy resulted in the recruitment of other MNI fellows with like interests, most notably Cosimo Ajmone-Marsan, John Van Buren, Choh-luh Li, and Igor Klatzo.[8]

Table 19.1
The MNI South: MNI fellows at the origin of the NINDB

Milton Shy	Clinical director, head of the Medical Neurology Branch
Maitland Baldwin	Neurosurgeon, head of the Surgical Neurology Branch
Cosimo Ajmone-Marsan	Head of EEG and Neurophysiology
Donald Tower	Head of Neurochemistry
Choh-luh Li	Head of Experimental Neurosurgery
John Van Buren	Neurosurgeon, neuroanatomy
Igor Klatzo	Head of Neuropathology
Anatole Dekaban	Developmental neurology
John Lord	Consultant neurosurgeon
Shirley Lewis-Baldwin	Operating room nurse
Maureen Benson-DeLemos	Chief EEG technologist

William Caveness (Neurology), Anthony Gorman (EEG and Neurophysiology), and Costa Stefanis (EEG and Neurophysiology) were also MNI residents and fellows who later joined the staff of the NINDB. See also H.H. Jasper, "Memoirs," MNI Archives; D.B. Tower, "The 1950s Clinical Program at the NINDB," in *Mind, Brain, Body, and Behavior*, ed. I.G. Farreras, C. Hannaway, and V.A. Harden (Amsterdam: IOS, 2004), 296.

Cosimo Ajmone-Marsan arrived at the MNI as a research fellow from Turin, Italy, in 1949 to study neurophysiology and EEG with Herbert Jasper. Ajmone-Marsan reminisced about his time at a the MNI, after he had arrived with his family at the end of January 1950, and of the annual Easter EEG Society Ski Meetings in the Laurentian hills:

A few days after we arrived in Montreal, we attended the first Eastern EEG Society Ski Meeting. I had never been north of the city, of course, and only had heard that the meeting was supposed to be held "up in the mountains." We were offered to be driven to the meeting by Dr Elliott … and without waiting for an answer he started his car. It was a nice, very small black car … with two windows – one with glass – and with-out heating … We arrived at Ste Marguerite about 12:30 A.M. and it took less than 30 minutes to defrost Rosy and get – finally – to our room, [which was] occupied by a young couple who turned out to be the McLeans.[9] Paul speeded up the defrosting process with a generous glass of scotch. The following day, after the usual scientific session, we were introduced to the sport of skiing. I had to rent a pair and found out that on Saturday, there would be a slalom race. A young unknown Canadian by the name of Bill Feindel beat me to win the race and I hated him for this forever.[10]

Cosimo Ajmone-Marsan left the MNI in 1954 to become chief of clinical neurophysiology at the NINDB. During his career in Bethesda he became a leading figure in epilepsy research and treatment.[11]

John Van Buren had trained in neurosurgery with Penfield and Elvidge and had done fellowships with Boris Babkin in neurophysiology and with Herbert Jasper in clinical encephalography.[12] His research interests at the MNI included cortical representation, the interrelationship between cortical and subcortical structures, and the use of metallic stains in the investigation of inflammation of the central nervous system. He obtained an MSc working with Babkin on a truly Pavlovian topic: "The Cortical Representation of the Feeding Reflex."[13] Van Buren was recruited to the NINDB, where he studied the anatomy of the temporal lobe and of the thalamus, and pursued his interests in the surgical treatment of epilepsy and of movement disorders. Van Buren was appointed head of Surgical Neurology at the NINDB after Baldwin's death. Of note, John Van Buren participated in the training of George Ojemann, who became an authority on the surgical treatment of epilepsy, and who joined the Department of Neurosurgery at the University of Washington, Seattle, headed by MNI fellow Arthur Ward.[14]

Choh-luh Li arrived at the MNI as its interests were migrating from the frontal to the temporal lobe and from the temporal neocortex to the mesial structures. He obtained a MSc with Herbert Jasper[15] and worked with him in recording single cortical cells with fine, individually handmade microelectrodes. The excitement that Jasper felt as he described Li's results to the staff of the institute was palpable: "The microelectrode studies with Dr Li have been most illuminating. It has been found that there is a veritable beehive of activity going on in the depths of the cortex, which is not detected by the usual methods of recording with the electroencephalogram from the surface … Gradually the true pattern of cortical activity is being revealed; it is organized in depth, and under the constant influence of to and fro currents from sub-cortical structures, the delicate balance of controlled function being lost in the explosive chain reaction of the epileptic discharge."[16] In was in this heady atmosphere that Li wrote his doctoral dissertation, "Microelectrode Studies of the Electrical Activity of the Cerebral Cortex,"[17] and it was the experience and expertise – and the ability to make beautiful microelectrodes – nurtured in Jasper's laboratory that brought Choh-luh Li to Bethesda in 1954, to head the Section on Experimental Neurosurgery of the NINDB.

Igor Klatzo was born in St Petersburg shortly before the outbreak of the Russian Revolution. His family escaped to Lithuania, where Klatzo obtained his medical degree. Like Chorobski, Klatzo was active in the Polish Resistance to Nazi occupation during the Second World War,[18] and at war's end, Igor Klatzo and Jerzy Olszewski joined Cécile and Oskar Vogt at their research institute in the Black Forest of Germany, where they had taken refuge after they had been dismissed from the Kaiser Wilhelm Institute by the Nazis. There, Klatzo studied neuroanatomy and the architectonic organization of the cerebral cortex.[19] With the Vogts' support, Klatzo and Olszewski both came to the MNI in 1948. Klatzo stayed at the institute until 1952, working mostly on malignant gliomas, then relocated a few steps down University Street to the Pathological Institute of McGill University, where he studied the anatomy of the brain stem.[20] Klatzo was recruited to head Neuropathology at the NINDB in 1956, where he did novel, fundamental work on the blood brain barrier and cerebral edema and on the neuropathology of slow virus diseases.[21] Igor Klatzo lived thirteen full years of active, joyful retirement, during which he completed a wonderful biography of Oskar and Cécile Vogt.[22]

Donald Bailey Tower matriculated at Harvard College in 1941 and graduated from Harvard Medical School in 1944. Following service in the Unites States Navy at Subic Bay, the Philippines, Tower came for an interview at the

MNI, with the intention of becoming a neurosurgeon. Good sense prevailed and he instead turned to research. Tower spent six and a half years at the institute, earning an MSc and a PhD from McGill University.[23] As Tower recounts his beginning at the MNI,

> When I initially met with Dr Penfield he stressed a basic tenet of the MNI training program: to combine clinical care with laboratory research. Each senior clinical staff member shared this philosophy by heading a ward service and by supervising a research laboratory. In view of my background in chemistry, Penfield proposed that I spend a year or so doing a research project in the Neurochemistry Laboratory, staffed by Donald McEachern as director and chief of the MNI Neurology Service and by K.A.C. Elliott, recently recruited as full-time neurochemist (incidentally, the first anywhere in the field to be so designated).[24]

Tower began two years of clinical service after completing his MSc, with part of his time spent with Penfield and Elvidge. The observations of such an insightful and clear-headed observer on two great neurosurgeons of the twentieth century are worth noting. Although most interested by Penfield's awake craniotomies and cortical mapping, Elvidge's demeanour, stamina, and skill in the operating room most impressed Tower: "I spent the year of 1948–1949 in the neurosurgical residency program. I still marvel at the many tours-de-force carried out by Arthur Elvidge: massive glioblastomas, formidable arteriovenous malformations, and horrendous head injuries with compound skull fractures. A high percentage of these cases survived and prospered – a tribute to Elvidge's surgical skills and unorthodox approaches to many of these seemingly impossible problems."[25]

Although he greatly admired him, Tower notes, "Penfield could be difficult." Tower relates an episode when he embarrassed "the Chief" during the presentation at Grand Rounds of a patient on whom Penfield, with some difficulty, had operated upon three days earlier. To Penfield's surprise, Tower elicited a post-operative aphasia that had gone unnoticed. Then, Tower relates, "I saw Dr Penfield sweep off his glasses – a sure sign of displeasure – and he stopped me and took over the presentation with the remark that the patient was not aphasic. That placed me in an uncomfortable position, reinforced by a meeting with Penfield in his office after rounds. The implication was that my future at the MNI was in grave difficulty." But all was not lost, Tower continues: "Shortly afterwards Penfield sent for me again and apologized, saying that he had re-examined the patient and confirmed my observation that he was aphasic. I was vindicated; the crisis was over."[26]

After two years of neurosurgical training, Tower faced an existential moment: to pursue the jealous mistress that is neurosurgery or to make a career as a research scientist. He chose the latter and was awarded a five-year Markle Foundation Fellowship to continue studies in neurochemistry with K.A.C. Elliott. As Tower recalled, "The course seemed clear: study ACh [acetylcholine] content and metabolism in the cerebrocortical samples being excised by Penfield at surgery for focal epilepsy. My year scrubbing with the Penfield team would stand me in good stead since I now knew the limitations under which the surgeon operated and the criteria used to characterize the brain samples. It became my habit to sit in the OR gallery to observe the results of cortical stimulation and EGG recordings and to personally pick up the excised cortical samples for immediate processing and study in the lab."[27]

Tower left the institute to pursue his career at the NINDB, where he established the first clinical neurochemistry research laboratory. He was appointed director of the NINDB in 1973, a post that he held until his retirement in 1981. Like his good friend Maitland Baldwin, who had married Shirley Lewis, operating room nurse at the MNI, Donald Tower also followed this MNI tradition by marrying Arlene Croft, assistant head nurse on the old Two East Ward of the institute.

20

The McConnell Wing

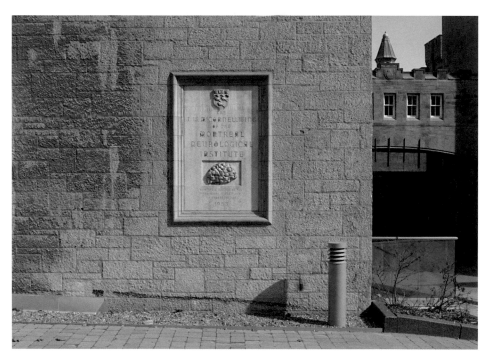

Figure 20.1: The McConnell Pavilion dedication plaque, designed by Galt Durnford, with Marjorie Winslow's bas-relief, *The Children of the Brain*. The path leads to the newest addition to the MNI, the North Wing, currently under construction. The Bronfman Bridge is visible at right. (Photographer Richard Leblanc)

The departure of fellows to Harvard, NIH, and other academic centres did nothing to dampen the enthusiasm of the Second Foundation ceremonies of the Montreal Neurological Institute and the opening of the McConnell Wing on 20 November 1953. Like the First Foundation, the Second Foundation was commemorated with a handsome volume,[1] its cover stamped with the Neurological Institute's first logo, the staff of Asclepius crossed by a reflex hammer and trephine over a section of the brain at the level of the temporal lobes.

Governor-General Vincent Massey was in attendance, as was Cyril James, principal of McGill University. Wilder Penfield acknowledged the generosity of those who had made the construction of the McConnell Wing possible and unveiled a plaque in their honour. In recognition of the Lily Griffith McConnell Foundation for Neurological Research, which provided a permanent endowment for basic science research in the MNI, a second plaque was unveiled as well with an inscription from Psalms, "Beauty and truth are met together," which greets all who enter the institute. A portrait of J.W. McConnell was hung in the corridor of the new wing, and a portrait of Lily Griffith McConnell was placed in the quiet seclusion of the Fellows Library, both still prominently displayed in the main corridor of the institute.

Allan Gregg, vice-president of the Rockefeller Foundation, gave the Second Foundation Lecture. Reflecting upon the MNI, Gregg commented, "If I were asked to name a single grant that the Medical Sciences Division of the [Rockefeller] Foundation has made since 1931, that I consider ideal in purpose, in performance, in local response and in national and international influence, and in the character of our relationships maintained from the very beginning, I would say without a moment's hesitation the grant to the Neurological Institute of McGill University."[2]

Gregg spoke knowingly on the role of medical institutes and stressed the need for orderly, planned changes in their governance. He suggested that as a matter of course, fellows should leave the institutes in which they had trained and be invited back, some time later, if they had proved their mettle elsewhere. Gregg's suggestion was acted upon and Theodore Rasmussen was invited back to the institute, to become neurosurgeon-in-chief, freeing Penfield for other pursuits.[3]

Children of the Brain

Some whimsy was introduced in the Second Foundation ceremonies when the governor-general unveiled a dedication plaque that featured a relief sculpture christened *Children of the Brain*.[4] Under the sculpture appeared Wilder Penfield's favourite quote from the Book of Job, "Where shall wisdom be found and where is the place of understanding?"

The origin of *Children of the Brain* goes back to 1932, when Wilder Penfield received a Christmas card with a drawing by Ludwig Edinger of the brain's convolutions as babies. Charmed by the image, Penfield commissioned Hortense Douglas Cantlie, his medical illustrator, to pose the infants to correspond to functional areas of the cortex. In the new version, an infant cupping a hand about the ear lay in the location of the auditory cortex. The faces and heads of

Table 20.1
Invited speakers, Second Foundation, 20 November 1953

Speaker	Topic
Roma Amyot (Montreal)	Research, Teaching, and the Care of the Sick
Claude Bertrand (Montreal)	The Parietal Lobe
D. Denny-Brown (Harvard)	Cortical Function
Joseph Evans (Cincinnati)	Reminiscences
G. Jefferson (Manchester)	Present and Future of Neurosurgery
Kristian Kristiansen (Oslo)	The State of Neurosurgery
Kenneth McKenzie (Toronto)	The Surgical Treatment of Spasmodic Torticollis
Theodore Rasmussen (Chicago)	Irradiation of the Hypophysis
Dorothy Russell (London)	Research in Neuropathology
E. Walker (Johns Hopkins)	Subcortical Epilepsy

two other babies were properly located at the lower end of the sensorimotor area. In the frontal pole a child pensively tapped an index finger to the temple as though straining for thought. On the basis of Cantlie's drawing, the bas-relief was created by Marjorie Winslow and incorporated by architect Galt Durnford into the plaque identifying the McConnell Pavilion. For Wilder Penfield, *Children of the Brain* symbolizes the fact that our understanding of the human brain is only in its infancy (figure 20.2).[5]

THE ADVANCE OF NEUROLOGY

Unveiling and Concealment

Still commemorating the Second Foundation, Mary Filer's evocative *Advance of Neurology* was unveiled by Premier Maurice Duplessis on 14 November 1954 (figure 20.4). Mary Filer had been an operating room nurse at the MNI from 1942 to 1946. She left the institute to work and study as an artist in Pennsylvania, New York, and England. She is increasingly recognized as one of the great Canadian artists of her time, mastering works on paper, canvas, and glass. Although Arthur Lismer and John Lyman were her principal influences as a burgeoning artist in Montreal, *The Advance of Neurology* is inspired by the great Mexican muralists of the last century. As Filer describes it,

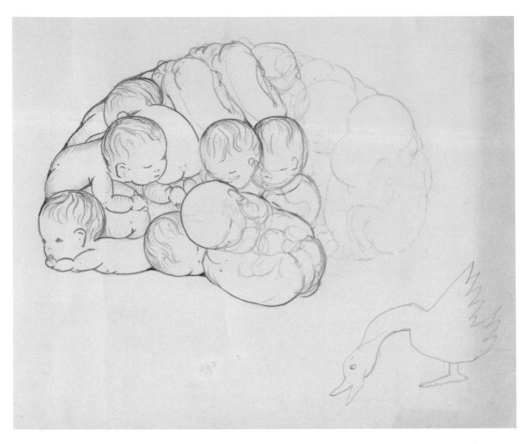

Figure 20.2: Hortense Douglas Cantlie sketch of *Children of the Brain*. Note the position of the faces at the bottom of the sensory-motor strips, and the baby holding its ear in the auditory area. (MNI Archives)

In 1953 Dr Penfield was concerned about the absence of any visual expression of his neurological advances in theory and practice. Sometime earlier he had been impressed by the murals he had seen in Mexico in which surgical procedures were depicted. He envisaged a great collage of notable neurologists surrounding him at a moment of perception in the diagnosis of epilepsy. When he found a bare wall at the end of the conference room in the new McConnell Pavilion he approached me on the possibilities of composing a mural based in his concept.

By 1954 the pursuit of Dr Penfield's vision quickened when Dr Francis McNaughton's influence came into play. It was decided that the Monday morning ward round should provide a setting for the "moment of perception" and that the collage of notable neurologists should convey a sense of the history of neurology as well as the presence of neurological genius at the Institute.[6]

In a letter to Francis McNaughton dated 7 April 1954, Filer cites other influences besides the Mexican muralists and reveals the artistic insight brought to bear in the creation of a great work of art and on the joy of creation itself:[7]

The general plan of the mural is taking shape now. I believe that simplification and change in scale is necessary to suit the dimensions of the conference room … After this long period of developing it I feel, more strongly than ever, that the subject lends itself to interpretation in the great tradition of group portraits and such compositions as Greco's "Burial of Count Orgaz," Hals' group of soldiers, Rembrandt's "Anatomy Lesson," etc. and I do so hope that we can represent various members of the Institute in idealized likenesses in the composition. I think, too, that this would be capitalizing, if you like, on some of my characteristic resources as an artist … in other parts, my delight in groups of odd-shaped objects and natural forms will lend style to the mural too where such little details occur. Of course I am mindful of the need for variety in the areas, and so much must be quiet and simple. Not only must there be strength and dignity, but also, the poetry of expression, which is peculiar to my work. I so look forward to bringing it to life on the wall.

Filer depicts neurology from pre-Columbian trephining with a flaked stone (figure 20.5), to the modern use of electroencephalography, to the shining light of future neurological discoveries.[8] The dominant figure of the mural is a likeness of Mary Filer herself as the patient. Filer also depicted herself as the nurse whose gentle hand comforts the patient on her sickbed. Above her, Eileen Flanagan looks on, satisfied that the patient is being attended to her exacting standard. Surrounding the patient in the background are the luminaries of nineteenth-century neurology. Close to her, in the forefront, are the great clinicians Charcot and Osler. Osler stands immediately above the patient, to Flanagan's right. Jean-Martin Charcot, reflective, is to her left. On the patient's bedside table rests a gloxinia.

Donald McEachern holds the patient's hand while Francis McNaughton, in white, stands at her side. Jean Saucier, holding a score of his beloved Brahms, and the kindly Roma Amyot frame McNaughton on either side. Looking on are

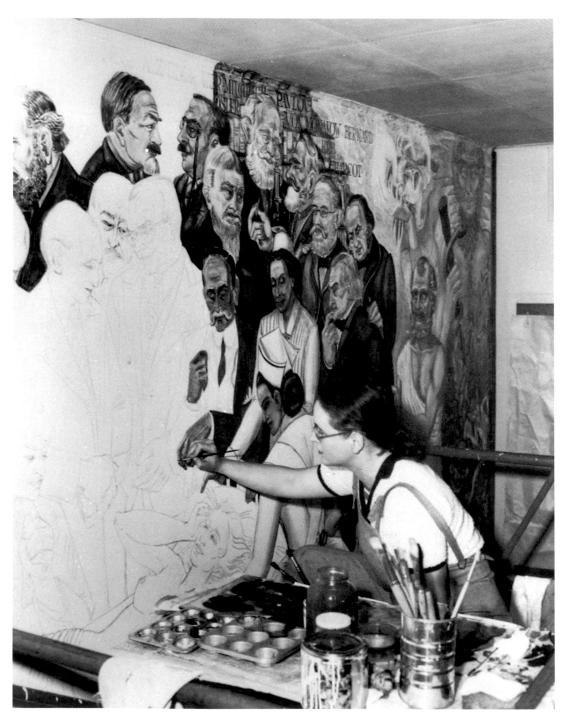

Figure 20.3: Mary Filer at work on *The Advance of Neurology*. (MNI Archives)

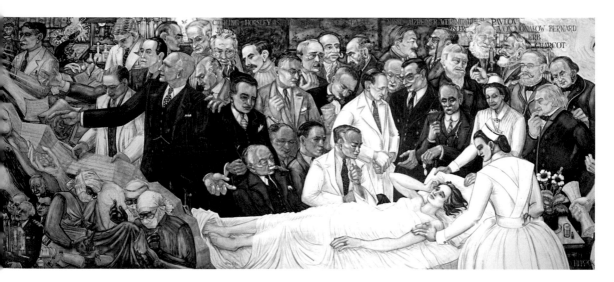

Figure 20.4: *The Advance of Neurology* (*detail*). Francis McNauthton is standing, in white lab coat. To his right, with distinguishing eyeglasses, stands Arthur Elvidge. Herbert Jasper is standing at upper left, in white lab coat and glasses, annotating an EEG print-out. The artist, Mary Filer, is depicted as the patient and the nurse in profile, attending her. To Filer's right are gloxinias, Filer's tribute to a departed friend.

Colin Russel, in brown suit and vest, and between him and McEachern sit Arthur Young and Preston Robb. Arthur Elvidge stands behind Young and Robb, and Cone, in blue, stands behind Russel. John Kershman, also in blue, stands opposite Cone. Edward Archibald stands between Penfield and Cone, his hand gently resting on both their shoulders.[9]

Rasmussen, the heir apparent, and Jasper, studious, are to Penfield's immediate right. Both he and Rasmussen look toward the future of neurology, shining brightly through open curtains. Elliott and McRae appear on either side of Rasmussen. Olsewski stands alone, the uppermost left figure, as if sequestered in his laboratory. At the left, assisting in the operating room are Penfield's assigned operating room nurse Phoebe Stanley, Mr Stanley Ellis, a beloved operating room orderly, and Penfield himself, bespectacled, intensely focused, holding a probe in his left hand, an instrument in the other.

Donors and dignitaries are depicted as a group at the lowermost left. Cyril James, principal of McGill University, is at the extreme left, in profile. John Wilson McConnell, Lily Griffith McConnell, and William Henry Donner are seen, to the right of Premier Maurice Duplessis, who is depicted in full face. Camillien Houde, mayor of Montreal, resplendent with his large bald pate, Allan

Gregg, representing the Rockefeller Foundation, and Paul Martin Sr, the federal minister of health, also appear.

To the right of the mural we see Hippocrates, who seems to be bringing enlightenment from the darkness of primitive trephining to rid the brain of evil spirits. His scroll reads, "Life is short, the art is long, opportunity fugitive, experience deceptive, judgement difficult."

Mary Filer's mural continues to reveal its secret, as in a letter from Filer to William Feindel dated 31 May 2007: "The pot of flowers is a gloxinia, one of my favorites. If you wonder about the choice of plant it is because it was introduced to me in my nursing training, by an admirer! And sadly, as I was just completing the mural, news came of his sudden demise – and I was moved to include it as a memorium."

Earlier, Filer had written, "It is not known who was first disturbed over the half-covered patient's body, but early in 1955 Dr Penfield asked me to repaint the covering sheet, extending it up to the neck and down to the ankle! Some years after, and probably because of the repainting of the sheet, the mural was declared an Historical Document of McGill University."[10]

EPILEPSY AND THE FUNCTIONAL ANATOMY OF THE HUMAN BRAIN

The opening of the McConnell Wing celebrations did not replace the MNI's other academic activities. Professor Théophile Alajouanine, from la Salpêtrière in Paris, gave the 1954 Hughlings Jackson lecture, "Verbal Expression in Aphasia." Sir Russell Brain, Churchill's last physician, presented "Encephalitis and Encephalopathy in Childhood." As chance would have it, in that same year the institute also hosted John Walton, who would edit Brain's classic textbooks *Diseases of the Nervous System*.[11] Roger Sperry, then at the University of Chicago, read "Cutaneous Sensibility." Sperry was awarded the Nobel Prize in 1981 for his work on cerebral dominance, sharing the prize with David Hubel, vice-president of the MNI Fellows Society that year, who was in the audience for Sperry's address.

The most significant academic event of 1954, however, was the publication of *Epilepsy and the Functional Anatomy of the Human Brain*, Penfield and Jasper's magnum opus.[12] It is encyclopedic in its coverage of epilepsy and its treatment; and represents the summation of every aspect of the work done at the MNI to the time of its publication. Notably, it illustrates for the first time the somatotopic organization of the thalamus.

THE CENTRENCEPHALIC INTEGRATING SYSTEM

As one reviewer of *Functional Anatomy* pointed out, the centrencephalic integrating system "runs like a silver thread of continuity through many chapters."[13] Although he had alluded to it in his 1936 Harvey Lecture, "The Cerebral Cortex and Consciousness," Penfield coined the term *centrencephalic integrating system* in an address at the December 1950 meeting of the Association for Research in Nervous and Mental Disease, after consultation with Herbert Jasper and Stanley Cobb. The address, published in 1952, was entitled "Epileptic Automatism and the Centrencephalic Integrating System."[14]

Although the centrencephalic system is unnamed in his 1936 address, Penfield's meaning is quite clear. When he speaks of consciousness and asks, "Where shall wisdom be found? And where is the place of understanding?," he is not speaking metaphorically. He is endowing his use of the word *consciousness* with the attributes of the mind: self-awareness, reason, judgment, the will to act – the mind. And where shall it be found? Not in the cortex:

> Finally, there is much evidence of a level of integration within the central nervous system that is higher than that to be found in the cerebral cortex, evidence of a regional localization of the neuronal mechanism involved in this integration. I suggest that this region lies not in the new brain but in the old – that it lies below the cerebral cortex and above the midbrain.
>
> Such localization does not signify that other parts of the brain play no role in this mechanism. All regions of the brain may well be involved in normal conscious processes, but the indispensable substratum of consciousness lies outside the cerebral cortex, probably in the diencephalon.
>
> This discussion has avoided the subject of the nature of consciousness. That is a psychologic problem. It has been concerned with the localization of the "place of understanding," and by "place" is meant the location of those neuronal circuits which are most intimately associated with the initiation of voluntary activity and with the sensory summation prerequisite to it.[15]

Penfield was more explicit in his 1950 address: "An understanding of the intellectual functions of the brain must wait upon clearer knowledge of the mechanisms which integrate the activity of the two hemispheres. With the beginning of this knowledge there is opening before us a new chapter in neurophsysiology, the chapter of the *mechanisms of the mind*."[16] The "mechanism which integrates the activity of the two hemispheres," as Penfield would have it, lies within the "intralaminar system of the thalamus and the reticular system," which has "widespread connections to both hemispheres, connections that would make possible the central organization of the function in the cerebral cortices."[17]

Penfield and Jasper elaborated on the role of the cortex within this construct in *The Functional Anatomy of the Human Brain*:

> It is obvious that the higher mental functions which distinguish man from lower animals, such as speech, the capacity for higher mathematics, and other abstract thought processes, are not possible without the cortex, particularly that of the frontal and temporal lobes. The vast interconnected network of cells and fibres in the cortical matrix must, therefore, constitute an essential part of the *machinery of the mind*. But without the constant selective activating influences of the reticular network of the higher brain stem, the cortical mantle lies dormant ... Highest level functions cannot therefore be strictly localized but result from the dynamic interaction between centrencephalic mechanisms and those areas of the cortex the function of which in momentarily being employed at a given time.[18]

INK BY THE BARREL

The identification of the mind with the integrative action of the upper brain stem and parts of the cerebral cortex did not meet with everyone's approval. Most notably, Penfield was severely criticized by his erstwhile friend Sir Francis Walshe, in the pages of *Brain*. "It seems scarcely credible," Walshe wrote, "that within this small and phylogenetically ancient part of the brain such numerous and complex functions could be carried out. How comes it that despite the great development of the cerebral cortex in man, the gamut of physiological and psychological activities characteristic of man, should still be carried on in these meagre collections of cells in the 'old brain,' as Penfield says?"[19] To which Penfield responded, in the same journal, "There is no room or place where consciousness dwells. But there is a place, a region of the brain, in which neuronal activity makes conscious thinking possible. Consciousness exists only in association with the passage of electrical potentials through ever-changing circuits of the brain-stem *and cortex*. One cannot say that consciousness is here, or there. But certainly, without centrencephalic integration it is non-existent."[20]

Penfield and Walshe had previously crossed swords over the homunculus. Now, there was a fresh bone to gnaw, the centrencephalic system. After restrained volleys in the pages of *Brain*, the exchange became more stinging in private correspondence,[21] which, tart as it is, has the virtue of succinctly expressing Walshe's – and others' – objection to Penfield's concept, and of clarifying Penfield's meaning. Walshe began with a letter to Penfield on 1 November 1958:

Let's be frank about all of this, you have never paid your readers the compliment of being consistent, and your repeated half-hearted emendations, made and unmade, and the wide variations of actual and hypothetical statement, have made of your hypothesis in its present state a thing of shreds and patches. It has never had a sure morphological foundation, and in effect you have dropped a unbodied hypothesis, like a cuckoo's egg, into Magoun's reticular activating nest – which is very hard upon his little family of ideas growing innocently therein, and not at all wanting this preposterous foundling foisted upon them.

Penfield's reply came on 16 January 1959:

You say I have never done readers the compliment of presenting them with grounds to support my conclusions regarding centrencephalic integration. Heavens above, man! What have I been writing about in recent years! All observations of the cortex are relevant to my conclusion … You don't seem to understand that I used the word centrencephalic only to emphasize the opinion that transcortical connections were less important for integration than those through the brain stem. Surely, the results of cortical excisions bore that out.

The letters became more vituperative, until, finally, on 3 February 1959 Penfield draws a close to the correspondence:

I suppose continuation of this correspondence serves no good purpose … My own work is drawing to a close. You call me the Emperor who "has no clothes." Well, he has no throne either. He never did sit on one, unless office administration and begging for money is that. Now he is preparing to work with his hands at a new job, as long as life's tether lets him carry on.

Penfield received a short note two days later: "Perhaps you are right … Let's call it a day and end our disputations … I am in my seventy-fourth year, and I ought to shut up. It can't be long before I do."

An unexpected request came to Penfield, on 6 December 1962, from Mc-Donald Critchley: "Many of us have thought that it would be a seemly gesture to secure a portrait [of Walshe] to hang in the National Hospital, Queen Square. It is with this object in mind that I am venturing to approach some of Walshe's friends and admirers … would you be good enough to send a cheque?" Penfield replied on 11 January 1963: "Your letter of 6 December has just come addressed to 'some of Walshe's friends and admirers.' It made me look back over the past – I'm glad to join the company and to enclose a contribution toward the painting of his portrait."

Francis Walshe died on 21 February 1973.

Figure 20.5 (*opposite*): The mythic and classical phases of neurosurgery. At the extreme right, a shaman is performing a ritualistic trepanning the skull with a sharpened flint, in an effort to rid a tribesman of the evil spirits afflicting him. Hippocrates, holding a scroll of his aphorisms, turns his back on the shamanistic practice of medicine, giding the way to the golden age of the Montreal Neurological Institute. Mary Filer, *The Advance of Neurology*, detail).

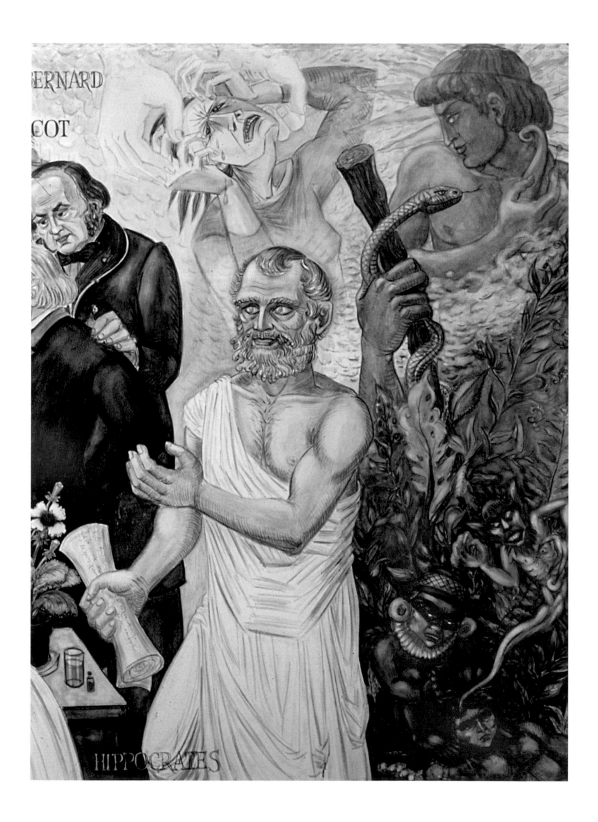

William Feindel's Departure

Reflecting his family's pioneer background, Penfield reviewed with satisfaction the Second Foundation's first year with an image worthy of Thomas Hart Benton: "We have just finished the first full year after the Institute's Second Foundation … A new harness has been fitted, strong young workers added, and each member of the team now pulls according to the strength the Good Lord gave him, knowing that the future of the common cause is secure for a season." Echoing McNaughton, twenty years earlier, Penfield continued, "It will be our policy to enlarge the permanent clinical staff still further, giving preference, in the immediate future, to men whose primary language is French until an appropriate balance is reached. It should be remembered that our objective is to demonstrate the fact that the Montreal Neurological Institute is a bilingual institute in a bilingual province."[1] Gilles Bertrand was appointed to the staff of the MNI in July 1955, as assistant neurosurgeon and assistant neuropathologist, both departments headed by Dr Cone.

DEPARTMENTAL ACTIVITIES

The Department of Neurophysiology continued charting the connections between the thalamus and the cortex, most notably through the efforts of John Hanbery and Blaine Nashold, working closely with Herbert Jasper, Cosimo Ajmone-Marsan, and Jerzy Olszewski.[2] John Hanbery was later appointed as head of the Division of Neurosurgery at Stanford University, in 1961. Nashold had a distinguished career at Duke University and was invited to give the 1984 Fellows Day Lecture during the MNI's fiftieth anniversary celebrations. Irving Heller's interests lay elsewhere, as he studied the genetics and metabolism of brain tumours in the Donner Laboratory.[3]

A significant event for all residents and fellows also occurred in the academic year 1954–55, as noted by Penfield, with an ever-watchful eye to the bottom line:

"This year the Royal Victoria Women's Auxiliary … has extended its field of service to include this Institute … and a generous anonymous donor made it possible for us to build a Coffee Shop."[4] The coffee shop, operated by the Friends of the Neuro, remained in operation into the twenty-first century, its profits, among other worthwhile endeavours, providing seed money to establish the endovascular service at the MNI.

ACADEMIA

Academic affairs continued to meet the high standards of previous years. The highlight of the academic year was the three-month tenure of Theodore Rasmussen's father, Andrew T. Rasmussen, emeritus professor at the University of Minnesota, as visiting professor of neuroanatomy.[5] Rasmussen gave the Annual Neuroanatomy Lecture, "The Cerebral Cortex." On a similar topic, but in the discipline of neurophysiology, Lloyd G. Stevenson, medical librarian at McGill University, presented "Historical Review of the Work of David Ferrier on Cerebral Localization." But perhaps the address that had the most impact on the invited *speaker* was Karl Pribram's "Temporal Lobe in Primates." Twenty tears after his visit, Pribram's interaction with Penfield on the human condition continued to resonate:

> Some twenty years ago, I addressed the Montreal Neurological Institute on the topic of temporal lobe function. My data were obtained from experiments performed with monkeys. Wilder Penfield was in the audience and opened the discussion with the question as to whether I believed that the difference between man and the nonhuman primates was quantitative or qualitative. My answer was that I believed the difference to be quantitative but of such an extent that qualitative changes emerged. I used the then new computer technology as an example. Vast increases in the capacity of the memory in central processors had changed computational power not only quantitatively but qualitatively. Penfield argued the case for a more fundamental distinction that distinguished man and we agreed to disagree.[6]

It is a monument to Penfield's insightful mind that an informal discussion in the steep tiers of the Hughlings Jackson amphitheatre set Pribram on a course of study and reflection on "What Makes Man Human,"[7] which is still commented upon today.[8]

ARRIVALS AND DEPARTURES

Theodore Rasmussen added a third neurosurgical service to the two headed by
William Cone and Arthur Elvidge. Penfield, first amongst equals, had the leisure
of choosing on which service he operated. Almost invariably, he chose Rasmussen's. Lamar Roberts returned to the MNI to continue his work on language localization, and a new resident, Charles Branch, joined the house staff.
Branch would have a major impact of the clinical and scientific activities of the
institute. Pierre Gloor also returned to the MNI from Switzerland, to become
assistant elecroencephalographer and eventually headed the department. These
arrivals, however, could hardly compensate for the many departures from the
institute to the University of Saskatchewan.

MNI ON THE PLAINS

The singular event of 1954 was the departure of William Feindel to become the
inaugural chair of the Department of Neurourgery at the newly opened Faculty
of Medicine of the University of Saskatchewan, in Saskatoon.[9]

Wilder Penfield received a letter from William Feindel on 8 October 1954
while he was travelling in Turkey, announcing his intention to leave the institute:[10]

Dear Dr Penfield,
I am writing to describe an offer which I have had for the position of
Associate Professor of Neurosurgery in charge of 20 beds at Saskatoon,
where, as you know, a new university hospital is about to open. Although
my interest in this at first was quite casual, Faith and I have been out to
look over the situation after discussing it with Ted Rasmussen, Francis
McNaughton and Dr Cone ... and provided the university out there
agrees to arrange certain clinical and research requirements, there is little doubt in my mind that I should accept the position ... The heads of
the various departments are rather unusual in that they are all young and
yet all, like Wendell MacLeod and Allan Bailey, have given up promising
positions in larger universities and hospitals to take on the challenge of
developing this new center.

Penfield responded urgently via a telegram from Istanbul stamped 22 October 1954: "PLEASE MAKE NO FINAL DECISION UNTIL YOU RECEIVE
LETTER SENT TODAY."

A very thoughtful letter from Istanbul dated 21 October 1954 followed this urgent plea.

Dear Bill,

I simply cannot think of the M.N.I. without you in the next ten years … My initial reaction is that if the University of Pennsylvania – California, Chicago, Ann Arbor, N.Y. – were to offer you a chair or even Toronto you would have to consider it. But short of that no.

Why is my initial reaction so violently against your going? … I suppose it is, first because I know the Institute needs you, second because I should miss you personally so much, third because you could do so much constructive work in the coming 5 or 10 years If you stay with us while your practice is gradually growing. You will not be able to do constructive work out there until you are organized and have developed another man to pull in equal harness with you and until you find a new Herbert Jasper and maybe a George Olszweski. [Feindel didn't need to, as Olszweski also made the trek to Saskatoon] … There is no other Institute like the M.N.I. anywhere. Nor will there be in the next 20 years, even in Saskatoon. You may develop a unit that will rival the other cities I have mentioned but you will not equal the set up in Montreal within the time of your greatest capacity … Other men finish their training and go out with our blessing. It is the normal thing but you are different. We need you and have counted on you as a permanent part of us … With Bill Cone and Arthur [Elvidge] on the job you and Herbert Jasper and Ted and I will have 5 or 10 years of scientific exploration and harvest that will mean much to each of us. Don't pass it up too lightly.

Wilder Penfield

Feindel responded on 10 November 1954, explaining his reasons for leaving.

I appreciate very much your reasons against my going although I am not sure that the Institute needs me in particular. I suppose it will continue to need young men but I do not see why others cannot do the job as well as I can (and be less demanding!) … I somehow feel that if you were in my shoes you would take the set-up at Saskatoon like a shot. It seems to me that it is what you and Dr Cone did in 1928 … I believe I have made my decision carefully and I hope wisely.

And so the die was cast and William Howard Feindel headed west, as did

Joseph Stratford. Penfield put on a brave face at the institute's loss of Feindel and Stratford and at Olszewski's imminent departure:

> Changes have occurred this year, changes sweet and bitter. The Medical School and Hospital of the University of Saskatchewan has taken Dr William Feindel from us to head the Department of Neurosurgery and Dr Joseph Stratford to be his assistant … A serious loss is that of Dr George [Jerzy] Olszewski, who will leave us this summer to go to the University of Saskatchewan. He has done brilliant work in neuroanatomy since he came from Poland eight years ago. Our best wishes go with him and all the others. It is good to realize that in leaving us they do not desert our common cause.[11]

William Feindel initiated the Department of Neurosurgery at the University of Saskatchewan, which he headed from 1955 to 1959, and his time there was in every way formative and innovative. But, as Alan Gregg had suggested during his Second Foundation address, those who have trained and worked for a time at an institute such as the MNI "ought to leave after a stipulated period of two or perhaps four years, and those that are wanted back can be called back."[12] William Feindel's callback came on 4 May 1959 with the passing of William Vernon Cone.

◆◆◆

Bill Feidel's departure was not the only loss sustained by the MNI early in this half-century: Colin Russel, a monument to Canadian neurology, died on 4 March 1956 (figure 21.1).[13] His colleagues and friends remembered him as a wise, kindly, dignified man with a pioneering spirit. He loved adventure, particularly in his youth. During his student years he joined a geological survey each summer and was among the first Caucasians to cross the northern Labrador Peninsula. Penfield, with his usual heartfelt eloquence, was moved to write, "We mourn the passing of Colin Russel, friend, companion, teacher, explorer, soldier and troubadour. He was the founder of Neurology in the Montreal Neurological Institute, a renowned leader in the field. Words seem inadequate to express the affection we felt for him, all of us. Principal James has said that the memory and tradition that cling to an institution may be immortal. So it will be with our first neurologist. I borrow the phrase we have heard him use so often, 'Bless you.' Bless you, Colin Russel."[14]

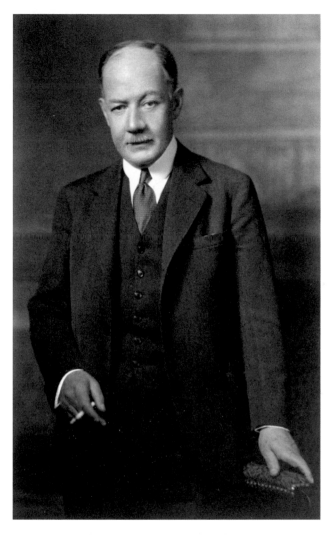

Figure 21.1: Colin Russel. (MNI Archives)

Hugh McLennan, who had carried out the early studies with Ernst Florey on gamma aminobutyric acid, left the institute to take a position at Dalhousie University, Halifax. Irving Heller, who was apointed assistant clinical neuro-chemist, replaced him. André Pasquet, who had "been indefatigable and conscientious in the extreme" in his leadership of Anaesthesia at the MNI, also moved to Dalhousie.[15] Maurice Héon also left the institute. His move was not as far eastward as Hugh McLennan's and André Pasquet's, but ended in the Eastern Townships of Quebec, as he became the founding professor of the Department of Neurosurgery at the Université de Sherbrooke.

THE LIFE OF THE INSTITUTE

A great institution mourns its losses but stays the course, replenished by bright young and devoted fellows. Mark Rayport and his wife Shirley Ferguson were of that group, as were Nicholas Zervas, Gordon Thompson, and Juhn Wada. Mark Rayport became professor and chief of Neurosurgery at the University of Toledo, Ohio. He and his wife were great friends and benefactors of the MNI, endowing a very generous fellowship in epilepsy.[16] Nicholas Zervas was later chief of Neurosurgery at the Massachusetts General Hospital. Gordon Thompson became chief of Neurosurgery at the Vancouver General Hospital, and June Wada – who introduced the carotid amytal test at the MNI – had a distinguished career at the University of British Columbia, where he pioneered the study of "kindling" in the genesis of epileptic seizures.[17] Frank Morrell was also interested in secondary epileptogenesis. Echoing Theodore Erickson's earlier work and as a foreshadowing of his contributions to secondary epileptogenesis, Morrell did important work at the institute on the connectivity of epileptic foci.[18] Frank Morrell became chairman of Neurology at Stanford University – at the age of thirty-three.[19]

Eighteen fellows and staff worked in the Neurophysiology Department in 1955, on projects ranging from microelectrode recordings of epileptic discharges to studies of the neurophysiological mechanisms of learning. Significant publications came from the pens of Gloor on the connections of the amygdala, Heller and Elliott on cerebral metabolism, and David Ingvar on the cerebral cortex.[20]

ACADEMIA

As in previous years, distinguished invited speakers visited the institute.[21] Amongst all the brilliant and celebrated visitors to come to the institute since its opening, one stands out as truly remarkable: Diana Beck, senior neurosurgeon from Middlesex Hospital. Beck had specialized in neurosurgery with Sir Hugh Cairns in Oxford in 1939, and she also worked with former MNI fellow Dorothy Russell, most notably on thrombosis of the superior longitudinal sinus.[22] She came into public prominence when she operated upon A.A. Milne, author of *Winnie the Pooh*.[23] Her address at the institute, "Acute Postoperative Compression in the Posterior Fossa," was probably the last one she gave, as she died in March 1956, aged fifty-four, from complications of a thymectomy performed for myasthenia gravis. Sir Geoffrey Keynes, who popularized thymectomy for this condition, discussed this procedure the following year as a guest speaker at the MNI.[24]

The Red Arrow Express

As in previous years, noteworthy publications originated from the institute, including a report of Wilder Penfield's second trip to the Soviet Union.[25] This was a whirlwind tour of showcased neurological institutes. Six were in Moscow, including the Burdenko Institute of Neurosurgery of the Academy of Medical Sciences. Penfield had met Burdenko in 1943 when he was chief surgeon of the Red Army. From Moscow, Penfield took the *Red Arrow Express* to Leningrad, where he visited four institutes, including two in which Pavlov had worked.

These institutions were all engaged in expanding the Pavlovian concept of reflex action of the central nervous system. Penfield seems to have been a hail-fellow-well-met in his visits and lectures, as he recounts: "In Leningrad a member of the audience startled me by asking how the patient K.M. was getting along! Fortunately, I recalled the case of K.M. which I published, with Professor Donald Hebb, in 1940, under the title 'Human Behaviour after Extensive Bilateral Removal from the Frontal Lobes.' I replied that K.M. was well and working full time, but that he proved to be irresponsible, shifting about from job to job. When I added that possibly they had known workmen like that in the U.S.S.R., even without operation, there was a general laugh."[26]

Perhaps it was the train trip from Moscow to Leningrad on the *Red Arrow Express* and the proximity of the Neva River that brought on a reflective mood, but Penfield's stay in Leningrad provides insight into the romantic aspects of his nature and his interest in the brain–mind relationship. At Pavlov's Institute of Physiology, Penfield's imagination took flight: "This institute is housed in a curiously curved building on the Neva River. From the front door a grand staircase of white marble leads upward to the second floor. As we climbed I could hear the faint echo of the barking dogs and I thought of how often Pavlov had himself climbed those stairs and savoured the familiar smells and sights and sounds. A superstitious dualist, if one had been present, might have fancied that the spirit of Pavlov was walking with us through the laboratory."[27] Penfield would continue to mull the two extremes at play in that statement, the materialistic conception of the mind as a series conditioned reflexes, and the idealist separation of the mind and brain. Penfield continued his reflection on this subject in the following year's annual report, where he seemed to favour the Pavlovian view: "The long-term project of this Institute is to fill the gap in knowledge between nerve impulse and the mind of man. The brain with its appendages constitutes man's master organ. We have made a beginning of study. In the years that lie ahead, workers will come, no doubt, to comprehend this master organ. Then, perhaps, they will understand the mind, and even man's behaviour. And, at last, when he is better acquainted with himself, who knows, Man may even understand the love of God."[28]

Penfield's recounting of his trip to Russia is telling of his naïveté toward the political situation at the time, as he ends his account of his travels in Russia: "As I look back on that busy fortnight I realize that there is much less difference than there was between life in the U.S.S.R. and our life in the West."[29] Coming barely a year before Russian tanks entered Budapest under Khrushchev, it is a striking statement. Added to the fact that much of the scientific work at the time was done by scientists and engineers in labour camps, the immensity of the statement enters the realm of fiction.[30]

The MNI made significant contributions to more traditional areas of Pavlovian physiology as Wilder Penfield and Murl Faulk studied the role of the insula in gastrointestinal function in patients in whom "gastric tone and motility were recorded by means of an inflated intra-gastric balloon ... connected to a ... manometer." Stimulation of the insula during surgery for the resection of an epileptogenic focus "demonstrated clearly that, in conscious men, the island of Reil can exert a control over gastric motility and stomach tone."[31]

Despite these forays confirming the brain's service to the gut, the most significant publication of 1955 – some would argue the most significant publication of the institute – was "The Effects of Hippocampal Lesions on Recent Memory" by Brenda Milner and Wilder Penfield, presented at the eightieth meeting of the American Neurological Association in Chicago in 1955. This communication was followed two years later by the more widely known "Loss of Recent Memory after Bilateral Hippocampal Lesions," which Brenda Milner wrote with William Beecher Scoville, on the case of Henry Gustav Molaison, patient H.M.

Neuropsychology at the MNI

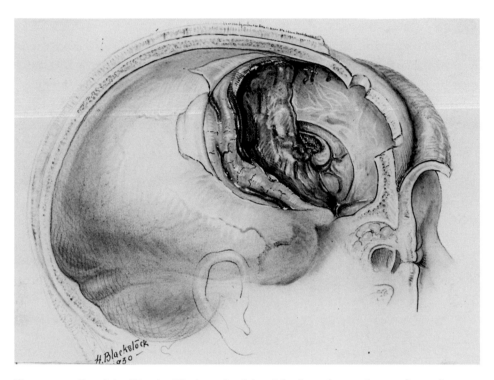

Figure 22.1: Sketch by Harriet Blackstock of the right frontal resection performed by Penfield on his sister Ruth Inglis. (W. Penfield and J. Evans, "The Frontal Lobe in Man: A Clinical Study of Maximum Removal," *Brain* 58 [1935]: 115–33.)

PENFIELD, EVANS, AND THE FRONTAL LOBES

To destroy a delicate instrument is not the best way of studying its function.
– Penfield and Evans

The psychological and behavioural effects of resection of cerebral tissue had been a concern from the earliest days of the institute, most notably large resections of the frontal lobes. This was first addressed in "The Frontal Lobe in Man: A Clinical Study of Maximum Removal" by Wilder Penfield and Joseph Evans, published in *Brain* in 1935.[1] The paper, a report of only three cases, is perhaps more touching than informative: one of the patients was Penfield's sister Ruth, whose frontal lobe had been invaded by a cerebral tumour.

As William Feindel recounted to the editor of *Brain*, Penfield "was urged to operate on Ruth by his neurosurgical colleagues Eddie Archibald and Bill Cone; Colin Russel, who provided neurological counsel, agreed with this decision. For the first time they used the arrangement of drapes allowing communication under local anaesthesia learned from Otto Foerster in Breslau … It was a harrowing experience since in attempting to remove the last part of the tumour deep in the mesial frontal region, and against Cone's advice, Penfield caused 'massive bleeding." Penfield referred to it as "a sharp haemorrhage."[2]

Penfield's sister recovered from surgery and the question arose of further treatment in the form of radiation therapy. Penfield wrote Cushing for his advice on 13 December 1929:

> Dear Dr Cushing,
>
> I wish to ask you a word of advice. The day before yesterday I removed most of the right frontal lobe of a patient who had an Oligodendroglioma … You will understand how much this case means to me when I tell you that it was my own sister … I had to leave some tumour behind in the vicinity of the corpus callosum; I do not know whether it goes across to the other side or not. She had a close shave of it, but is doing very well. Would you advise my using x-ray therapy, or would it be better just to let her go and if the symptoms occur again re-operate? … As a matter of fact I should have very much preferred bringing her to you, but the family, spurred on by a strange type of confidence, was anxious to have me do it. Will you please give me your advice about subsequent therapy?

Cushing replied on 15 December 1928:

> Dear Penfield:
>
> I am distressed to learn of your sister's malady and that circumstances forced you to take the case on yourself, but I am glad to have been spared the anxiety of operating on a member of your family and rejoice to learn that she is doing well. I don't believe I would recommend radiation. We have not had a great deal of experience in radiation on these particular tumours, and they are as a matter of fact as benign as any form of glioma … [Percival] Bailey is making just now a study of all our cases. They are

curiously much alike, and I would suggest your writing him to ask something about the prognosis. As he has gone into the matter more recently than I have, his information will be more valuable than any I could give you.

So for your own comfort do send him a couple of slides with an outline of the history, and ask him from our Brigham experience what you may expect; and then like a good man do let me know what he says – that is, whether he agrees with me or not about the radiation and with you as to the histogenesis of the lesion.[3]

The effects of extensive damage to the frontal lobes were largely unknown beyond the famous case of Phineas Gage, and there were concerns that similar alterations in personality would befall patients after a large frontal lobe resection. Gage was a railroad worker laying track in Vermont in 1848 when the spark from a ramrod ignited a powder charge that propelled a metal rod three feet long through his left cheek and out the top of his head, damaging both frontal lobes. Gage appeared well after he recovered from the immediate effects of the blow. However, some months later, from the kind and considerate man that he had been before his accident, it was discerned by his physician, John Harlow, that "the equilibrium or balance, so to speak, between [Gage's] intellectual faculties and animal propensities, seemed to have been destroyed." Gage became "fitful, irreverent, … impatient … capricious and vacillating, devising many plans of future operations, which [were] no sooner arranged than they are abandoned."[4] Gage rambled through the Americas as a sideshow attraction. His skull and the offending rod made their final appearance in the Warren Anatomical Museum of the Countway Medical Library at Harvard Medical School, where they remain. Concerned that a similar calamity might befall his sister, Penfield closely observed her following her operation while she was in hospital and later at home, tending to her daily chores. "There was no change in personality or capacity for insight," Penfield observed, "nevertheless the loss of the right frontal lobe had resulted in an important defect. The defect produced was a lack of capacity for planned administration. Perhaps the element which made such administration almost impossible was the loss of power of initiative."[5]

Penfield also recounts the subsequent course of his sister's illness: "Twenty-two months later, following a rather sudden reappearance of symptoms, she was re-operated upon at our request by Dr Harvey Cushing who found a recurrence of the tumour and removed it again without any further amputation of cerebral tissue. She continued to feel well but six months later died from hemorrhage into the tumour."[6]

The brain was removed at autopsy and two photographs of it, one from the top, one from the bottom, were published in Penfield and Evans's paper. Later, Penfield used samples from her tumour to illustrate the histological appearance of an oligodendroglioma.

Penfield and Evans's paper was not without flaw: there were only three patients upon which to draw ostensibly generalizable conclusions, the principal observer could in no way be considered objective, at least in one case, and standardized neuropsychological pre- and post-operative tests were not performed, let alone by a trained observer. These deficiencies needed to be corrected if subsequent observations on the effects of resection of the frontal lobes were to be of value. Nonetheless, the paper was greatly influential.

Penfield presented these three cases to the 1935 International Congress of Neurology in London, "at which Richard Brickner also reported on a patient in whom Walter Dandy had removed the frontal lobes, and Carlyle Jacobsen described the effects of bilateral frontal lobectomy in two chimpanzees. Antonio Caetano de Abreu Freire Egas Moniz – professor of neurology, contributor to the introduction of cerebral angiography, minister of foreign affairs, ambassador to Spain, later Nobel laureate, and near-fatal victim in his office of a gun-toting schizophrenic – listening in the audience, returned to Portugal and, on 12 November 1935, persuaded his neurosurgical colleague Almeida Lima to make a lesion in the frontal lobes of a psychotic individual, thereby initiating the discipline of psychosurgery. Donald Hebb, with whom Penfield later collaborated, considered that "Penfield changed the whole doctrine and theory of frontal lobe function and the basis of so-called frontal lobe signs."[7]

HARROWER AND HEBB

The First Department of Psychology at the MNI

Penfield and Evans's paper clearly indicated that the MNI was in need of trained psychologists to properly assess the cognitive, behavioural, and psychosocial impact of frontal resections. Penfield proposed two candidates to the Department of Psychology at McGill University to fill that need: Molly Harrower and Donald Hebb. Bringing them to the institute, however, was not without difficulty, and it is astonishing to read that the appointment of D.O. Hebb, one of the most influential psychologists of the last century, was "hanging fire," as clearly stated in a letter of 9 February 1938 addressed to Penfield from the Department of Psychology:

Dear Dr Penfield,
    I had the pleasure of a visit from Dr Molly Harrower. Like Dr Hebb I

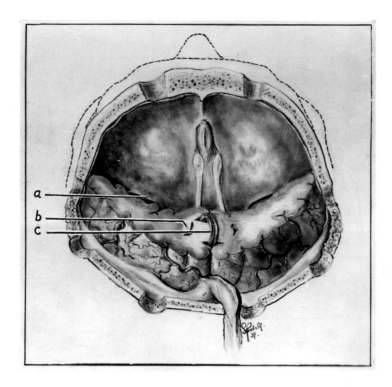

Figure 22.2: Harriet Blackstock's drawing of the extent of resection in patient K.M. (Penfield Archives) *A* represents the sphenoid ridge, *B* the tip of the frontal horns of the lateral ventricles, and *C* the pericallosal artery as it curves around the genu of the corpus callosum. (D.O. Hebb and W. Penfield, "Human Behavior after Extensive Bilateral Removal from the Frontal Lobes," *Archives of Neurology and Psychiatry* 44 [1940]: 425)

think that she is a very real addition to our little psychology community. I was very much impressed by her.

So far Dr Hebb's attachment to this department is hanging fire. Dean Hendel appears to be hesitant and perhaps a word from you would stir him into action. He asked for definite hours for Dr Hebb and I replied that was a matter between you and I. As the calendar matter is now in hand I would like to have his appointment settled as soon as possible so that his name could be included.

Sincerely yours

[Illegible]

Fortunately for the MNI and McGill University, Penfield was able to cut through the red tape, and Harrower and Hebb were appointed lecturers in clinical psychology at the institute. Had Penfield not prevailed, McGill would have

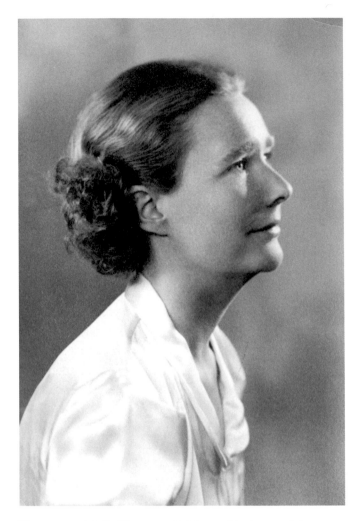

Figure 22.3: Molly Harrower-Erickson. (Archives of the History of American Psychology, the Drs Nicholas and Dorothy Cummings Center for the History of Psychology, University of Akron)

lost in Hebb a future chair of psychology and a chancellor of the university, and in Harrower the MNI its first head of Psychology.

Molly Harrower

Mary Molly Rachel Harrower was truly extraordinary: intelligent, well-educated, well-travelled, and infected with a spirit of adventure. She was born in Johannesburg and educated in London, Paris, and Switzerland. She studied psychology at the University of London and obtained a fellowship to Smith College in Massachusetts, where she studied Gestalt therapy with Kurt Goldstein. Allan Gregg, vice-president of the Rockefeller Foundation, directed her to Wilder Penfield and the MNI, where she arrived in 1937, in time to contribute a chapter on the psychological assessment of epileptic patients to Penfield and Erickson's "Epilepsy and Cortical Localization."

"It was incredible," she related in an interview. "I was really coping with being the only woman in the hospital, the only woman fellow, the only woman on the staff and the only psychologist. It was [a] very lonely and extraordinary time."[8] She was not "the only psychologist" for very long, because both she and Hebb are listed as lecturers in clinical psychology and both appear in the 1938 staff photograph. "During this time, working with colleagues such as Donald Hebb, Harrower began to come into her own as a researcher in clinical settings … most spectacularly, Harrower was the psychologist under the surgical tent when Penfield did his astounding open-skull direct brain stimulation studies."[9] Following the first of these nine-hour sessions, Harrower relates, she went back to her apartment and fell into bed. Before long she was in a deep sleep – with the bath water running![10] Despite this soggy beginning, Harrower quickly began adding to the breadth of the academic work of the institute by analyzing the effects of cortical lesions on perception.[11] Hebb left Montreal a few years after his appointment to the institute, but the Department of Psychology continued with Molly Harrower as clinical psychologist and Matilda Steiner as assistant clinical psychologist.[12] One of Harrower's major contributions at the MNI was in war research, assessing the fitness to serve of aviators and other recruits, which she did largely with the use of a modified Rorschach test of her own design.[13] Another psychologist who would have an immense impact on the activities of the institute, Brenda Milner, was doing similar work in Britain at the time.[14]

Molly Harrower had married Theodore Erickson in 1938 and left with him for the University of Wisconsin, Madison, in 1941. Of her stay in Montreal she would reflect that it "was very successful because it enabled me to have four years of establishing the first Psychology Department in a hospital." She and her husband "were very popular and had a great time."[15] However, Harrower and Erickson divorced in 1944 and Molly Harrower moved to New York City, where she established a successful psychoanalytic practice.[16] She returned to academic life in 1967 when she accepted a position as professor of clinical psychology at the University of Florida-Gainesville.

This Gaunt Maritimer

It can easily be argued that, after Penfield, one of the most influential people to have frequented 3801 University Street in the shadow of Mont-Royal was Donald Olding Hebb (figure 23.1). As Hebb scholar Richard Brown and one of Hebb's most distinguished students and colleagues, Peter Milner, succinctly put it, "Hebb's name is increasingly used as an adjective, so that we have the Hebb synapse, Hebbian synaptic plasticity, Hebbian learning rules, Hebbian neural networks," and as proof of the originality of his thinking, there is "even anti-Hebbian learning."[17] Donald Hebb was born in Nova Scotia in 1904. Like many great intellectuals, he had difficulty with his early schooling, some of which was in one room where a single teacher taught many grades. Perhaps this early experience influenced his later thinking on the importance of early learning on psycho-physiological behaviour.

Hebb first came to the Department of Psychology at McGill University in 1928, but he was dissatisfied with the Freudian bent that held sway in the department at the time, and with the poor quality of the research being done. His first stay in Montreal was also marked by personal tragedy with the death of his wife at an early age. Seeking a new start and a new discipline, Hebb embraced a physiological approach to psychology, a field in which he later conceived of the fundamental mechanism underlying learning and memory, as the result of repeated activity across a synapse leading to a permanent biochemical change in its constituents. This results in a facilitated synaptic response referred to as an engram.[18] Thus, Hebb left McGill for the University of Chicago to work with Karl Lashley and later moved with him to Harvard, which awarded him a doctorate in 1936. Donald Hebb returned to McGill in September 1937 and joined Molly Harrower as a lecturer in clinical psychology at the MNI.

Hebb's first task was an extension of Evans's work, the study of the psychological effects of frontal lobe resections.[19] Hebb reported on four patients who had undergone large frontal resections and whose IQ he had measured. One patient had been tested pre-operatively and his IQ scores were not affected by surgery. The other three patients were only tested post-operatively, but their IQs were in the normal range. Hebb concluded that "any effect of frontal lobectomy upon intelligence test performance must be relatively small." Nonetheless, Hebb commented that "the lack of symptoms in the individual case does not preclude the discovery of systematic group deviations from the normal, or deviations distinguishing temporal lobe cases, for example, from frontal lobe cases." He added that, to be valid, conclusions must rest on "the use of standard psychological measures" that can be collated and compared by different clinics. Further, he bemoaned the deficiencies of the psychometric tests available at the time. Brenda Milner and an ever-growing bevy of brilliant collaborators would later address these deficiencies.

Nociferous Cortex

Hebb's next paper was a report with Penfield on the case of a very well-studied patient, K.M., whose fame had preceded Penfield to Russia (figure 22.2). K.M.'s case was very similar to that of Phineas Gage. K.M. was a sixteen-year-old sawmill worker when an overhead carrier struck him on the head. The injury was so severe that he remained unconscious for ten days. The force of the blow was directed to the left frontal bone and orbit, but the resultant fracture extended bilaterally. Like Gage, K.M. was "irresponsible, childishly stubborn, restless and forgetful" after his injury, but it was recurring seizures that brought him to the MNI.[20] K.M. underwent the psychometric tests available at the time, and large, bilateral frontal lobectomies were performed. Much to Hebb's surprise, the patient's behaviour improved and his test scores increased postoperatively! Similarly, Molly Harrower noted a significant improvement in his pre-operative personality disorder. Hebb and Penfield introduced the concept of the *nociferous cortex* to explain these changes produced by surgery, suggesting that "abnormal cerebral activity in a region of pathologic change is capable of interfering with the normal activity of the rest of the brain."[21] Once the epileptic area was removed, the remainder of the brain, no longer bombarded by repetitive epileptic discharges, returned to normal activity. The idea of the nociferous cortex frequently recurs in Penfield's writings.

Hebb's stay at the MNI was short-lived. He left for Queen's University in 1939 and later worked with Lashley studying primates. Hebb returned to McGill as professor in the Department of Psychology in 1947 and was appointed chair of the department a year later. With Hebb and Harrower gone, the MNI was left without a designated neuropsychologist, an unfortunate situation that prevailed until 1950, when a young woman came to Montreal, ostensibly for one year, and stayed for the whole of her unparalleled career.

BRENDA MILNER AND THE RENEWAL OF PSYCHOLOGY AT THE MNI

Call Me Brenda

Brenda Milner, née Langford, was born in Manchester, England, in July 1918. She was taught French as a schoolgirl by her mother, a skill that would serve her well in her future career in Montreal. She entered Newnham College, Cambridge, in 1936, to study mathematics but soon realized that she would never excel in that discipline and transferred, much to her mother's chagrin, to psychology. The Department of Psychology at Cambridge had a strong physiological orientation and shared quarters with the renowned physiologist Lord Edgar Adrian, who, with Sir Charles Sherrington, had been awarded the Nobel Prize in 1932. Langford's supervisor at Cambridge was the distinguished psychologist Oliver Zangwill, who encouraged her in the study of the behavioural effect of brain lesions as a means of gaining insight into normal cerebral function. Langford married Peter Milner, a physicist – and later noted neuropsy-

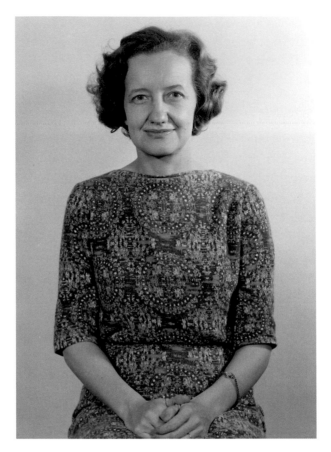

Figure 22.4: Brenda Milner. (MNI Archives)

chologist – and accompanied him to Canada, where he came to help in establishing atomic energy research at Chalk River, Ontario. Brenda Milner took an appointment in the Department of Psychology at the Université de Montréal under Father Noël Mailloux, "a Dominican priest whose somewhat unconventional approach to psychology combined the teachings of St Thomas Aquinas with those of Freud."[22] She joined D.O. Hebb as a graduate student at McGill University in 1949, and was assigned to the MNI to study patients operated upon for the treatment of focal epilepsy, while doing research for her dissertation, "Intellectual Effects of Temporal-Lobe Damage in Man."[23] Thus, in June 1950, Brenda Milner relates, "I began to carry out research at the MNI, and knew immediately that this was the kind of work I wished to pursue, whatever the practical difficulties. Meantime, the only advice Hebb gave me was to make myself as useful as I could and not to get in anyone's way. He also bequeathed me a few tests. The rest was up to me."[24]

Milner's initial experience with the effects of frontal lobe resections largely mirrored Hebb's and Penfield's. When, however, she applied a test that measures "the ability to shift from one mode of solution to another," she found that it was impaired in frontal patients.[25] Milner found the same deficiencies in K.M. in 1962 and concluded that well-chosen tasks designed to assess a specific function could reveal previously unsuspected frontal lobe deficits.[26] Thus, using appropriate tests, she was able to discern that left frontal lobe resections sparing Broca's area nonetheless limited spontaneous speech, and difficulty in generating abstract designs was found in patients with right frontal resections by Milner's student, Marilyn Jones-Gotman.[27] Over the subsequent years, others came to the MNI to study frontal lobe function, including Michael Petrides from Cambridge University, who would eventually succeed Brenda Milner as the head of the Department of Neuropsychology at the institute.

The importance of Milner's observations on frontal lobe function notwithstanding, the early part of her career is mostly remembered for her remarkable work on the temporal lobes' function and memory.

THE DUALITY OF MEMORY

Initially, the surgical treatment of temporal lobe epilepsy was limited to resection of the lateral neocortex because of the severe behavioural deficits reported by Kluver and Bucy following bilateral hippocampectomy.[28] However, clinical observations and experimental results suggested that mesial temporal structures might be involved in generating epileptic seizures.[29] Thus, gingerly, surgeons began to encroach on the amygdala and hippocampus. It was during this evolutionary period at the MNI that Brenda Milner came to examine Penfield's patients and found the seat of memory, or at least one of its haunts.

Examining patients of Penfield and his colleagues pre- and post-operatively, Milner was able to identify a deficiency in the appreciation of spatial relations in patients whose epilepsy originated in the right temporal lobe.[30] She later observed that patients with left temporal lobe epilepsy complained of poor memory. She found, upon further questioning, that "the examples they gave were always from the domain of verbal memory. They forgot what they heard and what they read. It seemed that, whether I liked it or not, I ought to begin investigating memory." The chance came earlier than she had anticipated when "in fairly rapid succession we [saw] two cases of severe memory loss following unilateral anterior temporal lobectomy."[31] Her encounter with patients P.B. and F.C., as they are referred to in the medical literature, would now localize short-term memory to the hippocampi.

Penfield's Cases

Patient P.B. had first been operated upon for left temporal lobe epilepsy in 1946, when Penfield's standard operation was limited to the lateral neocortex, leaving the mesial structures undisturbed. Although P.B. exhibited no memory deficiencies, his seizures remained poorly controlled. Thus, he underwent a second operation, in 1951, when the left mesial structures were removed. Unlike the first, lateral resection, the mesial resection was "followed by a severe, persistent, and generalized impairment of recent memory … The impairment was manifest clinically as a profound anterograde amnesia, such that the experiences of daily life were forgotten as soon as the patient's attention shifted to a new topic."[32] A second patient with left temporal lobe epilepsy, referred to as F.C., was later encountered. By this time, Penfield's standard temporal lobe resection included the mesial structures contained within the uncus (the amygdala and anterior hippocampus), and a varying extent of the hippocampus. It became immediately apparent post-operatively that F.C. exhibited the same memory deficits as had P.B. A review of both cases revealed that epileptic activity had also been recorded from the un-operated, right temporal lobe. Penfield and Milner concluded that although the resected mesial structures had been the most epileptogenic, the opposite structures must have also been damaged. Moreover, in previous operations when the amygdala had been removed and the hippocampus spared, there had been no memory impairment. Thus, bilateral hippocampal damage was felt to be the cause of the short-term memory loss. This hypothesis was later confirmed when patient P.B.'s autopsy revealed long-standing right hippocampal atrophy.[33]

Night Train to Hartford

A report of these two cases was read at the 80th Annual Meeting of the American Neurological Association in Chicago, on 13 June 1955, and later came to the attention of William Beecher Scoville. Scoville, a neurosurgeon in Hartford, Connecticut, contacted Wilder Penfield and told him that he had a patient, H.M., in whom he had performed bilateral hippocampectomies and who had memory deficits similar to those that Penfield and Milner had reported. So Brenda Milner made her first of many trips to Hartford to study H.M.[34]

As Milner recalled,

> Scoville had designed the operation of bilateral medial temporal lobe resection as an alternative to frontal lobotomy in the treatment of seriously ill schizophrenic patients. Because of the known connections between

the medial temporal region and the orbital frontal cortex, he had hoped that this procedure would prove psychiatrically beneficial, while avoiding the undesirable side effects of a frontal lobotomy. As it turned out, the operation did little to alleviate the psychosis, and any memory changes went undetected until much later, when I had the opportunity to examine eight of these patients. Although some were difficult to test, I did manage to establish the presence of anterograde amnesia in all cases where the removal had encroached upon the hippocampus and parahippocampal gyrus, but not where the removal was limited to the uncus and amygdala.[35]

H.M. – identified as Henry Gustav Molaison after his death in 2008, at the age of eighty-two – had long suffered from incapacitating, medically refractory seizures and underwent bilateral hippocampectomies in 1953.[36] After he had recovered from surgery, it became obvious that Molaison had severe recent and retrograde amnesia: "He could not remember what he had had for breakfast, and he could no longer find his way around the hospital or recognize members of the hospital staff."[37] Milner first met Mr Molaison at Scoville's request in April 1955 and immediately recognized that he suffered from the same deficits as the two patients she had encountered in Montreal.[38]

Milner observed that H.M. was able to remember information for thirty to forty seconds, after which he could not recall information or instructions given to him. This appeared to "support the distinction between a primary memory process with a rapid decay and an overlapping secondary process ... by which the long-term storage of information is achieved."[39] Specialized tasks from the McGill experimental psychology laboratory, however, showed that H.M. was able to accomplish complex visual-motor tasks, after prolonged, repeated instructions, although he had no recollection of having performed that particular task before.[40] This indicated that motor skills could be learned independently of the mesio-temporal structures, and pointed to "the existence of more than one memory system in the brain ... It was not until much later that the concept of multiple memory systems became widely accepted."[41]

Interestingly, magnetic resonance imaging has shown, as Milner had suspected, that the damage to H.M.'s brain extended beyond the hippocampi to include the perirhinal and entorhinal cortices, part of the para-hippocampal gyrus and the amygdala.[42] Henry Molaison donated his brain to science. And, just as Oskar Vogt studied Lenin's brain, H.M's brain will be studied with, it is hoped, more instructive results.

The Stream of Consciousness

Brenda Milner and Wilder Penfield agreed to disagree on the topic of memory, which Penfield based on his operative findings and the concept of the centrencephalic integrating system. Penfield had postulated that memory is stored in the brain as a chronological and continuous ribbon, or, as he affirmed, as "a strange tape recorder capable of bringing back sounds and sights and thoughts."[43] Penfield at first localized this narrative record of past events in the neocortex of the temporal lobes: "where local electrical stimulation can call back a sequence of past experience. An epileptic irritation in this area may do the same. It is as though a wire recorder, or a strip of cinematographic film with sound track, had been set in motion within the brain. The sights and sounds, and the thoughts, of a former day pass through the man's mind again."[44] Penfield later placed this "area" in the upper brainstem and proposed that "the lateral temporal cortex would then have ... an interpretive function rather than being itself the storehouse of memory traces," to which access is gained from the hippocampi. This formulation of the functional organization of memory is based on the larger concept of the centrencephalic system, as summarized in Penfield's 1974 paper with Gordon Mathieson, "Memory: Autopsy Findings and Comments on the Role of Hippocampus in Experiential Recall":

> I was forced to conclude that, in [the] case of experiential flashbacks, the stimulating electrode, placed on certain areas of the temporal cortex ... activated gray matter that was located at a distance in the diencephalon ... That centrally located target for activation with its connections must constitute the neural recording of consciousness ... If that is so, ... in the hippocampus of either side there must be a mechanism that is essential in the process of scanning the past and calling to mind selected material.
>
> Thus, we come to the conclusion that there are at least three functional units of gray matter involved in the act of scanning and recall of experience: (1) the interpretive cortex of the temporal lobe, (2) the hippocampi with their direct connections to the brain stem, and (3) the experiential recording within the higher brain stem ... The proposition is, then, that neuronal potentials do pass from the hippocampi to the centrally placed experiential record, activating it selectively.[45]

Penfield made no clearer statement on the functional organization of the centrencephalic integrating system and his concept of the workings of the mind.

If the centrencephalic system is involved with the storage and recall of memories, how are they laid down in the first place? Penfield's answer is Hebbian facilitation: "It may now be surmised that the hippocampi are involved with the interpretive cortex of both temporal lobes in the function of scanning and recall. It is the record of the stream of past consciousness that must be scanned. That record is a continuous pattern of neuron connections that have been permanently facilitated for the subsequent passage of neuronal currents. This continuous thread of facilitated passage is the experiential engram."[46]

In Brenda Milner's view, however, Penfield's formulation of the brain's memory system "will seem to most psychologists little more than a picturesque metaphor." Nonetheless, Milner recognized, in this, as in other things, "Penfield's speculative, inquiring mind; he was wishing right to the end to understand the baffling retrograde and anterograde amnesia in those patients who had taught him and all of us so much."[47]

Milner's point requires emphasis. Penfield may have gone beyond his reach in equating the centrencephalic system and the mind. Nonetheless, he was the first to stress the concept of the vertical integration of cerebral structures, which Jasper elucidated in his discovery of the reciprocal excitatory and inhibitory interrelationship of the cortex, thalamus, and upper brain stem. Penfield's error was not anatomical or physiological, but conceptual, in referring to the mind rather than limiting himself to *attention* and *arousal*.[48]

THE WADA TEST

Language Lateralization

Lamar Roberts and Wilder Penfield had shown that cortical language function resides in the supplementary motor area, as well as in Broca's area and within the posterior speech region encompassing Wernicke's area and the inferior parietal lobule. The lateralization of language, however, remained unclear. The lateralization of cerebral dominance for speech was eventually established with the introduction of the intracarotid amobarbital test devised by June Wada.

As Milner recalled in 1998,

I remember the occasion when he [Wada] first told us of the possibility of determining the side of speech representation by injecting a barbiturate, sodium amobarbital, into the common carotid artery of one side. It was during a preoperative EEG conference on a left-handed patient whose seizures arose from the left posterior temporal region, but who showed no postictal speech difficulty. Penfield had just remarked how wonderful it would be if only we had a means of determining ahead of time if the lesion was in the dominant hemisphere for speech, in which case he would not operate. Wada, sitting at the back of the room, suddenly spoke up, asserting that there was indeed such a way. Penfield removed his glasses (a sure sign of annoyance) and said that this was ridiculous. But Wada was quietly persistent, and soon he and Rasmussen embarked on rigorous testing of monkeys to establish the safety of the procedure.[49]

Removing his glasses and wiping them across his chest must have been a frequent occurrence, since everyone who trained at the MNI either saw Penfield do it or heard about it from someone who did. In this case it led to one of the most significant and clinically useful research programs ever undertaken at the institute.

Juhn Atsushi Wada graduated in medicine from Hokkaido Imperial University in Sapporo in 1946, and obtained a doctorate of science there in 1951.[50] Wada was then appointed to the academic staff of Hokkaido University, where his first scientific interests were spurred by the need to mitigate the side effects of electro-convulsive therapy in psychiatric patients.[51] Thus, Wada conceived of a way to isolate the language-dominant hemisphere from the generalized, convulsive effects of ECT by anaesthetizing it through the intra-carotid injection of a short-acting barbiturate, which caused temporary aphasia when the injection involved the hemisphere dominant for speech.[52]

Juhn Wada interrupted his work in Japan to come to the MNI in 1955 and 1956, where his first interest was in microelectrode studies of corticofugal projections to the thalamus and brain stem reticular formation.[53] But, as was often the case at the MNI, an interesting clinical observation by a fellow often sent him in the laboratory for the next six months, investigating the phenomenon that he had brought to the attention of the attending staff. So it was with Juhn Wada who, working with Theodore Rasmussen in 1956, was set to verify the safety of the intra-carotid injection of barbiturates in macaques.[54] This was followed over the next two years by a clinical trial in a restricted number of right- and left-handed patients who were to be operated upon for the relief of intractable seizures. Amytal was injected into each carotid artery on alternate days to establish which hemisphere was dominant for speech, and this was then verified by cortical stimulation at the time of surgery. In each case the results were concordant. Wada and Rasmussen's paper was submitted to the *Journal of Neurosurgery* in October 1958 but was published only in March 1960, indicative of an unusually long peer review period.[55] The safety and reliability of the Wada test thus established, Milner, Rasmussen, and Charles Branch studied the lateralization of speech in a large number of patients over the next two decades.[56] Branch, Milner, and Rasmussen also determined the hemispheric lateralization

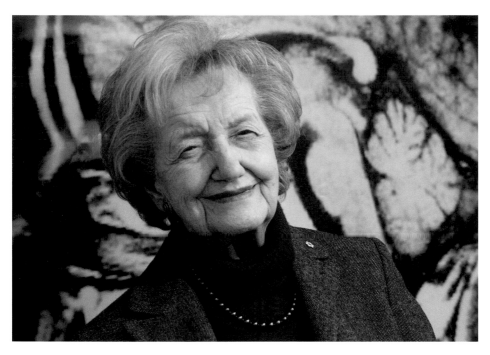

Figure 22.5: Brenda Milner. The MRI image in the background is that of William Feindel. (Photographer Owen Egan)

of each patient's language in relation to handedness. As was the case with Wada and Rasmussen, results obtained by amytal injections were confirmed at the time of surgery, and they were striking: speech was located within the left hemisphere in over 95 per cent of natural right-handers and in 70 per cent of natural left-handers.[57] The situation was more complex in individuals who had sustained left-hemisphere damage at birth or in infancy. In those cases the right hemisphere was dominant for speech in over half of the individuals but *only if* the injury involved the peri-sylvian speech regions defined by Dejerine.[58] (See figures 15.7 and 15.11.)

Amytal Memory Testing

As a result of the severe, disabling, short-term memory deficits in the patients studied by Penfield and Milner and by Scoville and Milner, surgery was withheld in individuals whose hippocampus contralateral to the side of the proposed surgery was suspected of being damaged. Thus, patients with intractable temporal lobe epilepsy who might well have befitted from surgery were denied operation for fear of damaging memory function.[59] This situation prevailed until Theodore Rasmussen suggested to Brenda Milner that she might devise a psychometric task that would indicate if memory function could sustain the resection of the hippocampus felt to be epileptogenic. This was not a simple request. The challenge was formidable: a task had to be devised that would test a patients' short-term memory while he or she may be rendered aphasic during the injection of the amytal, and this had to be done in less than three minutes, while other tests were being performed. Despite these unavoidable limitations, Milner was able to devise such a task based on the re-cognition of items presented to the patient as a multiple-choice series. The test proved to be very successful in predicting the safety of the removal of the epileptogenic hippocampus, and it has become a standard part of the MNI's psychometric armamentarium.[60]

23

A Tribute to William Cone

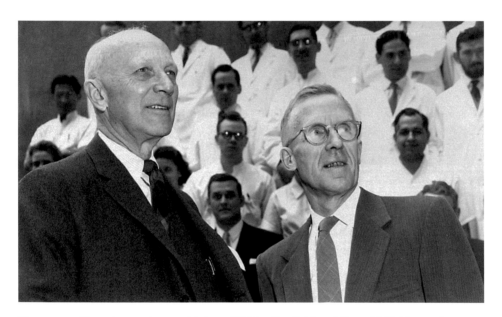

Figure 23.1: Two giants of neurobiology, Wilder Penfield and Donald Hebb, on the occasion of Hebb's 1958 Hughlings Jackson Lecture. Lamar Roberts is seen in dark jacket between the two. (MNI Archives)

The departure of so many MNI alumni to the National Institutes of Health a few years previously was not without unintended consequences, as the NIH awarded the MNI a grant in support of Americans training in neurology.[1] Not all departments were as fortunate as the Department of Neurology, and Theodore Rasmussen, impatiently echoing the complaint of all who have written a two-year grant application, lamented the uncertainty of research funding: "The lack of assurance of continued support creates serious difficulties in planning and carrying out long range and basic research programs. The time spent in writing progress reports and drafting new applications makes heavy inroads on valuable staff research time, which is subject to all too many unavoidable erosions from service functions, teaching commitments, administrative data, etc."[2]

Nonetheless, research continued apace: Brenda Milner on the role of the hippocampus and memory, and Hanna Pappius on cerebral edema.[3] John Blundell, Gilles Bertrand, and Jan Gybells, from Louvain, collaborated with Louis Poirier of Laval University in research on the basal ganglia and were preparing to apply stereotaxic techniques to the surgical treatment of Parkinson's disease and other dyskinesias.[4] Lamar Roberts was finalizing the text of *Speech and Brain Mechanisms*, in his last year at the institute. He also published an important paper on functional plasticity in cortical speech areas in an early use of the term *plasticity* in relation to cortical function.[5]

FELLOWS FROM BOTH SIDES OF THE IRON CURTAIN

The institute broke new ground by hosting a female neurosurgical fellow, Alexandra Georgievna Zemskaya, from the Leningrad Neurosurgical Institute. Zemskaya later headed the Faculty of Neurosurgery at the St Petersburg Academy of Postgraduate Education.[6] She and her colleague Yuri Savchenko, from Omsk, spent a few months at the MNI learning Penfield's approach in the surgical treatment of epilepsy.[7]

Two fellows came from Poland to study at the institute: Jerzy Majkowski and Miroslaw Mossakowski. Majkowski studied the role of the cortex, hippocampus, and brainstem in the elaboration of conditioned reflexes, basically repeating Pavlov's experiment with a cat, a bell, and a shock to the paw,[8] while Mossakowski studied the succinic dehydrogenase activity in glial tumours in relation to malignancy, as well as Parkinson's syndrome and metachromatic leucodystrophy.[9] His work predates current interest in the identification of enzymatic markers of malignancy in glial tumours by half a century. Mossakowski later presided over the Polish Academy of Sciences.

Jan Gybels, from Belgium, was another new arrival to the MNI, who worked with Gilles Bertrand and John Blundell on the development of stereotactic techniques for the treatment of movement disorders, and with Herbert Jasper on microelectrode studies of the cortex.[10] He returned to Belgium to take up a post at the Catholic University of Louvain, where he was a founder of the university's neurophysiology laboratory. Gybels achieved international attention for the investigation and the treatment of pain, and in the field of stereotactic surgery. Joseph Klingler, from the Anatomical Institute in Basel, demonstrated his technique of white matter dissection in a course to some fifty graduate students from the institute and other departments at McGill.[11] He and Peter Gloor produced a landmark paper on the connections of the amygdala.[12] Byron Cone

Pevehouse, a recipient of a National Science Foundation award from the United States National Academy of Sciences, arrived at the institute in 1958 to pursue a master's degree under William Cone.[13] Pevehouse had a distinguished career at the University of California, San Francisco, and later the University of Virginia, with John Jane, also an MNI alumnus.

The MNI's connection with China survived the 1949 Revolution and eventually flourished under the new regime. In 1956, however, the institute welcomed one of its most distinguished fellows, Chung Jen Shih, from Taiwan. Shih received a scholarship to study abroad from the China Medical Board, an organization founded by the Rockefeller Foundation to promote health care in China. Shih came to the MNI to train in neurosurgery and neuropathology. His training completed, Shih returned to Taiwan in 1958 where he had a brilliant career, eventually rising to the directorship of the International College of Surgeons.

PUBLICATIONS

K.A.C. Elliott, Alva Bazemore, and Ernest Florey published an important paper on GABA in *Nature*;[14] Gilles Bertrand published a novel paper on the distribution of efferent fibres from the supplementary motor area;[15] Arthur Elvidge published two papers on the MNI's experience with astrocytomas of the brain and spinal cord;[16] and Pierre Gloor published his doctoral dissertation on seizure discharges originating in the amygdala.[17] The neurobiology of woodland creatures was not ignored, as Richard Lende co-authored a whimsical paper with Clinton Woolsey on the sensorymotor localization in the cerebral cortex of the porcupine.[18]

RASMUSSEN'S SYNDROME

Most noteworthy, Theodore Rasmussen, Jerzy Olszewski, and Donald Lloyd-Smith published the highly influential "Focal Seizures Due to Chronic Localized Encephalitis."[19] Now universally known as Rasmussen's encephalitis, the condition is usually seen in children who exhibit inexorably progressing hemiplegia over months or a few years, associated with intractable focal epileptic seizures involving the affected limbs. Radiological investigations performed over the course of the illness reveal progressive atrophy of the hemisphere opposite to the weakened side. Histo-pathological analysis shows the characteristic findings of chronic encephalitis.[20] Little has been added to the description of the pathology of this condition and on its suspected viral etiology since Mary-Jane Aguilar's masterful thesis, "The Role of Chronic Encephalitis in the Pathogenesis of Epilepsy" addressing these issues.[21]

The investigation of this condition continued to occupy many at the MNI over the years. The individuals most involved, besides Aguilar, were Gordon Mathieson, Stirling Carpenter, and Yves Robitaille in neuropathology, Yannick Grenier, Kirk Osterland, and Jack Antel in immunohistochemistry, and, from the NIH, Carleton Gajdusek, who investigated the possible role of slow viruses in this condition. Despite the efforts of these and other workers, the etiology of Rasmussen's encephalitis remains unknown,[22] but the treatment is surgical and is quite effective.[23]

SPEAKERS

David Ingvar, from the Institute of Physiology in Lund, Sweden, was invited to the MNI to speak on a topic dear to Wilder Penfield, "Cortical Excitatory State and Cortical Circulation."[24] The distinguished biologist J.Z. Young, from University College, London, spoke on what must have seemed a very esoteric topic, "Memory System in Octopus."[25] Going from sea to air, Stanley Cobb, from Harvard, addressed "Some Problems in Avian Neurology."

Herbert S. Gasser, former director of the Rockefeller Institute and 1944 Nobel Prize recipient for his work on action potentials, gave the 1957 annual Hughlings Jackson Lecture, "The Properties of Unmedullated Nerve Fibers with Afferent Function,"[26] and D.O. Hebb gave the 1958 Hughlings Jackson Lecture, "Intelligence, Brain Function and Theory of Mind," which he published the following year in *Brain*.[27] As an insightful reconciliation of the brain stem arousal system with intellect, emotion, and free will, in thirteen pages, it is unsurpassed.

THE FELLOWS REUNION: TRIBUTE TO WILLIAM CONE

A special reunion of the MNI fellows was held in Montreal on 28–9 April 1957 to pay tribute to William Cone.[28] For most of the fellows this was the last time that they would be with him.

Theodore Rasmussen presided over Monday morning's scientific session, which consisted of eleven short papers delivered by returning fellows. The First Annual Fellows Lecture, delivered by Joseph P. Evans, professor of neurological surgery at the University of Chicago, was "Brain Injury." Evans expressed the feeling of all fellows, old and of more recent vintage, when he commented, "I wish that it were possible to transmit to younger men and women entering our specialty, something of the joy, heartache, and excitement of earlier years in our field."[29]

Table 23.1

Speakers at the reunion in honour of William Cone, 28–29 April 1957

Fellow	Title
George Austin and Grayson McCouch (Pennsylvania)	Intraspinal Sprouting of New Afferent Terminal as a Cause for Spasticity
Francis Echlin (NYU)	Observations on the Supersensitivity of Chronically, Neuronally Isolated and Partially Isolated Cerebral Cortex
Joseph Evans (Chicago)	Brain Injury: Present Concepts and Challenges*
William Fields (Baylor)	Spinal Epidural Hemangiomas in Pregnancy
William Grant (CME)**	Cerebellar Subdural Hygroma and the Post-traumatic Syndrome: Diagnosis and Treatment
Ira Jackson (University of Texas)	Observations on the Surgical Treatment of Cervical Carotid Artery Thrombosis
John Hunter (Boston City)	Major Neurosurgical Complications from Minor Surgery
Igor Klatzo (NIH)	The Relationship between Edema, Blood-Brain-Barrier and Tissue Elements in Local Brain Injury
Robert Knighton (Henry Ford Hospital)	A Simplified Technique for Chemopalldolysis for Parkinsonism, Illustrated by a Movie
Ed Lotspeich Jr (Cincinnati)	Cervical Spondylosis: Treatment by Removing the Offending Spurs, Illustrated by a Movie
Nathan Norcross (Pennsylvania)	The Role of Trauma in Disc Herniations
Robert Pudenz (HMRI)***	The Production of Hydrocephalus in the Experimental Animal

* First Fellows Day Lecture, 29 April 1957.
** College of the Medical Evangelist – later Loma Linda University.
*** Huntington Medical Research Institutes, Pasadena

24

Melancholia: 4 May 1959

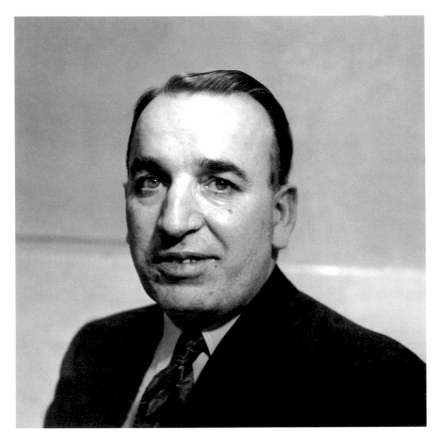

Figure 24.1: William Vernon Cone. (Penfield Archives)

On 4 May 1959, William Vernon Cone put an end to his life of sixty-two years, his head resting serenely on a pillow placed upon his office floor.[1] None have written more eloquently, revealingly, or lovingly of Bill Cone than his operating room nurse, Faith Lyman Feindel.

Much has been written about Dr Cone. All of us saw him in our own way. Physically he was short and stocky with a large head, the most enormous brown eyes I have ever seen and a deep rich baritone voice. As a person he was kind, gentle and softspoken. Sometimes he was sulky and petulant, sometimes patient, sometimes less so, and often very difficult; but a more lovable man would be hard to find. When he was pleased with your work his gratitude was almost overwhelming.

What stands in my mind is that Dr Cone really and truly respected nurses and was himself an excellent bedside nurse. He could make any patient comfortable by positioning and gentle handling.

We became good friends. Possibly my expertise was that I understood his moods, and could usually bring him out of his sometimes melancholy state of mind. He loved nurses, championed our work, encouraged us and always thanked us. If one followed him around radiology, the pathology laboratory, or anywhere else where he was working, he would teach. Naturally many of us were caught up in his enthusiasm and obsession for work, proud to be part of his entourage.

Sometimes he would sulk, like the time Bill Feindel, whom I later married, invited me to the Shriner's Circus at the Forum. It was my afternoon off and I was determined to go. Dr Cone booked a brain abscess and expected me to stay to take the case. I left him with the set-up ready, a quick and efficient nurse to take over and took off with my beloved date. Next morning, I was scrubbed as usual. It was a Saturday and Dr Cone had booked five cases, one after the other. Through all those cases he never uttered a word to me, not even "Good Morning." I was being punished for deserting him.

This must seem strange to present-day nurses, but to us these dramas affected us deeply. We worked hard, surgeon and nurse thrown together for hours on end right through the night. In my family, Dr Cone was a household word. My oldest sister, Beatrice Johnson, broke her neck riding and was in the Neuro for several years. She was not an easy patient but she loved all the nurses and remained close friends with many of them right to the end of her life.

Once when Bill and I had dinner at my family home, we brought along a visiting doctor. I cannot remember his name or what he said, but he made some derogatory remark about Dr Cone. But I do remember my brother's booming military voice in reply, "Are you speaking of Dr Cone? Do you realize that in this household we worship at that man's shrine?" I think there were and still are many of those shrines, at least in our hearts, in memory of a great man.[2]

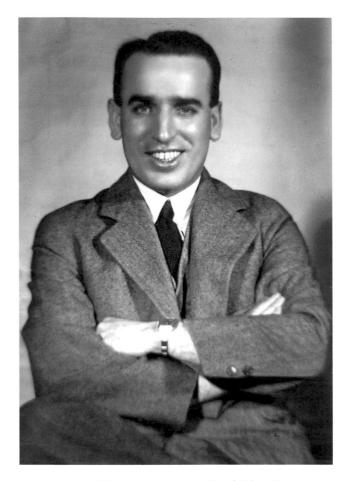

Figure 24.2: William Vernon Cone. (Penfield Archives)

The director of nursing, Eileen Flanagan, in her report for the academic year 1959–60, announced that Mrs Samuel Reitman had donated an annual bursary to the memory of Dr Cone. The first recipient was Jean McMillan, operating room nurse who had worked with him.

◆ ◆ ◆

Beyond the heartfelt words and eulogies that marked William Cone's passing, a more permanent memorial to the man, cast in bronze, remains in the halls of the institute. As Eileen Flanagan recalled,

Mrs Avis Cone was given an etching of the Sir George Frampton statue of "Peter Pan" which stands in Kensington Gardens, London, England. This statue personifies the Peter Pan of Sir James Barrie's play performed in 1904 and published as a book in 1911. Sir James bequeathed the copyright to the Great Ormond Street Hospital for Sick Children in London – over the years the royalties have been estimated to amount to several million dollars. Dr Cone suggested that it would be very interesting and entertaining for the children if we could acquire a statue for them.

Thereupon I wrote to the son of Sir George, Mr Meredith Frampton, in England and asked him if there was any replica in miniature in existence … Mr Frampton said that he knew of an owner of one of the models, Mrs Christine Bedam, the sculptor's daughter, living near Bournemouth, who wished to sell it on account of death duties [figure 24.4]. I wrote to her offering to buy the statue and she accepted …

In 1953 I left for England on my holidays and on arriving at Southampton I proceeded to the home of Mr and Mrs Summers. He was ill with chicken pox and was in isolation so we conducted the negotiations through the bedroom door. The little model was embedded in the centre of a beautiful old carved oak table. It stood in a glass basin of water filled with flowers. Mrs Summers said it had been in the family all her life and she could hardly bear to part with it. When I left she and the children were crying and I must say I almost did too.

When it finally arrived in Montreal in 1953 it lay on the dock for two or three weeks, as it was addressed to McGill University who disclaimed any knowledge of it. Cook's [Travel Agency] had omitted to put the Neurological Institute's name on the address.

We then had to find someone to sculpt a miniature base to match the original in Kensington Gardens, and were fortunate in finding the noted sculptress, Marjorie Winslow, who undertook the work. She did this in her atelier at her home on the Richelieu River … Mrs Winslow then executed a plaster model of the intricate base you see under the statue. All the little figures and little animals were copied perfectly. We found an artisan who worked in bronze, Mr B.J. Aerts, up in Côte-St-Michel. This took almost two years to complete at a cost of $900.00.

The statue was placed in the children's ward to the great pleasure of countless children. Twice the flute was taken from the statue but fortunately it was recovered each time. The cost of the whole endeavor was over $2000.00 covered by many friends of the institute, the Nursing and

Medical staff and with great assistance from Dr Cone. The inscription on the base reads: "Dedicated to the children of the MNI in memory of Dr William Vernon Cone whose devotion, interest and skill were given to them in such unselfish measure."[3]

Peter Pan was located in various places during renovations of the building, not an easy task since the bronze statue weighs over five hundred pounds. During one of the moves, his flute was lost again, never to be found. A replacement was made and is now firmly held in place, protected from music lovers and souvenir hunters. Peter now plays his flute on the first floor just inside the doors of the University Street disabled patients' entrance, where it is the subject of much interest and admiration, and marks William Cone's devotion to his patients.

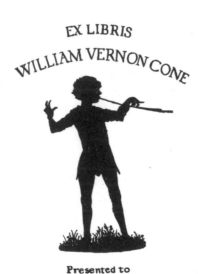

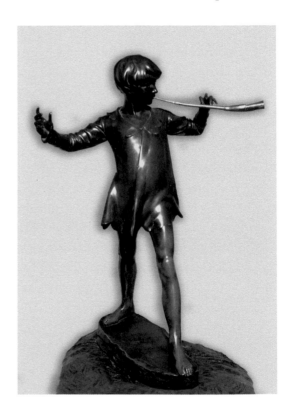

Figures 24.3 and 24.4: (*Left*) William Cone's *ex libris*. (MNI Archives). (*Right*) The MNI's *Peter Pan*, before alighting on his base. (MNI Archives)

PART THREE

The Second Director
1960–1972

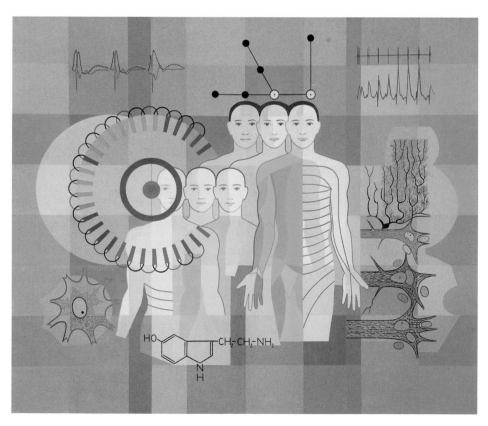

Luba Genush, *The World of Neurology* (*centre panel*), highlights the electrical activity of the brain and a montage of the technology of positron emission tomography, and is bordered on the right by a network of nerve cells.

25

Twenty-Five Years on University Street

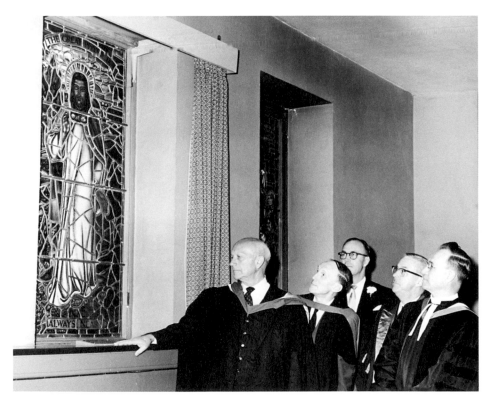

Figure 25.1: Stained glass window of *The Great Physician, Always Near*, in Saint Andrew's Church, Montreal, dedicated to Dr William Vernon Cone. In attendance at the dedication are (*left*) Drs Penfield, McNaughton, and Robb. Also in attendance are Dr Gerald W. Halpenny, president of the Canadian Medical Association, and Reverend Dr D.M. Grant, minister. The church was lost in a conflagration and this photograph is all that remains of *The Great Physician*. (W. Penfield, McNaughton, Robb, etc., at St Andrew's United Church, 26 June 1961. Lloyd Blackham, *Montreal Star*)

STAY THE COURSE

Wilder Penfield paid tribute to his departed friend, but cloaked the circumstances of William Cone's death in metaphor (figure 25.1):

> This is not the time for obituaries nor is it the place for tears. But I must report the death of Dr William Cone … He was a dreamer and a worker, a friend, a man of infinite kindness. He had an unshakable determination to realize perfection in our Art. He was a surgeon excelled by none. He, more than any other, has made this Institute what it is.
>
> In the early morning hours of May 4th, shortly before his 62nd birthday, when his resident assistants thought that he was working in his office preparing his report for this meeting, he dropped over the side of the ship and set off in the pilot's boat, heading for the unknown shore. We, who remain, will hold this ship to its course.[1]

For Herbert Jasper, the course had been charted in 1934 by "the close interweaving of devotion to the healing of the sick and the advancement of science,"[2] made possible by the unique symbiotic relationship of the disciplines at the MNI. This was nowhere more evident than in the collaboration of Neurology and Neurosurgery. "I doubt," Francis McNaughton reflected, "If many Departments of Neurology are as fortunate as we are at the M.N.I, in the invigorating contact at every level of experience with our neurosurgical brothers-in-arms. This interchange of thought and experience is a most important part of the training of both neurologist and neurosurgeon, which we would not want to diminish, but rather increase. The lack of it is a serious defect in a great many training centers around the world today. For the good of the Neurology and Neurosurgery of the future, I only hope that our experience will be copied elsewhere."[3]

Francis McNaughton was promoted to professor of neurology, and Donald Lloyd-Smith was appointed to the permanent staff. Lloyd-Smith's task was to bring the work of the EEG laboratory more closely in touch with the clinical neurological service and expand its use to general medical problems to which EEG studies were proving to be useful. Pierre Gloor, Theodore Rasmussen, and Richard Rovit were also developing specialized EEG techniques for clinical applications, which included the ever-increasing use of sphenoidal electrode recordings of the basal surface of the temporal lobe.[4] Richard Rovit was a driving force in these endeavours, which would serve as the basis of his MSc thesis.[5]

Gilles Bertrand and John Blundell, a newcomer to the institute, began carrying out stereotaxic procedures for Parkinson's disease.[6] Blundell was a young

British neurosurgeon who had worked with Percival Bailey on his and Schaltenbrand's stereotactic atlas.[7] Blundell came to the MNI in 1957 and spent the first six months of his appointment in Sweden with Lars Leksell, to study his technique in stereotactic neurosurgery. He and Gilles Bertrand performed the first pallidotomy at the MNI in 1958, and the first thalamotomy at the institute was performed a year later.[8] Blundell was named head of Neurosurgery at the Montreal Children's Hospital when pediatric neurosurgery was relocated there. He was highly respected as a teacher and mentor to all residents who worked on his service.

As in the previous year, the institute welcomed guests from behind the Iron Curtain. Lucjan Stepien, Chorobski's associate and eventual successor at the Medical Academy of Warsaw, studied the effect of cortical and amygdalo hip pocampal lesions on recent memory.[9] Georgii Donatovich Smirnov, from the Laboratories of Neurophysiology of the Academy of Sciences in Moscow, also came to the MNI to work with his friend Herbert Jasper,[10] who warmly introduced Smirnov to the staff of the MNI:

> We are particularly pleased to be able to welcome to our laboratories George Smirnov, an old friend and colleague from Moscow, who is engaged in electrophysiological studies of sensory mechanisms of attention and is incidentally a most congenial coworker, devoted as well to the cause of international co-operation in brain research. He was one of the principal organizers for the Soviet Academy of Sciences of the International Colloquium which I had the pleasure of attending in October, out of which has developed an International Brain Research Organization now known as IBRO, working under the auspices of UNESCO.[11]

Wilder Penfield renewed his acquaintance with Smirnov a few years later, at the bedside of Russia's most prominent nuclear physicist, Lev Landau.

Jasper also welcomed Geneviève Arfel-Capdevielle from the Université de Paris, where she held positions as electroencephalographer at Hôpital Foch and at La Pitié, two hospitals renowned for their care of epileptic patients. While at the institute she shared her extensive experience with coma and studied the prognostic aspects of EEG following the resection of an epileptic focus.[12]

Residents and Fellows

The resident staff of the academic year 1958–59 includes a score of individuals who would ascend to leadership in their discipline. Three would become president of major neurosurgical associations, one an editor of the *Journal of*

Neurosurgery, and another, Arthur M. House, would be appointed lieutenant governor of Newfoundland and Labrador.[13]

Max House graduated from Dalhousie University Medical School in 1952 and came to train in neurology at the MNI, where he was befriended by Francis McNaughton. House left the institute in 1959 for St John's, Newfoundland, where he began his practice as the first neurologist in the province. He was active in the creation of Memorial University, eventually becoming professor of neurology, and held many administrative positions during his thirty-year academic career. Falah Maroun, a neurosurgeon who had also trained at the MNI, joined House at Memorial in 1967. Maroun rendered inestimable service to the people of Newfoundland and to Memorial University during his long and distinguished career.[14]

By its twenty-fifth year, 350 individuals from thirty-seven countries had trained at the institute for one year or more, while others had come for shorter periods. The current resident staff and fellows were not different: their stay at the MNI was supported by scholarships and grants ranging from the Colombo Plan to the Swiss Academy of Medical Sciences. Among the new arrivals was Prakah Narain Tandon of New Delhi, a teaching fellow on the Neurological Service who had trained in neurosurgery in Oslo with former MNI fellow Kristian Kristiansen. Tandon returned to India to become chief of Neurosurgery at the All India Institutes of Medical Sciences, New Delhi, and quickly gained fame not only for his surgical skills but also for his talent as a teacher and scientific investigator. The lessons that he learned at the MNI were passed on to students who founded Neurosurgery departments throughout India, including Srinagar, Delhi, and Mumbai. Patients came to him from across India, as well as from neighbouring Nepal, Bangladesh, Afghanistan, and Sri Lanka. Foreign governments flew him in for emergency consultations. During his long career, Prakah Narain Tandon co-authored India's first textbook on neurosurgery.[15] Among his national and international awards and distinctions, he was the only clinician to be president of the National Academy of Sciences, India.

The most notable new member of the house staff was George Karpati, assistant resident on the Neurology Service, who would eventually head the Neuromuscular Research Laboratories at the institute and be recognized for his outstanding research in diseases of muscles and nerves.[16] Two fellows, Luigi Sperti of Padua, Italy, and Christian Vera from Santiago, Chile, joined Pierre Gloor's laboratory to study the mechanisms of hippocampal discharge during experimentally induced seizures[17] and produced important papers on this topic.[18]

Table 25.1
MNI class of 1959

Jesse Barber	Howard University; president, National Medical Association
Gilles Bertrand	McGill University, Montreal Neurological Institute
Perry Black	Hahnemann University
John Blundell	McGill University, Montreal Children's Hospital
Charles Branch Sr	University of Texas, San Antonio
Henry Garretson	University of Louisville; president AANS*
Jan Gybels	Université catholique de Louvain
Jules Hardy	Université de Montréal
Arthur M. House	Memorial University; lieutenant-governor, Newfoundland and Labrador
John Jane	University of Virginia; editor, *Journal of Neurosurgery*; president SNS**
M. Mossakowski	Polish Academy of Sciences
Jewell Osterholm	Thomas Jefferson University
Phanor Perot	Medical University of South Carolina; President SNS
Byron Pevehouse	University of California at San Francisco; president AANS,* vice-president WFNS***
Richard Rovit	New York University School of Medicine
Georgii Smirnov	Brain Institute, Academy of Medical Sciences, Moscow
Lujian Stepien	University of Warsaw
Prakah Tandon	All India Institutes of Medical Sciences

* American Association of Neurological surgeons
** Society of Neurological Surgeons
*** World Federation of Neurosurgical Societies

There were also notable departures from the institute in this twenty-fifth year: Gordon Thompson completed his residency and left Montreal for the University of British Columbia, where he became head of Neurosurgery, while Anton Tarazi returned to Jordan to become its first neurosurgeon and practised at St Augusta Hospital, Jerusalem.[19]

Among the fellows who stayed in Montreal were Bernard Graham and his wife Shirley Fyles, most dedicated physicians; Israel Libman, who became a senior neurologist at Montreal's Jewish General Hospital; Alan Morton, neurologist; and Emile Berger, neurosurgeon. Jules Hardy was foremost among the fellows who stayed in Montreal. His renown, however, is worldwide.

Sir Geoffrey Jefferson again visited the institute and shared his touching "Recollections of Sir Hugh Cairns" with the staff and fellows.[20] Sir Geoffrey sustained a myocardial infarction the following year on his way to California. He convalesced first at the home of Thomas Hoen and, later, at Francis Echlin's, before returning to England.[21] Jefferson died in 1961. It is of some comfort to us that his last hosts in America were two MNI fellows.

A RETIREMENT IS ANNOUNCED

Wilder Penfield marked the MNI's twenty-fifth anniversary by affirming his gratitude to the people of Canada and his faith in the permanence of the institute. The MNI, he said, would "continue as long as Montreal institutions stand, serving society and the cause of science. It will repay our debt of gratitude many times, not to those who gave but to those who inherit. The ultimate aim of those who spend their working lives in this Institution is carved in stone outside on the corner of the building, 'Dedicated to relief of sickness and pain and to the study of neurology.'" It is in the latter half of that statement, the study of neurology writ large, that Wilder Penfield revealed a loftier goal: "This Institute is dedicated to a vast project of exploration and the hope that, through understanding of the human brain, man may come in time to understand himself and his own mind. It is my belief that when that day of understanding does dawn we shall no longer 'see through a glass darkly but know at last the nature of the spirit of man and of God.'"[22]

Penfield then continued his address with the news that all were anticipating: he announced his retirement as director of the Montreal Neurological Institute in favour of his long-time friend, student, and collaborator, Theodore Brown Rasmussen: "At the same time, seven years ago, I handed in my resignation as Professor of Neurology and Neurosurgery. My successor was chosen then … It brought Theodore Rasmussen back to us from the University of Chicago … He is wise, modest, kind, firm, as well as being a brilliant neurosurgeon. On his arrival in 1954, Dr Rasmussen took up the academic responsibility. Today, by leave of Principal and University Governors, he becomes Director. With Francis McNaughton as full Professor of Neurology and with Jasper, Elliott, Mathieson in scientific neurology, the future is filled with exciting promise."[23]

Penfield also reported that the first William Cone Professor of Neurosurgery would be William Howard Feindel, late of the University of Saskatchewan: "I am delighted to report that the University Governors have appointed Dr William Feindel to be the first Cone Professor of Neurosurgery. Dr Feindel, who was born in Nova Scotia, has had a distinguished career as Rhodes Scholar, neuroanatomist, neurophysiologist, neuropathologist and neurosurgeon … He returns to Montreal after building up a most successful neurosurgical clinic at the University Hospital in Saskatoon."[24]

The Cone Professor benefited from the William Cone Memorial Research Fund, substantially enriched through the efforts of Colin Webster, a great patron of the institute and admirer of William Cone. William Feindel's task was to establish a radioisotope laboratory, the tenth research laboratory at the institute, and his first priorities were the study of the cerebral circulation utilizing radioactive tracers and the development of an upgraded model of the automatic scanner developed in Saskatoon.[25]

In the reorganization that followed Penfield's resignation, Arthur Elvidge became neurosurgeon-in-chief, Gilles Bertrand associate neurosurgeon, and John Blundell and Charles Branch were made clinical assistants in neurosurgery. Roméo Éthier joined the Department of Neuroradiology, which he eventually led, and Pierre Gloor took the helm of the Department of EEG from Herbert Jasper, who was on sabbatical in Paris as executive secretary of IBRO.

SILVER ANNIVERSARY CELEBRATIONS, 5–8 OCTOBER 1959

The academic highpoint of Penfield's retirement year was the elaborately prepared twenty-fifth anniversary of the founding of the MNI.[26]

Activities began on the evening of Monday, 5 October 1959, with a short symposium on neurosurgical education. Theodore Rasmussen chose the topic because McGill had just gone through a lengthy process that resulted in changes in the curriculum that affected the teaching of neurosurgery at the university. Kristian Kristiansen, perhaps with a wink, said that medical education in Norway was financed from the government's stake in football pools! The following morning Lyle Gage, Joseph Evans, and Keasley Welch spoke of times gone by at the institute. The newly appointed Cone Professor of Neurosurgery, William Feindel, highlighted the probing of brain function, which was the mainstay of research at the MNI at the time, into structures where "angels would have feared to tread": the hippocampus, the thalamus, and the basal ganglia.

Tuesday afternoon was reserved for conferring honorary degrees. Initially, it had been proposed that there would be four, awarded to Yi-cheng Chao, Jerzy Chorobski, Dorothy Russell, and Sir Charles Symonds. Unfortunately, Chao could not make his way to Montreal from the People's Republic of China, and his doctors forbade Sir Charles to travel. Thus the two honourees were Russell and Chorobski. Jerzy Chorobsky's address, "Pathogenesis of Involuntary Movements," focused on patients with brain tumours.[27]

On the following morning there was a symposium on what participants found most intriguing in the fields of neurology and neurosurgery. Martin Nichols, from Aberdeen, discussed the more radical approach for the treatment of cerebral aneurysms that was going through its growing pains. He did not, however, minimize the challenges faced by the newly emboldened aneurysm surgeons in those heroic times: "No surgeon can ever plead lack of interest when an aneurysm comes off in his forceps," he related, "when the sucker is clearly inadequate to deal with the floods coming up from below and when the delicate handling of the operative field is interrupted for the necessity of opening the chest for a little cardiac massage."[28] Less sanguine, Robert Pudez showed a movie depicting the development of the new Pudenz-Heyer system for the ventriculo-atrial shunting of cerebrospinal fluid in the treatment of hydrocephalus.

Wednesday's most insightful speaker was C. Miller Fisher. "To carry out fresh observations of abnormal cerebral functions in human brain disease – describing and analyzing, trying to discern new correlations and generalizations – is the most exciting facet of neurology. Closely allied to this subject is the prospect that knowledge of aphasia, or apraxia or agnosia and the rest, will allow an analysis of all human mental faculties," he said, unabashedly flying his locationist colours. "To understand aphasia is to comprehend much about thinking; to understand memory would tell us much about learning; a knowledge of agnosia would give us clues concerning insight, awareness, and even psychopathic proclivities."[29] Fisher's highly materialistic view of the cerebral cortex as the substrate of thinking, learning, insight, and awareness was at odds with Penfield's centrencephalic system that Jasper described in his Hughlings Jackson later that afternoon. Jan Droogleever-Fortuyn, from Groningen, The Netherlands, went further than Fisher, speculating on the brain as a computing system: "The brain as a biological entity can be considered as an instrument of homeostasis … If now our body including our brain may be considered as an instrument, we might envisage the possibility that a number of distinctions we make find their origin, not in the world around us, but in our own organization. In this respect, modern viewpoints on cybernetics and information theory deserve our full interest."[30] Webb Haymaker, from Washington, DC, also in a speculative mood, discussed how space travel and radiation might affect brain function.[31] Cosimo Ajmone-Marsan, from Bethesda, was less inclined to philosophize on cybernetic theory as a conceptual model of the brain and how a rarefied atmosphere in a pressurized suit would affect the brain. Rather, he discussed the more down-to-earth subject of the effects of repetitive cortical stimulation on the refractoriness of membrane depolarization.[32] Similarly, Jerzy Olszweski looked within. The study of architectonics, which had occupied anatomists for half a century, had run its course, he said, unabashedly. "Future research," he felt, "will be most fruitful in the study of intrinsic intra-neuronal connections, that is, of synaptology and electron microscopy."[33]

The afternoon ended with Herbert Jasper's twenty-fifth Hughlings Jackson Lecture. Undaunted by talk of inner or outer space, computing machines and cybernetics, his subject was "The Evolution of Concepts of Cerebral Localization since Hughlings Jackson."[34] This seemingly non-contentious topic gave Jasper the opportunity to review the concept of the centrencephalic integrating system and the hierarchical organization of the brain. His construct rested on two pillars: Hughlings Jackson and Ramón y Cajal. For Jackson the highest level of brain function "was a vast, widely distributed neuronal system located in the association areas of cortex in both hemispheres."[35] But Jasper also recalled that Cajal had been "impressed with the complexity of the organization in the brain stem reticular system and presumed that it must have some highly *integrative* function."[36] For Penfield, the reticular formation of the diencephalon and its reciprocal connections with the cortex constituted the cenetrencephalic integrating system,[37] and Jasper left it to Penfield to explain how this system gave rise to consciousness and the will to act by quoting Penfield himself: "The circuits of this system run out into the various functional area of the cortex and back again. In a very real sense there is no 'higher' and no 'lower' in this system. The place of understanding is not walled up in a cell or in a centre of grey matter. It is to be sought in the perfect functioning of all these converging circuits."[38]

A well-filled afternoon!

The Lasting Presence of William Cone

Thursday morning was given over to ward rounds, and guests observed Theodore Rasmussen as he performed surgery and electro-cortical stimulation while Herbert Jasper read the electrocorticogram. Thursday afternoon was devoted to William Cone and the areas in which he had the greatest influence. Ira Jackson, from the University of Texas at Galveston, discussed Cone's contributions to the treatment of hydrocephalus. As Cone never published his work on the subject, Jackson went into some detail:[39]

> As early as the mid-thirties, [Cone] had contemplated using the venous system as an absorbing area and, in 1945, actually carried out a shunt from the lateral ventricle to the superior sagittal sinus. In the following years, he also anastomosed the ventricle to the jugular vein in the neck. Some of the infants thus treated were helped, but, in every instance,

blockage of the tube occurred when the ventricular pressure became lower than the venous pressure. In recent years this method has been revived and, as a result of valves in the tube, which prevent backflow of blood, very encouraging results are now obtained … Dr Cone constantly experimented with tubes of different types of plastics and rubbers. When the ventriculojugular shunts continued to fail, Dr Cone shifted to the peritoneal shunt, in which the cerebrospinal fluid is taken from either the lateral ventricle or the lumbar subarachnoid space and diverted through a tube into the peritoneal cavity, where it is absorbed. In 1948, Dr Cone carried out his first anastomosis of this type in a patient with a lumbar myelomeningocele, leading a tube from the meningocele sac into the abdomen. Subsequently, the tube was shifted to the lumbar subarachnoid space when the patient showed evidence of communicating hydrocephalus after resection of the meningocele sac.[40]

Jackson summed up, perhaps with a furtive look in the direction of Robert Pudenz, by stating that William Cone's "greatest contribution in the field of hydrocephalus, however, was probably the interest that he stimulated in others concerning the surgical treatment of an affliction that had been regarded as quite hopeless up to the middle forties."[41]

Cod Liver Oil and Honey

Guy Odom, from Duke University, spoke of Cone's treatment of brain abscesses before the introduction of antibiotics. After evacuation of the abscess, usually through a burr hole, "a large, soft rubber tube was inserted into the abscess cavity, which was packed with gauze soaked in Alphamel, a mixture of cod liver oil and honey. Then, the scalp was closed around the rubber tube and wet dressings were applied."[42] Dressings were changed daily and the cavity repacked until the abscess was healed. This situation prevailed until the advent of chloromycetin, which replaced cod liver oil and honey and was used to irrigate the cavity once the abscess had been drained. The day ended with the Annual Fellows Dinner, where Dorothy Russell gave the third Fellow's Day Lecture, "Reflections on Neuropathology," a fitting after-dinner topic.

The twenty-fifth anniversary celebrations gave Theodore Rasmussen, the institute's director-in-waiting, the opportunity to formulate his vision, centred on research, patient care, and teaching. This required, in his view, not only specialized researchers but also the "cross-fertilization between the clinic and the laboratory." The latter, he felt, was the essential reason for an institute. Rasmussen ended his address on a more than positive note, stating, "Among man-made institutions, universities and hospitals have proven to be among the most enduring. The Institute, being both hospital and department of a university, should have a future without a foreseeable end."[43]

Table 25.2
Silver Anniversary Celebrations, 5–8 October 1959

Speakers*	Topic
Jacob Chandy (Vellore)	Neurosurgical Education in India
Kristian Kristiansen (Olso)	Neurosurgical Education in Norway
Lloyd Stevenson (McGill)**	McGill's Medical Curriculum
Jean Saucier (Montreal)	Evolution of Neurology in Montreal
Francis McNaughton (McGill)	Neurology Coming of Age
Lyle Gage (West Virginia)	Neurosurgery at the MNI before 1934
Joseph Evans (Chicago)	The MNI: First Years
Keasley Welch (Denver)	The MNI: Middle Years
William Feindel (McGill)	Neurosurgery Today
Eileen Flanagan (McGill)	The Nursing Service and the Graduate Teaching Program
Theodore Rasmussen (McGill)	The Institute Looks Forward
Wilder Penfield (McGill)	Down the Stream of Time
Claude Bertrand (Montreal)	The Pneumotaxic Guide and Basal Structures of the Brain
Eduardo Palma (Montevideo)	A New Method for the Exposure of the Posterior Fossa
Arthur Ward (Seattle)	Microelectrode Studies of the Activities of Single Cells in the Human Brain
Sloan Robertson (Scotland)	Surgery of Pituitary Tumours
Ed. Boldrey (San Francisco)	The Place of Neurosurgery in Medicine
Lamar Roberts (Gainesville)	The Department of Neurosurgery at the University of Florida
Doros Oeconomos (Athens)	Organization of a Unit for the Study and Treatment of Epileptic Patients
Martin Nichols (Aberdeen)	The Surgical Treatment of Aneurysms
Fuad Haddad (Beirut)	The Surgical Treatment of Intracerebral Echinoccocal Cysts
Robert Pudenz (Pasadena)	Ventriculo-atrial Shunt for the Treatment of Hydrocephalus
Miller Fisher (Boston)	Aphasia, Apraxia, and Agnosia

Table 25.2 (*continued*)
Silver Anniversary Celebrations, 5–8 October 1959

Speakers*	Topic
David Daly (Rochester)	Narcolepsy
Kenan Tükel (Istanbul)	Clinical and EEG Findings in Hypoinsulinsm***
Milton Shy (Bethesda)	Periodic Paralysis
Jerzy Olsweski (Toronto)	Future of Neuroanatomy and Neuropathology
C. Ajmone-Marsan (Bethesda)	Unit Analysis of the Electrical After-Discharge
Jan D-Fortuyn (Groningen)	Comparative Anatomy of the Brain
W. Haymaker (Washington)	Neurologic Hazards of Space-Travel
Jerzy Chorobski (Warsaw)	The Pathogenesis of Involuntary Movements
Herbert Jasper (McGill)	Evolution of Conceptions of Cerebral Localization since Hughlings Jackson****
Donald McRea (McGill)	The Symptoms of Abnormalities of the Cervical Spine
A. Ortiz-Galvan (Mexico)	Upper Cervical and Foramen Magnum Abnormalities
Ira Jackson (Galveston)	Dr Cone's Contribution to the Treatment of Hydrocephalus
Igor Klatzo (Bethesda)	Dr Cone as a Neuropathologist
Guy Odom (Duke)	Dr Cone's Method of Treatment of Brain Abscess
Gilles Bertrand (McGill)	The Twist Drill in Neurosurgery
Dorothy Russell (London)	Reflections on Neuropathology*****

* In order of presentation
** Dean, McGill Medical School
*** Kenan Tükel was detained in Istanbul, but Peter Gloor presented his paper
**** Hughlings Jackson Lecture
***** Fellows Society Lecture

26

Theodore Rasmussen

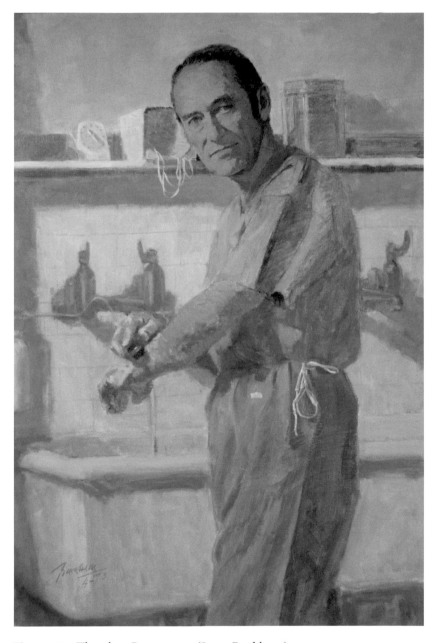

Figure 26.1: Theodore Rasmussen. (Lynn Buckham)

Theodore Brown Rasmussen was born in Provo, Utah, in 1910, the son of Andrew Rasmussen, professor of neuroanatomy at the University of Minnesota. A lover of jazz, Rasmussen supported himself through medical school by playing saxophone in a jazz band (figure 26.2). He headed for New York City after graduation in 1935, to King's County Hospital in Brooklyn, not for the jazz clubs but for the proximity to Madison Square Gardens, where he could indulge his other interest, track and field. It was this latter interest, as William Feindel recounted, that cemented their relationship. "I first came to know Ted Rasmussen in June 1942, when I came from Dalhousie Medical School for two weeks at the Neuro to learn techniques for examining peripheral nerves. Dr Penfield assigned Dr Rasmussen as my mentor … A bagpiper appeared for several nights in Molson Stadium [abutting the institute], practicing vigorously. By the third night, Ted could stand it no longer and said 'Let's go to a movie.' On the way down University Street he recited the records to the minute and second of the main track and field champions at that time. We became good friends for the next sixty years."[1]

Theodore Rasmussen took a decisive turn towards neurosurgery while at King's County when he came under the influence of Jefferson Browder, a neurosurgeon who had trained with Harvey Cushing. His course thus set, Rasmussen, a no-nonsense type, contacted Wilder Penfield directly and soon found himself on a Greyhound bus to Montreal, where he spent the next five months. With Rasmussen's first tour at the MNI coming to an end, Penfield advised him to seek further training in neurology at the Mayo Clinic. Soon thereafter, Rasmussen was back on a bus to Rochester, Minnesota, where he spent the next three years training in neurology and earning an MSc for his thesis, "Experimental Intracranial Ligation of the Cerebral Arteries of the Dog."[2]

Rasmussen returned to the MNI for his neurosurgical training, from 1939 to 1942, joining a carefree band of fellow American neurosurgical trainees that included Edwin Boldrey, Warren Brown, Theodore Erickson, Lyle Gage, Wolfgang Klemperer (the conductor's son), Guy Odom, Robert Pudenz, and Walter Stuck. America had not yet entered the war, and these must have been exhilarating times of research and discovery for these young men not yet called to duty.

For Theodore Rasmussen, the call came in 1942, just nine months short of the end of his residency. He served with distinction in Burma, attending wounded GIs and Chinese nationals fighting the Japanese.[3] Rasmussen returned to the MNI upon his discharge from the Army, not to finish his training, for the war had seen to that, but to join his mentors as assistant neurosurgeon at the

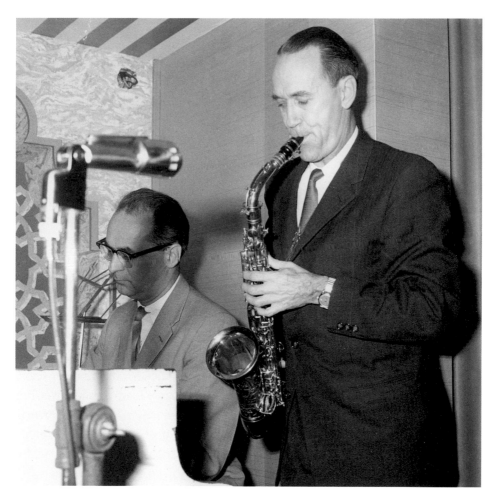

Figure 26.2: Bill Feindel (*left*) at the keyboard and Ted Rasmussen, second director of the MNI, on saxophone during the Fellows Day Dinner at Ruby Foo's Restaurant in 1959. (MNI Archives)

MNI and lecturer in neurosurgery at McGill University. During that time, he collaborated with Wilder Penfield on the writing of *The Cerebral Cortex of Man*.[4] Rasmussen stayed two years at the institute before moving on to head the Department of Neurosurgery at the University of Chicago. As one of his successors at Chicago put it, "As was usual for Dr Penfield's trainees during that era, he went from being a junior staff man at the Montreal Neurological Institute to become the Professor of Neurological Surgery elsewhere."[5]

Theodore Rasmussen's major interest in Chicago mirrored Penfield's: the relationship between cerebral ischemia and electrocortical activity. Rasmussen and his colleague John Harvey observed that the brain could tolerate short periods of ischemia without producing EEG changes, but that prolonged ischemia had pronounced effects on the EEG, which were, "on the whole," proportional to the duration of the occlusion.[6]

They also observed that manipulation of the middle cerebral artery could produce spasm of such severity that the artery was sometimes difficult to identify with the naked eye. Richard Lende later performed similar experiments at the MNI, which ultimately led to his beautifully illustrated paper "Manipulation Hemiplegia."[7]

Theodore Rasmussen left the University of Chicago in 1954 and returned to the MNI as professor and chairman of neurology and neurosurgery. He was appointed director of the institute in 1960, inheriting a clinical and research staff second to none in the world.

HOSPITAL NUMBER 19

Change was also occurring outside the institute as the new premier of Quebec, Jean Lesage, and his minister of health, Alphonse Couturier, lost no time in enacting the newly elected Liberal Party's ambitious socio-economic reforms. Thus, "on 1 January 1961 the Quebec Hospital Insurance Plan came into being and [the MNI] became Hospital Number 19."[8] Theodore Rasmussen, a practical man, saw both opportunity and danger in this numerical reassignment: "This is an important and perhaps critical year for the hospital side of the Institute ... since there is now visible a beacon of hope for future financial stability. Vision, foresight and cooperation will be needed from political authorities, the public, doctors, nurses, hospital administrators and other hospital personnel, to insure that this financial stability is not achieved at the cost of lowering the standards of patient care."[9] As the MNI became the MNI-H, Theodore Rasmussen emphasized that this would in no way alter the close cooperation between the clinical and research activity of the institute or weaken its ties with McGill University. Hospital services, however, were another matter, as Preston Robb reported, contrary to Rasmussen's expectations, "The budget for 1962 has been submitted and reviewed by Quebec. There was a 30% cut. In a word, this is ridiculous."[10] Still, Robb remained resolute: "The reputation of this Institute is built on the best in medical, surgical, and nursing care. It has always been expensive. I want to assure you, that regardless of the pressures to reduce costs, we shall not lower our standards."[11] In this, Robb found his most stalwart support in Bertha Cameron, the new director of nursing.

Table 26.1
Clinical staff, 1960–61

Francis McNaughton	Neurologist-in-chief
Preston Robb	Neurologist
Donald Lloyd-Smith	Associate neurologist
J.B.R. Cosgrove	Assistant neurologist
Bernard Graham	Assistant neurologist
Irving Heller	Assistant neurologist
David Howell	Assistant neurologist
Reuben Rabinovitch	Assistant neurologist
William Tatlow	Assistant neurologist
Arthur R. Elvidge	Neurosurgeon-in-chief
Gilles Bertrand	Neurosurgeon
William Feindel	Neurosurgeon
Theodore Rasmussen	Neurosurgeon
John Blundell	Assistant neurosurgeon
Charles Branch	Assistant neurosurgeon
Richard Rovit	Assistant neurosurgeon
Donald McRae	Radiologist
Roméo Ethier	Associate radiologist
Herbert Jasper	Neurophysiologist
Pierre Gloor	Electroencephalographer
Donald Lloyd-Smith	Assistant electroencephalographer
Richard R. Gilbert	Anaesthetist
G. Frederick Brindle	Associate anaesthetist
Ronald Millar	Associate anaesthetist
K.A.C. Elliott	Neurochemist, Donner Fellow
Hanna M. Pappius	Associate neurochemist
Leonhard S. Wolfe	Associate neurochemist
Gordon Mathieson	Neuropathologist
Brenda Milner	Research psychologist

Note: Gilles Bertrand also functioned as assistant neuropathologist and Irving Heller as clinical neurochemist. Francis McNaughton was the head of the Department of Neuroanatomy, J.B.R. Cosgrove was head of research in multiple sclerosis, and Charles Hodge and Jean Garneau were the photographers.

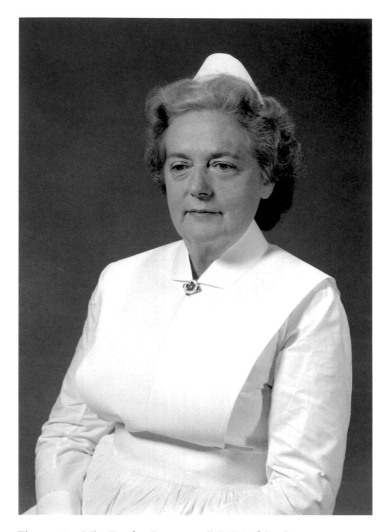

Figure 26.3: Miss Bertha Cameron. (MNI Archives)

A PLAIN WHITE DRESS AND A STIFF STARCHED BIB

Eileen Flanagan retired from nursing in September 1961 and Bertha Cameron was appointed the MNI's second director of nursing. Cameron had come to Montreal to train in nursing at the RVH, then began her career at the Vic after graduating in 1931 and was made head nurse on Wilder Penfield and William Cone's ward. She was chosen to be night supervisor when the MNI opened on University Street in 1934, and was later appointed assistant director of nursing. Cameron "always wore the Royal Victoria Hospital regulation white, crisply-laundered uniform: a plain white dress covered by a stiff starched bib and a gathered apron. The collar and cuffs were also starched. Her RVH cape was folded in the correct manner to a point."[12]

Bertha Cameron was well spoken, poised, and dignified. She was knowledgeable and, like all successful nursing administrators, she was helpful and supportive of younger nurses, even in the face of the social changes that affected nursing and society during her tenure: "the era of the Beatles, Medicare, union development, miniskirts, teenage expressiveness, and beehive hairdos. Changes were coming fast. One of the post-basic (Nursing program) groups wanted their photograph taken in street clothes!"[13] (figure 26.4).

Table 26.2
Montreal Neurological Institute nursing staff, 1961–62

Bertha Cameron	Director of nursing
Louise Hall	Assistant director of nursing
Eleanor Carmen	Administrative assistant
Annie Johnson	Supervisor dressing rooms
Irene McMillan	Educational director
Maureen E McIntosh	Clinical director
Elizabeth Barrowman	Night supervisor
Helen Kryk	Assistant night supervisor
Lillian McAuley	Assistant night supervisor
Marilyn Manchen	Assistant night supervisor
Phoebe Stanley	Operating room supervisor
Evelyn Bain	Assistant operating room supervisor
Evelyn Adam	Head nurse
M. Agnew	Head nurse
Alice Cameron	Head nurse
Mary Cavanaugh	Head nurse
Helen Danaher	Head nurse
Audrey Kimberley	Head nurse
Delta MacDonald	Head nurse
Viola Store	Head nurse

Despite the whimsical accompaniment of the British invasion led by the Beatles, the early 1960s was a difficult time for the newly appointed director of nursing. Quebec society underwent political and social change affecting all spheres of public and private life overnight with "in the Quiet Revolution" that

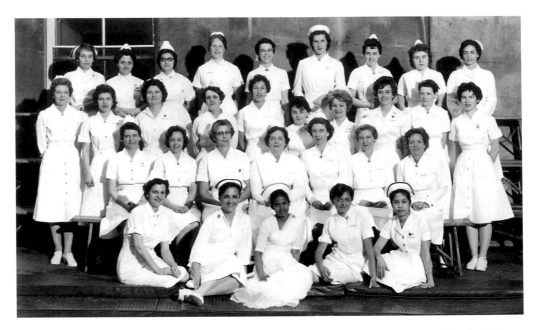

Figure 26.4: 1961 MNI nursing staff photograph. No street clothes, no beehive hairdos, nary a miniskirt in sight. Bertha Cameron is in the second row, fourth from the left. Her sister Alice, who had come with her from Nova Scotia to train in nursing in Montreal, is at the extreme left in the third row. Alice Cameron was the head nurse on Four South. Mary Cavanaugh is in the same row as Alice, ninth from the left. Mary Cavanaugh was head nurse on Two South, William Cone's ward, and until Paediatric Neurosurgery was relocated to the Montreal Children's Hospital, the Paediatric Ward, where Peter Pan first alighted. (MNI Archives)

followed the Quebec general election of 1962. Some of the revolutionary changes that the MNI had to accommodate were trade unionism and the forty-hour workweek. This was the first issue that Bertha Cameron had to face, as she reported to the staff:

> Since the 5-day (40-hour) work week began and added personnel were needed to plan for time off, we have been unable to get the desired number of general staff nurses to carry out the quality of nursing we consider essential. To overcome the shortage, we found it necessary to employ General Staff Relief nurses paid on a daily basis and more nursing assistants … Although we do have many nursing assistants on our staff who are well trained (most of them trained on the job), we found that many of those newly employed had little or no training. Training nursing assistants on the job means an added load on the nursing staff.[14]

The need for nurses trained in the specialized care of neurological and neurosurgical patients was paramount, but the solution to the shortfall was not obvious. The RVH and the Montreal General Hospital had their own highly regarded nursing schools. However, with the continued consolidation of the Quiet Revolution, the provincial government took responsibility for training nurses.[15] The challenge that Bertha Cameron faced was therefore twofold: to find English-speaking nurses who were also specialized in the care of neurologically impaired patients, when both were dwindling commodities. The postgraduate course in Neurological and Neurosurgical Nursing was thriving despite these difficulties, Cameron noted, and offered a partial solution: "Graduate nursing students from many parts of Canada and all over the world enter our classes in April and October … and I am pleased to say that a goodly number remained with us to gain further knowledge and experience."[16]

Bertha Cameron oversaw a first at the institute, the awarding of named prizes in recognition of nursing excellence. The first Eileen Flanagan prize, from a scholarship fund established by nurses who had worked with her, was awarded to Shirley Jaskari, of the postgraduate class. Two other prizes would have far-reaching consequences on the Neurological Institute. Caroline Robertson received the Mrs Samuel Reitman Nursing Bursary, in memory of William Cone, and the Women's Auxiliary Nursing Bursary was awarded to Patricia Murray. These bursaries allowed Robertson and Murray to pursue their education at the School for Graduate Nurses at McGill University, and both would play a prominent role at the institute, Caroline Robertson as successor to Bertha Cameron and Patricia Murray as operating room supervisor.

◆◆◆

If the MNI faced a new beginning, it also saw the loss of many residents and fellows who, having finished their training and their research projects, carried the traditions of the institute as nearby as a few blocks down Sherbrooke Street to Hôpital Notre-Dame and as far away as the Punjab. André Barbeau left to become assistant professor of experimental neurology at the Université de Montréal, where he became a leading figure in elucidating the role of dopamine in Parkinson's disease. He was also appointed to the Outpatient Staff of the MNI, where he pursued his interest in extra-pyramidal disorders.[17] John Blundell relocated a few blocks west, to the Montreal Children's Hospital. John Hunter, after a few years at the MNI, went farther in the opposite direction, to start a neurosurgical service in Hong Kong. Richard Rovit left the institute for Jefferson Medical College in Philadelphia, as head of its Division of Neurosurgery, and Jesse Barber returned to Howard University, Washington, DC, as assistant professor of surgery.[18] Des Raj Gulati, "a man with a large heart, a broad warm smile and gentle, soft speech," also left Montreal to head the newly formed Department of Neurology and Neurosurgery at the Postgraduate Institute for Medical Education and Research, Chandigarh, Punjab, India. Raj Gulati did pioneering work with Hanna Pappius on cerebral edema and wrote a seminal paper with Theodore Rasmussen on the use of cortisone in postoperative brain swelling.[19]

HIT THE GROUND RUNNING

Despite these departures, MNI research not only continued apace, but was enhanced by the coming of William Feindel, Leon Wolfe, and Allan Sherwin.

The Cone Laboratory

William Feindel wasted no time in putting the Cone Laboratory on productive footing. The new automatic contour brain scanner – a much-improved version of the scanner that he and his colleagues had developed in Saskatoon[20] – was put in full operation, and 235 brain scans were performed in its first year. It proved useful in detecting and localizing neurological lesions and in providing information on the vascularity of brain tumours and other pathologies.[21] These were the toddling steps of a laboratory that would evolve into the McConnell Brain Imaging Centre, a world leader in neurological imaging.

Brain Tumours

Henry Garretson also began his study on the growth and metabolism of gliomas in cell culture, a project that would occupy him for the next few years. In this, he followed in the steps of Keasley Welch and his work on the growth and vascularization of glioblastoma multiforme cells implanted in the anterior chamber of the guinea pig eye.[22] Garretson observed, "Glioblastoma multiforme appears to possess a remarkable ability to induce new vessel formation in even such avascular structures of the cornea,"[23] but these observations would not be fully exploited for another generation and more.[24] Charles Branch and his associates continued their work on the intra-arterial infusion of chemotherapeutic agents in monkeys,[25] and this approach also would not be exploited in clinical cases either for another two decades.

Neurochemistry

Allan Sherwin advanced from his post as senior neurology resident to join the staff of the Department of Neurology, and wasted no time, publishing a paper in *Science* within his first year on staff.[26] He would be a stalwart at the Neurological Institute for the whole of his career. The Donner Laboratory was strengthened by the recruitment of Leonhard Scott Wolfe, a fellow of the Elizabeth Kenny Foundation. Wolfe would eventually replace K.A.C. Elliott as head of the Donner Laboratory, where he achieved international renown.

ACADEMIA

Visitors: Gap Junctions and Absolute Zero

Perhaps inspired by the newly arrived New Zealander Leon Wolfe, the invited lecturers of the academic year 1960–61 were heavily weighted in favour of the Commonwealth. Sydney Sunderland, from Melbourne, presented "The Effect of Stretch and Compression of Peripheral Nerves." Walpole Lewin, from the Radcliffe Infirmary, Oxford, discussed "Closed Head Injuries." Lucien Rubenstein, Dorothy Russell's collaborator from the London Hospital, offered "Growth and Spread of Intracranial Gliomas." The first of many editions of his and Russell's landmark *Pathology of Tumours of the Nervous System* had just recently been published. The lecture of John Marshall, from Queen Square, was "Cerebrovascular Disease," an area on which he spoke with authority. The highwater mark of this British wave was Sir Charles Symonds's 1960 Hughlings Jackson Lecture, "Memory Disorders Following Brain Damage." Sir Charles had been the first to diagnose a cerebral aneurysm pre-operatively during a fellowship on Harvey Cushing's service in 1923. Guy L. Odom, professor of neurosurgery at Duke University, who gave the fifth annual Fellows Lecture, "Vascular Lesions of the Spinal Cord," held the American end.

As it often did, the MNI hosted a contingent from Harvard. The most influential Bostonian was undoubtedly Francis O. Schmitt from the Department of Biology at the Massachusetts Institute of Technology. Schmitt, a founder of the Neurosciences Research Program, delved deeply into neurobiology with "The Molecular Biology of the Neuron."[27] The influential Paul Yakovlev combined his vast knowledge of embryogenesis and of the limbic system for the annual Neuroanatomy Lecture, "The Limbic System and the Hippocampus," and Raymond D. Adams gave the 1961 Hughlings Jackson Lecture, "Thiamine and the Human Nervous System." David Robertson, associate biophysicist at McLean Hospital, Boston, presented "The Ultrastructure of Unit Membranes and Their Contact Relationships in Synapse" – later known as gap junctions – which he had just described in the goldfish brain.[28]

David Keith Chalmers MacDonald, fellow of the Royal Societies of Edinburgh (1954), Canada (1958), and London (1960), Division of Pure Physics, National Research Council, Ottawa, gave the most incongruous lecture, "'The moving finger writes' … (The Irreversibility of Time)." Few visitors to the MNI delved into Persian poetry and near absolute zero in their talk.[29]

T for Texas

The University of Texas at Austin published the very timely and informative *Electrical Stimulation of the Brain*, in which, among contributions from the MNI staff, Herbert Jasper and Cosimo Ajmone-Marsan published their influential atlas, "Diencephalon of the Cat."[30] Jasper also wrote an authoritative chapter, "Thalamic Reticular System," as did William Feindel, titled "Response Patterns Elicited from the Amygdala and Deep Temporo-Insular Cortex." Lamar Roberts's "Activation and Interference of Cortical Function" was based largely on *The Cerebral Cortex of Man* and *Speech and Brain Mechanisms*.

CONSCIOUSNESS

Wilder Penfield gave two prestigious lectures based on his experience with cortical stimulation. The Alexander Welsh Lecture of the Royal College of Surgeons of Edinburgh was "A Surgeon's Chance Encounters with Mechanisms Related to Consciousness," and the Lister Oration of the Royal College of Surgeons of England was "Activation of the Record of Human Experience."[31] Penfield, in collaboration with Phanor Perot, also published the influencial "Hallucinations of Past Experience and Experiential Responses to Stimulation of Temporal Cortex."[32] A fuller version, at 102 pages and with a new title, "The Brain's Record of Auditory and Visual Experience," was published three years later in *Brain*.[33] Consciousness, psychical phenomena, and recall as studied in patients with temporal epilepsy had long been of interest to Penfield, and the *Brain* paper is the summation of his experience in these spheres of neurology.[34] His concept of a continuous stream of experience localized within the temporal neocortex that he formulated from these experiences has not been met favourably by contemporary neuropsychologists, but these papers record the first instances of the recall of music by the brain, an area that would begin to be exploited only in the next century, with the MNI's Robert Zatorre in the lead.

27

Penfield in Russia

JEKYLL AND HYDE

Theodore Rasmussen had been anxious to reassure the staff that the Quebec Hospital Act would not interfere with the MNI's mission of clinical care, research, and teaching. His assurance was made possible by combining clinical practice at the newly created Montreal Neurological Hospital with an active research program in the laboratories of the Montreal Neurological Institute, both sited in the same building. But not all were confident that this would be a tranquil relationship, as Francis McNaughton pointed out: "It is a difficult feat to combine the smooth Dr Jekyll of clinical practice with the shaggy Mr Hyde of the research laboratory – but we hope that a reasonable balance can be maintained."[1] A reasonable balance was what was achieved.

The Epilepsy Clinic was supported largely by a federal-provincial rehabilitation grant. Nonetheless, there was great need "for wider public understanding of epilepsy, and more social aid for those people of all ages who suffer from it."[2] This challenge was met by l'Association pour les Épileptiques du Québec (The Quebec Association for Epileptics) and the opening of new offices in Montreal. The social integration of patients suffering from epilepsy was a major preoccupation of Cynthia Griffin, director of Social Services at the MNI. She coordinated the efforts of her department with those of the Université de Montréal School of Social Work, who assigned a student to French-speaking young adult seizure patients. Further, four McGill social work students were completing master's theses or papers on the problems of employment and of payment for medication of epileptic patients.[3] The Multiple Sclerosis Clinic, under the direction of Bert Cosgrove, was assuring care to over 500 patients afflicted with this condition, while Irving Heller, despite his demanding clinical responsibilities, pursued his investigation of the biochemistry and metabolism of neuronal tissue, with generous support from the Multiple Sclerosis Society of Canada.[4] Allan Sherwin developed a clinical immunochemical program addressing neurological and muscular disease, which resulted in the development of enzyme assays and other methods for the identification of autoantibodies as aids in the diagnosis of central and peripheral nervous system disorders.[5] The study of immune mechanisms in neurological diseases gained strength in other departments of the institute through the work of many clinician-scientists. Especially noteworthy were advances in ataxia-telangiectasia.[6] These endeavours and other activities were made possible largely by a bequest from the Walter Chamblet Adams Memorial Endowment, whose income was earmarked for clinical activities not covered by the Quebec Hospital Insurance Service. Allan Morton was in charge of anatomical demonstration at the institute, while doing graduate work on the hypothalamic nuclei.[7]

McNaughton's unfortunate Jekyll-and-Hyde metaphor also applied to neurosurgery, as three new residents joined the team caring for patients while pursuing graduate degrees. Robert Hansebout continued the investigation of intracarotid chemotherapy begun by Charles Branch. Phanor Perot and Bryce Weir investigated the manner in which specific structures of the midbrain, thalamus, and cortex participate in generating electrographic seizure activity – work begun by Martin Nichols in 1938.[8]

Weir wrote two classic papers while at the MNI, one on tuberous sclerosis with Perot and Rasmussen and the other on oligodenrogliomas with Arthur Elvidge.[9] Hansebout and Perot remained on staff after their residencies, and Bryce Weir left the institute to join Guy Morton and Tom Speakman, also former MNI fellows, at the University of Alberta. All three eventually headed their own university departments, Robert Hansabout at McMaster University, Phanor Perot at the Medical College of South Carolina, and Bryce Weir at the University of Alberta and later at the University of Chicago. Most notably, Theodore Rasmussen and Charles Branch, despite carrying heavy clinical loads, established a highly fruitful relationship with Brenda Milner in the elaboration of hemispheric dominance for speech.

THE NEW DEPARTMENT OF NEUROPSYCHOLOGY

The recognition of the importance of Brenda Milner's work with Wilder Penfield and William Scoville's patients breathed new life into psychology at the MNI. Theodore Rasmussen, aware of the intricacies of psychometric testing, began coordinating the timing of his surgeries with Milner's availability to allow her the time necessary to properly study his patients pre- and post-operatively. It was also under Rasmussen's tenure that a new Department of Psychology was created at the MNI, with Milner as director.[10] Milner set out the priorities of the new department with her usual clarity: "The main programme of this department has continued to be the study of perception, learning and memory in patients with focal cerebral seizures, who are tested extensively before and after unilateral cortical excisions and in long-term follow-up. This work has a dual aspect: first, the application of tests of proven diagnostic usefulness to aid in the localization of areas of cerebral dysfunction; secondly, the development of new methods to throw further light on human temporal and frontal-lobe function and on the problem of cerebral dominance."[11]

Laughlin Taylor, that most perfect of gentlemen, had joined Brenda Milner as a graduate student in 1957 and stayed at the MNI for the remainder of his career. He obtained his MSc from McGill for his work with Pierre Gloor on reading and electrocortical activity, and worked with Gilles Bertrand on the psychological assessment of patients with Parkinson's disease.[12] Cooperation with neuropsychology was greatly strengthened by the appointment of Taylor as a full-time research assistant, and Taylor had the distinction – with Charles Hodge – of being referred to as *Mister*, which set him apart and enhanced the respect that all felt for these wonderful and talented men.

Doreen Kimura also joined the new department. She published her doctoral dissertation, "Visual and Auditory Perception after Temporal-Lobe Damage," in 1961, and two highly influential papers on cerebral dominance using the Broadbent dichotic listening test.[13] In these publications she reported the astounding discovery that "regardless of the site of the damage, preoperative recognition of spoken material is more efficient for the ear contralateral to the dominant hemisphere."[14] As a consequence, the dichotic listening test became part of the MNI's standard armamentarium in the determination of hemispheric dominance for language. With time, a veritable catalogue of psychometric tests was added to EEG and radiological findings to identify the epileptogenic area before surgery, thus assuring a remarkable improvement on the results of temporal lobectomy. Donald Shankeweiler replaced Kimura as research associate when she left the MNI for Zurich, to establish a neuropsychological unit with Professor Krayenbuhl. Shankweiler came to the institute after a post-doctoral fellowship with Professor Zangwill, who had also been Brenda Milner's mentor at Cambridge.[15] Suzanne Corkin obtained a PhD in the Department of Neuropsychology[16] and later relocated to the Massachusetts Institute of Technology. Corkin assured the long-term study of H.M., to whom she was introduced by Milner.[17] Milner and Corkin continued their ongoing characterization of H.M.'s memory deficit, in collaboration with Professor H.-L. Teuber of the Massachusetts Institute of Technology. Meanwhile, the

Department of Neuropsychology continued to make inroads on hemispheric specialization and language, perception, and memory.[18] Philip Corsi correlated the effects of dominant and non-dominant hippocampal resection on verbal and non-verbal memory in his master's thesis, "Human Memory and the Medial Temporal Region of the Brain."[19] Corsi observed that verbal memory is affected by extensive hippocampal resection of the left, speech-dominant hemisphere, and that conversely, spatial, non-verbal memory is affected by large resections of the right hippocampus. A similar verbal–non-verbal dichotomy was observed in frontal lobe function and the ability to remember the order in which a stimulus was presented.[20] By the mid-1960s, so much information had accrued from correlating post-operative test results to the areas resected that neuropsychological evaluation could now be used in pre-operative patients to help lateralize and localize structural brain lesions, such as a brain tumour or vascular malformation.[21]

Donald McRea, Charles Branch, and Brenda Milner explored morphologic cerebral asymmetry related to cerebral dominance in an important but largely neglected paper, "The Occipital Horns and Cerebral Dominance,"[22] which was first read at the annual meeting of the American Society of Neuroradiology in 1966 and was published in *Neurology* in January 1968. McRea, Branch, and Milner found that cerebral dominance, as reflected by handedness, correlated with structural asymmetries of the brain as reflected by ventricular size. Geschwind and Levitsky published their own paper demonstrating morphological asymmetry – in their case involving the planum sphenoidale – six months later.[23] Graham Ratcliff, Carl Dila, Laughlin Taylor, and Brenda Milner returned to morphological asymmetries of the cerebral hemispheres in 1980.[24] They correlated the results of language lateralization demonstrated by bilateral amytal testing to differences in the geometry of the arterial architecture in the posterior Sylvain region. They concluded, "The general picture which emerges is that of a complex and interrelated set of differences in the anatomy of the posterior Sylvian region in the two hemispheres … These include differences in the position of the Sylvian fissure and development of the parietal operculum as well as in the size of the planum temporale. Accordingly, we will use the term 'posterior Sylvian asymmetry' to refer collectively to the set of morphological differences in this part of the brain, recognizing that they are interrelated and avoiding the implication that any member of the set is more significant than the others."[25]

The institute's expertise in assessing cerebral dominance caught the notice of Roger Sperry, who invited Brenda Milner and Laughlin Taylor to join him at the California Institute of Technology to study patients who had undergone sectioning of the corpus callosum to control intractable epileptic seizures. This would be the beginning of a decade-long collaboration bridging the two coasts as the corpus callosum bridges the hemispheres.[26]

Table 27.1
Department of Neuropsychology, 1962–63

Brenda Milner	Clinical research psychologist
Doreen Kimura	Research associate
Donald Shankeweiler	Research associate
Laughlin Taylor	Research assistant
Suzanne H. Corkin	Graduate student

TWO LORDS

The institute was host to well-regarded American neurosurgeons during the academic year 1962–63: Edgar Kahn from the University of Michigan, Ann Harbor; Donald Matson from the Children's Hospital, Boston; Guy Owens from the Roswell Park Memorial Institute, Buffalo; J. Lawrence Pool from the New York Neurological Institute; and Alan Rothballer from the Albert Einstein College of Medicine. Rothballer had obtained his MSc at the MNI with Herbert Jasper on the reticular activating system.[27]

From the British Isles came Ritchie Russell, later Lord Russell, of the Radcliffe Infirmary, Oxford, to present a lecture titled "Some Aspects of Aphasia." His compatriot, Lord Russell Brain, gave the 1963 Hughlings Jackson Lecture, "Reflections on Brain and Mind," which was published, appropriately, in *Brain*.[28] Lord Brain also gave an after-dinner talk, "Dr. Samuel Johnson and His Doctors," who, despite their efforts, lived to the ripe old age of seventy-five.

SNOW ON CHERRY ORCHARDS

Professor Lev Davidovich Landau, a Russian theoretical physicist, was awarded the Nobel Prize in 1962 "for his pioneering theories for condensed matter, especially liquid helium."[29] Helium was necessary to build the Soviet hydrogen bomb, and Landau has been referred to as the Russian Oppenheimer for his role in the Soviet Union's thermonuclear program. Landau was a promising young physicist in 1929 and won a travel fellowship to Niels Bohr's laboratory in Copenhagen.[30] On the same trip he met and befriended Pyotr Kapitsa, a fellow Russian, who had been working with Rutherford at the Cavendish Laboratory, Cambridge, for ten years. This friendship may have ultimately saved Landau's life. Kapitsa left Cambridge in 1934 to visit his parents but was not allowed an exit visa to return to England, so Kapitsa founded the Institute for Physical Problems.[31] Landau became Kapitsa's protege, but Kapitsa could not prevent Landau's arrest in April 1938 for suspected counter-revolutionary activities. Landau was taken to KGB headquarters at the Lubyanka Prison where, after two months of interrogation, he confessed to the charges held against him but was released on parole on May Day 1939, through Kapitsa's influence. Landau's friend and co-accused, Yuri Rumer, was sentenced to ten years in a *sharashka* – a scientific and engineering penal facility where the inmates performed scientific research as forced labour.[32] Landau continued his own work in physics until a road traffic accident plunged him into a coma. Like Foerster's call to Moscow to attend a dying Lenin in 1922, Penfield was called to Moscow, four decades later, to attend Lev Landau. Penfield thought the events important enough to commit twenty-nine handwritten pages of his diary to it while at Moscow's Hotel Ukraine on 28 February 1962, and en route from Moscow to Amsterdam on 1 March 1962.

Penfield recalls that Sunday morning, as he was leisurely reviewing a few pages of an address that he was to give to the Canadian Education Conference, a phone call came from the Soviet Embassy, rapidly followed by a call from Moscow. Professors Boris Yegorov and Propper Graschenko, who had been at the MNI, had requested an urgent consultation on a distinguished theoretical physicist, Professor Lev Davidovich Landau. "Never mind visas," Penfield was told.[33] As instructed, Penfield wasted no time with preparations, save a note left for his secretary to find upon her arrival at the institute Monday morning:

> Miss Dawson:
>   Prof. Landau a physicist working under Prof. Kapitzka (!spelling) had an automobile accident 7 weeks ago. Not speaking but not unconscious. Seen by Yegorov and by Graschenko … My address? Care of Acad. Sciences or NeuroSurg Inst. + Prof Yegorov. Those address are in my Russian reprints. I'll be back Thursday I hope.
>   W.P.

Penfield was met at the Moscow airport "by two Academy representatives" and brought directly to the city hospital, staffed by "robust nurses in white dresses more like shrouds than uniforms." There, Penfield became acquainted with the patient and the circumstances that brought him to his bedside: "The patient, Prof. L.D. Landau, (I was to learn later) was one of the first five or ten physicists in the field of theoretical physics in the world, a foreign fellow of the Royal Society, in Kapitza's Institute."[34]

Penfield saw Landau in City Hospital, in Moscow, on 26 February. Landau's car had been struck by a truck while he attempted to pass another vehicle idling on the side of the road and was rendered unconscious. "Professor Yegorov made a trephine hole in the left frontal region, [and] reported that he found no blood and no increase of brain pressure," Penfield noted.[35] Penfield was called to see Landau seven weeks after the injury and found him to be "unconscious and paralyzed on the right side." In view of the patient's apparent unconsciousness, Penfield initially suggested that a diagnostic ventriculogram should be performed. Raymond Garcin, a neurologist from La Salpêtrière, and Gerard Guiot, a neurosurgeon from Hôpital Foch, had come from Paris and were in a small room. With them were Graschenko, who had visited the MNI in 1937, and Smirnov, who had worked with Jasper in 1958, among others.[36] Garcin "with typical scholarly exactness outlined the location of two lesions deep in the hemispheres … Finally I could only say the anatomy described by Garcin must be correct but since there might be a round clot still making some pressure near [the] midbrain … I would transfer him to [the] neurosurgical Institute and carry out a ventriculogram at once." Penfield's suggestion was met with awkward silence and the first consultation came to an end.

"The phone wakened me at 10" the next morning, Penfield confided to his diary. He and Evgeny Lifshitz, Landau's collaborator,

> drove along the riverbank of the frozen Neva to Kapitza's Institute. The gates swung open mysteriously. At the right of the gate were two houses side-by-side, homes of Lifshitz and Landau … The cherry orchard below was covered with snow. Lifshitz rang, and a shrill barking resulted. Finally a man opened the door and stood waiting with a little Pekingese dog … Kapitza led me through a bare hall into an enormous study and library. Large windows looked onto the river on one side and onto the orchard on the other. An enormous desk was heaped with books and papers. There were two of the largest over-stuffed chairs I have ever seen in front of a stone fireplace. [Kapitsa] motioned me to one and he collapsed into the other. "These chairs were brought from England. They don't make comfortable chairs anywhere else … That wild Russian, they used to call me at Cambridge" …

"If an operation is necessary who will do it?" You have authority. They will do what you say. Will you? They are afraid to touch him. If they did and Landau should die! Yegorov [Boris Grigorevich Yegorov, director of the Bordenko Neurosurgical Institute], well, young men are sometimes better."

Kapitza's son drove Penfield to the hospital.

Outside Landau's room [were] two women. One was tall, blond, with attractive deep-set eyes. She might have been crying … She entered the room with me. A nurse stood aside. The patient's left arm was making slow sinuous movements; the right hand was clenched against his side … She took his left hand and bent over him, and I leaned close over her shoulder. Landau's eyes turned slowly [and] focused on her. She spoke in Russian. He nodded slightly and looked then at me, focussing. I moved my head and the eyes followed. Then his head turned away, out of contact again. Outside the room the other woman joined us. "Is this his wife?" "Yes." The wife took my hand and held it. The friend said, "She says she believes in you as though you were God" … Back in conference … I looked around at the silent people and finally at Graschenko; "Now speak," he said.

"The man is better. He knew his wife and understood something. Since he seems better. I withdraw my suggestion of ventriculography." Yegorov nodded violently, his face all smiles …

"I think he will steadily improve … The brain's machine is not broken but there is interference deep in the brain, trouble with communication from the highest level to the cortex."

Landau's case left Penfield wondering, "Has the brain explained the mind?"[37] He devoted the rest of his life attempting an answer.

Landau did regain consciousness and was able to function but never at the level at which he had before his injury, and passed away a few years later, at the age of sixty. Smirnov relayed the results of Landau's post-mortem examination to Penfield on 9 December 1970. Landau's brain showed widespread damage to both hemispheres – as Garcin had diagnosed – and damage to the lower brainstem – as Penfield had surmised.[38]

For Penfield then, Landau's case was a critical experiment devised by nature, which confirmed to him that the interplay of the upper brainstem and cortex is essential to consciousness and to the attributes of the mind. It is in this that Landau's case justifies its telling, of self-awareness lost, regained, and recalled with an evolving lesion of the centrencephalic integrating system.

28

Penfield in China

Wilder Penfield was well travelled in 1962. Not only was he called urgently for a whirlwind consultation to Landau's bedside, he also had a momentous visit to the People's Republic of China, at Mao Zedong's request. Unlike his trip to Moscow, Penfield's trip to the PRC took substantial planning and the invocation of Norman Bethune. Although they were at polar opposites on every spectrum except dedication to duty, the destinies of Penfield and Bethune intersected nonetheless, and Bethune's memory helped Penfield slit the Silk Curtain and enter Red China.

1928: THE MONTREAL DECLARATION

Edward Archibald recruited two surgeons to the Royal Victoria Hospital in 1928. One, Wilder Penfield, achieved world renown in his profession. The other, Norman Bethune, achieved fame as a battlefield surgeon on the Republican side of the Spanish Civil War, and iconic status with Mao Zedong on the Long March during the Chinese Revolution. Under constant attack from the Nationalist Chinese forces, Bethune operated from dawn to dusk, sometimes without gloves when supplies ran out. During one of these operations he contracted gangrene and died shortly thereafter, in full knowledge of his inexorable fate. Mao Zedong wrote an essay in tribute to his fallen comrade, the only document that Mao, a prolific writer, ever wrote about a foreigner.[1]

Bethune spent five years as a thoracic surgeon at the Royal Victoria Hospital and relocated to Sacré-Coeur Hospital in Montreal as chief of thoracic surgery after he left the Royal Victoria in 1933.[2] Bethune attended the Fifteenth International Physiological Congress in Leningrad and Moscow in the summer of 1935.[3] Shortly after his return to Montreal, Bethune joined the Communist Party of Canada, and, with Francis McNaughton, Jean Saucier, and others, he founded the Montreal Group for the Security of the People's Health. The group, under Bethune's pen, wrote the "Montreal Declaration" during the 1936 Quebec provincial election, promoting compulsory health insurance and medical care for the unemployed.[4] Disillusioned at the hostility with which the declaration was received, Bethune left for Spain, where, in charge of a medical evacuation unit, he was the first to use blood transfusion on the battlefield. McNaughton stayed in Montreal, where, with others, he was a founding member of the Norman Bethune Foundation and remained a supporter until he passed away in 1986.[5] But Penfield's connection with China was more direct than through Francis McNaughton's friendship with Norman Bethune, and began in 1938, with the MNI's first Chinese fellow, Yi-cheng Chao.

YI-CHENG CHAO, 1938

Yi-cheng Chao graduated from Yanjing University and received his medical degree in 1934 from the Peking Union Medical College. A Rockefeller Scholarship brought him to the MNI in 1938, where he trained in neurosurgery with Wilder Penfield and the other neurosurgeons at the institute. Chao returned to China in 1940, where he and his family faced hardship during the war against Japan, but after the war, he worked with renewed vigour, setting up a neurosurgical department at the Tianjin General Hospital and then at the Tong-Ren Hospital in Beijing. The latter became the Beijing Neurosurgical Institute in 1960, the largest neurosurgical centre in China. Penfield recollected Chao's stay in Montreal and his contributions to nascent Chinese neurosurgery (figure 28.1):

> In 1940, after 2 years of work in Montreal, Y.C. Chao (Yi-cheng) returned to China and went back to the Peking Union Medical School, where he had qualified in medicine. But the Japanese invasion forces closed that school and hospital in 1942. From then until sometime after the Communist regime took over in 1949, there was chaos as far as medical practice was concerned. During the confusion Chu Hsien-yi … gathered a group of bright young Chinese doctors around him in Tientsin [now Tianjin Northern China]. In 1952 Chao joined them and immediately inaugurated a program of residency training in neurosurgery.
>   About 1954, … [O.I. Arutiunov] director of the Kiev Neurosurgical Institute, was brought from the U.S.S.R. to plan the development of the specialty. After 6 months in China he returned to Kiev, recommending that a Neurosurgical Institute be created in Peking, and that Y.C. Chao be brought back from Tientsin to direct it. This was done. Today [1963] the Peking Neurosurgical Institute in the new Hsuan Wu Hospital has 120 beds devoted to the specialty and a remarkably skilled medical staff.[6]

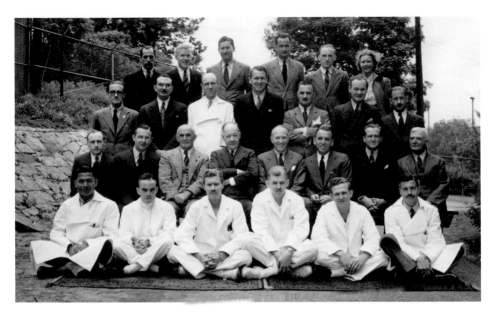

Figure 28.1: 1938 MNI staff photograph. Chao is at the extreme left of the front row. To his left are W. Klemperer (the conductor's son), O.W. Stewart, E.B. Boldrey, G. Odom, F. Echlin. (*Second row*) J.N. Petersen, A. Barbeau, N. Viner, C.K. Russel, W. Penfield, W.V. Cone, D. McEachern. (*Third row*) P. Prados, J. Kershman, J. McCarter, T.C. Erickson, J. Saucier, A.W. Young, H.H. Jasper. (*Top row*) M.D. Cardenas, D.O. Hebb, A.R. Elvidge, A. Cipriani, F.L. McNaughton, M. Harrower. (W. Feindel, "Brain Physiology at the Montreal Neurological Institute: Some Historical Highlights," *Journal of Clinical Neurophysiology* 9 [1992]: 176–94)

Yi-cheng Chao's research interest at the MNI lay in the development of a membrane to cover the brain that would not cause an inflammatory reaction or the formation of adhesions. The topic continued to interest Chao into the 1960s and served as a conduit for some of his correspondence with Penfield after the Chinese Revolution.[7] Their friendship eventually led to Penfield's visit to China, in 1962, and in a sororal relationship between the MNI and the PRC that persists to this day: "Beginning this year [1963]," Penfield announced, "an annual alternating exchange lectureship will be inaugurated between the Chinese Medical College and McGill University in Montreal. It is called the Norman Bethune lectureship after Norman Bethune, who lost his life in 1939 while serving as a surgeon in the Communist Army."[8]

MAO ZEDONG, 1962

Penfield's 1962 visit to the PRC resulted from a directive issued by Mao Zedong to Fu Lien-Chang, president of the Chinese Medical Association. Penfield recounts how it came about in a letter dated 15 November 1961, addressed to Norman Robertson in the Office of the Undersecretary for External Affairs of Canada:

In the autumn of 1956, a Chinese graduate student who was working with me in Montreal, wrote without my knowledge to Mr Mao Tse Tung suggesting that Mrs Penfield and I should be invited to China for a lecture tour in connection with our projected trip to India under the Colombo Plan scheme in the spring of 1957. Mao, I gather, sent the letter on to Dr Fu Lien-Chang, president of the Chinese Medical Association. The latter wrote, offering to pay our expenses from Montreal and return. I refused the invitation, however, because of lack of time.[9]

Despite this first refusal, Penfield accepted an invitation to visit China as a guest of the Chinese Medical Association in 1962. He thus contacted Fu Lien-Chang, president of the CMA, and found it politic to mention Norman Bethune: "Professor Edward Archibald at the Royal Victoria Hospital here in Montreal was both a neurological surgeon and a thoracic surgeon. He was the chief under whom Norman Bethune worked and I worked. We were comrades, he working on the chest diseases and I on the brain. I shall be glad to learn as much as I can of Bethune's last days, devoted so heroically to China."[10]

That Penfield would refer to himself and Bethune as "comrades," beside the political charge of the word, would be surprising to those who knew both men.[11] Nonetheless, Penfield took on the responsibility of bringing a short film, *The Heart of Spain*, produced in New York in 1937, with him to China.[12] The film is of great historical interest because Paul Strand, the influential American photographer, was one of the film's editors, and it shows Bethune and his comrade, Hazen Sise, in cinéma vérité style, with their mobile transfusion unit at the front during the Spanish Civil War.[13] Sise, who had served at the National Film Board of Canada, brought the short 16 mm film to Penfield's attention. Bringing in a 16 mm film into Red China required some preparation. Penfield thus wrote to Fu Lien-Chang on 20 June 1962: "There is a Canadian here, Mr Hazen Sise, who was assistant to Norman Bethune all through his time in Spain during the Spanish Civil War. He has told me of 16 mm moving picture film which lasts about 20–30 minutes and which presents the activity of Bethune in Spain during that struggle. I am planning to bring that film with me and would like to present it to you for the Chinese Medical Association."

Chang responded on 4 August 1962: "I wish to express my thanks for the moving picture that you will bring here. We appreciate much the precious material about his activities in Spanish Civil War of Dr Norman Bethune, the great fighter of internationalism, who devoted his life to the cause of Chinese revolution."[14]

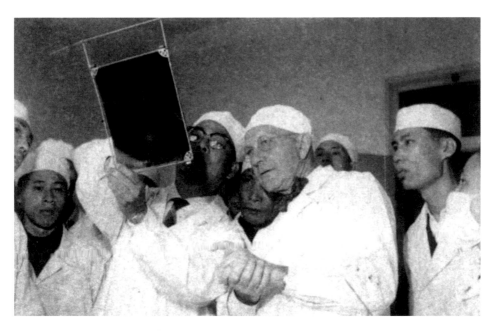

Figure 28.2: Chao and Penfield examining a skull X-ray. (MNI Archives)

Penfield's visit to China in the fall of 1962 was a great success, as he reported in the pages of *Science*.[15] The publication of Penfield's observations in such a prestigious and scientifically rigorous journal is but an indication of the opacity of the Silk Curtain that had been drawn over Chinese scientific affairs since 1949.

Penfield, Chao, and their wives maintained a cordial correspondence in which they exchanged holiday greetings and other pleasantries, as well as small gifts, and discussed cultural matters. But the correspondence between Penfield and Chao also dealt with professional issues. Most significantly, Penfield advised Chao at a critical time in his professional life, in a letter dated 9 January 1963, when Chao was asked to be the head of department at both Peking and Tientsin: "I feel that no man can actually be the Director of two units in different cities ... In my experience, it is not necessarily the best operator or the most impressive scholar that makes the best leader. Above all, you need a man who is honest in his criticism of scientific work, who is keen and enthusiastic about it and who is unselfish in his treatment of his confreres. It is usually true that a man who will make a good leader is the man to whom a small group of younger men are loyal."[16]

No man was more loyal to Penfield than Yi-cheng Chao.

1978–1980

As a result of Penfield's 1962 visit to China an academic exchange program was instituted between McGill and Peking University, and K.A.C. Elliott was the first Bethune exchange professor in 1964.[17] Francis McNaughton was later invited to be a member of Canada's delegation to China for the fortieth anniversary of Bethune's death, held at Shih-Chia Chung in November 1979, the site of Bethune's International Peace Hospital.[18] William Feindel had preceded McNaughton in China by a month or two. Feindel, with Donald Tower, director of the National Institute of Neurological and Communicative Diseases and Stroke, and Elana Bolis of the World Health Organization secretariat in Geneva, had been invited to visit China and observe some of its most prominent medical institutions.[19] As a result of their visit, Feindel and Tower "strongly recommended that two WHO neurosciences centres be established, one at the Peking Institute of Neurosurgery and the other at the Neurological Institute in Shanghai."[20] Further, "with the blessing of the Bethune Foundation," they announced, "the MNI will establish two Bethune-Chao fellowships to enable Chinese neurological and neurosurgical scientists to study here."[21] Ke-ming Chao, the son of Yi-cheng Chao, was the first Bethune-Chao Fellow.[22]

In 2004 the MNI received a delegation of friends, physicians, and administrators from the PRC, and they were welcomed with an address by William Feindel who recalled the rich and productive history of the institute and China. At the conclusion of the visit, the MNI and the Tianjin Neurological Institute formally agreed to become sister institutions.

29

Red Cerebral Veins

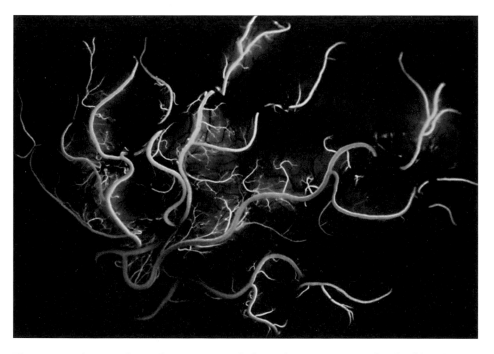

Figure 29.1: Fluorescein angiogram, arterial phase. (Marcus Arts, Richard Leblanc)

Attempts to foster better relationships between scientists behind the Iron Curtain and the MNI continued with Ruben Ashotovich Durinian, a visiting scientist of Armenian origin from the Union of Soviet Socialist Republics, and Tadeusz Bacia, Chorobski's collaborator from Poland. Bacia studied sensory evoked responses in epileptic patients with the help of Kenneth H. Reid, who was instrumental in developing the first computer system for the MNI's neurophysiological laboratory.[1] The exchange of scientists from countries under Communist rule went both ways, as K.A.C. went on sabbatical to the Chinese Medical College at Peking as the first Norman Bethune Exchange

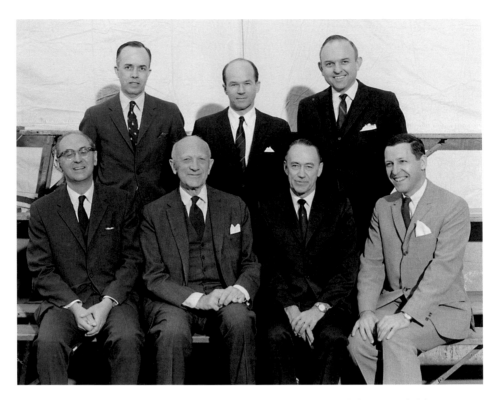

Figure 29.2: MNI neurosurgical staff 1964. (*Front row*) W. Feindel, W. Penfield,
T. Rasmussen, G. Bertrand. (*Back row*) C. Branch, P. Perot, H.D. Garretson.
(MNI Archives)

Professor. For Jasper, "Such activities must be viewed in the perspective of
improved international relationships in all fields of endeavor … which is by no
means restricted to our clinical or scientific specialties."[2] Penfield, however,
was perhaps expecting too much from the study of the brain under any
political system, which he felt would lead to insight into the mind, social
harmony, and world peace: "Increased understanding of the human brain
must certainly lead in time to better understanding of the human mind, and,
ultimately, of human society which may point the way to harmony among
men that is so badly needed throughout the world today."[3] It was a tall order
for a small institute on the side of Mount Royal.

CLINICS AND CLINICAL RESEARCH

Despite these lofty goals, the more mundane activities of the institute continued apace. The Department of Neurosurgery was divided into three services,
each with two attending neurosurgeons: the first with Theodore Rasmussen

and Charles Branch and the second with William Feindel and Henry Garretson. Gilles Bertrand became head of the third neurosurgical service upon Arthur Elvidge's retirement, and was joined by Phanor Perot (figure 29.2). Each service had a special interest: Rasmussen and Branch worked closely with Brenda Milner on the lateralization of language, Feindel and Garretson pursued their work on cerebral blood flow in the Cone Laboratory, and Bertrand was active in surgical treatment of Parkinsonism. Perot was working closely with Wilder Penfield on experiential phenomena related to the brain's record of auditory and visual experience.[4] Most notably, Bertrand and Jasper perfected techniques for microelectrode recording from the human thalamus and basal ganglia during stereotaxic operations for Parkinson's disease. Besides uncovering "a local group of cells which participate actively in the generation of certain forms of involuntary movement, … [the] technique has made possible the guidance of stereotaxic neurosurgery by the sound of the firing of cells … as heard in the loudspeaker, providing a new dimension to scientific neurosurgical methods."[5] This technique is now universally used in the stereotactic treatment of Parkinson's disease.[6]

Table 29.1
Neurological and neurosurgical staff, MNI, 1963–64

Francis McNaughton	Neurologist-in-chief
Preston Robb	Neurologist
Donald Lloyd-Smith	Neurologist
Bert Cosgrove	Associate neurologist
Reuben Rabinovitch	Associate neurologist
Bernard Graham	Assistant neurologist
Irving Heller	Assistant neurologist
Allan Sherwin	Assistant neurologist
William Feindel	Neurosurgeon-in-chief
Gilles Bertrand	Neurosurgeon
Theodore Rasmussen	Neurosurgeon
Charles Branch	Associate neurosurgeon
Henry Garretson	Assistant neurosurgeon
Phanor Perot	Assistant neurosurgeon

TIGER COUNTRY

The function of the insula had remained unexplored until it was occasionally observed that its electrical stimulation caused abdominal sensation and gastrointestinal motility.[7] Boris Babkin and his associates pursued these clinical observations in the laboratory and confirmed the role of the insula in gastrointestinal function.[8] Since a rising epigastric sensation sometimes preceded a psychomotor attack, the insular cortex was resected in some cases of temporal lobe epilepsy. This was done after the temporal structures had been removed, thus exposing the insula, and the resection was carried out between the branches of the middle cerebral artery spread over the insula. Wilder Penfield, Richard Lende, and Theodore Rasmussen raised doubt on the safety of working between these fine, reactive arterial branches. Herbert Silfvenius, a fellow from Helsinki, Pierre Gloor, and Theodore Rasmussen undertook to clarify the situation by reviewing all cases at the MNI in which the insular cortex had been resected along with the temporal structures.[9] Their findings were striking: hemiplegia or hemiparesis had resulted in over 20 per cent of patients in whom the insular cortex had been removed, but only one patient developed a temporary hemiparesis in those patients in whom the insula was left intact. Further, the result of post-operative seizure control was the same in both groups. Thus, resection of the insular cortex for the control of temporal epilepsy was largely abandoned.

New residents were also kept busy with research projects. Robert Ford learned intracranial ultrasonography with James Ambrose, the radiologist at Saint George's Hospital, London, who developed computerized axial tomography (CAT) scanning with Sir Godfrey Hounsfield. Ford joined Joseph Stratford at the Montreal General Hospital after graduation, where he remained throughout his career.

ACADEMIA

The Sex of Neurons

Invited speakers reflected the institute's interest in the physiology of the thalamus and the treatment of Parkinson's disease. McGill Professor Theodore Sourkes presented "Biochemistry of Basal Ganglia Disease," and Gérard Guiot, from Hôpital Foch, Paris, who had been at Landau's bedside with Penfield, gave a lecture titled "Electro-physiology and Stereotaxy of the Thalamus."

Other celebrated neurosurgeons also visited the institute. Dr Charles Drake form the University of Western Ontario presented the first report of a large series of surgically treated basilar aneurysms.[10] Murray Falconer returned to the MNI to present "Some Observations on the Pathogeneses of Temporal Lobe Epilepsy," in which he confirmed Penfield's findings of incisural sclerosis as the commonest cause of temporal lobe epilepsy.[11] This pathology would eventually be referred too as *medial temporal sclerosis*, a term less reflective of its putative etiology.

Former fellow David Hubel of the Department of Neurophysiology, Harvard Medical School, spoke on the physiological effects of visual deprivation in kittens. Denise Albe-Fessard of the Collège de France presened "Organization of Sensory System in the Monkey." The subject of her talk was elaborated upon in a paper co-authored with Yves Lamarre, then a post-graduate fellow at the MNI and later co-recipient of the 1994 Wilder Penfield prize awarded by the government of Quebec. As a sign of the times, Dr V.G. Longo, from the Istituto Superiore di Sanita, Rome, discussed neuropharmacological investigations of hallucinogenic drugs.[12]

Malcolm B. Carpenter of Columbia University, coauthor of the classic *Human Neuroanatomy*, gave the annual Neuroanatomy Lecture on the vestibular system. Dr Murray Barr, professor of microscopic anatomy at the University of Western Ontario, gave the 1964 Hughlings Jackson Lecture, entitled "Some Principles and Examples in the New Field of Human Cytogenetics." Barr was the discoverer on the "Barr body" which identified the sex of neurons.[13]

Reflecting William Feindel's growing influence at the institute, Donald Bates of the Johns Hopkins Institute of the History of Medicine gave a paper titled "Thomas Willis and the Epidemic of 1661." Dr Bates later relocated to McGill, to become the Osler Librarian of the History of Medicine.

À tout prendre

The Eighth Annual Fellows Society Lecture was dedicated to the memory of Jerzy Olszewski, who had died at the tragically young age of fifty-one. The lecture, "Vasomotor Control of Cerebral Circulation," was given by Kristian Kristiansen of Oslo. The annual Fellows Society Dinner was held on 20 May 1964 at the National Film Board of Canada studios, with Claude Jutra, film director, as guest speaker. Jutra spoke on his recent film *À tout prendre* (Take it all).[14] *À tout prendre* is one of the most significant Canadian postwar films, telling the story, in the style of the French New Wave, of a troubled love affair set in the effervescent and turbulent times of post–Quiet Revolution Montreal. That the Fellows Society would invite Jutra to discuss his film at their annual dinner speaks volumes on their awareness of the artistic fervour, political activism, and social ferment that surrounded their Scottish-baronial enclave at the top of University Street.

RED CEREBRAL VEINS AND THE CEREBRAL
STEAL SYNDROME

The Cone Laboratory for Neurosurgical Research

The buzz of electronic instruments and the presence of yellow and black hazard signs as one approached the Cone Laboratory did not fail to attract the notice of Herbert Jasper, head of the institute's Graduate Studies and Research, as he noted, "The Cone Laboratory of Neurosurgical Research under Dr Feindel has been tooling up with a most impressive array of electronic equipment for the application of radio-isotopes to studies of cerebral circulation."[15]

The usefulness of radioisotope scanning of patients harbouring a brain tumour and other intracranial lesions had been firmly established with the introduction of the Mark III model of the Contour Brain Scanner at the institute in 1960.[16] Early studies with this machine had begun in collaboration with Richard Rovit and continued with Henry Garretson and Lucas Yamamoto.[17] A method was also developed for measuring cerebral blood flow during surgery, directly from the exposed cortex. The technique depended upon the use of miniature radiation detectors placed on selected areas of the exposed brain and the rapid injection of a radioactive tracer through a catheter placed in the internal carotid artery. With this technique it was possible, for the first time, to get quantitative measurements of the cerebral circulation as temporarily radio-emitting blood flowed through selected regions of the brain. This new method was augmented by the use of coloured dyes that gave a striking visual picture of the blood flowing through the surface of the brain. These techniques were especially well suited for the study of hyper-vascularized intracranial lesions often associated with red draining veins, a phenomenon first noted by Wilder Penfield some thirty years before. Penfield had discovered early in his career that alterations in cerebral blood flow were sometimes associated with epileptic seizures. On occasion, he observed the presence of arterialized veins, which he felt was due to a "reactive hyperemia" in the postical phase. The investigation of red cerebral veins and their relationship to cerebral metabolism would be of great interest to the Cone Laboratory well into the twenty-first century. Lucas Yamamoto, who joined William Feindel in the Cone Laboratory shortly after its inauguration, played a major role in this area of research.

Yasokasu Lucas Yamamoto was born in Shibetsu, Japan, and received his medical education at Hokkaido University Medical School. From 1954 to 1958 Yamamoto trained in neurosurgery at Georgetown Medical Center and in neuropathology at the Armed Forces Institute of Pathology, the latter under former MNI fellow Webb Haymaker. He was then at the Medical Research Center of the

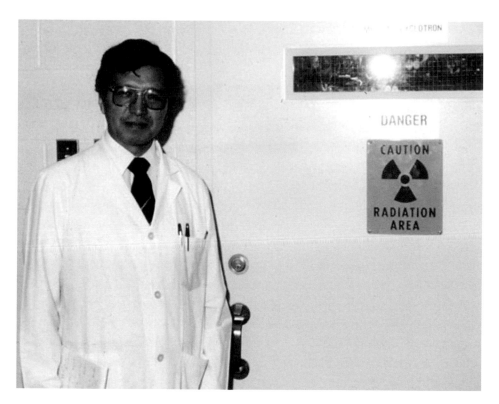

Figure 29.3: Yazokazu Lucas Yamamoto. (MNI Archives)

Brookhaven National Laboratory from 1958 to 1961, where he was involved with the treatment of brain tumours using boron-10. Yamamoto was awarded a doctoral degree for his participation in this work from Yokohama University in 1961, the year that he came to the MNI.[18] Yamamoto had a stellar career at the institute, one facet of which was his development, with William Feindel, of a novel method of measuring intra-operative cerebral blood flow using radioisotopes. Feindel had already made a foray into this field with the medical physicist Sylvia Fedoruk, during his tenure at the University of Saskatchewan. The technique that they had developed consisted of the intravenous or intra-carotid injection of radioactive iodinated human serum albumin in patients who had radiation detectors placed over the head and neck. Changes in the time of appearance of peak radiation count between the carotid artery and the brain, and between the brain and the jugular vein, provided an estimate of the cerebral transit time.[19] Although ingenious, this method was inaccurate and did not provide an assessment of regional cerebral blood flow, so its use as a diagnostic tool was severely limited. Feindel relocated to the MNI soon after he and Fedoruk reported this technique, and, with the arrival of Lucas Yamamoto, the

Cone Laboratory made great strides in the study of cerebral circulation. Feindel and Yamamoto were joined in this work by a talented duo of neurosurgeons, Henry Garretson and Phanor Perot.

Lucas Yamamoto is remembered as a kind, considerate man and as a bold and imaginative researcher. He advanced the careers of many who worked with him in the Cone Laboratory, including a score of Japanese fellows, many of whom have gone on to distinguished careers in their homeland (appendix 1).

In the Absence of a Better Term, We May Call This a "Cerebral Steal"

Phanor Perot graduated from Tulane Medical School in 1952, then served as a lieutenant in the United States Navy from 1954 to 1956. Perot trained in neurosurgery at the MNI and was awarded a PhD for his studies on spike and wave epilepsy during his residency, after which he joined the attending staff of the institute, in 1961.[20] Besides his work in the Cone Laboratory, Perot is especially remembered for his monumental paper, co-authored with Wilder Penfield, on the localization of experiential phenomena within the temporal lobes.[21]

William Feindel and Phanor Perot reviewed a series of cases whose scientific interest lay in the presence of red cerebral veins draining an epileptogenic lesion.[22] Some of the lesions were cysts and infarcts, some were tumours, and others were arteriovenous malformations. The explanation for the occurrence of the rapid shunting of arterialized blood through the lesion and into one or more early filling draining veins was obvious in the case of arteriovenous malformations. In the case of infarction, the explanation would come later, as the "luxury perfusion syndrome" was elucidated by positron emission tomography. In the case of tumours, Feindel and Perot suggested that "the local distribution of red veins evidently indicates vascular and metabolic features which are distinct from the surrounding normal brain." This concept was addressed explicitly in Feindel and Perot's discussion of blood flow alterations associated with epileptic seizures: "The blood through the local region could flow at normal speed but appear as red arterial blood in the veins because of the lack of uptake of oxygen by neurons exhausted by the epileptic discharge. It is also possible that the accumulation of metabolites, especially carbon dioxide, within the tissue involved in the epileptic discharge could cause dilatation of the regional blood vessels and a temporary opening up of the local vascular bed. Arterial blood, flowing at an increased rate, would thus provide oxygen in excess of that which could be utilized by neurons even at normal metabolic rates."[23] Feindel and Perot's great insight was thus to relate complex metabolic alterations and microcirculatory changes. Full exploration of hemodynamic-metabolic coupling was beyond the technology of the times and would have to wait another three decades to be confirmed with positron emission tomography. But for now, some conclusions could be drawn, especially on arteriovenous malformations, which resulted in the first formulation of the cerebral steal syndrome: "Finally, radioisotopic studies indicate that the vascular shunt through an angioma is associated with a reduction in the circulation through the surrounding normal cortex. In the absence of a better term, we may call this a 'cerebral steal.'"[24]

Feindel and Perot first coined the term *cerebral steal* by analogy with the recently described subclavian steal syndrome. As described by William Feindel, Lucas Yamamoto, and Charles Hodge in a magisterial paper, cerebral steal is present when "excessive blood flow is diverted through an arteriovenous malformation at some expense to the circulation of the surrounding brain."[25] More specifically, "The cerebral steal syndrome includes a short circulation time, early uptake [of the angioma] on the brain scan, turbulent flow in the red [draining] veins and a dramatic conversion of shunt flow to perfusion flow after the arterial obliteration of the feeding vessel. On this basis it is suggested that production of progressive symptoms in these patients such as focal seizures, neurological deficits and memory impairment, may be related to the non-nutritional shunt flow rather than to recurrent haemorrhages."[26]

Coomasie Blue Dye

William Feindel, Phanor Perot, and Lucas Yamamoto were joined by Henry Garretson in 1968. Garretson trained in neurosurgery at the MNI from 1959 to 1963, after graduating from Harvard Medical School. Like Phanor Perot, Garretson obtained a PhD during his training, on the growth rate of malignant gliomas. He then served for five years on the staff of the MNI as an assistant professor of neurosurgery and as a member of the Cone Laboratory for Neurosurgical Research.[27] Garretson and his colleagues adapted the amytal injection method as an aid in the diagnosis of complex partial seizures and developed the technique for the intracarotid injection of innocuous colour dyes into the cerebral vessels to aid in the surgery of aneurysms and angiomas.[28] The first dye used was coomasie blue, which visually identified areas of abnormal regional cortical blood flow and guided the placement of small regional scintillation detectors. This method provided "consistent quantitative data on transit times and relative volumes of blood flow through the human cerebral cortex. The circulation through the complex network of pial vessels on the surface of the exposed brain [could] be separated into flow patterns which appear distinctive for arteries, veins and capillaries. In this way, quantitative measurements of arterial, capillary and venous flow patterns were obtained."[29]

Garretson presented this work at the annual meeting of the Harvey Cushing Society – now the American Association of Neurological Surgeons – in 1964. The importance of the published paper was highlighted by the editor of the *Journal of Neurosurgery* who, quite unusually, also published commentaries on it by the distinguished neurosurgeons Paul Crandall, from the University of California at Los Angeles, and Lyle French, from the University of Minnesota. Crandal wrote, "One of the most intriguing aspects of this group's work is the opportunity presented to compare the pre-operative angiographic studies with the direct isotopic measurements of the region of involvement. Similarly, for those of us engaged in external monitoring techniques, these direct studies of the cortex are of fundamental importance."[30]

Clinically, the injection of coomassie blue dye was especially useful in separating feeding arteries from oxygenated, red draining veins in cases of arteriovenous malformations and helped identify which vessels to avoid during the resection of the lesion. The injection of dye was also useful in aneurysm surgery, assuring that the artery on which the aneurysm arose remained patent after the aneurysm was clipped, and that the cortical circulation remained unaffected.[31] This technique has been revived, half a century later, and is now at the forefront in the microsurgical treatment of cerebral aneurysms.

The Cone Laboratory extended its activities to include a collaborative project with visiting scientist Richard Saunders and his associate Victor Carvalho of the Department of Anatomy of Dalhousie University. Their efforts, with those of the Cone Laboratory staff, produced fascinating work on the microarchitecture of the cortical vasculature of the brain, which had a direct bearing on the interpretation of the laboratory's cortical radioisotopic circulation studies.[32]

Mr Hodge

Coomassie blue, as useful as it was in its time, was not ideal. The contrast it produced in arteries was sometimes fuzzy, and the capillary and venous phases were poorly detailed. A better method of evaluation of the cortical circulation was inspired by the use of fluorescein dye in ophthalmology, but it required a master of photography, at the summit of his art, to make it routinely applicable during craniotomy. Such a person was Charles Hodge, known as Mr Hodge to those who were fortunate enough to be allowed down the short flight of stairs that led from his darkroom to the inner sanctum of his office overlooking University Street.

H.S. Hayden was the first photographer at the MNI. He left his position in 1945 and Charles Hodge was asked to take over his duties, initially as an unpaid volunteer.[33] Thus, at the age of twenty-one, Charles Hodge became head of the

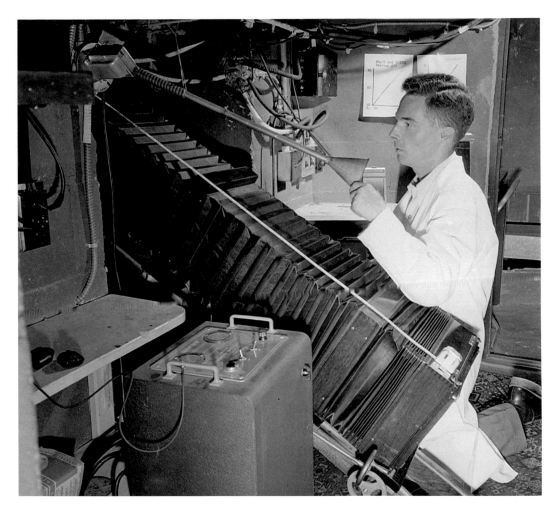

Figure 29.4: Charles Hodge beneath the operating room gallery, taking a photograph of the exposed cerebral cortex through a mirror suspended above the operative field. (MNI Archives)

Department of Neurophotography at the MNI. His only credential for this responsible and exacting job was his enthusiasm for photography acquired a few years earlier through the use of a Kodak box camera. However, he certainly had a protracted exposure to medicine in general. From the age of twelve, Hodge spent three years as a patient in the RVH after he was severely burned by a fire in a model airplane shop. During his recovery he went through agonizing skin grafts and reconstructive surgeries. Hodge gave himself a crash course in medical photography, stimulated by the exacting demands of Wilder Penfield for intraoperative photographs of his epileptic cases, and by the usually urgent requests of William Cone for illustrations of pathological specimens, surgical instruments, and operative procedures. During his half-century of dedicated service to the institute, Hodge became well known to all staff

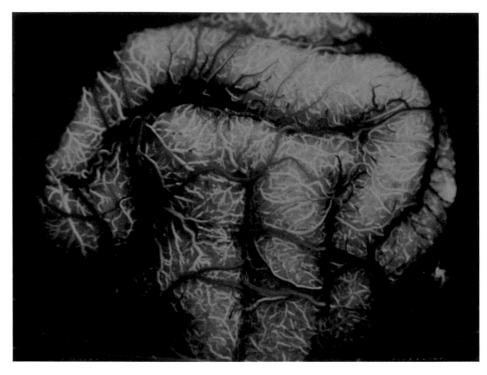

Figure 29.5: Fluorescein angiogram, early venous phase. (Marcus Arts, Richard Leblanc)

members, nurses, and particularly the residents and research fellows. He provided them with endless teaching materials for rounds and conferences and for their research publications. When shown at national and international meetings, slides and posters from the Neuro set a standard of excellence.[34] "Beyond all that, we will recall his warmth to his friends and his cheerful fortitude in overcoming substantial handicaps to become one of the best scientific photographers of his era."[35]

Fluorescein Angiography

Charles Hodge showed great interest and tenacity in developing new photographic techniques. His best-known innovation was the invention of cerebral fluorescein angiography to replace the use of coomasie blue dye for the demonstration of cortical circulation.[36] The technique involved the intra-carotid injection of the fluorescent dye fluorescein, flooding the operative field with blue light, and recording the flow of fluorescein in the cortical vessels through a series of filters attached to still and video cameras, while a strobe light was flashing. The results were immediately available for playback on a stop-motion video screen in the operating room. The whole process took less than twenty seconds. The technique was applied in the Cone Laboratory for many experimental studies of cerebral occlusion and ischemia, arterial anastomosis and vasospasm, and in the operating room as an aid in the resection of arteriovenous malformations.[37]

Continuum

By 1970s, the investigation of the cerebral steal syndrome, and indeed of cerebral blood-flow under a variety of clinical and experimental conditions, largely reached the limits of contemporary technology. Better methods for measuring cerebral blood flow would be developed, but the insights of the major contributors to the Cone Laboratory and the association of cerebral blood flow with cerebral metabolism would have to wait further technological advance, and ultimately the development of positron emission tomography, to progress. This then became the major focus of the Cone Laboratory for Neurosurgical Research and eventually led to the formation of the McConnell Brain Imaging Centre of the Montreal Neurological Institute. It was with positron emission tomography that the cerebral steal syndrome associated with arteriovenous malformations of the brain was confirmed and further characterized.[38]

Herbert Jasper's Departure

Despite the Cone Laboratory's exploration of the cortical circulation in health and disease, the Donner Laboratory's great advances in neurochemistry, ground-breaking work on language and memory in neuropsychology, and not the least, the exploration of brain stem and cortex at the single cell level, Herbert Jasper felt, inexplicably, that "with a few notable exceptions … participation of senior clinical staff has not been sufficiently active, for one reason or another, to make possible the close coordination of basic and clinical work which has been hitherto the hallmark of our Institute."[1] After a conversation with Theodore Rasmussen, Jasper wrote an aide-mémoire dated 23 June [1964] that ended, "Confirm in writing – letter of resignation. Going to basic research."[2] He sent Rasmussen his letter of resignation on 24 June 1964, and it was accepted the following day. At the next opportunity, Rasmussen informed the MNI staff, with "keen regret," of "Herbert Jasper's move … to the other side of the mountain to accept a Research Professorship in the Department of Physiology at the University of Montreal, where he hopes the blandishments of clinical neurophysiology will not interfere so much with his increasing involvement in the more basic aspects of experimental neurophysiology."[3] Wilder Penfield was more candid in recounting Jasper's departure in a letter to Kristian Kristiansen, dated 10 May 1965.

> Herbert Jasper had been feeling that there was, at the Neurological Institute, too much attention and time given to the neurosurgeons and not enough to basic physiological research. He seemed to believe that some of the funds which came to the Institute for academic and scientific work went into the salaries of the neurosurgeons. Ted and I tried to explain to him the working of the ceiling in relation to neurosurgery. As you well know, what comes in above the ceiling in our scheme comes back into the Institute to be used for academic and research purposes at the discretion

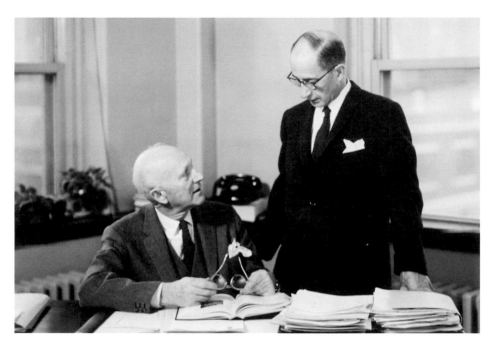

Figure 30.1: Penfield and Jasper. (MNI Archives)

of the Director. Thus there is no reduction in the money available for basic research.

Ted is hopeful that he will continue to cooperate with us. Actually his departure for the work at the University of Montreal was delayed a month or two by the fact that Ted carried out a disc operation on him and he was rather slow in getting on his feet.[4]

Herbert Jasper later expressed his own view on this issue:

Following the retirement of Dr Penfield ... the support for basic research at the Neuro had become untenable. The Medical Research Council in Ottawa was giving research support by means of "Block Grants" given to the Director of the Institute to distribute as he saw fit. I would be awarded grants for my research project but I would not receive the money because it went directly to the Director who used it mostly to pay salaries to neurosurgeons ... to try and induce them to do more research ... I would receive some research funds only if there was money left over. Furthermore, basic science was considered by the new director, a neurosurgeon, to be a waste of time and money if it did not contribute directly to clinical neurology and neurosurgery. This attitude, together with the lack of funds, made it impossible for me to continue the research program I had under way.[5]

Jasper invoked another reason that facilitated his departure: the prospect of creating, with Jean-Pierre Cordeau, who had been a research fellow in Jasper's laboratory, "a series of research laboratories in the neurological sciences working toward a first class research program with adequate support from the University and from the Medical Research Council."[6]

Jasper's leaving the institute was not, in his telling, without consequence: "When the Medical Research Council discovered that one main reason for my leaving McGill was the 'block Grants' they were giving to the director of the MNI they ceased giving such grants. These grants were replaced by 'program Grants' which were distributed to the research workers themselves … During the first year of our Program Grant … we received two million dollars for the support of five senior staff and their assistants … From then on I never regretted moving from McGill."[7]

Pierre Gloor, now the new head of Neurophysiology, commented on his predecessor's departure as a "great loss to this Institute, for few have contributed more than he did to its scientific activities and fame; all of us who worked with him will never cease to remember how much we owe him and how rich his contributions in research and teaching have been."[8]

REJUVENATION

Herbert Jasper's departure, if not quite tectonic, caused an aftershock that had a significant effect on the institute's future activities as Pierre Gloor became director of the Department of Neurophysiology and Frederick Andermann was appointed assistant electroencephalographer. Under Gloor, the Neurophysiology Department moved forward in its investigation of the interactions of the amygdala and hippocampus with other limbic structures and published an important paper in *Science* on the subject.[9] K.A.C. Elliott became chair of the Department of Biochemistry at McGill and Leonhard Wolfe became head of Neurochemistry at the MNI. Most importantly, two MNI fellows, whose activities in neuromuscular research would bring them international recognition, retuned to the institute.

Stirling Carpenter, a quiet, dignified man, was always willing to share his vast knowledge of neuropathology with young, ambitious neurosurgery residents, even as he chided them for misspelling his given name. He returned to the institute from the University of California at Los Angeles to join Gordon Mathieson in the Department of Neuropathology, to take charge of the newly created electron microscopy unit.[10] Carpenter began working with the newly acquired electron microscope and made new observations on axonal lesions in motor neuron disease.[11]

Carpenter found a kindred spirit in George Karpati. Karpati had trained at the MNI and, having spent two years of research on neuromuscular disease at the National Institute for Nervous Diseases and Blindness in Bethesda, he returned to the institute with generous support from the Muscular Dystrophy Association.[12] He and Carpenter gained international recognition for their insight into diseases of muscles and nerves.[13] George Karpati was a brilliant scientist and scientific administrator.[14] Under his direction the Neuromuscular Research Group collaborated with half a dozen senior research scientists with overlapping interests, and his students and fellows have gone on to prominent posts in other leading institutions.[15] One of them is Guy Rouleau, current director of the MNI. George Karpati's most significant contribution was localizing the Duchenne muscular dystrophy gene product to the sarcolemma of skeletal muscles.[16] To Ken Hastings, his collaborator at the MNI, George Karpati "had extremely broad interests but especially in clinical issues, where he was famous for knowing everything. He reacted to all new information with unbelievable enthusiasm. But he always thought in terms of the patient first, then the disease, then the molecule. When he was looking at cells, the patient was informing what he saw. The patients delivered insights."[17] No higher praise can come to a physician-scientist.

To some he was a taciturn man, an impression perhaps born of humility. The most one could expect if one crossed him in the hall was a small nod of the head, with eyes partially closed, looking downwards. Eventually, some gave up and greeted him the same way, and it was fine like that. One of the photographers, whose studio was across the hall from George Karpati's office, recalls an encounter that was out of the ordinary:

My baby daughter and Jerry Lewis changed my relationship with Dr Karpati forever. As an infant, my daughter was not a sleeper. It was a Labor Day weekend around 1992 or 93. I know it was a Sunday night, because the Jerry Lewis MDA Telethon was on. I was on the sofa, cradling my daughter, watching, half awake, when I spotted a familiar face. There, on my television, on stage with Jerry Lewis, was Dr Karpati. He seemed a little shy, but he was certainly beaming.

Several days later, back at the Neuro, I ran into Dr Karpati as he stepped out of the elevator. I said good morning, as he walked by, head hung low. He grumbled something under his breath as he walked past me. Until that day, this was the most he had ever said to me. Quickly, I stopped and called to him.

"Dr Karpati, I have a bone to pick with you."

He stopped, turned to me and asked me what I was referring to. I explained that I saw him on television with Jerry Lewis, and was quite upset that he didn't bring back an autograph for me.

He chuckled a little, smiled then approached me.

"Did you really see me? Jerry Lewis is such a nice man. How did I look?"

We spoke for several minutes afterward, and from that day forward, he always smiled and said good morning to me. Often, we would just talk about random subjects in the hallway. One could almost say that we had become friends. He would often ask me to help him with his presentations. Sometimes, we would sit together in his office discussing his frustration that Napster had been taken offline. That one sleepless night afforded me the opportunity to see the warm side of him that very few saw.[18]

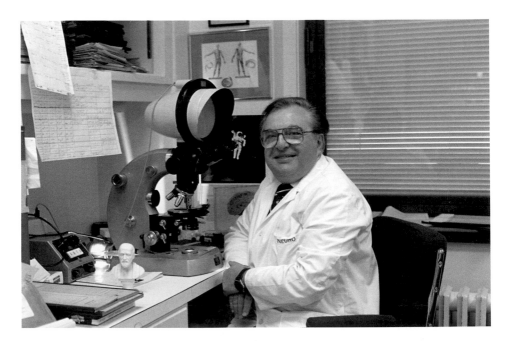

Figure 30.2: George Karpati. (MNI Archives)

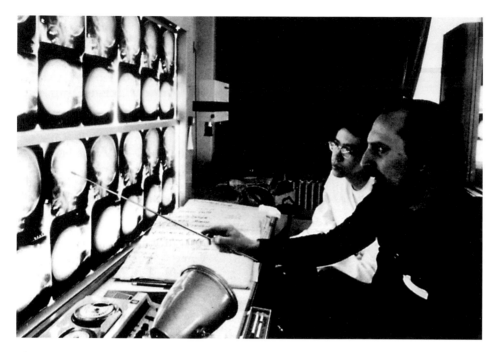

Figure 30.3: Roméo Ethier, sans ascot, teaching a resident the subtleties of neuroradiology. (MNI Archives)

Working in the Dark, Looking at Shadows

Roméo Ethier's appointment as head of Neuroradiology was as important to the MNI as those of Stirling Carpenter and George Karpati.[19] Under Ethier's leadership the governance of the department remained stable for over two decades and saw the introduction of computed tomography (CT) scanning and magnetic resonance imaging (MRI) in North America. Denis Mélançon and Jean Vézina were associate radiologists in the department. Both, like Ethier, had trained in neuroradiology at the MNI. Mélançon, a superb teacher, like Ethier, remained at the institute for the whole of his career, gaining great expertise in the diagnosis of brain tumours. Vézina eventually joined Jules Hardy at Notre-Dame Hospital, where he became internationally known for describing the radiological diagnosis of pituitary tumours.

ACADEMIA

Not all advances in molecular neurobiology came to the MNI via the Jerry Lewis Telethon, as an especially accomplished group of invited speakers continued to make their way to the MNI. Among them were John A. Simpson, from the University of Glasgow, famous for establishing myasthenia gravis as an autoimmune disease,[20] and D.A. Brewerton, who discovered the association of ankylosing spondylitis and HLA B27.[21] Krešimir Krnjevic, from Cambridge University, spoke on cholinergic pathways in the cerebral cortex. Krnjevic relocated to McGill University the following year and eventually became chairman of its Department of Physiology.[22]

The Neuroanatomy Lectures focused on subcortical structures, as Walle J.H. Nauta, from MIT, described in "Connections of Corpus Striatum," and Professor J. Auer, of the University of Ottawa, presented "Reticular Formation of the Thalamus." Paul C. Bucy, of Northwestern University, was the 1965 Hughlings Jackson lecturer. Despite an intriguing title, "The Delusion of the Obvious," which promised insight into the cognitive function of the brain, Bucy addressed the pyramidal tract in human and monkey.[23] Roger Sperry, from the California Institute of Technology, gave the wonderfully titled 1966 Hughlings Jackson Lecture, "Mental Unity and Surgical Disconnection of the Cerebral Hemispheres."[24] David Hubel, from the Department of Neurophysiology at Harvard University, was also a guest of the institute that year and offered "The Visual Cortex and Perception." Hubel and Sperry woud later again share the podium, in Stockholm, when they were awarded the 1981 Nobel Prize in Physiology or Medicine, Hubel for his work with Torsten Nils Wiesel on the columnar organization of the visual cortex, and Sperry for his work on cerebral dominance.

For Peardon Donaghy, from the University of Vermont, the trip to the MNI was only a two-hour drive north along I-89. Donaghy had established one of the first micro-neurosurgical laboratories, where Gazi Yasargil, the ablest of neurosurgeons had trained.[25] Donaghy described the use of magnification in neurosurgery in his talk at the institute. Richard Leblanc recalls that hosting Donaghy was one of his more pleasant duties as senior resident at the MNI, during one of Donaghy's frequent visits. At the time, the new Penfield Wing was under construction, and there was scaffolding in the main entrance and down the corridors through which I, apologetically, guided him. "Don't worry son," Donaghy said, "I've been coming to the MNI since it opened and its always expanding.

1967, CANADA'S CENTENNIAL YEAR

The major event at the institute in Canada's centennial year was the conversion of the Four North wing into a twelve-bed Intensive Care Unit, which also served as a post-operative recovery room. Although a great asset to the MNI, the new ICU made it all too obvious that the institute was once again outgrowing the building. As Theodore Rasmussen highlighted, "In 1954, the first year after the

McConnell Wing was opened, the expanded M.N.I. housed, just comfortably, 22 senior staff members and 40 Fellows, including all rotators. Now, the senior staff has increased to 38, nearly double the 1954 roster, and the Fellowship and Resident groups, including the rotators, has increased from 40 to 66."[26] The increased number of researchers had to be addressed. When Penfield and Cone had faced this problem in 1928, Jonathan Meakins had solved it in true Gordian fashion by putting room dividers in the laboratories, thus doubling the work space, but this was not an option in 1967 and it would be some time before the situation could be remedied. Nonetheless, even in cramped quarters, research continued without interruption.

Pierre Gloor, head of postgraduate education, spoke of the importance of individual and collaborative effort in the clinic and in the research laboratory as

> a bridge between basic science and clinical medicine. Much of our past pioneering in such fields as the surgical treatment of epilepsy can be regarded as the embodiment of this tradition; in recent years too we have progressed further along this road, as testified … by the elegant, single cell recording in the human thalamus carried out by Dr Bertrand in the operating room, by the biochemical identification of complex, but clearly definable cerebral lipids in certain lipidoses which have been performed in Dr Wolfe's laboratory and by the application of immunochemical techniques to the study of neurological problems performed in Dr Sherwin's and Dr Karpati's laboratories.[27]

This was high praise indeed, coming from Pierre Gloor, but warranted: these and other efforts resulted in publications in *Nature*, the *Proceedings of the National Academy of Sciences*, and *Science*, including an early paper on the dual brain authored by Brenda Milner, Laughlin Taylor, and future Nobel laureate Roger Sperry.[28] George Karpati and King Engel, director of clinical and laboratory research in neuromuscular diseases at the National Institutes of Health, Bethesda, published extensively on muscle ultrastructure, neuronal trophism, and myopathies. The localization of creatine phosphokinase in human skeletal muscle was identified for the first time, and the lactic dehydrogenase profile of common brain tumours was investigated.[29] Work on prostaglandins was proceeding at a rapid pace in the Donner Laboratory, and work on neurolipidoses was also producing interesting results.[30] Hanna Pappius and her collaborators studied the effects of dexamethasone in experimental spinal trauma and on experimental middle cerebral artery occlusion. Allan Sherwin and Andrew Eisen also took up the study of cerebral ischemia, evaluating the role of creatine phosphokinase in stroke.[31]

The thalamus remained the focus of other investigators, who studied its interconnections with the amygdala, its function as a modulator of pyramidal tract activity, and its role in Parkinson's disease. The role of the hypothalamus in thermoregulation was also investigated.[32] Pierre Gloor's contributions to the understanding of generalized forms of epilepsy were recognized by an invitation to present his laboratory's work to the New York Academy of Sciences.[33] Charles Needham and Carl Dila, under Phanor Perot's guidance, took advantage of the epileptogenic properties of cobalt powder when applied to the cerebral cortex, and observed that electrical stimulation of the reticular formation could activate these sensitized cortical areas.[34] Similarly, the excitatory and inhibitory events in and about an artificially created epileptic focus were elucidated.[35]

Much to the credit of the nursing staff of the MNI, the Barrow Neurological Institute, in Phoenix, Arizona, invited Helen Kryk, assistant director of nursing, to advise it on development of a teaching program for nurses. This was a great testimonial to the Postgraduate Nursing Program that had, by then, graduated over 800 nurses from thirty-seven countries.[36] It was also another instance of the close links of the MNI and the BNI, the first having been forged by former MNI fellow Harry Steelman, who joined John Green, founder of "The Barrow," in Phoenix after leaving the MNI.[37]

Fred Brindle left the institute to become professor and chairman of the Department of Anesthesia of the newly created medical school at the University of Sherbrooke, and three new physicians joined the Department of Neuroanesthesia at the MNI: Georges-Henri Sirois from the Université de Montréal and Laval University, Alexander Straja from Bucharest, and Davy Trop from Ghent, Belgium.[38] Trop later became head of the department, a position he held until his retirement.

ACADEMIA

Centennial Year Lectures

The Fellows Society initiated the Penfield Award for Excellence, a tradition that has been observed intermittently over the years. The first recipient was Robert Nelson and the second was George Matthews.

J. Clifford Richardson of the University of Toronto, was the Centennial Visiting Professor. He addressed the staff and fellows with "The Late Assessment of Brain Injury." Fred Walberg, of Oslo, gave the 1968 Neuroanatomy Lecture on the microscopic appearance of cerebellar relay nuclei, and Louis Poirier, of Laval University, gave the lecture the following year on the rubro-olivary tract.

Influential zoologist, anatomist, and neurophysiologist John Zachary Young, from University College, London, gave the 1967 Hughlings Jackson Lecture, "Information Storage in the Nervous System,"[39] and K.A.C. Elliott gave the 1968 lecture, "Neurochemistry: An Aspect of the Interdisciplinary Basis of Neurology," two topics close to his heart. Most noteworthy, perhaps, of all the invited lecturers was Holger Hyden, from Gothenburgh, Sweden, who gave the 1969 Hughlings Jackson Lecture, "Neural Plasticity of Learning." Hyden was the first to confirm Hebb's theory of altered synaptic connectivity in memory by demonstrating alterations in neuronal RNA with learning.[40]

Clinical Neurosurgery

The Congress of Neurological Surgeons held its 1968 annual meeting in Toronto, where the MNI had a substantial representation. Laughlin Taylor spoke on the localization of cerebral lesions by psychological testing, and Donald Lloyd-Smith discussed the electroencephalogram as a diagnostic aid in neurosurgery. Fred Brindle, from the Department of Neuroanesthesia, spoke on the use of neuroleptic agents in a neurosurgical unit, and Theodore Rasmussen described the role of surgery in the treatment of focal epilepsy. Gilles Bertrand and colleagues reported their work on microelectrode recording during stereotactic surgery, while Donald L. McRea spoke on the radiological assessment of bony abnormalities at the cranio-spinal junction, his forte.[41]

The Cerebral Microcirculation

The Fourth Canadian Congress of Neurological Sciences was held in Montreal in June 1969. William Feindel took the opportunity to organize an international symposium, "Recent Research on the Cerebral Microcirculation," which was published in the *Journal of Neurosurgery*.[42] Wilder Penfield gave an informative, insightful summary on his early studies with Chorobski, Gage, Cobb, and Forbes. Members of the Cone Laboratory described the biochemical control of the cerebral circulation and the effects of ischemia on microregional blood flow, and elaborated upon the cerebral steal syndrome as witnessed by red cerebral veins. Gazi Yasargil, from the University of Zurich, described the adrenergic innervation of cerebral blood vessels. Other participants came from Dalhousie University and the University of British Columbia, and discussed micro-cortical angiography and the circulation of the spinal cord.

THE BRAIN IS WIDER THAN THE SKY

Despite the entente cordiale between the francophone and anglophone neuro-logical communities, all was not well in the rest of the province. At a time of un-rest, when the Front de libération du Québec was setting off bombs and many were shouting "McGill français!" in the streets of the city, Penfield was moved to write,

> At this moment in Quebec history, it is well to recall that McGill Uni-versity is the major contribution which English-speaking citizens and scholars have made to the people of this Province, from the time of the fur-traders down to 1969. This Institute and Hospital are the same. We are bilingual in our work, bicultural in our allegiance. We serve all who need our help here and in the world of science beyond. This is the time to say that we are proud of the English-Canadian tradition of service and schol-arship. We are proud of our relationship to this great university.[43]

William Feindel also responded to the nationalist fervour by taking an in-ternationalist approach: "Today, neurosurgery, like its sister-specialty neurol-ogy (and indeed, all branches of medical science) is irrevocably international. Canada now has almost twice as many neurosurgeons as either Great Britain or France. This Institute and Hospital is an outstanding example of the liaison which we Canadians have with our professional colleagues in the United States, Great Britain, France and many other countries."[44]

A decade after the launch of the *Sputnik 1* in 1957, and now, with Neil Arm-strong's footprints on the moon, Feindel elevated the discussion above poli-tics by recalling a passage from an address that he had given while he was still in Saskatoon: "In 1959 at a Symposium ... on 'Memory, Learning and Lan-guage' at the University of Saskatchewan, I said, 'We hear much to-day of stars and planets and outer space has captured the imagination of man. But per-haps we would do well to remember that each of us has in his possession the most remarkable of galaxies – twelve billion nerve cells with their myriads of subconstellations in the compact universe of the human brain. It is this inner space of the mind which surely, of all our natural resources, offers the most exciting potentialities."[45]

Matter that Thinks

The Pontifical Academy is not usually where one looks for insight into neuro-science, but that is where Wilder Penfield was invited, in 1964, to participate in a symposium titled "Brain and Conscious Experience." Although his assigned topic was "Speech, Perception and the Uncommitted Cortex," and perhaps inspired by his surroundings, Penfield broadened his address to include his conception of the brain and consciousness.[46] In so doing, he betrayed his broad, catholic reading habits by quoting from Pierre Teilhard de Chardin's recently translated *Le Phénomène humain* (The phenomenon of man): "We have seen and admitted that evolution is an ascent toward consciousness. That this is no longer contested even by the most materialistic, or at all events by most agnostic of humanitarians. Therefore it should culminate forwards in some sort of supreme consciousness."[47] Teilhard de Chardin expressed this concept more succinctly as "*tout ce qui monte converge*" (all that rises converges). As he would in his later work, *The Mystery of the Mind*, Penfield rejected a materialistic and deterministic concept of human consciousness in favour of Cartesian dualism, stating, "We must use the terminology of dualism in science, [when] speaking of the brain and the spirit or mind."[48] Penfield's address to the Pontifical Academy is a reflection of a deep meditation that led to his ultimate statement of the subject of the brain, the mind, and the spirit, his 1975 monograph, *Mystery of the Mind*.[49]

Hans Berger and the Mystery of the Mind

Wilder Penfield was not the only one at the MNI concerned with the brain and mind. Pierre Gloor, having translated all of Hans Berger's papers on human electroencephalography into English,[50] published a highly insightful essay on Berger's motivation for his study of the electrical activity of the brain: the reconciliation of brain and mind as a single entity.[51] In his essay, Gloor shows how strikingly similar to Berger's was Penfield's conceptualization of the mind and of the putative role played by the upper brain stem as the driver of cortical integration.[52] As Gloor relates, "[Berger's] search for the electroencephalogram of man was motivated by his desire to find a physiological method that might be applied successfully to the study of the age-old problem of the relationship between the mind and the brain … Berger conceived of the electroencephalogram as a rhythmic sequence of activity cycles of large groups of cortical neurons. He believed that this activity was controlled by a regulatory center in the upper brainstem region, presumably in the thalamus."[53] Gloor's translation of Berger's papers and his rediscovery of Berger's purpose in inventing electroencephalography – the reconciliation of the brain and mind – was part of a chain of events that ultimately lead Penfield to *The Mystery of the Mind*.

Wilder Penfield received an invitation from George W. Corner of the American Philosophical Society to speak at the society's annual meeting of April 1973, in Philadelphia, on a topic of his choice. Penfield accepted the invitation and suggested "The Place of Understanding: A Discussion of the Brain and the

Mind," and prepared a thirty-page typescript for his talk.[54] Shortly thereafter Pierre Gloor proposed that the MNI host a symposium on the brain–mind relationship – "the question which was uppermost in Hans Berger's mind throughout his whole career from his medical student days to his death" – to be held at the institute in May 1973, the centennial of Hans Berger's birth.[55] Gloor was the first participant to speak at the MNI symposium with an address entitled "Hans Berger, Psychophysiology and the Discovery of the Human Electroencephalogram."[56] Wilder Penfield gave the keynote address, the same that he had given in Philadelphia, which he used "for further working toward 'The Mystery of the Mind.'"[57]

Figure 30.4 (*opposite*): Penfield's file folder for his notes on *The Mystery of the Mind*, whose index tab reads "Brain Mechanism + Mind of Man." (Penfield Archives.) ΝΟΟΣ (*noos*) is an ancient Greek word that to some refers to the mind, to others the soul. For Plato the *noos* "is there that true being dwells, without color or shape, that cannot be touched; reason alone, the soul's pilot can behold it, and all true knowledge is knowledge thereof." (R. Hackforth, "Phaedrus 247," in *The Collected Dialogues of Plato*, ed. E. Hamilton and H. Cairns [Princeton: Princeton University Press, 1978], 494)

SOURCE OF ENERGY

NOO

SYMBOLS—
MAN'S BEING
A BUSY BIT OF DOODLING
1972 — 1973

MYSTERY
FIGURES MYSTERY OF THE MIND

BR. + MIND —

31

A Rainbow of African Violets

With the coming of a new decade, the director of the MNI, Theodore Rasmussen, was moved to reflect on the decade just past and found it to be a decade of progress, expansion, and change.

> The beginning of the sixties saw Dr Penfield completing his transition to a second career. Dr K.A.C. Elliott, Dr Herbert Jasper and Dr Fred Brindle moved from the Active to the Consulting Staff. Dr Ronald Millar and Dr Donald McRae moved on to bigger posts. Dr Francis McNaughton handed the baton of Neurologist-in-Chief to Dr Preston Robb. Dr Elvidge retired and turned his neurosurgical service over to Dr Gilles Bertrand. Miss Eileen Flanagan passed on the leadership of the superb nursing corps she had fashioned to her long-time associate and co-worker, Miss Bertha Cameron, who immediately had to grapple with the problems of building up the nursing staff, to cope with the transition to the 40-hour week …. Death claimed two of Quebec's and Canada's best-loved and most colourful neurologists, both long associated with the M.N.I., Dr Reuben Rabinovitch and Dr Jean Saucier, and also Mrs von Nida, whose gay and energetic supervision of the Registrar's office will be long remembered.[1]

Academic achievements were singled out: by the end of the decade, some 250 fellows had studied at the MNI for periods of one to five years, of which twelve were on the staff of the institute, and many of the others held major academic and clinical appointments elsewhere.[2] The institute had accommodated itself to the Quebec Hospitalization Insurance Service and was none the worse for it.

Space posed a greater problem: the inner structure of the building had been altered to accommodate the ever-increasing needs of established laboratories

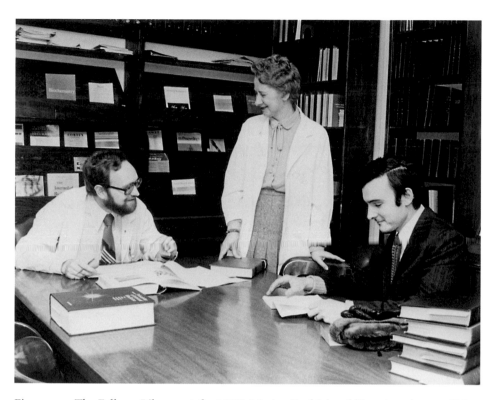

Figure 31.1: The Fellows Library at the MNI. Marina Boski, head librarian, shares a light moment with Peter Herscovitch (*left*) and Serge Gauthier (*right*). Their studiousness bore fruit: Peter Herscovitch became chief of the Positron Emission Tomography Department at the National Institutes of Health, and Serge Gauthier became a professor in the Department Neurology and Neurosurgery at McGill University. (MNI Archives)

and for the creation of new ones, and the hospital had lost a clinical ward with the conversion of Four North into the new ICU. The MNI was bursting at the seams. As Penfield had done before him, Rasmussen looked to the only solution for the problems created by increasing clinical and academic demands: build.

And, as ever, the friends of the institute rose to the task in this time of need. Generous donations were received from R.S. McLaughlin, from Thomas Henry Pentland. Hartland Molson, and from "an energetic anonymous Western friend," which were matched by two other anonymous benefactors. When added to the Robert Bruce and Walter Adams Bequests, the momentum was irresistible and the government of Quebec issued Order-in-Council No. 4084, on 17 December 1969, authorizing preliminary plans for the creation of a new wing, while the Federal Health Resources Fund assumed the remaining costs. After this lengthy master class in fundraising, Theodore Rasmussen affirmed, perhaps over-optimistically, "Barring expected delays, the time-table now indicates that the construction of the new wing, to be located between the M.N.I. and the Pathological Institute, should be under way early next spring."[3]

The institute could not stand idle, waiting for completion of the new wing. If patient care, teaching, and exploration of the mysteries of nature reluctantly revealed were to continue apace, new technology would be required. The Department of Neurophysiology had ventured down this road with the work of Douglas Skuce, a Killam Scholar from the University of Miami, who, "with the collaboration of Dr Levine of the Department of Mathematics at McGill University … has started a project of applying highly sophisticated computer methods to the study of some EEG phenomena."[4] This would require more computing power than was currently available in-house. The institute thus successfully turned to the federal government for a solution: a state-of-the-art PDP-12 computer system,[5] and Christopher Thompson was recruited from Atomic Energy of Canada to be in charge of the computer laboratory. John Ives, a biochemical engineer, soon joined Thompson and Skuce.[6] Pierre Gloor welcomed Thompson with an understated hope that he would "assist us in turning this system into a powerful research tool."[7] His hopes were more than fulfilled: by the following year, Gloor could report, "We have … taken our first hesitant steps in applying computer technology to the analysis of the EEG … Mr Thompson has written a program which allows the computer to locate spike and wave discharges in a prolonged tape-recorded EEG … Mr John Ives has applied other computer programs to these records in order to assess the degree of synchronization of spike and wave discharges. Mr Thompson has written a program which allows the computer to recognize epileptic spikes and to cross correlate them. It is hoped that this may ultimately help to determine the leading side in apparently bilateral, independent temporal lobe foci."[8]

Other clinical researchers were also innovating. Francis LeBlanc began work with Ronald Melzak in developing novel methods of pain control based on Melzak and Wall's "gate theory." Robert Hansebout, former MNI fellow Eric Peterson at the University of Ottawa, and the scientific staff of the National Research Council of Canada took advantage of miniaturization in the field of cold temperature physics, and together they designed a small saddle-like device for local cooling of the spinal cord in the hopes of mitigating the effects of spinal injury.[9]

Marina Boski replaced Sandra Duchow as the MNI librarian. Boski and her able, ever-cheerful assistant Claudia Ugolik, created a calm, welcoming refuge from the day-to-day grind of residency, the more so with the rainbow of African violets that adorned her desk and every sunny windowsill.

MEDICARE

The Medical Assistance Act of 1966 had assured that all individuals receiving social assistance were eligible for government-funded medical care. In the same year, the government of Quebec mandated Claude Castonguay, minister of heath and social services, to chair a commission on the ways and means of implementing comprehensive and universal health care in the province, and the Castonguay Commission tabled its report in 1967. In accordance with the commission's recommendations, the Quebec National Assembly gave assent to Bill 30, establishing the Régie de l'assurance maladie du Québec (the Quebec Health Insurance Plan).[10] With the plan due to come into effect on 1 July 1970, the provincial government halted all hospital construction effective May 1970, and the plan for a new wing for the institute came to a crashing halt. This development was not met with alacrity at the MNI:

> Some … aspects of the blueprint for changes in the delivery of health care … hint at reduced support for the major teaching hospital centres, in order to concentrate on facilitating the entry of the patient into the health-care orbit via less costly and elaborate community health centres. There is concern lest the Province's teaching hospitals may be discouraged or even prevented from updating and improving their facilities, in many instances already years out-of-date. The pace of medical research has quickened enormously, and translation of this growing fund of knowledge and new techniques into more effective, safer and more comfortable medical care is dependent, in large part on the strength and effectiveness of the teaching hospitals.

Put in his own Midwestern plain talk, Theodore Rasmussen summed it all up: "There is concern lest this new blueprint serve to level off the standard of health-care, by cutting off the peaks, rather than by filling in the valleys."[11]

NEUROLOGY AND NEUROSURGERY

Change was not all administrative, but also affected the staff. Frank LeBlanc accepted an offer from the University of Calgary to inaugurate the Department of Neurological Sciences, to be joined by MNI neurosurgery resident Terry Myles and Albert Pace-Floridia, a neuroanesthetist at the institute. André Olivier replaced Frank LeBlanc on Gilles Bertrand's service, where he pursued his interest in functional neurosurgery. Olivier came fully formed to the department, with a PhD from Laval University for his thesis "Chemoarchitecture of the Primate Thalamus," and postgraduate training with Louis Poirier, at Laval, and with Professor Hassler, at the Max Plank Institute, Frankfurt am Main. Olivier eventually succeeded Gilles Bertrand as the Cone Professor of Neurosurgery and head of the Department of Neurosurgery at MNI, all the while becoming the world authority on the surgical treatment of epilepsy.

Change was also felt in neurology as Lloyd-Smith left for Toronto. Ivan (John) Woods replaced him and became the youngest member of the department. Woods gave unparalleled service to the MNI as a neurologist, electroencephalographer, and medical administrator. With the recruitment of Woods, the Department of Neurology remained at full strength, operating three services headed by Preston Robb who was also neurologist-in-chief, Francis McNaughton, and Irving Heller. A new Department of Electromyography was created, headed by Andrew Eisen.

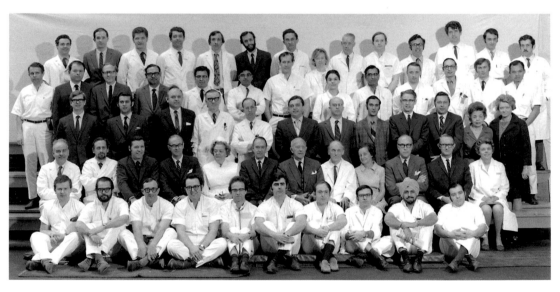

Figure 31.2: MNI staff photograph 1969–70. (*Front row*) P. Murray, M. Lewin, H. Tutt, D. Mercer, J. Lavigeur, A. Olivier, R. Hollenberg, L. Ravvin, R. Sidhu, E. Garcia-Flores. (*Second row*) P. Gloor, R. Ethier, G. Bertrand, W. Feindel, B. Cameron, T. Rasmussen, W. Penfield, F. McNaughton, B. Milner, P. Robb, C. Gurd, C. Griffin. (*Third row*) J. Woods, F. LeBlanc, H. Garretson, B. Cosgrove, B. Graham, G. Karpati, G. Mathieson, A. Eisen, D. Lloyd-Smith, R. Hansebout, C. Strauss, H. Pappius. (*Fourth row*) B. Krysztofiak, F. Andermann, L. Taylor, G. Thomas, L. Yamamoto, P. Khare, J. Peden, L. Prescott, B.Nangia, P. Langevin, A. Sherwin, H. Laurelli, G. Chong. (*Top row*) J. Clarke, D. Fewer, E. Daigle, J. Bulke, C. Dila, S. Nutik, F. Kekesi, R. Curtis, L. Henderson, T. Miles, M. Lechter, J. Armstrong, C. Pace-Asciak, J. Nowik. (MNI Archives)

Table 31.1
Neurological service, Montreal Neurological Institute, 1970–71

Preston Robb	Neurologist-in-chief
Francis McNaughton	Senior consultant
Donald Lloyd-Smith*	Neurologist
Bert Cosgrove	Associate neurologist
Irving Heller	Associate neurologist
Frederick Andermann	Assistant neurologist
Andrew Eisen	Assistant neurologist
Bernard Graham	Assistant neurologist
George Karpati	Assistant neurologist
Allan Sherwin	Assistant neurologist
John Woods	Assistant neurologist

*To December 1970

Table 31.2
Neurosurgical service, Montreal Neurological Institute, 1970–71

William Feindel	Neurosurgeon-in-chief
Gilles Bertrand	Neurosurgeon
Theodore Rasmussen	Neurosurgeon
Henry Garretson	Associate neurosurgeon
Robert Hansebout	Assistant neurosurgeon
Francis LeBlanc*	Assistant neurosurgeon
André Olivier	Assistant neurosurgeon

*To December 1970

NURSING

The Department of Nursing also went through major changes, as Joy Hackwell succeeded Bertha Cameron as director of nursing. The first problem was recruitment. Hackwell had the unfortunate distinction of presiding over the last undergraduate nursing class from the RVH to receive part of their training at the MNI. In 1972, hospital-based nursing schools were closed, and students who wanted a nursing education were now directed to the newly established general

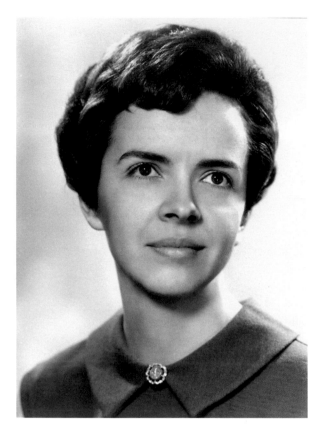

Figure 31.3: Joy Hackwell. (MNI Archives)

and vocational college system, known by the French acronym CEGEP. Although the MNI had been successful in recruiting nurses from all over the world – at the time Joy Hackwell took the reins, over half of the institute's nurses were originally from outside of Canada – it had not fared so well with the recruitment of French-Canadian nurses. To meet this challenge a bilingual recruitment brochure was created. This, and other efforts, resulted over time in a doubling in the recruitment of CEGEP and university graduate nurses, and the retention of many postgraduate students who had taken the Clinical Neurological Nursing Course. To free nurses from administrative duties, the position of ward secretary was created, with a secretary assigned to each nursing unit. This allowed the institution of the primary nurse concept in which "a nurse takes total responsibility for planning and directing nursing care for a number of patients," allowing "individual nurses to assume a professional level of responsibility in the nursing care of patients."[12]

Other measures that Hackwell instituted are still in place, such as the OR-ICU Committee, which assures optimal coordination between these two critical units. Having seen the institute through these and other challenges, Joy Hackwell resigned her post in 1974 to undertake postgraduate nursing studies[13] and was replaced by Caroline Robertson.

Table 31.3
Nursing staff, Montreal Neurological Institute, 1970–71

Joy Hackwell	Director of nursing
Irene MacMillan	Assistant director of nursing
Elizabeth Barrowman	Assistant director of nursing (night)
Roberta Clegg	Nursing supervisor (night)
Lillian McCauley	Nursing supervisor
Anne Carney	Nursing supervisor (day)
Annie Johnson	Nursing supervisor (day)
Cecilia Largo	Nursing supervisor (evening)
Barbara Petrin	Nursing supervisor (evening)
Helena Kryk	Assistant director of nursing education
Judith Trainor	Clinical coordinator
Geraldine Hart	Clinical instructor
Patricia Murray	Operating room supervisor
Alice Cameron	Head nurse
Mary Cananaugh	Head nurse
Lucy Dalicandro	Head nurse
Marion Everett	Head nurse
Delta MacDonald	Head nurse
Flora McCormack	Head nurse
Ursula Steiner	Head nurse

MOVEMENT DISORDERS

Gilles Bertrand, André Olivier, and Chris Thompson, taking full advantage of the PDP-12 computer system, developed a computerized brain atlas that could be matched to an individual patient's brain using mathematical transformations.[14] The PDP-12, the size of two Coke machines side-by-side, was wheeled into the operating room, along with a smaller high-resolution monitor. The anatomical target and the proposed path of the stereotactic probe

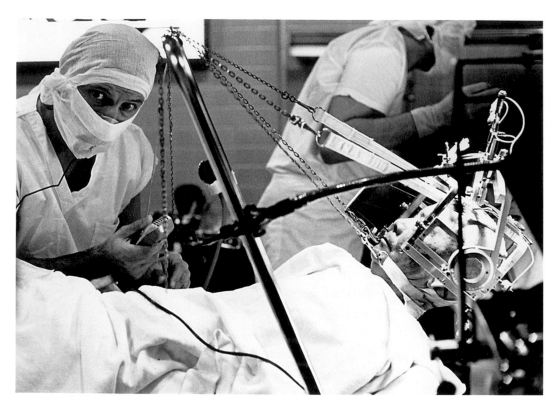

Figure 31.4: Gilles Bertrand (*left*) looks at the computerized atlas formatted to the patient's anatomy on the console (*not visible*) during stereotactic stimulation and thalamotomy for Parkinson's disease, while an assistant studies a conventional atlas. (MNI Archives)

were displayed on a monitor during the treatment of patients with movement disorders, most notably Parkinson's disease.[15] This approach proved useful not only for the treatment of patients afflicted with uncontrolled movement disorders; it also provided new neuroanatomical and neurophysiological data on the thalamus and associated structures[16] and remained influential into the twenty-first century.[17]

ACADEMIA

Visitors to the institute reflected its burgeoning interest in the pathophysiology and treatment of movement disorders. The neuroanatomist Alf Bordal of the University of Oslo crossed the Atlantic to address the question, "Where is the extrapyramidal system?" André Barbeau, increasingly prominent for his research in the treatment of Parkinson's disease, trekked west along Sherbrooke Street from Hôpital Notre-Dame to discuss L-DOPA in extrapyramidal disorders. Barbeau was echoed by the 1970 Hughlings Jackson lecturer H. Houston Merritt, from Columbia University, who gave the address "Pathophysiology of Parkinson's Disease and the Response of Symptoms to Treatment of Levodopa."

But the most distinguished speaker that year was a frequent visitor to the MNI, Sir John C. Eccles, awarded the 1963 Nobel Prize for his work on synaptic transmission. Eccles spoke on his most recent interest, the role of the cerebellum in the control of movement.[18]

Other speakers included Norman Geschwin on apraxia, David Hubel on the striate cortex, Gilbert Glaser on the ionic environment in epilepsy, and Clarence F. Gibbs on transmissible viral encephalopathies.

The 1970 Annual Fellows Day Lecture was given by Donald Tower at the Annual Fellows Banquet. The banquet must have been a great success as no one present was left able to record the topic of Tower's address.

A DEAR FRIEND

A great and distinguished friend of the MNI, Ruth Reitman, passed away on 19 December 1969. Reitman had been a patient of William Cone and, like most of his patients, she was very grateful for the care and treatment she received from this kind and gentle man. As a token of her gratitude, and entirely in keeping with the concept of the "Neuro family," Reitman planned a party for the institute staff at Christmas 1947, and the Reitman family dinner has continued uninterrupted since. "The party was held in the kitchen on Two South, Mrs Reitman presided as the gay hostess, and Dr Cone carved the turkey. It was a great success, so great, in fact, that it was repeated in 1948, and inevitably Mrs Reitman's party became an annual Hospital event. Each year the Christmas party grew in size as the Staff of the Hospital and the Institute expanded, but it was always planned with the same happy, personal touch, and with Mrs Reitman's friendly presence."[19]

Francis McNaughton expressed the feeling of all at the Neurological Institute when he wrote, "Our pleasure in remembering her last party is mixed with sadness and a sense of loss, for we have all lost a dear friend."[20]

JET PROPULSION LABORATORY

The institute was greatly interested in elucidating the characteristics of epilepsy in children whose seizures were so frequent or so severe that they had to be admitted to hospital for their care. Preston Robb entrusted this project to the youngest member of the Department of Neurology, Ivan Woods.[21] This assignment proved to be more daunting than one would have expected because the period of time over which EEG recordings could be performed was very limited. There seemed to be no solution to the problem, and the project was in jeopardy until a fateful night in 1969, as Woods recalls:

When I joined the MNI family on 1 January 1970, EEG technology had advanced since Jasper's time and Pierre Gloor was now Chief of the Department. It was still, however, restricted to being performed on patients attached to the EEG machine by many short wires. This limited recordings to immobile patients for no more than a couple of hours. This was very useful to confirm a diagnosis of epilepsy in many patients, although a negative recording was not conclusive.

Some patients had many brief seizures during the day and even more frequent bursts of epileptic activity on the EEG. Also, epileptic activity was known to be accentuated during the brief periods of sleep, which we could record. What we did not know was how certain activities during the day and also the various stages of sleep affected the epileptic activity in the brain. We had no way of recording the EEG on a freely mobile individual carrying on normal daily activities and during a normal night's sleep. I thought we might learn a lot more about epilepsy if we could do that.

One evening I was sitting at home fascinated, as were millions of others, watching grainy TV pictures of astronauts walking on the moon. The voice-over describing the scene mentioned that the Jet Propulsion Laboratory in California was monitoring the astronauts' EKG, respirations and EEG! That got my attention! People at JPL could monitor 24-hour EEG recordings of men on the moon and we could not do that at a Neurological Institute here on earth! I thought about it for a while and decided to write to JPL.

I explained to them what we hoped to do with 24-hour EEG recordings. They were very receptive to the idea and after a few weeks correspondence, they agreed to help. Shortly after that, I had on my desk the actual EEG transmitter from the astronaut's helmet and the receiver from the lunar lander. It was a small 4-channel transmitter (figure 31.5) but what a big world of opportunities it opened up! The unit had been developed by the Hughes Corp in California in 1967 for NASA.

We were fortunate to have on staff a gifted biomedical electronics engineer, John Ives. John fully deserves the credit for making the unit functional in our laboratory and developing it further. He was eventually able to split the signals so we could get 8 channels of EEG instead of 4. We started with 6 hour recordings on children with very active generalized epilepsy to find the best way to deal with the large amount of data generated over many hours. John devised a program for the 8K computer we had at our disposal to recognize epileptic discharges and record only those on paper.

Having the patient mobile was a wonderful advance. We soon found however that there are significant differences between the surface of the moon and earth. For one thing, there are no walls on the moon. On the moon, there could be several hundred meters between the transmitter and receiver. If our patient left the room with the receiver, the signal quickly deteriorated. We therefore were limited on how mobile our patient could be. This of course was no problem for sleep recordings, in which we were particularly interested. Since the patient had to be in the same room as the receiver, Mr Ives developed a thin cable, like a telephone cable. This was light and had the great advantage that we could now record 8 and eventually 16 clear channels. Thus we could perform 24-hour EEG recordings at the MNI as NASA had done on the moon. They are now of course standard procedure in all EEG labs. John Ives later moved to Harvard and helped them develop their system.[22]

Further innovation would come as the MNI kept pace with evolving technology in this field, as in others. By the beginning of the 1980s Ives and his coworkers had developed "a 16-channel portable EEG cassette for ambulatory EEG recordings. The use of a walk-man type tape recorder integrated with the 16-channel cable telemetry system … produced an EEG data acquisition system that could be used on a completely ambulatory patient."[23]

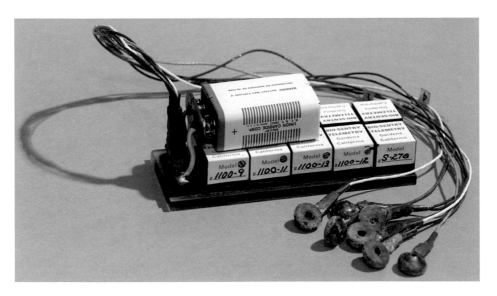

Figure 31.5: Transmitter package showing 9 V battery, modular construction of amplifiers, voltage-controlled oscillators, and electrodes for EEG telemetry. (Figure 1 from Ives, Thompson, and Woods, "Technical Contribution." MNI Archives)

PART FOUR

The Third Director
1972–1984

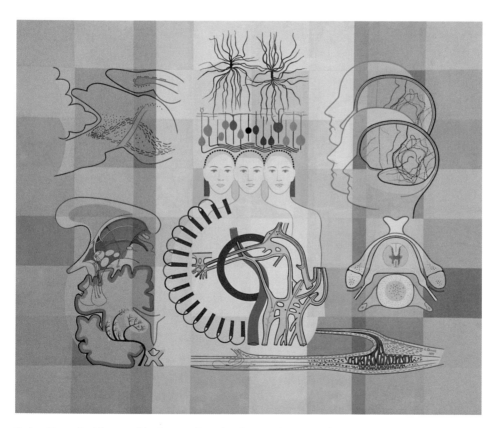

Luba Genush, *The World of Neurology* (*right panel*), which "displays networks in the brainstem and the brain's blood vessels; rows of brain cells above a stylized positron emission tomography scanner; the solar nerve plexus; brain maps of epilepsy surgery; the spinal column and nerves; a sensory-motor 'spiral' ending located in all our muscles which gives us feed-back signals that allow us to play Bach, Baseball or the Bard." (W. Feindel, *Images of the Neuro* [Montreal: Montreal Neurological Institute and the Osler Library of the History of Medicine, 2013])

32

A Fair Trial Followed by a Hanging

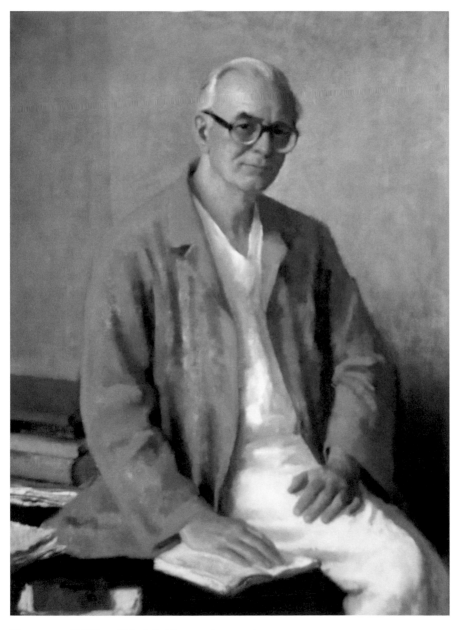

Figure 32.1: William Feindel. (George Augusta)

Theodore Rasmussen reflected on change in his last report as director of the MNI: "All human institutions must reckon with two forces. Their resulting conduct represents a sort of parallelogram of forces. One is the inherent intent to supply stability of purpose and effort, the other is to be promptly and delicately responsive to changes in the environment and even changes in objectives. It is the task of the team and its new leader to strike the proper balance between these two main forces that will be required to meet the needs and opportunities of tomorrow."[1] Rasmussen then explained how the reconciliation of change within continuity had been applied in his own case and in that of his successor as director of institute:

> A special plan of administrative continuity was set up in 1954, when I returned from the University of Chicago to take over the teaching and research administrative responsibilities from Dr Penfield. Continuity, but of a different sort, seemed to me to be required now, with the end of my statutory tenure as Director beginning to come into view. Accordingly … I asked the Dean and the Principal to initiate the statutory steps required to select a new Director, to guide the Institute and Hospital through the shoals and narrows of the years that lie ahead. Following the tradition of Western Frontier Days – "give the man a fair trial, then hang him" – I urged the Selection Committee to thoroughly survey the field and then nominate Dr Feindel.[2]

William Feindel then took the podium as the director-in-waiting of the MNI, and was able to announce,

> Just recently, Mr Howard Webster has informed me that the members of the Webster family … have arranged for a very substantial donation which will extend over a five-year period to establish what we propose to call the Webster Brain Research Fund. They wish this to be dedicated to the memory of the late Senator Lorne C. Webster and Mrs Webster, their parents. This will provide increasing endowment to support the search for new knowledge to treat patients with disorders of the brain and nerves due to causes which are now unknown. The first returns of this fund will be applied to the expansion of our work on the circulation of the brain, particularly those aspects of cerebrovascular occlusive disease and the role of the circulation in epilepsy.[3]

Other generous donations were received, most notably from George Maxwell Bell, who bequeathed a sum to be used towards the costs of the Penfield Wing and another to support a special brain research fund.[4] Beyond generous gifts from individuals in support of specific projects, the research budget of the MNI came from its endowments, research grants, and scholarships.[5] The Izaak Walton Killam Memorial Endowment had awarded ten Killam Scholarships to MNI basic or clinical researchers since they had become available in 1967. This, Feindel reported, had "enabled a number of projects to be initiated with topics ranging from the investigation of Muscle Disease to Electronic Computer handling of E.E.G. data, telemetering of brain wave potentials in epileptic patients, neurophysiological investigation of the complex, deep connections within the brain, chemical analysis of transmitting substances in nervous tissue, and anatomical studies of intracerebral pathways."[6] Most importantly, Feindel noted what appeared to be a favourable attitude of the provincial government towards the construction of a new wing, as had been proposed in 1969. Feindel also announced, with a modicum of pride, "We are in a position to contribute the cornerstone which I propose can be made from part of the memorial stone of Dr Thomas Willis which we have obtained from Westminster Abbey when the three-century-old stone was replaced some ten years ago."[7]

Gilles Bertrand, the newly appointed neurosurgeon-in-chief, welcomed the new director of the institute, William Feindel, in true Neuro family style, by removing a recalcitrant lumbar disc … on Father's Day.

Richard Gilbert stepped down from his position as head of Neuroanesthesia. He had joined the staff of the institute in 1950 as associate anaesthetist and became head of the department in 1955, a position that he held for twenty years. Gilbert was appointed chairman of the Department of Anaesthesia at McGill University in 1957. He was an outstanding leader and a superb teacher.[8] Davy Trop was promoted to replace Gilbert as the head of Anaesthesia at the institute, in a department that included Mounir Abou-Madi, Jennifer Barnes, Luis Cuadrado, and David Thomas.[9] Elizabeth (Lisa) Wilkinson had come to the institute as a fellow in 1970 and had joined the department the following year. She left the institute in July 1974 to head the Department of Neuroanesthesia at the Barrow Neurological Institute.[10]

DEPARTURES

There were other personnel changes, perhaps not as momentous, but nonetheless significant for the future course of the institute. Henry Garretson left the snowy streets of Montreal for the blue grass of Kentucky and the University of Louisville. Jean Vézina walked a few blocks east, to Hôpital Notre-Dame and the Université de Montréal. Derek Fewer returned to the institute to complete his training in neurosurgery after a year with Charles Wilson in San Francisco, then

established himself in Winnipeg. Patrick Murray began his training in neurosurgery at the MNI, then later also journeyed westward, to Vancouver. With
LeBlanc, Myles, and Weir in Alberta, Fewer in Manitoba, Paine in Saskatchewan,
and Murray in British Columbia, the western provinces were well stocked with
MNI fellows.[11] Eastern Canada was not left bereft of MNI-trained neurosurgeons, as Steve Nutik, after stellar work on the hypothalamus, left the institute
and joined MNI fellow Maurice Héon as assistant-professor in the Department
of Neurosurgery at the University of Sherbrooke.[12]

   A great loss was incurred to the MNI with the death of Arthur W. Young in
February 1973. Young had been on the staff of the Royal Victoria Hospital as
neurologist and psychiatrist since 1927 and had been appointed as associate
neurologist at the opening of the institute in 1934. A superb clinician, Arthur
Young had been a valued colleague of John Kershman, Francis McNaughton,
and Preston Robb.[13]

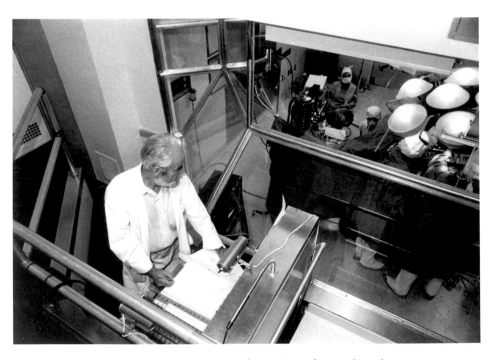

Figure 32.2: Pierre Gloor observing a cortical resection after reading the
electrocardiogram. (MNI Archives)

NEUROGENETICS

Collaborative research directed at a specific neurological disease was a hallmark of the MNI, as exemplified by a Neurological Grand Rounds held in 1971.[14] The rounds, held in the steep tiers of the Hughlings Jackson Amphitheatre, concerned a child with Krabbe's disease. The topic was introduced by quoting at length from Krabbe's original paper, and by presenting the clinical history. Roméo Ethier reviewed the radiological findings, which revealed a featureless skull suggestive of cerebral atrophy, and Pierre Gloor demonstrated the characteristic EEG of diffuse white matter encephalopathy, findings that he and his co-workers had recently described.[15] Needle electomyographic and motor evoked potential studies performed by Andrew Eisen were indicative of a segmental demyelinating neuropathy. George Karpati and Joe Clarke found segmental demyelination and galactocerebroside deposits on nerve and muscle biopsies. These findings confirmed the diagnosis of Krabbe's disease, which, Stirling Carpenter pointed out, could have previously been done only at autopsy. Eva Andermann discussed aspects of the genetic counselling of individuals in whose family the condition is present,[16] and George Karpati looked towards the prospects of enzyme replacement for its treatment. Fred Andermann, as was often the case, had the last word: "Prevention and rational treatment are the challenge for the future," he concluded. Joe Clarke and Leon Wolfe in the Donner Laboratory, whose efforts eventually led to the "prenatal diagnosis of this disease by the analysis of glycolipids from cultured amniotic cells," took up the challenge.[17] Similar approaches proved useful in the diagnosis of other conditions, such as Fabry's disease.[18]

After the great success of the interdisciplinary approach to the investigation of Krabbe's disease, E. Andermann, F. Andermann, S. Carpenter, A. Eisen, G. Karpati, L. Wolfe, and their collaborators applied their combined efforts to a panoply of conditions.[19] The interdisciplinary approach had notable success in the ultrastructural and neurochemical characterization of Batten's disease – which resulted in reports in *Brain* and in *Science*[20] – and in Friedreich's ataxia.[21] The collaborative efforts of neurogenetics, neurology, neuroradiology, and neuropathology produced a striking result in the discovery of a new syndrome – Andermann's syndrome – characterized by agenesis of the corpus callosum, mental retardation, and progressive sensimotor neuropathy.[22] The syndrome was elaborated upon and, although it was found to have a high prevalence in the Charlevoix region of Quebec, it is now known to occur worldwide. The Department of Neurogenetics further characterized the syndrome and was able to report, a few years after its discovery, that "45 patients in 24 sibships have now been identified, all originating from Charlevoix County, where the consanguinity rate is known to be markedly elevated. Recognition of the autosomal recessive nature of this hitherto described syndrome is important for genetic counselling and prevention."[23] The Department of Neurogenetics also made great strides in elucidating syndromes affecting the cerebellar vermis, including Joubert syndrome characterized by agenesis of the vermis, episodic hyperpnoea, abnormal eye movements, ataxia, and mental retardation.[24]

Other interests of the Department of Neurogenetics did not suffer from these activities: it was following more than forty families with Friedreich's ataxia, and it was designated as a Centre for Treatment and Research of this condition. Investigations into the teratogenic effects of anticonvulsants continued apace, with the new and distressing finding of "a significantly increased frequency of major congenital malformations in offspring of epileptic women taking anticonvulsant medication during pregnancy."[25] Pre-pregnancy counselling of epileptic patients became a major clinical service of the department.

The achievements of the neurogenetics group did not escape Pierre Gloor's attention as head of Graduate Studies and Research, who put a human face on familial neurogenetic conditions:

Much anguish and suffering is generated in a family when a happy and thriving infant begins to develop signs of a relentlessly progressive disease of the brain which inexorably leads to major neurological disability, mental retardation and ultimately death. The knowledge that such a tragedy could recur in another child of the family, because the hereditary origin of the disease is known or suspected, adds to the anguish and bewilderment of the parents. Research has been carried out on a number of these diseases in our Institute during the last year. Progress has been made on two fronts: for some of these conditions the mode of inheritance and the possibility to detect the carrier state in healthy relatives has been investigated by Dr Eva Andermann and her collaborators; the genetically determined biochemical derangement ultimately responsible for the clinical manifestations has been studied with considerable success by Dr Wolfe and his associates. He received invaluable assistance from Dr Carpenter who, with the help of the electron-microscope, was able to define the submicroscopic characteristics of the abnormal chemical material which accumulates in brain cells and which the biochemists were interested in identifying. The practical consequences of this type of research are that it is now possible in some of these conditions, at least, to detect healthy carriers, to determine in the early stages of pregnancy whether the fetus is affected by the disease and thus relieve much suffering and anxiety by well directed genetic counselling.[26]

COMPLEXITY

New discoveries and the access to new devices resulted in greater complexity in the investigation and treatment of patients. Thus, the operating microscope resulted in an increase of the number of operations for the treatment of ruptured aneurysms; and fluorescein angiography, which aided in resection of arteriovenous malformations, resulted in an increased number of operations for these lesions. Robert Hansebout began a clinical study of myelotomy to treat spasticity in multiple sclerosis, adding a new type of operation to the surgical roster. Stereotactic thalamotomy for the treatment of patients with Parkinson's disease whose symptoms were refractory to the recently introduced L-DOPA continued, with the aid of a computerized atlas and novel instruments.[27] The stereotactic insertions of indwelling depth electrodes for the evaluation of patients whose epileptogenic focus was not obvious to scalp EEG recordings increased in number.[28]

Diagnostic procedures, such as activation of epileptic seizures with pentylenetetrazol, computer-aided analysis of sixteen-channel cable telemetry EEG recordings, and prolonged recording from implanted depth electrodes also added to the complexity of the investigation of epileptic patients.[29] Although EEG recordings from the base of the skull had been introduced at the MNI by Jasper and Kershman by the early 1940s, the introduction of hair-fine sphenoidal electrodes developed by John Ives was a major technological advance that set the standard for all other epilepsy centres.[30] The clinical and research activities of the epilepsy program benefited greatly from the recruiting of Luis Felipe Quesney and Jean Gotman. Felipe Quesney had obtained a PhD under Pierre Gloor's supervision and joined him in the Department of Neurophysiology.[31] His major contributions at the institute were in the field of experimental generalized epilepsy, photosensitive epilepsy, and pre-operative depth electrode recordings in epileptic patients.[32] Jean Gotman came to the institute as part of a French cooperative exchange program and joined Christopher Thompson and John Ives as assistant computer systems engineer in the Computing Laboratory.[33]

Allan Sherwin demonstrated the critical role of monitoring anticonvulsant drug levels in the management of epileptic patients. His laboratory provided this service to hospitals in Quebec and the Maritime Provinces, and it became the reference laboratory for quality control sponsored by the American Epilepsy

Foundation and the National Institutes of Health, Bethesda. Allan Sherwin also embarked on a study of the biochemical characteristics of epileptic and non-epileptic cortex removed at surgery, an interest that he would pursue for the next two decades.[34]

The effect on the clinical services was that an ever-increasing number of patients with complex neurological and neurosurgical problems, and for whom investigation was prolonged and treatment difficult, sought consultation at the MNI. Nonetheless, basic research was not forgotten, as the Department of Neurophysiology pursued its investigations of cortico-reticular epilepsy, the interaction of the amygdala and the temporal cortex, and penicillin-induced generalized seizures.[35]

Table 32.1
Electroencephalography and clinical neurophysiology, Montreal Neurological Institute, 1975–76

P. Gloor	Electroencephalographer and neurophysiologist
F. Andermann	Associate electroencephalographer
E. Andermann	Assistant electroencephalographer
M. Aubé*	Assistant electroencephalographer
I. Woods	Assistant electroencephalographer
J. Ives	Biomedical engineer
C. Thompson	Computer system engineer
J. Gotman	Assistant computer engineer
K. Crystals	Chief technician

* Recipient of the 1974 Penfield Award for Excellence

NEUROPATHOLOGY OF EPILEPSY

Gordon Mathieson published two landmark neuropathological studies while on sabbatical leave.[36] The first study, of over five hundred cases, stressed the role of birth injury and febrile convulsions in frontal and temporal epilepsy.[37] The second included over eight hundred specimens obtained for the temporal lobe exclusively.[38] The commonest histo-pathological findings associated with temporal lobe epilepsy were neuronal loss and gliosis, gliosis with hippocampal sclerosis, and hippocampal sclerosis in isolation. On a similar topic, Wilder Penfield and Gordon Mathieson published a significant paper on patient P.B., whose case Penfield had previously published with Brenda Milner in 1958, and who had suffered severe memory loss after a left hippocampal resection.[39] Penfield and Milner had suggested that the opposite hippocampus must also have been affected to explain the patient's amnesia.[40] Penfield and Mathieson confirmed this hypothesis at post-mortem examination in 1974.[41]

Guy Remillard, Roméo Ethier, and Fred Andermann also published an interesting report of eight patients with temporal lobe epilepsy and hemianopia associated with partial occlusion of branches of the posterior cerebral artery.[42] Five of the patients reported had a history of difficult birth, suggesting a mechanism – hippocampal herniation – analogous to that proposed by Earle, Baldwin, and Penfield in 1953 as a cause of incisural sclerosis.

INNOVATION: THE EMI SCANNER

William Feindel, in his first report as the director of the Montreal Neurological Institute, announced that the Quebec government had requested a revised plan and cost estimates for what was now referred to as the Penfield Wing, based on the 1969 proposal that had been postponed in 1970. Further, the Ministry of Social Affairs had approved the purchase of a computerized axial tomographic (CAT) scanner manufactured by Electric and Musical Industries Limited (EMI), based on a prototype built by Godfrey Hounsfield, and put in clinical service by James Ambrose, a neuroradiologist at Atkinson Morley Hospital, Wimbledon. Hounsfield was knighted by Queen Elizabeth II and awarded the Nobel Prize for Medicine or Physiology in 1979. William Feindel described how the MNI acquired the EMI computed tomography (CT) scanner:

> In the fall of 1972 while at a neurosurgical meeting in Oxford, James Ambrose showed me some images from the prototype EMI scanner. I later visited to the EMI factory accompanied by Roméo Ethier, Head of Neuroradiology, Chris Thompson and Howard Webster, a friend of the Institute. After the visit, where Chris Thompson unnerved the EMI engineers by peering too closely into the workings of a scanner under construction, the group went to see Ambrose at Wimbledon. On the way back, Howard Webster asked me "Well, what do you think of the machine?" I answered enthusiastically, and Webster asked, rhetorically, "Well, don't you think you'd better get one?"

The deal was closed on their return to EMI headquarters that same day.[43]

James Ambrose delivered the MNI's first Thomas Willis Lecture a few months later, on computerized axial tomography of the brain, based on the first

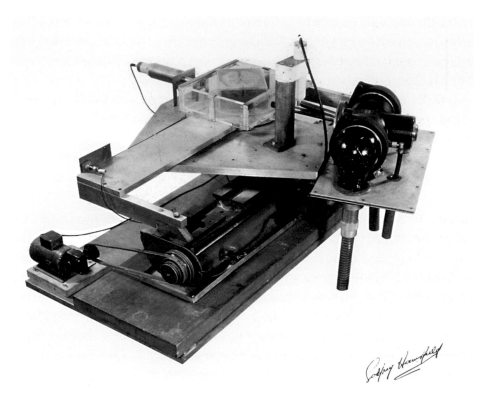

Figure 32.3: Hounsfield's first operational prototype of a computerized tomographic scanner, number five of a limited edition of ten, presented by Hounsfield to Dr Roméo Ethier. Hounsfield's signature is visible in the lower right corner. (Roméo Ethier)

150 patients examined with the scanner.[44] The institute took delivery of its EMI scanner in the summer of 1973, at the same time as the Massachusetts General Hospital and the Mayo Clinic, the 3Ms.

The EMI scanner became operational in October 1973, and its impact was revolutionary, immediately affecting the diagnosis and treatment of neurological patients. The nature of a stroke, ischemic or hemorrhagic, was previously a vexing and inaccurate exercise, even for experienced neurologists, but it immediately became apparent with CT scanning. The same was true of other hemorrhagic conditions, such as epidural and subdural hematomas, a diagnosis previously made, often inaccurately, by angiography. It was no longer necessary to perform a PEG to diagnose hydrocephalus.

Each CT examination produced eight tomographic images from the skull base to the vertex of the head. Each 60 x 60 pixel image was projected onto a cathode ray monitor. Each of the eight images was captured individually on instant black-and-white Polaroid film, and each print was affixed onto a cardboard chart, like photographs in the family album.

The EMI scanner rapidly became the busiest piece of equipment in the Department of Neuroradiology, and, although it operated twelve hours a day, this hardly met demand and the first thousandth examination was soon performed. The EMI scanner soon operated eighteen hours out of every twenty-four.[45] Very rapid technological advances and increased pixel grids would make the tool even more useful in short order.

THE FIRST INTERNATIONAL SYMPOSIUM ON COMPUTERIZED AXIAL TOMOGRAPHY

The First International Symposium on Computerized Axial Tomography was held at the MNI on 31 May and 1 June 1974. Outside participants included Godfrey Hounsfield and John Ambrose, while other participants represented the elite of neuroradiology in America and the United Kingdom. Juan Taveras and Paul Pew, from Harvard, spoke on the appearance of intra- and extra-vascular blood and infraction. Gordon Potts from Cornell University, and John Marshall and George DuBoulay from Queen Square compared computer to-mography to conventional methods of neuroradiological investigations, most notably in the diagnosis of intracranial tumours. Representatives from the Mayo Clinic and from the Cleveland Clinic described their initial experience with the new technology, and Ayoub Ommaya, from the National Institutes of Health, discussed the CT investigation of experimental neuropathology.

William Feindel, Denis Mélançon, Gary Bélanger, and Dan Galloway from the MNI discussed their experience with focal epilepsy, and Roméo Ethier, Allan Sherwin, Saul Taylor, Ilo Leppik, and Chris Thompson described the novel use of diatrizoate M-60% to enhance the aspect of vascularized lesions.[46] The use of contrast material greatly expanded the number of conditions that could accurately be diagnosed with CT scanning to include tumours, inflammatory conditions, and vascular lesions, and eventually led to the development of computed tomographic angiography.

33

Ars Longa

One of the first challenges faced by William Feindel was the erosion of funds for patient care, teaching, and research. The new director reviewed the relationship of the institute and hospital with the Ministry of Social Affairs and of the relationship of the institute with McGill University in all their byzantine complexity.[1] Under an agreement with the Ministry of Social Affairs, the institute and hospital shared the operation costs of the laboratories and other services. The budget of the institute, however, was maintained through endowments, as Feindel pointedly remarked: "The Director of the Institute has the clear responsibility to the donors or their executors and heirs, to ensure that these funds support research activities for which they were originally intended. They are not used to relieve the responsibility of the Government for the Operation of the Neurological Hospital," nor are they to be "considered as a means of relieving the responsibility of the Faculty of Medicine in regard to teaching activities in the academic Department of Neurology and Neurosurgery." The latter point was felt to be important enough to be belaboured: "Originally … teaching at the medical school in the basic neurosciences and in clinical neurology and neurosurgery was carried out by the staff of the Neurological Institute in order to bring this important subject to medical students and to develop post-graduate residency training programs … We have recently estimated that … almost half of the total annual income from the Institute's research endowment funds is encumbered within our budget for teaching as contrasted to research." Feindel hoped that the dean of the medical school and the principal of the university would "ensure that the activities of our teaching Department of Neurology and Neurosurgery [would] be increasingly supported from the Faculty budget, rather than from Institute research funds."

William Feindel identified four areas that threatened to affect the institute's ability to carry out its mission. The overall budget of the Medical Research

Council of Canada, from which the institute obtained one-third of its operating funds, had levelled off; reverses in the stock market had affected income from the endowment fund; these financial setbacks were compounded by a rise in inflation, while cost projections for the construction of the new wing were constantly escalating. "But," Feindel concluded, "despite these difficulties, we believe that this project must go forward. The alternative would be to lose the scientific and clinical momentum which has been built up here over the past forty years and to become a second rate establishment."[2] Feindel was right to persevere and to push ahead with planning for the new building: the following year, on 23 July 1975, Order-in-Council No. 3415-75 of the government of Quebec was passed and authorized the financing and construction of the Wilder Penfield Wing of the Montreal Neurological institute.[3]

In preparation for the expansion of the institute, McGill University's Department of Urban Planning reviewed some demographic features of the MNI's patients.[4] Almost half were francophone, 60 per cent originated from Montreal, 20 per cent came from other parts of Quebec, and the remainder came from outside the province. William Feindel appreciated the significance of such a large percentage of out-of-province patients as a reflection of the high regard in which the institute was held, as well as their contribution to the bottom line. "These latter patients contributed more than a million dollars a year, or almost one-fifth of our total hospital budget. They provide in a sense an indication of the quality of work carried out at the Neuro and our special facilities for dealing with complex problems of the brain and nerves."[5]

GOVERNANCE

Neurology and Neurosurgery

Preston Robb expressed a desire to retire within the academic year 1975–76 and Joseph B. Martin was asked to take the position of neurologist-in-chief at the MNI.[6] Martin had joined Donald Baxter in the Division of Neurology at the Montreal General Hospital in 1970 and was highly regarded in the field of neuro-endocrinology. As noted by William Feindel at the time, "with the appointment of Dr Joseph Martin as Neurologist-in-Chief, the study of endocrine changes during seizure activity and sleep has been started and a closer liaison has been made with the neuroendocrine research groups at the Montreal General Hospital and the Royal Victoria Hospital."[7] Martin was named chair of the Department of Neurology and Neurosurgery at McGill in 1977. The following year he was recruited to Harvard University as the Bullard Professor of Neurology. While at Harvard, Martin nurtured the career of Guy Rouleau, who became director of the Montreal Neurological Institute in 2013. Preston Robb once more answered the call to service and agreed to come out of retirement to be interim neurologist-in-chief at the institute after Martin's departure and until Donald Baxter accepted the position.

A graduate of Queen's University, Baxter first came to the institute for a period of two months during his internship and returned in 1952–53 as a research fellow and collaborated with Jerzy Olszewski on the classic atlas *Cytoarchitecture of the Human Brain Stem.*[8] Donald Baxter left Montreal in 1954 for Harvard's Boston City Hospital to train in neurology with Derek Denny-Brown. After an interlude in Saskatoon with William Feindel and Joseph Stratford, Baxter returned to Montreal in 1963 to head the Division of Neurology at the Montreal General Hospital. With Joseph Martin's departure, Baxter also became the chairman of Neurology and Neurosurgery at McGill University. He became director of the Montreal Neurological Institute in 1984 at the end William Feindel's term in office, a position that he held untl 1992.

With CT scanning replacing PEG and the availability of portable four-channel EEG cassette recorders, which the patient could wear outside the hospital, Preston Robb suggested that Neurology should shift its emphasis from in-patient to outpatient services. A new Ambulatory Daycare Centre and improvements in the clinical laboratories accommodated this change in orientation. Outpatient diagnosis of spinal problems was greatly facilitated by a CT scanner that could image the spine, in whose development the MNI had participated with engineers from EMI.[9]

Nursing

A most significant change in the day-to-day operation of the MNI came on 1 January 1975, when Caroline Elizabeth Robertson replaced Joy Hackwell as director of nursing, a position she held until 1989.[10] Robertson came to her position as an experienced head nurse on Two East at the MNI and as director of nursing at the Sherbrooke Hospital in Quebec's Eastern Townships. Her term as director at the institute was characterized by dedication to care, education, and leadership. Robertson was also a visionary and a progressive, implementing a more active role for nurses in the function of the hospital and in the care of patients. She empowered the nurses under her charge to develop specialty interests in rehabilitation, respiratory care, oncology, infection control, and spinal injury, so that they could become resource persons for patients and their loved ones. Most successful of this type of "specialized care in a specialized hospital" was the "Spinal Team" headed by Robert Hansebout and Lucy Dalicandro, whose broad brilliant smile brought joy to everyone she encountered. Ever aware of quality improvement, Robertson instituted a system of audits to track indicators of nursing care, which resulted in the

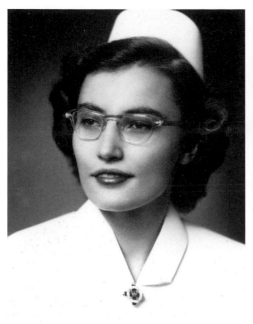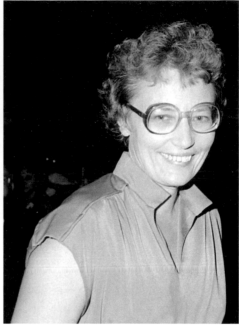

Figures 33.1 and 33.2: Caroline Robertson. (MNI Archives)

development of an Organization for Quality Assurance Manual and the creation of a Nursing Practice Committee.

ACADEMIA

Meetings of the Montreal Neurological Society became less frequent as the Université de Montréal developed its own highly regarded neuroscience programs. Nonetheless, the MNI continued to host prominent speakers throughout the decade. The Department of Neuropsychology took the lead with weekly seminars. The first of these visitors included such neuroscientists as Mortimer Mishkin from the National Institutes of Health, and Professor Hans-Lukas Teuber from the Massachusetts Institute of Technology. Three fellows of the Royal Society (London) were also hosted by the department: Professors Elizabeth Warrington of University College London, an authority on semantic memory; Lawrence Weiskrantz of Oxford University; and Oliver Zangwill, who had been Brenda Milner's thesis supervisor at Cambridge University. Weiskrantz and Warrington had made major contributions to the understanding of the phenomenon of "blindsight," the unconscious response to stimuli in an otherwise blind visual field.[11]

Elwood Henneman was foremost among former fellows hosted by the MNI. Henneman, the Walter B. Cannon Professor of Physiology at Harvard Medical School, was known internationally for his fundamental contributions to neurophysiology, and most notably for the formulation of "Henneman's law," which

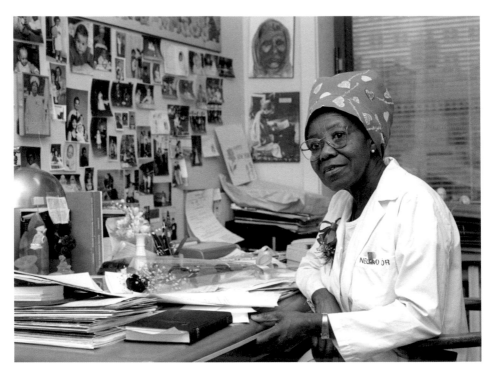

Figure 33.3: Norma Isaacs, operating room suprevisor, in her office. (MNI Archives)

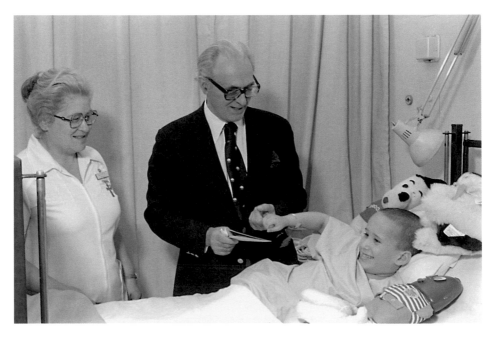

Figure 33.4: Ursula Steiner, head nurse, William Feindel, and a young patient. (MNI Archives)

Table 33.1
Nursing administration, Montreal Neurological Institute, 1974–84

C. Robertson	Director of nursing
I. MacMillan	Assistant director of nursing (days)
E. Barrowman	Assistant director of nursing (nights)
L. McAuley	Nursing supervisor (nights)
M. Smeaton	Nursing supervisor (nights)
C. Largo	Nursing supervisor (evenings)
L. Maruska	Nursing supervisor (evenings)
A. Johnson	Nursing supervisor (days)
A. Carney	Nursing supervisor (days)
H. Kyrk	Assistant director of nursing education
G. Hart	Coordinator of inservice education
F. Skretkowicz	Coordinator of inservice education
E. Roll	Nurse clinician (teaching)
L. Robbins	Nurse clinician
N. Isaacs	Operating room supervisor

Table 33.2
Head nurses and nursing coordinators, Montreal Neurological Institute,
1974–84

E. Andrews	M. Everett	F. Murphy	U. Steiner
I. Boucaud	P. Furlong	B. Nattucci	W. Watson
M. Cavanaugh	G. Jotic	C. Negus	
L. Dalicandro	D. MacDonald	B. Petrin	
M. de Guzman	N. McGuire	A. Saumtally	

relates the size of a motor neuron to its electrical activity. His topic was "Some Aspects of Control of Movements."

The academic year 1973–74 saw the institute's amphitheatre upgraded with funds bequeathed by Dean Cronan, of McGill University, to accommodate an increasing number of medical students, residents, fellows, and staff, and the amphitheatre was christened the Hughlings Jackson Amphitheatre at a ceremony hosted by Wilder Penfield.[12] Walle Nauta, institute professor at the Massachusetts Institute of Technology, inaugurated the newly christened space with his 1974 Hughlings Jackson Lecture, "The Frontal Lobe." Professor Ragnar Granit, former director of the Nobel Institute of Neurophysiology in Stockholm and 1967 Nobel laureate for his discoveries on the visual system, gave the lecture in 1975, "Muscle Spindle," which was published in *Brain*.[13]

PUBLICATIONS

The mid-1970s were especially rich in noteworthy publications by MNI staff in areas where they had achieved international prominence.

Epilepsy

Theodore Rasmussen published an influential paper on superficial hemosiderosis, a previously unknown, potentially fatal complication of complete hemispherectomy, performed for the treatment of some forms of intractable epilepsy.[14] Hemosiderosis was the result of the slow, progressive accumulation of hemosiderin in the linings of the resection cavity, causing hydrocephalus. Replacing the technique of complete hemispherectomy by one that disconnected the diseased hemisphere from the healthy one, Rasmussen found, could prevent the complication. This was a major technical advance in the surgical treatment of epilepsy, and it was adopted worldwide.

The Epilepsy Advisory Committee of the National Institute of Neurological Diseases and Stroke sponsored the publication of *Neurosurgical Management of the Epilepsies*, and of *Complex Partial Seizures* in 1975.[15] The topics covered extended for pre-operative diagnosis and psychological assessment pre- and post-operatively, to medical management, surgery, pathological analyses, and outcome. MNI staff and fellows contributed to the bulk of the volumes, while members of the institute also contributed key chapters to *The Epilepsies* for Vinken and Bruyn's authoritative and encyclopedic *Handbook of Clinical Neurology*.[16]

Pierre Gloor was an organizer of a symposium on the amygdala, at Jackson Laboratories in Bar Harbor, Maine, in June 1971. His paper for the symposium developed a "holistic view of temporal lobe function, to further our understanding of the relationship between neocortical and limbic physiology."[17] Gloor's studies in these areas would culminate in his monumental *Temporal Lobe and Limbic System*.[18]

Brain Edema

Hanna Pappius organized the Third International Workshop on Dynamic Aspects of Cerebral Edema, held in Montreal in May 1976, and published as *Dynamics of Brain Edema*.[19] There was strong participation from the MNI. Other participants were prominent in the field and came from major universities and institutions in America and Europe. Hanna Pappius and Robert Katzman, of the Albert Einstein College of Medicine, edited the influential *Brain Electrolytes and Fluid Metabolism*.[20] Klatzman, Pappius, and MNI fellows Igor Klatzo and John Sterling Meyer were later part of a study group on brain edema in stroke for the Joint Committee for Stroke Resources of the American Health Association.[21]

Pharmacology

Allan Sherwin co-edited *Clinical Pharmacology of Anti-Epileptic Drugs*,[22] and Andrew Eisen, Alllan Sherwin, Stirling Carpenter, George Karpati, and their collaborators contributed to *Recent Advances in Myology* on the effects of pharmacological agents on muscle fibers, on creatinine kinase in skeletal muscles, and on polymyositis.[23]

Psychology

Marilyn Jones-Gotman was awarded an MSc for her work on visual imagery and memory, and a PhD for her dissertation on certain effect of right hemisphere lesions in humans.[24] Brenda Milner published an extraordinarily detailed account of recent progress in the localization of higher mental functions in light of the work at the MNI and with the study of callosotomized patients with Roger Sperry at Cal Tech.[25] This was followed by a most informative chapter on hemispheric specialization for the Third Study Program on the Neurosciences organized by the Massachusetts Institute of Technology.[26]

HONOURS

Michael Dogali and Ilo Leppik were awarded the 1975 Wilder Penfield Prize, while Michael Dogali, Kenneth Laxer, and Jean-Guy Villemure were awarded the prize in 1976.[27]

Brenda Milner and Leon Wolfe were elected fellows of the Royal Society of Canada, and Milner was elected to the National Academy of Sciences of the United States. Charles Hodge was presented with the Louis Schmitt Award, the highest honour of the Biological Photographic Association of North America.

COMPUTER YEARS

One of the hallmarks of the MNI is change within continuity, as reflected in the image of the parallelogram to which Theodore Rasmussen alluded in announcing William Feindel's ascent to the directorship of the institute. Continuity was at the fore in early December 1975 when the MNI celebrated fifteen

Table 33.3
Notable speakers, 1971–76

Speaker	Topic
B. Arnason (Harvard)	Nerve Growth Factor and Its Relationship to Brain Tumours
Claude Bertrand (Montreal)	Contributions to Stereotactic Neurosurgery and Its Applications to Neurological Diseases (1973 FDL)
T.H. Bullock (University of California, San Diego)	Noise in the Neurons: Some Distinctions among Issues and Controversies on How Brains Work
F. Buchthal (Copenhagen)	Conduction along Sensory Nerve Fibers in Normal and Diseased Nerves
A.G. Engel (Mayo Clinic)	Motor End-Plate Fine Structure with Special Reference to Neuromuscular Transmission Defects
Miller Fisher (Harvard)	Some Clinical Pathological Aspects of Cerebral Vascular Disease (1976 HJL)
R. Gilliatt (London)	The Thoracic Outlet Syndrome and the Neurologist
Ragnar Granit (Karolinska)*	The Functional Role of the Muscle Spindles: Facts and Hypotheses (1975 HJL)
E. Henneman (Harvard)	Some Aspects of Control of Movements
S.K. Hilal (New York)	Therapeutic Embolization of Cerebral Arteriovenous Malformations
D. Kreiger (Mount Sinai)	The C.N.S. Etiology of Cushing's Disease
T.A. Lambo (WHO)	The World Health Organization Program in the Neurosciences
G. McKhann (Johns Hopkins)	Studies of Myelin Formation
J.S. Meyer (Baylor)	Measurement of Regional Cerebral Blood Flow in the Diagnosis of Migraine, Epilepsy and Dementia
H.Y. Miller (Newcastle)	Simulation and Malingering in Relation to Injuries to Brain and Spinal Cord
Walle H. Nauta (MIT)	The Problem of the Frontal Lobe: An Interpretation Based on Neuroanatomical Findings (1974 HJL)
T.H. Newton (UC San Francisco)	Arteriovenous Malformations

Speaker	Topic
J. Ochoa (Dartmouth)	Pathologic Changes in Acute and Chronic Nerve Compression
G.L. Odom (Duke)	Cerebral Vasospasm
W.H. Oldendorf (UCLA)	Blood-Brain Barrier Permeability and the Distribution of Drugs to the Brain
Theodore Rasmussen (MNI)	Some Dynamic Aspects of Focal Epilepsy (1973 HJL)
N.P. Rosman (Boston University)	Effects of Hypothyroidism and Malnutrition on Developing Brain and Skeletal Muscle
L.C. Scheinberg (St Barnabas)	Cerebellar Stimulation for Epilepsy and Motor Disorders
J. Sever (NIH)	Multiple Sclerosis Revisited
M. Victor (Case Western)	Disorders of Memory in Man and Their Anatomical Basis
A. Earl Walker (Hopkins)	Man and His Temporal Lobes (1972 HJL)
K. Welch (Harvard)	Dynamics of the Cerebral Spinal Fluid (1976 FDL)
Clinton Woolsey (Wisconsin)	The Cortical Motor Maps of Monkey and Dog after Section of the Medullary Pyramid (1971 HJL)

* 1967 Nobel laureate
FDL: Fellows Day Lecture
HJL: Hughlings Jackson Lecture

individuals who had served the institute since its opening. There were nine nurses – Betty Barrowman, Mary Cavanaugh, Sainada Chernikoff, Annie Johnson, Lillian McAuley, Delta MacDonald, Hilda Richards, Helen Sala, Norma Siddons-Grey; two operating room attendants – Walter Droz, Winifred Webb; two housekeepers – Irene Bergeron, Mildred Shaw; one orderly – Simon Katschurick; and one administrator – Joan Mallory. The PDP-12 was included with those celebrated, although it had been at the institute for less than five years, which corresponds to two decades in computer years.[28] The PDP-12 was asked to record its activities, which it did, in letters, not in zeroes and ones:

A DAY IN THE LIFE OF A COMPUTER
PDP-12

I am a PDP-12 computer. I am 5 years old and live on the 7th floor of the Neuro. People come in to look at me and they wonder what I do all day.
My day starts off at about 8 a.m., although often at that time I am still

doing work from the night before. My first visitor is "Marcia" who comes up from the EEG lab. She gets me to look at some of the EEGs that were recorded the day before. I am quite good at this now and can distinguish "theta waves" from "alpha waves" and both of these from "eye movement" artifacts. I can draw a diagram of the head and indicate on it where the most abnormal area is. I like doing this as I get to see a lot of patients.

Then "Chris" comes in. He is usually writing programs to get me to do new things. This used to be fun but now I think I know enough and don't want to learn any new tricks. He and "Jean" think otherwise. "Chris" showed me how to draw maps of the brain on the screen of my terminal. Recently "Ty" has been making millions of copies of these maps to show which parts of the thalamus contain cells corresponding to all the sensations people feel or movements they make.

"Jean" is trying to get me to recognize "spikes" in EEGs. This is really hard work because unlike people I can't see the tracings on paper, so must look at them as a lot of numbers. There are so many of them – over 3000 every second. I'm fast but that's really too much. But I am trying hard and soon, "Jean" hopes, I will be able to distinguish epileptic spikes from all the things that "look" like them but aren't, and draw a little diagram to show their distribution on the patient's head.

Sometimes I see what is going on in the operating room. During operations for Parkinson's disease, I can show where in the brain the surgeon will make the lesion which stops the patient's tremor. When I was younger, I used to go into the operating room myself, but one day I got stuck in the elevator so now I just send "Terminal" down. Besides, they used to wash me before going in and I don't like getting wet. Now I have cables going to the EEG lab, the operating rooms, and (for public relations purposes) the conference room.

I forgot – I talked about my "Terminal" – perhaps you don't know who he is. He is like a TV screen with a typewriter keyboard in front of it. He is my main contact with people – they type on the keyboard and I can draw things for them on the screen. Usually this "interaction" works just fine! You see, I can't talk (but I have a little loudspeaker and I can whistle some tunes!).

At lunchtime, if I am lucky, I get half an hour's peace and rest for a while. As you probably know, we computers don't eat, we just use electricity – about as much as the oven in your stove at home. From this you may think I get very hot – not really, as I have 23 fans to keep me cool.

This afternoon "Lucas" and "Ernst" are doing an experiment next door and I will help them. They are trying to understand what effect certain drugs and lesions have on blood flow in the very small vessels in the brain of a dog. They will put small detectors of radioactivity on the surface of the brain and inject a radioactive gas. With these, I can measure the differences in radioactivity before and after the experiment and tell them how much things changed. It takes a long time to do these experiments, so I will be busy until 6 o'clock.

I am hardly ever switched off to rest at night. I used to be switched off, but now I stay up all night, recording the EEG from patients who might have epileptic seizures. This staying up business started last year when "John" made up a gadget which fits on the patient's head to amplify his EEG. This thing (it's called an EEG telemetry multiplexor) chops up the 16 channel EEGs into little pieces, so they all squeeze onto one cable. This cable goes into all the hospital wards and ends up in my room. So now I spend most of my nights splitting this chopped up EEG into 16 channels and saving it on my disk. Patients connected up to me at night are usually candidates for surgery and before the operation, the surgeon wants to be quite sure where the epileptic "focus" is. A good way to do this is to record one of his seizures. Often these patients have their EEGs recorded all day, but don't have a seizure. Previously they couldn't be recorded all night. What I do is to save the last 2 minutes of EEG on my disk, so that I can give an instant replay of it. (This is just like the replays of goals in hockey games on TV for those who were getting another beer from the "fridge" when the goal was scored.)

The instant replay is done by switching on one of the EEG machines in the basement, and writing out the brain waves that happened 2 minutes ago. I can also save the seizure on tape because "John" thinks that "Chris" and "Jean" will one day teach me to recognize the "seizures" all on my own. I just don't have time now, since I spend all night unscrambling "chopped up" EEGs.

Before I realize it, it's morning and people start coming in to see me again. I have no time to get lonely or bored even though they turn the lights out at night. In one way it's nice to be a research computer as I am always up to something new. I would hate to work in a bank figuring out how much money everyone didn't have, or in a big store writing pay cheques and sending out bills. Life is really much more fun at the "Neuro."

34

Vita Brevis, *5 April 1976*

On 4 April 1976 William Feindel visited Wilder Penfield at the Ross Pavilion of the Royal Victoria Hospital, where he was hospitalized during his last illness.[1] Feindel

> took a Polaroid photo of the gap in the stone wall on the south-west corner of the Neuro, where the stonemasons, a few days before, had removed the dedication plaque to allow for the abutment of the new Penfield Pavilion then underway, despite the fierce competition with many Olympic projects going on at the same time. I took another Polaroid of the lovely white marble statue of "La Nature" that has graced the front foyer of the Institute since it was founded in 1934. Dr and Mrs Penfield had arranged to have this copy made when they were visiting Paris in 1932.
>
> In his room at the Ross Pavilion, Dr. Penfield was sitting up, looking frail; but he welcomed me with a smile. I showed him the photo of the hole from which the plaque had been removed, to convince him that the work on the Penfield Pavilion had started. He seemed pleased at that. Then I showed him "La Nature." He looked at it and said wistfully, "She's beautiful, isn't she?" He seemed very tired … He gave up the ghost the next day, while the staff members were making morning rounds.

There were many eulogies in the wake of the great man's death, but the most heartfelt was Pierre Gloor's.

> Dr Penfield had a dream, and the dream came true. It was like the answer to a prayer perhaps best expressed in one of Dr Penfield's favorite biblical quotations, the famous passage from the book of Job: "Where shall wisdom be found and where is the place of understanding?" I like to

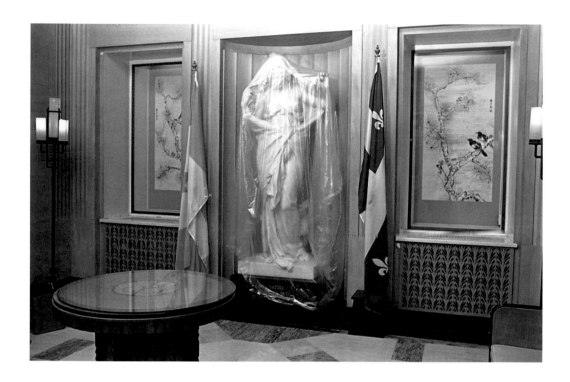

think that when Dr Penfield quoted this passage, as he did quite often, his thoughts turned to this Institute and that it expressed his hope that its noblest function was to be a place of wisdom of the true physician in the Hippocratic and Oslerian tradition, a wisdom nurtured in compassion and in the understanding that comes to those who have learned to ask Mother Nature the right questions with discernment and critical judgment, be it by the bedside or in the experimental laboratory. Whether we have been true to this ideal and fulfilled the hope, is for others to decide, but there is no question that we are heirs to a legacy that embodies great expectations. Dr Penfield, wherever your spirit may now dwell, let us assure you that we want to keep your dream alive. You have passed on to us the torch. May we tend this flame you have entrusted to us with the kind of wisdom and understanding that has always been yours.[2]

NO MAN ALONE

The institute held a memorial for Wilder Penfield, where reminiscences and addresses reviewing aspects of his life and work were presented, and which were later published, *in extenso*, in the *Canadian Medical Association Journal*.[3] Most notable of these essays is Herbert Jasper's unabashed defence of the concept of the centrencephalic integrating system, inspired by a fresh reading of *The Mystery of the Mind*. Jasper reviewed the circumstances that gave rise to the centrencephalic system, its evolution over the course of Penfield's life, its precedence over Maruzzi and Magoon's reticular activating system, and aspects common to both. Jasper ended with an insightful commentary: "Penfield's lifelong search for a better understanding of the functional organization of the brain and its disorders during epileptic seizures is symbolized, in a way, by his hypothesis of the central integrating system. It is never to be localized in any specific area of gray matter but in 'wider ranging mechanisms.' It is a sort of conceptual bridge between the brain and the mind. He concluded that we shall never be able to cross that bridge. Perhaps he is right, but many have been inspired by his efforts."[4] But the final word must come from Sir Charles Symonds, Penfield's life-long friend, who had composed a reflective commentary for *The Mystery of the Mind*, and who wrote to him six months before his death: "We shant I suppose meet again in our present fleshy garb, but if you are right [we] may yet communicate."[5]

35

The Third Foundation

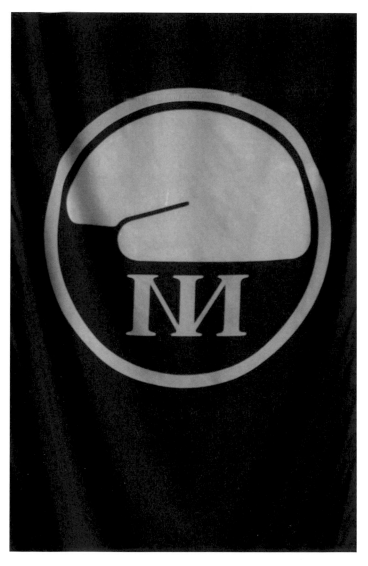

Figure 35.1: Third Foundation logo, the left hemisphere of the brain over the letters spelling *MNI* and the Roman numeral *III* on an MNI-blue banner, which hung in the Jeanne Timmins Auditorium during the Foundation ceremonies, 14–17 September 1978. (Photographer Richard Leblanc)

THE PENFIELD PAVILION

Jules Léger, governor-general of Canada, in the presence Monique Bégin, federal minister of national health and welfare, and Denis Lazure, Quebec minister of social affairs, officially opened the Penfield Pavilion on 15 September 1978, fifty years after Wilder Penfield and William Cone first came to Montreal. Thomas Lambo, deputy director general of the World Health Organization, and John Knowles, president of the Rockefeller Foundation, were in attendance, as were David Hubel, professor of neurobiology at Harvard University, and Henri Hecaen, director of the Neurolinguistic Research Institute in Paris.[1]

William Feindel, director of the institute, met the inauguration of the Penfield Pavilion with great excitement and optimism: "The pavilion doubled the space available for research, teaching, and clinical work, permitting enlargement of well-established research laboratories for neurophysiology, neurochemistry, neuroanatomy, and for neuromuscular, neuropsychological, neurological, and neurosurgical research. The facilities of the Penfield Pavilion also made it possible to launch new research units for neurogenetics, neuro-ophthalmology, neuropharmacology, and to provide certain common operating centres accessible to research teams, including computer units, tissue culture laboratories, temperature control rooms, and modern animal quarters, all of which are basic resources for scientific operations."[2]

The Penfield Pavilion extended south, along University Street. The third and fourth floors would accommodate two new nursing units – Three South, under Lucy Dalicandro, and Four South, the new Intensive Care Unit, under Barbara Petrin. And three new operating rooms were added to the fifth floor, two side-by-side and separated by a small intervening glassed-in room, containing an electroencephalograph, through which the electrocorticographer, the neuropsychologist, and their students could participate and observe two epilepsy surgeries at the same time. The two senior residents, David Dubuisson and Richard Leblanc, often looked at each other through the glass panes separating their operating rooms, while Peter Gloor, in white lab coat, or Felipe Quesney, impeccably dressed in an elegant business suit, analyzed the EEGs, looking for spikes. Brenda Milner, always accompanied by a throng of visitors, fellows, and students, was frequently present to enquire about the operative findings as she correlated them to the pre-operative neuropsychological test results. This was heady stuff for two young men about to start their careers in neurosurgery. Wilder Penfield's operating room, theatre number one, was kept intact but modernized. The viewing gallery and the photographer's cubby,

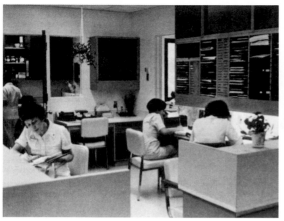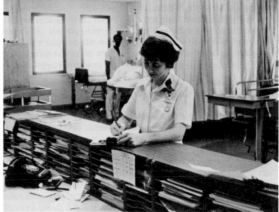

Figure 35.2: Miss Lucy Dalicandro (*left, seated*) in the new Three South nursing unit. (MNI Archives)

Figure 35.3: Mrs Barbara Petrin, in the new Intensive Care Unit on Four South. (MNI Archives) Nursing education was assured by L. Desbiens, G. Fitzgerald, G. Imbeault, and M. Manchen.

however, were kept unchanged and remain as they were on the opening of the institute in 1934 (figure 32.2).

SINGULAR FELLOWS

The Department of Neuroradiology was host to three singular fellows: Guy Breton, who would become rector of the Université de Montréal, Giuseppe Scotti, who became chairman of Neuroradiology and dean of medicine at the Università Vita-Salute San Raffaele, and Karel Terbrugge, from the University of Toronto, who would become a renowned expert on the endovascular treatment of cerebral aneurysms and arteriovenous malformations.[3] The department also hosted Tian-zhu Yang, a Bethune-Chao Scholar from Hebei Medical College, who studied the brainstem reticular formation.[4]

MNI residents and fellows won the trifecta of awards given by the Canadian Association of Neurological Sciences at its annual meeting in Vancouver in 1978: Richard Branan, from the Cone Laboratory, won the Kenneth Mackenzie Award in Neurosurgery for his studies on computer imaging of cerebral blood flow; Kenneth Nudleman won the Herbert Jasper Award for his project on cortical and cervical somatosensory responses in suspected multiple sclerosis, that he completed in Andrew Eisen's laboratory; and Serge Gauthier won the Francis McNaughton prize for his work with Theodore Sourkes, director of the Biochemical Laboratory at the Allan Memorial Institute, on the neural regulation of adrenal tyrosine hydroxylase. Howard Blume won the American Academy of Neurological Surgeons' award for his paper, "Peptides in the Hypothalamus," on work that he performed with Leo Renaud at the Montreal General Hospital Research Institute. John Wells, recipient of the 1977 Penfield Award, won the McKenzie Prize of the Canadian Neurosurgical Society for experimental work on the effect of hypothermia on spinal cord trauma.[5] John Stewart received the 1978 Penfield Award in neurology. José Montes and James Nelson won the award for neurosurgery and for neurology, respectively, the following year.

The director of the institute noted that a quota had been imposed for non-Canadian residents and fellows, and that "the overall restriction of the number of residency posts in the Province of Quebec have made the planning for residency programs in neurology and neurosurgery extremely precarious."[6]

Nonetheless, Rick Holmberg, from the University of Calgary, Richard Leblanc, from the University of Ottawa, and Mohammed Maleki, from the University of Tehran, were accepted as junior residents in neurosurgery, starting 1 July 1978.[7]

INVITED SPEAKERS

Notable visitors to the institute were H. Richard Tyler of Harvard Medical School and a bibliophile of world stature,[8] who spoke on motor neuron disease, Anders Bjorklund, of the University of Lund, Sweden, and who discussed regeneration in the central nervous system.[9] Phanor Perot gave the 1978 Annual Fellows Day Lecture, "Somatosensory Evoked Potentials in Spinal Cord Injury," and Charles Branch gave the 1979 lecture, "The Complications of Chymopapain Injection for the Treatment of Lumbar Disc Disease."

Henry Barnett, chairman of clinical neurosciences at the University of Western Ontario, gave the 1978 Thomas Willis Lecture on recent advances in stroke. The 1979 Willis Lecture was given by Andrew Schally, who had been awarded the Nobel Prize in 1977 for his work on neuroendocrine homeostasis and releasing factors, the topic of his Willis Lecture.

Hughlings Jackson Lectures

Norman Geschwind, from Harvard, gave the 1977 Hughlings Jackson Lecture, "Left Inattention: A Paradox Resolved." Vernon Mountcastle of Johns Hopkins University, the dean of American neurophysiologists, gave the 1978 Lecture, "A New Paradigm for Cerebral Function," based on the columnar organization of the cerebral cortex, in which he made the compelling argument that "the manner in which local cortical columns, as processing and distributing units, operate upon their inputs to produce their output is qualitatively similar in all neo-cortical areas and is basic to the carrying out of high-order functions of the brain … Although older parts of the brain may play a significant role, the key to any fruitful theories of higher brain function must be the unique structure and properties of the cerebral cortex."[10] In this Mountcastle echoed Pavlov who wrote, *"The cerebral hemispheres are the organ of conditioned reflexes."*[11]

Brenda Milner, recently elected fellow of the Royal Society of London, gave the 1979 Hughlings Jackson Lecture, "On the Duality of the Brain," and was later invited to speak on the same topic at the Pontifical Academy of Sciences.[12] Theodore Rasmussen and Brenda Milner were invited to address the New York Academy of Sciences on early left-brain injury and speech lateralization, and the paper that resulted became a classic in the field.[13]

POSITRON EMISSION TOMOGRAPHY

With computed tomography scanning well entrenched in the diagnosis of structural brain lesions, the MNI looked to the development of a different kind of imaging device, one that would reveal the metabolic activity of individual brain structures and pathologies: the positron emission tomography scanner. Thus, William Feindel made a momentous announcement in his 1974 annual report: "Recently, we have begun clinical trials with another unique device that measures blood flow in quite small areas of the brain by a method in which the patient breathes a microscopic amount of a radioactive tracer. This sophisticated instrument, which is called a positron emission tomograph (PET), has been developed by Dr Yamamoto with the scientific team at the Brookhaven National Laboratory."[14]

Starting in 1966, Lucas Yamamoto had worked at the Brookhaven National Laboratory on Long Island, New York, on a device to measure cerebral blood flow in animals using positron-emitting tracers. The Brookhaven scanner was upgraded at the MNI by 1970 and christened "the Positome." Based in the Cone Laboratory, the Positome was used to measure cerebral blood flow in a clinical situation and within experimental protocols. It remained in use until 1978, when a significant upgrade was unveiled.

The First International Symposium on Positron Emission Tomography
Positron emission tomography had attracted enough interest throughout the world for the institute to host the First International Symposium on Positron Emission Tomography, 1–3 June 1978. The symposium, with some 100 attendees, was a great success and the abstracts of the papers presented were published in the new *Journal of Computer Assisted Tomography.*[15] The highlight of

the meeting was the presentation of the Positome II to an international audience. Developed by Chris Thompson, Lucas Yamamoto, and Ernst Myer, it was the first PET scanner to use an array of sixty-four bismuth germanate oxide crystals detectors. The Positome II was further modified by Atomic Energy of Canada and was the origin of most clinical PET scanners over the next decade.[16] The influence of the first PET symposium and the development of the Positome II had far-reaching consequences, as William Feindel recalled: "The significance of PET as a research tool for investigating brain chemistry became evident to Donald Tower (then Director of the National Institute of Neurological Diseases and Stroke) and his colleagues when they attended the First International Symposium … On the advice of its council and staff, the NINDS promptly allotted 10 million dollars to create eight PET centers. The members of the PET team at the MNI played a prominent role on the review committees for this initiative." MNI fellow Peter Herscovitch was later appointed chief of the Positron Emission Tomography Department at NIH.

A problem remained: although positron emission tomography could measure the metabolism of radio-labelled compounds, the isotopes had to be generated by the cyclotron at McGill's Foster Radiation Laboratory, across Pine Avenue from the MNI. Thus, these short-lived compounds had to be transported "hot from the oven," post-haste, to the Cone Laboratory where the scanning took place. The solution was obvious to William Feindel and Lucas Yamamoto: the institute would buy its own cyclotron and put it in its basement. Referred to as the "Mini Cyclotron" or the "Baby Cyclotron," it was capable of producing carbon-11, fluorine-18, nitrogen-13, and oxygen-15, all the biologically important isotopes. This would allow the correlation of cerebral blood flow and blood volume, and oxygen and glucose metabolism in humans, in normal and disease states.

The miniature cyclotron arrived at the institute in October 1980 and became operational the following year. Mirko Diksic, a radiochemist, and Leo Nikkinen, a cyclotron engineer, joined the staff of the Cone Laboratory to wean the baby cyclotron.

In keeping with the MNI's commitment to PET, Marcus Raichle, of Washington University at St Louis, was invited to give the first K.A.C. Elliott Lecture in Neurosciences, on the topic of positron emission tomography. Louis Sokoloff of the National Institutes of Health and recipient of the Lasker Award, often a prelude to the Nobel Prize, gave the second K.A.C. Elliott Lecture in 1980. Sokoloff's pioneering work in deoxyglucose autoradiography would soon become applicable to humans through further advances in PET, thereby coupling blood-flow measurements and cerebral metabolism in normal and disease states.[17]

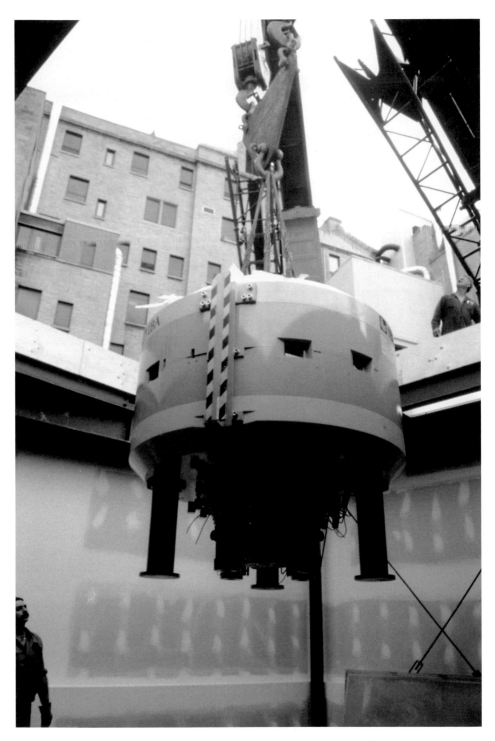

Figure 35.4: Mini-cyclotron being lowered into the basement of the MNI under the watchful eye of Mr Jean-Paul Bonhomme (*left*). (MNI Archives)

Functional Imaging

Ernst Meyer, in the Cone Laboratory, devised more accurate methods to evaluate regional blood flow and blood volume, the fraction of oxygen extracted by the brain, and the regional cerebral oxygen and glucose metabolism. As part of these efforts to improve methodology, Meyer began evaluating the role of the so-called water-bolus technique, the continuous infusion of oxygen-15 labelled water. This technique opened a new field of investigation, namely the functional imaging of eloquent regions of the brain activated by such tasks as movement, sensation, and speech. The feasibility of functional scanning was demonstrated at the MNI by Per Roland, who was on sabbatical from the Karolinska Institute, Ernst Meyer, and their co-workers, who showed that sequential movements of the fingers produce focal increases in cerebral blood flow in the contralateral, anatomically appropriate structures.[18] Richard Leblanc and Ernst Meyer later demonstrated the clinical applicability of the labelled water method as an adjunct to surgery in patients with a structural brain lesion.[19] The institute's use of positron emission tomography was greatly aided by the recruitment of Alan C. Evans from Atomic Energy of Canada, a most significant appointment for the future of brain imaging at the MNI.

36

The Last Half-Decade

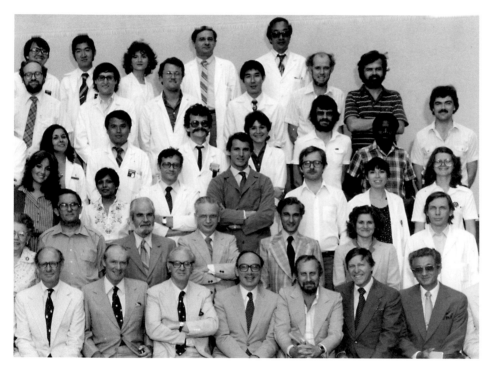

Figure 36.1: MNI staff 1980 (*detail*). (*Front row, left to right, 3, 5, 6*) W. Feindel, R. Ethier, and G. Bertrand. (*Second row, 2–6*) P. Gloor, D. Baxter, A. Eisen, J. Arpin, and J. Wells. R. Leblanc is in the third row (*4*), in the neurosurgical resident's distinctive green lab coat. In the fourth row are R. del Carpio, R. Ochs and T. Peters (*1, 4, 5*). In the fifth row we see P. Herscovitch, B. Zifkin, and C. Thompson (*1, 2, 5*). (MNI Archives)

NEW STAFF

A number of new appointments, both on the clinical services and in research laboratories, were made under William Feindel's directorship, which would have a lasting effect on the MNI and its activities.

Clinical Appointments

Neurology
Peter Herscovitch, George Elleker, Gordon Francis, Elizabeth Matthew, Daniel Gendron, and Serge Gauthier joined the Department of Neurology. Each had a special interest: Francis in multiple sclerosis and Matthew in developmental neurobiology and epilepsy. Francis and Matthew eventually moved on after rendering important service to the institute and its patients. Peter Herscovitch later took the now-familiar route to Bethesda, Maryland, to head the Department of Positron Emission Tomography at the National Institutes of Health. George Elleker took on responsibility for electromyography at the MNI after Andrew Eisen left for Vancouver in September 1980. Elleker introduced plasma exchange at the institute, for patients with Guillain-Barré syndrome.[1] Daniel Gendron became director of the EMG Laboratory upon Elleker's departure for the University of Alberta.[2] Serge Gauthier eventually led a multi-centre, multidisciplinary team dedicated to the investigation of Alzheimer's disease as the director of the McGill University Research Centre for Studies in Aging. Ghislaine Savard, trained in neurology and psychiatry, joined the neuropsychiatry staff.[3]

Neurosurgery
Jean-Guy Villemure replaced Carl Dila when he left for Connecticut. Villemure would have a distinguished career in four major universities on two continents. He was recruited to the institute in 1978 and established the first MNI program for the investigation and treatment of patients with normal pressure hydrocephalus. He is most remembered at the MNI for his pioneering work using positron emission tomography in the investigation of patients harbouring a malignant glioma, and for the intra-arterial chemotherapeutic treatment of malignant gliomas in conjunction with disruption of the blood-brain barrier. Villemure left the institute in 1997 to become chairman of the Department of Neurosurgery at the University of Lausanne and professor of neurosurgery at the University of Geneva. He returned to Montreal in 2007 as professor and chairman of the Division of Neurosurgery at the Université de Montréal, a position he held until his retirement in 2011. Kathleen Meagher-Villemure joined Stirling Carpenter and Yves Robitaille in the Department of Neuropathology.[4]

There were two departures from the Department of Neurosurgery: Joy Arpin relocated to Dallas, Texas, and John Wells joined Robert Hansebout at McMaster University.[5] As the neurosurgeon-in-chief, Gilles Bertrand reported,

> These departures would have been very demoralizing had it not been for the arrival on our staff of Dr Richard Leblanc. Dr Leblanc is a graduate of the University of Ottawa. He completed his four years of neurosurgical residency at the MNI. He has research interests that date back to the early years of his medical school in Ottawa and which have continued here in the Cone Laboratory where his work on cerebral vasospasm is supported by a fellowship from the Medical Research Council of Canada. He is most welcome in our ranks as a neurosurgeon and as a scientist.[6]

Richard Leblanc's interest in cerebrovascular disease was the result of his work on cerebral vasospasm as a medical student in Eric Peterson's laboratory at the University of Ottawa. During his residency, Leblanc trained with Theodore Rasmussen and William Feindel, then, being particularly interested in problems of the cerebral circulation, Leblanc took a fellowship with Charles Drake at the University of Western Ontario.[7] Leblanc then worked in the Cone Laboratory under Feindel, Yamamoto, and Meyer, and obtained an MSc from McGill University for his thesis "Calcium Antagonism in Cerebral Vasospasm."[8]

Research Appointments

Anatomy

Barbara Jones and Alain Beaudet joined the Department of Neuroanatomy. Jones attended the University of Delaware and did her doctoral thesis on the role of catecholamines with Michel Jouvet, a pioneer in sleep research, in Lyon, France. Jones then did postgraduate work in Paris before taking a position first at the University of Chicago, and then at the MNI to pursue her interest in the role of monoamine neurons in the sleep-wake cycle. Her studies centred on the dorsolateral pontine tegmentum, and combined rigorous experimental design with beautiful 3-D colour graphic representations of her data.[9] Alain Beaudet, a graduate of the Université de Montréal, did post-doctoral work at the Centre d'études nucléaires in Paris and at the Brain Research Institute in Zurich, on the distribution of serotonin in the forebrain. Baudet investigated the ultrastructure of dopaminergic and serotoninergic neurons at the MNI.[10] Beaudet has been influential in the scientific life of Quebec and Canada, as president and chief executive officer of the Fonds de la recherche en santé du Québec, and later, as president of the Canadian Institutes of Health Research. Edith Hamel joined the Department of Anatomy as an MRC post-doctoral fellow, where she worked with Alain Beaudet on opiate receptors.[11] She and Peter Herscovitch would later be successive presidents of the International Society for Cerebral Blood Flow and Metabolism.[12]

Cerebrovascular Disease

Antoine Hakim joined the neurological staff in July 1979, after working with Hanna Pappius on thiamine deficiency. Hakim's interests evolved from lack of vitamins in the diet, to lack of oxygen supply to the brain, as he replaced Lucas Yamamoto as head of the McConnell Brain Imaging Centre. Hakim made important contributions to the study of stroke, especially in the quantitation of blood flow and metabolism within the ischemic penumbra about an infarcted area.[13] Richard Leblanc, Jane Tyler (a fellow in the McConnel Brain imaging Centre), Lucas Yamamoto, and Tony Hakim quantitated the hemodynamic and metabolic effect of internal carotid artery stenosis and occlusion, especially as they affect the anterior borderzone between the anterior and middle cerebral artery distributions.[14] Hakim left the MNI in 1990 and became director of the Neuroscience Research Institute at the University of Ottawa. Ronald Pokrupa, a neurosurgeon trained at the University of Ottawa with MNI alumus Eric Peterson, took a fellowship in the Department of Neurochemistry, where, with Antoine Hakim, he studied the metabolic effects of stroke. Pokrupa joined the Department of Neurosurgery at the MNI after his fellowship, and later took a position at Queen's University, Kingston.

Neurophysiology

Daniel Guitton was recruited to the MNI in 1974. Guitton, a neurophysiologist, and Trevor Kirkham, a neuro-ophthalmologist recruited to the institute in the same year, shared a common interest in eye movements.[15] Guitton's early work addressed the role of the superior colliculi on the coordination of head and eye movements,[16] and he later established the Gaze Control Laboratory at the MNI. Robert Dykes joined the Department of Neurophysiology at the MNI in 1977, where his major interests lay in the exacting, detailed study of the somatotopic organization of different sensory modalities, the role of GABA in the sensory receptive fields of the cerebral cortex, and the reorganization of the somatosensory cortex after peripheral nerve injury.[17] Massimo Avoli was the newcomer in the group. He was appointed to the MNI after completing his PhD in Pierre Gloor's laboratory in 1982.[18] Avoli's interests initially centred on the study of neocortical and hippocampal epileptic activity *in vitro*, and on the interplay of excitatory and inhibitory influences in the genesis of epileptic seizures.[19]

Neuropsychology

The recruitment of Michael Petrides to the Department of Neuropsychology added new vigour to the study of frontal lobe function.[20] Gabriel Leonard, Alain Ptito, and Robert Zatorre also joined the neuropsychology group, adding greater dimension to the department's activities.[21]

Neuromuscular Disease

Heather Durham joined the MNI to pursue her interest in neurotoxicology.[22] She applied herself to the study of amyotrophic lateral sclerosis – Lou Gehrig's disease – and became a world leader in translational research into this condition.[23] Paul Holland also joined the research staff. His major interest was in the cellular biochemistry and development of skeletal muscle cells, which complemented the interests of Carpenter and Karpati.[24] Sergio Pena inaugurated the biochemical genetics laboratory at the MNI and joined the neuromuscular group in their efforts to identify the defective gene in Duchenne muscular dystrophy using techniques of biochemistry and cell biology new to the institute. The major event for the neuromuscular laboratory, however, was undoubtedly the publication of the magisterial, comprehensive, and authoritative *Pathology of Skeletal Muscle* by Carpenter and Karpati.[25]

NEW TECHNIQUES

Interventional Neuro-Radiology

Interventional neuro-radiological procedures were first developed at the MNI by Denis Mélançon – not for vascular diseases, for which they are most currently performed today – but for lesions of the spinal cord.

Mélançon graduated from the Faculty of Medicine of the Université de Montréal in 1960 and completed his training in neuroradiology at the MNI in 1967, after a time in general practice. He then joined the Department of Neuroradiology at the institute and was its director from 1995 to 1999. He remains a greatly valued neuroradiologist at the institute to this day. Many will remember his weekly morning brain-cutting sessions designed to teach residents and fellows how to visualize in three dimensions the structures revealed by shadow and light on flat X-ray films and monitors. Mélançon's dedication to teaching and service have been recognized by the creation of the Denis Mélançon Neuroradiology Conference and Annual Lecture, one of the most well-attended conferences at the MNI.

The development of image-guided, percutaneous puncture of the spinal cord was developed to aid in the diagnosis of focal spinal cord swelling of undetermined etiology before the advent of high-resolution CT scanning and to

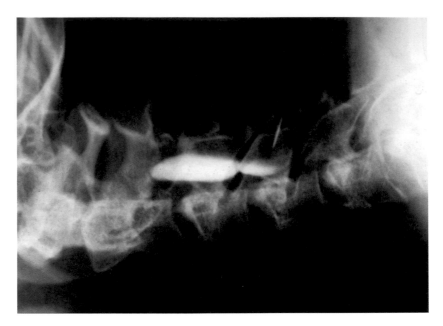

Figure 36.2: X-ray-guided percutaneous cervical cord puncture showing the puncture needle and the contrast material filling a syringomyelic cavity. (Courtesy Denis Mélançon)

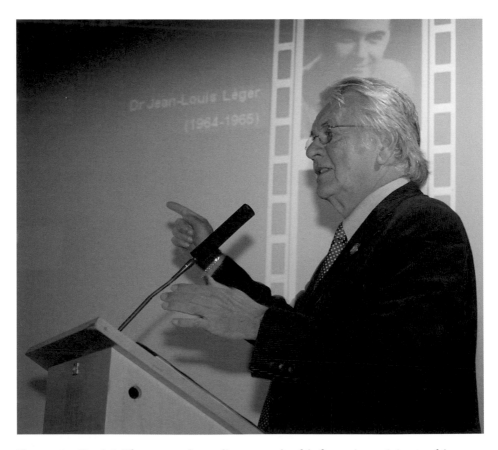

Figure 36.3: Denis Mélançon at the podium pursuing his favourite activity, teaching. (MNI Archives)

drain cysts of the cord as a therapeutic measure. Denis Mélançon and his colleagues first reported the results of this procedure in 1978.[26] As Mélançon recalls, the technique required "a posterior approach and two spinal needles, as for discography. The first needle, a number 20 lumbar puncture needle, accommodated a second, much smaller number 25 LP needle. The number 20 needle entered the subarachnoid space but stopped short of spinal cord, which was then easily punctured by the smaller needle."[27] If a cyst was entered, it was aspirated and its fluid analyzed to determine if it was tumoural or hydromyelic. Symptomatic relief was achieved most often within twenty-four hours if the cyst was under pressure. The extent and contour of the cyst could be imaged after the injection of a contrast material. The puncture hole(s) were not obvious to inspection in those patients who were subsequently operated upon." Donatella Tampieri, who replaced Mélançon as head of the Department of Diagnostic and Therapeutic Neuroradiology, now occasionally performs the procedure.

Pharmacokinetics and Intra-Arterial Chemotherapy

Jacques Théron, from Caen, France, came to the institute in 1983. A pioneer in the field in Europe, he was one of the first vascular interventional neuroradiologists in North America. Théron introduced numerous intravascular procedures to the MNI, most notably angioplasty for the treatment of extra-cranial arterial stenosis and the use of detachable balloons for the treatment of carotido-cavernous fistula. In collaboration with Jean-Guy Villemure, Mirko Diksic, Lukas Yammamoto, and Jane Tyler, a protocol was elaborated to study the pharmacokinetics of bis-chloroethyl nitrosourea (BCNU) within malignant tumours and the surrounding brain. The accumulation of labelled BCNU and measurements of cerebral blood flow and of oxygen and glucose metabolism provided valuable information on the metabolism of malignant gliomas and of the brain substance under its influence.[28]

Stereotaxy and Depth Electrode Implantation

Advances in computer technology, the refinement of instuments, and the development of digital subtraction angiography added new impetus to stereotactic neurosurgery, mainly due to the efforts of André Olivier and Terry Peters.[29] Further advances were anticipated with the delivery of Canada's first magnetic resonance scanner in 1985. This would allow neurosurgeons "to target deep cerebral structures with enough precision to carry out functional procedures without having to resort to ventriculography and other indirect methods of visualization."[30]

Epilepsy

Bitemporal Epilepsy

A major advance in the care of epileptic patients resulted from stereotactic implantation of depth electrodes in patients with bitemporal epilepsy.[31] In many cases of putative bitemporal epilepsy, prolonged depth electrode recording and video-telemetric analysis of seizure patterns identified a dominant focus responsible for the patient's seizures. With improved definition of the laterality of seizure onset, patients who would previously have been denied operation could proceed to surgery. Further, these studies confirmed the primary role of the temporal mesial structures in temporal epilepsy, and helped to elucidate the interplay of the amygdala, hippocampus, and lateral temporal neocortex in this condition.[32]

Experiential Phenomena

The depth electrodes could not only record epileptic phenomena arising from the structures in which they were implanted, they could also be used to stimulate them. In this way the psychical phenomena that often accompanies temporal epilepsy could be studied and localized to a specific structure within the brain. As the joint effort of the Departments of Neurosurgery and of Neurophysiology in the investigation of experiential phenomena was being readied for publication, Pierre Gloor gave an unedited report of the paper's conclusions: "Complex visual and auditory hallucinations, memory flash-backs, mnemonic illusions like *déjà vu*, and ictal emotions all were intimately linked to activation of limbic structures, either by seizure discharge or by electrical stimulation. Neocortical activation by itself was incapable of producing these phenomena. The amygdala in particular seemed to be implicated in the elaboration of these psychic phenomena."[33] The implications, he felt, were clear: "In conjunction with the earlier findings published many years ago by Dr Penfield and associates, these data suggest that the evocation of these epileptic phenomena as well as normal human subjective experience in the visual, auditory, mnemonic, and affective spheres depend upon a close interaction between neocortical and limbic mechanisms."[34]

Secondary Epileptogenesis

While they were on sabbatical at the MNI, Frank Morrell, professor of neurology at the Rush Presbyterian–St Luke Medical Center in Chicago, and his wife, Leyla de Toledo Morrell, studied the phenomenon of secondary epileptogenesis. The Morrells observed that nearly 40 per cent of patients operated upon for the resection of a tumour in a *temporal* lobe had "secondary [epileptic] foci in homotopic areas contralateral to the primary lesion." A secondary, independent focus was present, however, in fewer than 20 per cent of patients with a *frontal* tumour.[35] Frank and Leyla Morrel concluded from these observations that "secondary epileptogenesis … seems to represent a significant aspect of the pathophysiology of human epilepsy" and that the temporal lobes seemed to be more intrinsically susceptible to this phenomenon than other areas of the brain. Frank Morrell later wrote an insightful review of secondary epileptogenesis based in part on the patients he studied at the MNI.[36]

NEW DIGS

The World of Neurology

The academic activities of the MNI continued in the new decade. The Penfield Award for 1980 went to Douglas Arnold, resident in neurology, and to Richard Leblanc, resident in neurosurgery. The following year these awards went to David Dubuisson and Thomas Staunton in neurosurgery and neurology, respectively; and a special award was presented to Edith Hamel for her progress in scientific research. Upon graduation from the Neurosurgery Program, David Dubuisson took a position at the Beth Israel Hospital of Harvard University. Tom Staunton worked in Toronto and at McMaster University before returning to the United Kingdom, to the Norfolk and Norwich University Hospital.[37]

Two distinguished fellows inaugurated a new decade of Hughlings Jackson Lectures. The 1980 lecture was delivered by Donald Tower, just returned from the People's Republic of China, titled "Prospects and Challenges for Neurology and Neuroscience." David Hubel, the 1981 Nobel laureate in medicine or physiology, delivered his first post-Nobel address, "The Eye, the Brain, and Perception," at the MNI, as the 1982 Hughlings Jackson Lecturer. Hubel was the eighth Nobel laureate to give the Hughlings Jackson Lecture since its inauguration by Wilder Penfield in 1935, but he wasn't the only Nobel laureate to address the institute that year: John Vane, from the University of London, gave the 1982 K.A.C. Elliott Lecture, "Neurochemistry on Prostaglandins in Health and Disease," and was awarded the Nobel Prize a few days later.

William Feindel organized a symposium on 26 January 1983, with the assistance of the Osler Society of McGill University, in celebration of Wilder Penfield's birthday. Feindel discussed "Penfield the Oslerian," and Theodore Rasmussen recalled "Penfield the Surgeon."[38] The distinguished academician William Carleton Gibson, chairman of the Universities Council of British Columbia, addressed "Penfield the Physiologist and Cytologist."[39] The final event of the day was the vernissage of Luba Genush's triptych *The World of Neurology*, which depicts the human form in all of its vulnerability yet in harmony with twentieth-century technology.[40] Initially hung in the Izaak Walton Killam Conference Room, the mural now greets patients and visitors entering through the lobby of the Webster Pavilion.

The Webster Pavilion

With the coming of the new decade, Willam Feindel had announced, "In keeping with the MNI's interest in brain scanning over the past twenty years, we recently evaluated the role of nuclear magnetic resonance, another new technique for picturing the brain and for analyzing changes in phosphorous compounds in the metabolism of brain and muscle. Based on information gathered at scientific symposia, on visits to other research centres, and on the splendid Willis lecture given here by Dr George Radda, head of the NMR unit at Oxford, we have decided it would be valuable to introduce this method at the institute."[41]

An added advantage of nuclear magnetic technology was the possibility of performing spectroscopy and biochemical studies of the brain. Douglas Arnold, a neurologist, and Eric Shoubridge, a research biologist, went to Oxford to work with George Radda in preparation for their role in the development of the nuclear magnetic resonance unit,[42] which was installed at the institute in September 1983 and became operational in 1985. It, the mini-cyclotron, the new Positome III scanner, the computed tomography body scanner, and all computers and laboratories necessary for their operation would be located in close proximity to each other at the McConnell Brain Imaging Centre. The BIC would be located in the newest addition to the institute, "called the Webster Pavilion in appreciation of the magnificent support Howard Webster, Colin Webster, and other members of the Webster family have given over the past decade to develop these advanced imaging systems."[43]

The Webster Pavilion, Feindel continued,

> was assigned space in the north corner of Molson Stadium. Extensive excavation of bedrock gave an almost ideal location for the powerful new magnetic resonance unit designed for brain and body imaging. The second level of this pavilion will be used to house the positron emission tomography research unit closer to the cyclotron and radiochemistry laboratory. The third and fourth levels, already partly occupied by the EEG laboratory, will also provide space for research and clinical offices. On the top two stories, the 350-seat auditorium will provide the only

large conference centre in the entire RVH–Pathology Institute–Neuro complex. The foyer space on two levels has been designed as a centre for displays on the normal and disordered brain. The footing sand columns of this pavilion are designed to support, in the future, an additional four levels.[44]

The auditorium was named in honour of Jeanne Timmins in gratitude for a generous gift from her estate, as appreciated as it was unexpected. With the Penfield and Webster Pavilions, the square footage of the institute had doubled in the past decade.[45] The pavilion was officially inaugurated during the fiftieth anniversary celebrations of the Montreal Neurological Institute, in September 1984.

SYNAPSE 50: THE FIFTIETH ANNIVERSARY OF THE MNI

The fiftieth anniversary of the opening of the MNI was celebrated on 23–26 September 1984. Former fellows and nurses, distinguished guests, and guest speakers attended. Caroline Robertson, director of nursing, and Verna Bound, director of social services, organized a program of lectures, workshops, and discussions, which were held on Sunday, 23 September.[46]

Monday, 24 September

The inaugural ceremonies of the Webster Pavilion were held on Monday morning, 24 September, as the new pavilion was officially dedicated by Colin and Howard Webster, and McGill University held a special convocation conferring a doctor of laws on Colin Webster and honorary degrees of doctor of sciences on William Feindel, C. Miller Fisher, and Donald Tower.

With subsequent events the title under which the fiftieth anniversary celebrations were held, SYNAPSE 50, revealed its meaning: a reflection of the contacts that had been created over its first fifty years between the MNI and numerous academic institutions spanning the globe through the fellows whom it had trained, and the facilitated communication of scientific ideas made possible by advanced technology.

Through the collaboration of Bell Canada, Teleglobe, the Ministry of Communications, and the Canadian Broadcasting Corporation, a live television link was set up with other neurological centres in Washington, London, Paris, Santiago, Belgrade, and Kyushu. This allowed a "lively exchange with Dominique Comar's group in Paris on dopamine receptors and between Michael Walker in

Washington and [the MNI group] on recent advances in the chemical treatment of brain tumours. The opening ceremonials were followed over the next two days by the established named MNI lectures, and other lectures in honour of MNI staff."[47]

Table 36.1
SYNAPSE 50 named lecturers

Named lecture	Lecturer	Lecture title
Theodore Rasmussen Lecture	Charles Drake, University of Western Ontario	The Surgeon Investigator
Hughlings Jackson Lecture	David Kuhl, UCLA	Emission Imaging: An Emerging View of the Functioning Brain
Donald McRae Lecture	George Radda, Oxford University	From Molecules to Man: Looking into the Cell with Nuclear Magneticresonance
K.A.C. Elliott Lecture	Igor Klatzo, NIH	Reaction of the Brain to Injury
Francis McNaughton Lecture	Stanley Appel, Baylor University	Neurotrophic Factors in Neurologic Disease: An Approach to Neuromuscular and Brain Degeneration
William Cone Lecture	Gazi Yasargil, University of Zurich	Cerebrovascular Surgery
Herbert H. Jasper Lecture	David Prince, Stanford University	Focal Epilepsy and Cortical Neuronal Function
Thomas Willis Lecture	Miller Fisher, Harvard University	Cerebrovascular Update
Fellows Lecture	Blaine Nashold, Duke University	The DREZ (Dorsal Root Entry Zone) Operation for Pain Relief

Of Note, George Radda, whose Willis Lecture the previous year had reinforced the institute's determination to purchase an MRI scanner, described the potential uses of MRI to identify chemical elements in living tissue that could be used to provide a "chemical biopsy" of the brain. This technique was later applied at the MNI for the non-invasive diagnosis of cerebral tumours, based on their nuclear magnetic spectrum, a world first.[48] Current MNI fellows Stephen Strother and Jane Tyler gave the Fellows Prize essay on cerebral glucose metabolism studied by PET.

A FELLOW'S REMINISCENCE

An informal address was given at a dinner held at the University Club on Wednesday evening by one of the fellows who had attended the opening of the institute five decades earlier. He relived some light-hearted moments, as when Arne Torkildsen, perhaps succumbing to a deep-seated Nordic prudishness, hung his academic robes on the marble statue, *La Nature*. Or the story of the two surgical interns returning from the Nurses Ball and still in top hat and top form, persistently ringing the night doorbell and being greeted by Miss Flanagan, who was not amused in the least. Or of the two residents "who were assisting the Chief at an operation under local anaesthetic. At his request that *one* should drop out of the sterile field and, under the drapes, observe the patient, both dived for the opportunity to rest. A stern word suggested that *one* was enough! Cortical stimulation seemed to produce no reported movement in the patient. Whereupon it was found that the observer had fallen asleep on the patient's chest!" Still under Archibald's spell, the Old Fellow ended on a more elevated tone, undoubtedly reflecting the sentiments of all those present, recalling Archibald's word: "To gather knowledge and to find out new knowledge is the *noblest* occupation of the physician. To apply that knowledge – with sympathy, born of understanding, to the relief of human suffering, is his *loveliest* occupation."[49]

And so our story ends where it began, with Archibald, and his commemorative address at the opening of the institute:[50] "Finis is not written here. It marks truly the end of one stage, but it marks the beginning of another."

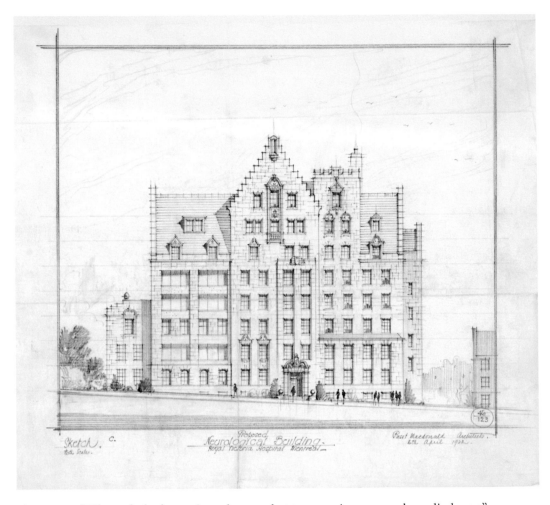

Figure 36.4: "Whereof what's past is prologue; what to come, in yours and my discharge." – Antonio, *The Tempest* (Architectural drawing of the MNI, 1932, Ross & Macdonald, Montreal Neurological Institute, elevation of the main facade, 1932, ARCH33365, Ross & Macdonald fonds, Collection Centre Canadien d'Architecture)

Epilogue

The Boy from Bridgewater:
William Howard Feindel, 1918–2014

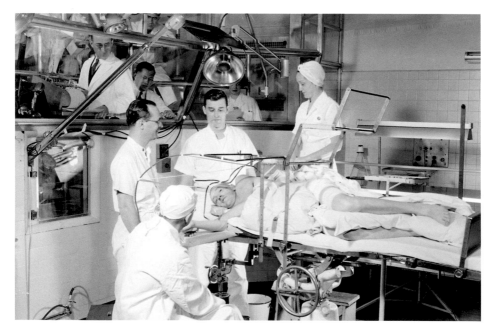

Figure 37.1: William Feindel, junior resident (*standing, left*). To his left are Lamar Roberts and Phoebe Stanley, assistant operating room supervisor. Sitting is André Pasquet, anaesthetist. Herbert Jasper (*standing*) and Choh-luh Li are in the gallery. (W. Penfield and H.H. Jasper, *Epilepsy and the Functional Anatomy of the Human Brain* [Boston: Little, Brown, 1954], 751.)

William Howard Feindel passed away quietly at the Montreal Neurological Institute and Hospital of McGill University on 12 January 2014, following a brief illness. He was ninety-five years old.

William Feindel was one of the world's most distinguished neurosurgeons and a brilliant neuroscientist. As the MNI's third director he proved to be a singular medical and scientific administrator. Indefatigable, Feindel remained a daily presence at the MNI up to the last, attending grand rounds and conferences, taking notes in his ever-present pocket diary. The comment "Good question," spoken in a quizzical tone by first-year residents and distinguished professors alike, was heard from the podium at every conference that William Feindel attended. At the MNI's annual Feindel Lecture, a few weeks before his passing, he officiated at the launch of his most recent book, *Images of the Neuro*. He left us an unfinished book – taken up by his friends and colleagues – that is now in the reader's hands.

William Feindel was born on 12 July 1918 in Bridgewater, Nova Scotia. He graduated from Acadia University in 1939 and was awarded a Rhodes Scholarship to Merton College, Oxford. Feindel obtained an MSc in physiology from Dalhousie University in 1942 and an MDCM from McGill University in 1945. He went up to Oxford at the end of the Second World War to take up his Rhodes Scholarship and was awarded a PhD in neuroanatomy from Oxford University in 1949. His thesis examinor was J. Godwin Greenfield.

While in England, Feindel attended the National Hospital, Queen Square, where he studied with Sir Hugh Cairns, the dean of British neurosurgery at the time, and Sir Charles Symonds, the distinguished neurologist who, as a young man, had studied with Harvey Cushing, the father of American neurosurgery.

William Feindel returned to Montreal for his neurosurgical training at the Neurological Institute, with Wilder Penfield, William Cone, and Arthur Elvidge, whom he joined in clinical practice at the end of his training. It was during this time that Feindel made his first significant contribution to neurology, when he discovered the role of the amygdala in temporal lobe epilepsy. This finding opened a new field in neurophysiology and revolutionized the surgical treatment of patients with medically intractable psychomotor seizures.

William Feindel left the MNI in 1955 to become the first director of the Department of Neurosurgery at the University of Saskatchewan. While there, he was instrumental in developing Canada's first radioisotope contour brain scanner for the detection of intracranial lesions. He and Joseph Stratford, who would later be neurosurgeon-in-chief at the Montreal General Hospital, described the clinically relevant anatomy of the cubital tunnel and developed a technique of decompression of the ulnar the nerve at the elbow for the treatment of tardy ulnar palsy.

William Feindel returned to the MNI in 1959 to become the first William Vernon Cone Professor of Neurosurgery at McGill University, a position that he held until 1988. During that time Feindel was neurosurgeon-in-chief at the Montreal Neurological Hospital and at the Royal Victoria Hospital, director of the Montreal Neurological Institute, and chairman of the Department of

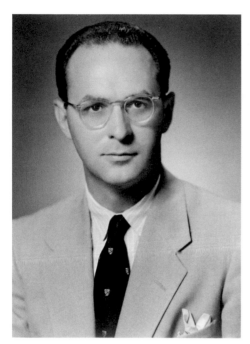
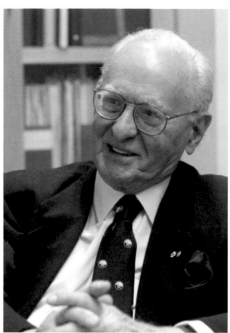

Figures 37.2 and 37.3: Dr William Howard Feindel as a young man with a Merton College tie, and in later life, mirthful and inquisitive, in his dapper blue blazer, characteristic vibrant red pocket-handkerchief, and his MNI Third Foundation tie. The Order of Canada and the National Order of Québec medals are neatly pinned to his lapel. (Left: MNI Archives; right: Owen Egan photographer)

Neurology and Neurosurgery of McGill's Faculty of Medicine. A visionary in the field of neuroimaging, William Feindel assembled a team that, evolving over time, pioneered in the applications of neuro-isotope brain scanning and the study of cerebral blood flow; and the introduction of computed tomography, magnetic resonance imaging, magnetic resonance spectroscopy, and positron emission tomography in North America. Established under his guidance, the MNI's McConnell Brain Imaging Centre continues to be a world leader in the field.

William Feindel was a fellow of the Royal Society of Canada and governor and chancellor of Acadia University. He was a consultant to the World Health Organization, the Medical Research Council of Canada, and the National Institutes of Health, Bethesda. He was a fellow of the Royal College of Physicians and Surgeons of Canada and a member of the American Association of Neurological Surgeons. William Feindel was also a diplomate of the American Board of Neurosurgery, the American College of Surgeons, and the American Academy of Neurological Surgery, of which he was vice-president. He was also

vice-president of the Society of Neurological Surgeons, and president of the
Canadian Neurosurgical Society, the Montreal Neurological Society, and
l'Association des neurochirurgiens du Québec. The William Feindel Chair of
Neuro-Oncology at McGill University was created in his honour.

William Feindel was awarded the Order of Canada and he was made a Grand
Officier de l'Ordre national du Québec. He was inducted into the Canadian
Medical Hall of Fame, and was honoured with the J. Kiffin Penry Award for Ex-
cellence by the American Epilepsy Society.

Having a passion for medical history, Feindel was honorary librarian and
member of the Board of Curators of McGill University's Osler Library, cura-
tor of the Wilder Penfield Archives, and recipient of the John Neilson Award
from the Hannah Institute for the History of Medicine. He published over 500
articles, 300 in peer-reviewed scientific and medical journals, and wrote or edited seven books.

Dr Feindel was a true gentleman and a caring mentor to those of us who
were fortunate enough to have come under his influence. His professional life
began with the pioneers of our profession and continued with the eminent neurosurgeons of our age, most of whom he knew on a first-name basis. With his
passing the MNI lost one of its brightest lights and most ardent champions.

Theme 1

Building the Institute[1]

ANNMARIE ADAMS AND WILLIAM FEINDEL

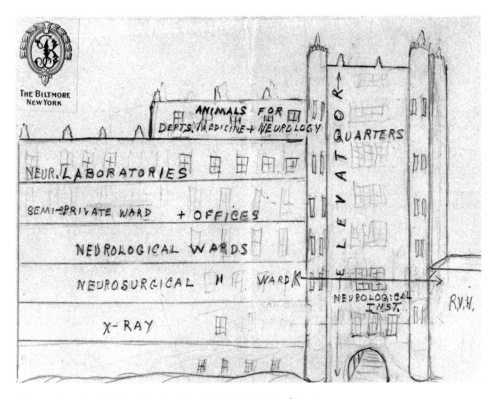

Figure T1.1: Penfield's sketch of the MNI. (MNI Archives)

Wilder Penfield's sketch from 1929 on the letterhead of the Biltmore Hotel in New York clearly expresses his architectural vision for the MNI.[2] The drawing of the seven-storey hospital, amateurishly rendered by Penfield as an elevation with some suggestion of perspective, shows the program of the new building as a series of vertical relationships. From the ground up, these are an unidentified ground floor, another for X-ray, two floors of wards for neurological patients, above which were two floors of laboratories for brain research. Indicated with an arrow, Penfield's third level shows a continuous relationship with Ward K of the adjacent RVH. This vision of the MNI was connected to the RVH, rather than occupying the current site across University Street.

By the summer of 1932,[3] however, the site at the RVH had proven unsuitable. Among other problems, Hospital Superintendent William Chenoweth worried that the neurological extension behind the west wing of Henry Saxon Snell's 1893 hospital might block the view of paying patients in the Ross Memorial Pavilion, directly above it. University Principal and Vice-Chancellor Sir Arthur Currie describes the situation in a letter to Allan Gregg, dated 27 November 1931:

> Plans were immediately discussed, and it was decided to liberate space in the Royal Victoria Hospital for neurology and neuro-surgery, by removing the resident staff from the central building of the Hospital and erecting a special home for them on a piece of land outside the main building.
>
> This new home was erected and has been completed recently. Further study of the situation, however, convinced us that the space thus afforded would be insufficient to meet the requirements of Dr Penfield.[4]

Currie subsequently convinced the McGill University Board of Governors to give the site currently occupied by the MNI, owned by the university, opposite the RVH on University Street, just north of the Pathological Institute, and next to the Percival Molson sports field-house. This separate-but-connected location ensured that the institute would be identified with McGill University for building maintenance, utilities, and communications, though still dependant on the RVH for hospital services. The change of site from the cramped space at the back of the RVH to upper University Street also offered options for future expansion.[5] It provided a clearer architectural and functional autonomy and resulted in future ownership of the MNI by McGill University, rather than the RVH.

Not surprisingly, the University Street building echoed the spirit of Wilder Penfield's Biltmore sketch intended for the earlier, never-used site. Despite his relatively deep investment in architecture as a client, however, Penfield always saw the building as a mere container for what happened within, rather than as an integral part of the MNI's mission or identity: "But the significance of the building lies in the things which it houses. The building is only a shell," Penfield said at the opening.[6]

Equally influential in the architectural development of the MNI was the first, unbuilt scheme, as delineated by a set of drawings held at the Canadian Centre for Architecture. This earlier, little-known, and unbuilt project established the general architectural character of the MNI as built: the close connection with RVH, inspiration of architect Henry Saxon Snell's Scottish-baronial design of 1893, and certain aspects of the program. Subsequent architectural additions, too, took their cues from adjacent buildings rather than from neurological hospitals elsewhere. It was an innovative and international hospital with a thoroughly Montreal-inspired design.

Why Ross & Macdonald? By 1930 the partnership of George Allan Ross (1879–1946) and Robert Henry Macdonald (1875–1942) had designed icons of Canadian architecture, with particularly outstanding work in hotel and commercial architecture. Toronto's Royal York Hotel (1928–29) and Montreal's Mount Royal Hotel (1921–22), the T. Eaton Department Stores in both Toronto (1929–30) and Montreal (1925–27) are among their best-known work. Perhaps because of this commercial specialization, Wilder Penfield was surprised that Principal Currie had engaged the architectural firm of Ross & Macdonald for the project. Sir Herbert Holt, president of the RVH, had, in fact, chosen the architects when the building was envisioned as an annex to the existing hospital. Currie's decision to remain with Ross and Macdonald after the change of sites was justifiable. The firm had proven itself in health-care design in the past, having designed McGill University's biology building (presumably today's James Administration Building, designed 1922),[7] and they were also designing the Interns Residence (1930) and the laundry, garage, and workshop (1931), located across from the eventual site of the neurological institute.

Ross & Macdonald's Interns Building was closely linked to the first project for the MNI, both physically and aesthetically.[8] A plan dated 26 November 1931, the day before Currie's letter to Gregg, shows the proposed layout of the new hospital wing, including new tunnels leading directly to the Interns Building and the Ross Memorial Pavilion.

Indeed, the main entrance to the new Neurology Department also faced the Interns Building, connecting through a parking lot just outside its door. Inside the never-built, *L*-shaped plan appear many aspects of the eventual MNI building: a square entrance hall inside a small vestibule, and a corridor leading to two operating rooms, including one with a viewing gallery. The west elevation of this early scheme, too, foreshadows the subsequent scheme built on University Street a few years later. Like the Interns Building and older Nurses Home by the architects Edward and William Maxwell,[9] the Neuro at the RVH appeared strangely domestic, mostly through the inclusion of features like crenellated gable ends, dormers, and chimneys. The entrance boasted classical detailing; windows, terraces, and certainly the picturesque, gabled rooflines looked wholly domestic.[10]

Adding to Penfield's bewilderment on the choice of designers, a bevy of alumni from the McGill University School of Architecture wrote to Currie protesting that he had not given other architectural firms an opportunity to bid on this important McGill contract.[11] Currie responded by pointing out that the architects had already spent considerable time and effort working on plans for the Neurological Institute as an annex to the RVH, a fact borne out by the multitude of plans now held at the Canadian Centre for Architecture. Students also wrote to Currie about the choice. On 31 May 1932, Currie answered Homer M. Jaquays, president of the Graduate Society, explaining the decision:

> I suppose there will be a good deal of criticism concerning the decision that has been made, but I do not think there was anything else to do. Ross & Macdonald had been chosen architects in the first place, by the Hospital it is true and not by the University; they had done a great deal of work on the job and had many consultations with those most directly concerned. Only an accident made it necessary to change the location to University property, and I wonder if it would have been ethically fair to dismiss them and choose a University architect? Of course, any money that Ross & Macdonald have already been paid will be deducted from their bill – and I assure you that we have no money to waste in these days.[12]

In the same letter, the former military-general-turned-principal cannily points out a strategic element in his decision involving Holt: "There was another factor, and that was that in conversation with Sir Herbert Holt, who is contributing $100,000 towards the building, I learned that he felt very strongly that Ross & Macdonald should continue as architects. He had chosen them, of course, when the building was to be put on the Royal Victoria Hospital, and Sir Herbert is very sensitive when his wishes are disregarded." Thus, in Currie's estimation, Ross & Macdonald were both a practical and political choice, and the firm was subsequently invited to continue with the commission. This freed Currie from the tedious, costly, and time-consuming process of receiving new bids and approving additional contracts. Despite initial misgivings about the choice, Penfield later described Australian-born architect Robert Macdonald as a "creative genius"[13] and spent long hours with him planning every aspect of the institute.[14] The planning began in earnest as soon as the Rockefeller grant was confirmed in April 1932. And over the next year designs were gradually developed in close collaboration with Penfield.

PROBLEMS WITH CHENOWETH AND RVH BOARD

Some time in late 1931 and early 1932 Currie found that negotiations and communications with Chenoweth, at the RVH, became increasingly difficult.[15] Among other things, Chenoweth seemed very reluctant to cooperate in the planning and provision of hospital services within the MNI. The problems began in earnest with a letter from Chenoweth to Holt on 17 November 1931. Voicing grave concerns[16] over the financial viability of the proposed institute, Chenoweth observed, "It should be borne in mind that if we commit ourselves to this project it means that we will be unable to bring up other fundamental departments in the Hospital to a higher standard of efficiency than now exists for the reason that the proposal will swallow up all our possible resources for some considerable time to come." Chenoweth went on to decry the costs associated with maintaining the Institute, particularly those that would be borne by the RVH. After an exhaustive iteration of costs,[17] Chenoweth added a postscript, perhaps designed to cast doubt on Penfield's commitment to Montreal: "Dr Penfield leaves for Philadelphia tonight to study their proposal. Then on to Rockefeller to try and find what they are prepared to do."[18]

In response to Chenoweth's letter, two days later, on 19 November 1931, Holt sent a clear message to McGill's chancellor, Edward Beatty: "I am enclosing you a letter from Chenoweth in reference to the Neurological Institute and thus showing what Dr Penfield says is the least he will require. I asked Chenoweth to make up an estimate of what the Institute would cost the Hospital and I think you will probably come to the same conclusion as I have – that it is out of the question for the Royal Victoria Hospital to take on this obligation."[19]

Unbeknownst to Penfield, 26 November 1931 would prove to be a critical day that would determine the fate of the MNI. In the early morning, Chenoweth, having previously contacted Ross & Macdonald, received an update on the project's costs, which included "an enlargement of the 2nd and 3rd floors at the West End, an addition of one and a half stories in the height, and interior rearrangement on all floors, resulting in an increase in cube quantity of 40%."[20] Ross & Macdonald noted an increase in costs from an estimated $244,800 to $344,672.[21] Chenoweth was not amused, and called an emergency meeting of the RVH Board of Governors. The purpose of the meeting was clear: to put an end to the proposed MNI. Fortunately, Currie, aware of the significance of the meeting, had prepared a five-page address to the Board of Governors.[22]

Currie opened with high praise and gratitude for the work of Wilder Penfield and William Cone, noting to the board, "There can be no doubt whatever about their importance to McGill University and the Royal Victoria Hospital."[23]

Currie then continued pitching the building campaign as a way to keep top doctors in Montreal:

> It is with great satisfaction that we have noted the success of doctors Penfield and Cone. Dr Penfield heads up an important and independent department, which embraces all medical diseases of the nervous system, of surgical injuries to nerves throughout the body, of brain operations, the treatment of injured spines, and of fractured skulls. They have both been here three years, and have proven their worth, both as personalities and men, diagnosticians, surgeons and consultants. There is no practicing physician in Montreal, or indeed, in Canada, nor is there any clinical teacher in our University, who would feel otherwise than that it is of capital importance to keep them here, and that it would be a tragic loss to have them go. Dr Penfield personally is one of our greatest drawing cards. He has attracted patients from all over the continent. He has himself brought $75,000 in money for his department. He has a prestige which places him in the very front rank of neurological surgeons.

Having passionately outlined Penfield's and Cone's impressive credentials and surgical success rates,[24] Currie pointed out the wastefulness and folly of abandoning the project so near to its realization: "We have already accumulated and spend [*sic*] on this Department, since June 1, 1928, more than $75,000. Are we now going to throw this sum into the discard, after such a promising start, a start universally recognized as one of great value and importance and of unlimited promise for the future?" Currie, continuing with a note of foreboding, observed,

> If we lose doctors Penfield and Cone, and if we neglect to take advantage of the interest of the Rockefeller Foundation, we shall place such a black mark on the record of our Medical School that it will take long years to erase it, and it will be many, many years before such an institute, with all its attendant advantages to students and patients, will be available in our country. If these men now leave Montreal we will not be able again in a generation to start new men upon this road, and our work in Neuro-Surgery will be placed where it was ten or fifteen years ago, that is, in a position of utter mediocrity. It is men, and not buildings, that make a hospital and a medical school.

It is clear that, without Currie's passionate intervention, the future of the project would have been called into serious jeopardy and may never have been realized. What is not so clear is whether Penfield was aware of how tenaciously Currie had pleaded his case. Over the years, Penfield's recognition of Currie's contribution to the project was muted at best. Had Penfield been aware of Currie's letter to the RVH board, he may well have viewed McGill University's principal in a different light.

THE BUILDING BUDGET

In addition to ongoing tensions with Chenoweth, Currie and Penfield were at odds more than once, being two strong-willed men, each with a sure sense that his own view was the right way to get things done. Penfield had worked tirelessly on the plans, going over myriad details with the architect and considered the design to be "the perfect little building"[25]

But Currie, concerned about costs, noted that in the revised plans, as compared to those submitted to the Rockefeller Foundation, a second elevator would be installed, another clinical floor added, and the lecture theatre doubled

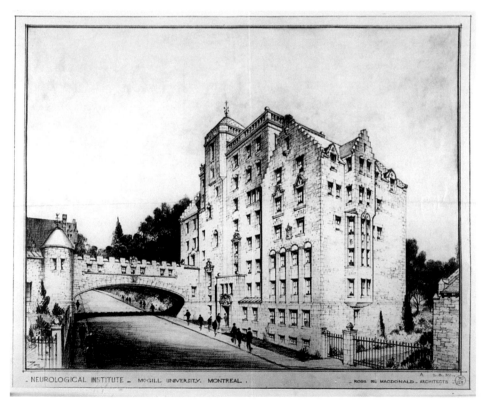

Figure T1.2: Perspective view of the MNI looking north up University Street toward Mount Royal. (MNI Archives, Ross & Macdonald Architects)

in size. A squash court had also appeared on an earlier set of plans, which Penfield justified the need for as recreation for his fellows. On 17 August 1932, Currie wrote to Penfield to express his concerns. He estimated that these alterations would add "probably 225,000 dollars"[26] to the estimated cost of the institute. Currie then continued, "I have not the heart to go to the Building committee with the plans in their present condition. I have no idea where the increased money called for could be found. I have always said that as far as the building costs were concerned, we could not exceed the $344,672, of which the Foundation agreed to pay half … You will see that we must reconsider these plans, eliminating enough to bring the cost down to the original estimate. Do you think any good would come of approaching the Foundation again?"[27]

Currie kept a close eye on the budget, and when Penfield's plans went beyond the estimated costs, he called on Penfield to cut the expense. The problem came to a boiling point one afternoon in late January 1933, when Penfield, abruptly summoned by Currie's secretary, cancelled his patient appointments and hurried to Currie's office. Currie had plans on the table to delete the two top floors, intended for laboratories and animal quarters. This would have wiped out the research potential of the institute. "We must cut the coat," Currie said firmly, "to fit the cloth."[28] Penfield, writing later to his mother, recorded his own angry retort, "You will have to go ahead with this project without me … No one will want this coat as you have cut it."[29]

As Penfield recalled, Currie brought his enormous closed fist crashing down on the table and exclaimed, "Damn it! They told me you would say just that." He laughed and then added, "We can't go on without you whether we like it or not. The university will have to take a chance that you know what you're talking about, and that you and Cone and Russel and others can run your own show and keep us out of debt after the building is built."[30] Penfield calmed down somewhat and reassured Currie, "If our work is any good at all, the university will never be called upon for funds.[31] This institute will pay its way with money that comes to it for that purpose."[32] Penfield even pledged the research funds from Mrs Madeleine Ottmann, the mother of a former patient, and the first instalment from the Rockefeller Foundation of almost $50,000 against any overrun in the construction cost. After tense discussion, it was agreed that strict budget controls would be set up by the architects in order to trim costs.[33] One such saving, for example, was the omission of one of the two elevators planned to go in the double shaft. For a decade, medical and support staff, patients going to and from the operating room, meal trolleys and animal feed and litter, as well as all the transport engendered by hospital activity were transported by one slow freight elevator. The architects also left one large laboratory unfinished, which served for a decade as a squash court, then in 1945 the space was converted into the world's first laboratory of neurochemistry through help from the Donner Canadian Foundation.

The design of the MNI was described in the *Royal Architectural Institute of Canada Journal* in October 1934, accompanied by four photographs showing the building's main characteristics. Like the nearby RVH, to which it linked by an overhead bridge, the new MNI resembled a high-rise, fortified castle. Constructed of grey limestone walls, the institute boasted a picturesque, variegated silhouette. At its centre was a narrow tower of about ten storeys, topped by a gable roof and distinctively crenellated gables. Minimal windows in this tower make it reminiscent of Italian medieval dwellings. Stepped back from the tower and at varying heights, the sections of the MNI appear almost as if they were constructed at different times, since some are capped by a flat roof and balustrade, another with a pitched copper roof, like the central tower. In general, the form of the building shows a remarkable in-and-out form, which broke down its massive scale. Since the MNI was most often seen at an obtuse angle, this ziggurat-like section would have been even more exaggerated on site.

Although the materials and castle-like features were clearly inspired by the Royal Victoria Hospital's original design, another important influence for the architects may have been their own stunning designs for high-end apartment blocks in Montreal. The firm's designs for the Chateau Apartments (1924–25) and Glen Eagles Apartments (1929–30) showcase the same skill in using a complex cross section and multi-faceted facade to make a massive, high-rise building appear more humanly scaled. Although constructed in brick rather than limestone, the design of the Glen Eagles, in particular, shares much with the new MNI. Both are constructed on a difficult, sloped site, and both projects use a technique of breaking the massing into sections of different heights to achieve a picturesque effect.

Adding to the romanticism of the MNI's design was the addition of stone carvings on the facade, articulating the building's unique place in the history of medicine. As Penfield described them, they are "the staff and serpent of Aesculapius, the Greek God of Medicine who became so proficient in the healing art that he was accused by Pluto of producing a shortage of shades in Hades. For this venture into 'state medicine' he was destroyed by a thunderbolt from the hand of Zeus. This emblem, together with the representation of the brain over the entrance, is intended to symbolize the field of neurology."[34] In addition, Penfield instructed the architects to include carvings of devices called trephines, that medieval surgeons had used to make holes in the skull. And over the lintel of the front entrance of the building is a model of the brain. These gave the building a historical touch that emphasized the history of neurology going back to two famous Greek physicians, Hippocrates and Galen.

PLANS AND INTERIOR FEATURES

A beautiful set of architectural plans, drawn in pencil at the scale of 1/8″ = 1 foot and dated 10 August 1932, illustrate the architects' proposed arrangement of the building.

The ground floor plan featured a deeply set entry with stairs leading to a Reception Room. To the north is a double-loaded corridor of small study spaces; to the south is this level's major space, a 150-seat amphitheatre. Between this theatre and the street was an elaborate photographic department that we know from Penfield's description was arranged by H.S. Hayden, an English medical photographer.[35]

The second, third, and fourth floors contained patient wards. Floors two and three were for public patients and had identical plans, though differentiated by being named after J.W. McConnell and Sir Herbert Holt, the first two donors to the McGill fund to match offers from the Rockefeller Foundation. Floor four had semi-private and private rooms. On the wards, the nursing station had large glass panels so the nurse could observe a single ward of twelve patients (note that the plans show ten and Penfield notes in the opening day brochure that the number had to be increased to fourteen during the first year). This direct surveillance was especially important for the nurses to monitor patients who might have seizures.

The fifth floor contained an operating room, with a glassed-in row of seats for viewers, and in a pit beneath the seats, a fine Ross telephoto camera, which was protected through a glass window facing upward to an overhead mirror that reflected the operative field. This ingenious setup allowed Penfield and other surgeons to make precise recordings of the places on the surface of the brain where a gentle electrical probe produced positive responses of movement in the hand or face, or induced tingling, which could be used to map out the sensorymotor cortex. The patient, who was awake during this entire procedure under local anaesthesia, would be presented with a series of simple objects on cards, such as scissors, lamp, comb, etc., thus stimulating the brain, so that the patient's speech area could be identified. This was critical in allowing the surgeon to remove a brain tumour or scar tissue without encroaching on this es-

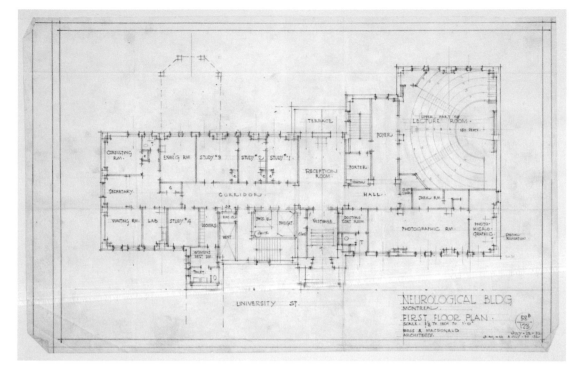

Figure T1.3: Plan of the first floor of the Montreal Neurological Institute. The Amphitheatre and the photography laboratory are at upper and lower right, respectively. They adjoin the porter's office and the doctors' cloakroom. The vestibule and reception room, later renamed the Feindel Foyer, are seen to the right of center. The reception room's east wall sheltered *Nature*. From the vestibule and reception room, a corridor leads to offices and examining rooms. (Ross & Macdonald, Montreal Neurological Institute, first floor plan, 1932, ARCH33375, Ross & Macdonald fonds, Collection Centre Canadien d'Architecture / Canadian Centre for Architecture, Montreal)

sential language area. Over the years many patients with speech difficulty, due to a nearby tumour, who might not be operated upon elsewhere, were referred to the institute. Penfield and his surgical colleagues were able to treat many of these patients, using the brain-mapping techniques, to help safely remove tumours without damaging the patient's language functions.

This fifth-floor operating room, which was given special articulation in the massing of the building by the architects, provided the setting for 6,000 operations of the special type to treat epilepsy. The resulting surgical records, photographs, dictation of the stimulation responses, and description of the electrical changes recorded from the operative site, together with the patient's medical history and psychological evaluation, made up a corresponding file of the same magnitude. This is, without doubt, the largest and longest-standing collection of records on human neurophysiology. It will continue to

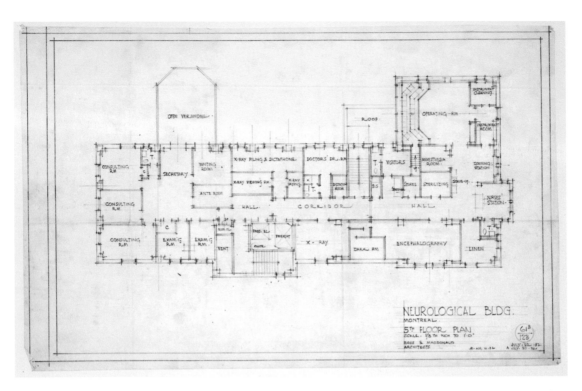

Figure T1.4: Plan of the fifth floor illustrating relationship of the operating room to the adjoining anaesthesia induction room, the visitor's gallery, the EEG laboratory, and the X-ray Department. (Ross & Macdonald, Montreal Neurological Institute, fifth floor plan, 1932, ARCH33372, Ross & Macdonald fonds, Collection Centre Canadien d'Architecture / Canadian Centre for Architecture, Montreal)

serve as an enormous database from which the staff of the Neuro and visiting scientists can access information on the long-term results of the surgical treatment of epilepsy.

On the sixth floor were labs, library, and Penfield's corner office. Research labs were critical to the scientific mission of the institute. As expected from Cone's passionate interest in neuropathology, the laboratory for gross and microscopic analysis of the brain and spinal cord and peripheral nerves was superb. Special stone sinks and draining boards were used to prevent any damage from the acidic chemicals used in the staining techniques. A long room with a long table, presumably the Fellows Lab, served as an ideal place to have the weekly neuropathology conferences attended by the staff and fellows. Within the same room there were half a dozen "Madrid" cubicles, partitioned off partly by tall cupboards for books and papers, and with utility services, electricity,

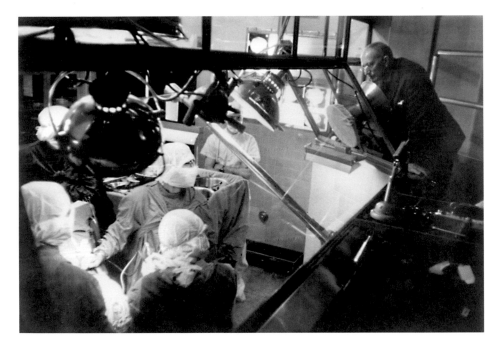

Figure T1.5: William Feindel, the newly appointed Cone Professor (*left of centre, wearing glasses*) during an intra-operative discussion with Wilder Penfield in the gallery (*right*). The surgical team is wearing the trademark MNI hair covering. Penfield is speaking through a two-way, megaphone-like apparatus whose protrusion into the operating room is covered with cloth. A set of opera glasses, affixed to a light chain and stored in a small open box, was available for those wanting a closer look at the operative field. The operating room was modernized for the opening of the Penfield Pavilion, but the gallery was kept intact. (MNI Archives)

suction, oxygen, and a small water basin to use in histological preparations. Each cubicle was also provided with a Zeiss binocular microscope.[36] The seventh floor hosted animal quarters and physiology labs, and on the top floor were five bedrooms for residents on duty, described by Penfield as "a monastic atmosphere important in their education."[37]

Four features of the building's interior deserve attention: the surgical theatre (described above), lecture theatre, lobby, and bridge. Penfield took a special interest in the lecture theatre, which included a pit where patients could be brought in their beds for presentation. A projector could display X-ray films on a large screen. Theatre seating was raked at a slope of 45 degrees, rather like the medieval anatomical theatres in Padua and Liege. This sharp angle made it somewhat risky for senior members of staff to come in at the top and walk down the steep aisles without rails to seats in the front rows. Some time later it

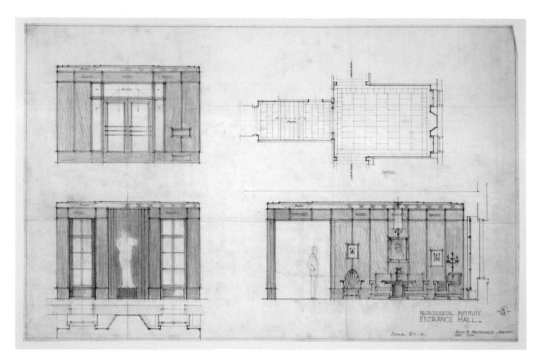

Figure T1.6: Large-scale elevation and plan of the lobby. At upper left is the view upon exiting the building. The upper right illustration shows the continuity of the vestibule with the lobby, separated by the doors illustrated in top left. The recess in the lobby was for *La Nature*, as illustrated in lower left. The lower right illustrates the north wall of the lobby. The circular table with a fanciful, inlaid cross section of the brain is still there. (Ross & Macdonald, Montreal Neurological Institute, interior elevations and plan for entrance hall, 1933, ARCH33404, Ross & Macdonald fonds, Collection Centre Canadien d'Architecture / Canadian Centre for Architecture, Montreal)

was named the Hughlings Jackson Amphitheatre, and a bronze bust[38] of the famous neurologist, a copy of the original at Queen Square, London, was placed on a pedestal in the theatre.

The most interesting architectural space in the Neuro's interior was the entry lobby, also known as the Hall of Neurological Fame. Decorated by Barnet Phillips,[39] this relatively small room was the setting for a marble copy of a statue of a female figure by Ernest Barrias.[40] Phillips used the brain as his main inspiration for the decoration of the lobby. The ceiling features the neuroglial cells within the cerebellum after a drawing by Camillo Golgi. A ram's head is at the ceiling's centre, with four hieroglyphic figures that are intended to symbolize the brain. Even the iron gratings over the radiators represent a nerve fibre by neuroanatomist Nageotte. The furniture too was especially designed to express the

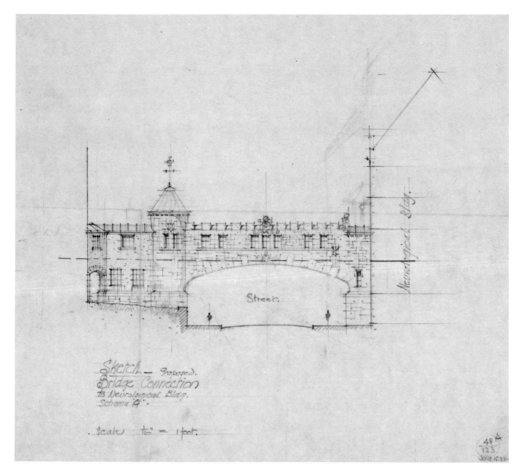

Within the image:
- Sketch — Proposed. Bridge Connection to Neurological Bldg. Scheme "A".
- Scale — 1/6" = 1 foot.
- Street.
- Neurological Bldg.
- 48 A / 123 / JUNE 1933

Figure T1.7: South elevation of the Bronfman Bridge linking the MNI (*right*) to the RVH (*left*). (Ross & Macdonald, Montreal Neurological Institute, elevation of bridge connection, 1932, ARCH33367, Ross & Macdonald fonds, Collection Centre Canadien d'Architecture / Canadian Centre for Architecture, Montreal)

significance of research on the brain. Penfield explained at the opening that the lamp stands were based on drawings of the spine, the inlay on the table was "the form of a cross-section of the human hemispheres," and the room was topped by a ring of names of influential neurologists.[41] Four large-scale drawings done by Ross and Macdonald in December 1933 indicate the special care taken in the design of the space.

A third distinctive feature of the Neuro's architecture is the overhead bridge across University Street, which is completely anomalous in the context of Montreal architecture and did not truly function until long after the MNI's opening. Like other special features of the final building, it caused some friction between Penfield and others, especially Chenoweth. Penfield reports that the hospital superintendent sent a strongly worded message, supposedly from Holt, when he learned of plans to connect the two institutions: "If they build a Goddamn bridge across University Street into our hospital, I won't give a cent to construction."[42] The bridge was constructed after further tempestuous correspondence on the topic, connecting the third floor of the MNI to the corresponding floor of the Royal Vic, which ended in the Children's Ward and then continued by way of two elevators into the general corridor of the main hospital. At the MNI's opening, Penfield spoke of it as one of the building's shortcomings: "Most urgent of all," he said, "a direct passage from the bridge to the main corridor of the Royal Victoria Hospital, as originally promised, is essential to promote full co-operation both here and in the wards of medicine and surgery with the other departments of medicine."[43] The design of the bridge plays up the MNI's romantic character in its reference to famous European precedents such as Oxford University's Hertford Bridge, or Bridge of Signs, which joins two parts of Hertford College over New College Lane, constructed in 1914. Cambridge University's Bridge of Sighs is older, constructed in 1831, and provides passage cross the River Cam for St John's College. Both British bridges refer back to Venice's much older Bridge of Sighs, so named for prisoners who were said to sigh before going to prison. In architectural design, the bridge at the Neuro most closely resembles the Venetian bridge.

GROWTH

The institute doubled in size in 1953, again in 1978, and expanded four times between 1983 and 2012. During wartime, the government built a temporary military annex to sustain the influx of returning soldiers into the hospital. This annex was later demolished in order to build a new wing to the MNI, the McConnell Pavilion of 1953. It was also during wartime years that the firm Fetherstonhaugh and Durnford was invited to extend the seventh floor to make two new labs and an office. The firm was joined by Bolton and Chadwick in 1946, and there is evidence of the firm designing an addition to the MNI from as early as 1949. This extension doubled the floor space and thus increased the number of beds from 49 to 135. The McConnell Pavilion continued the same architectural language as the 1934 pavilion, with the use of Montreal limestone for its facade.[44]

The next addition to the MNI was in the 1970s, to the south of the original building and next to the Pathological Institute. Designed by Ellwood & Henderson, floor plans date to October 1977, and the pavilion opened 18 September 1978. This third pavilion displayed a bold, new architectural language, standing out from the rest of the Neuro: brutalism. Recognizable by its use of

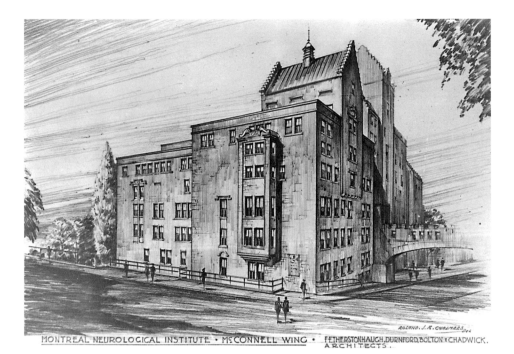

MONTREAL NEUROLOGICAL INSTITUTE · McCONNELL WING · FETHERSTONHAUGH,DURNFORD,BOLTON×CHADWICK. ARCHITECTS.

Figure T1.8: Perspective view of the McConnell Wing, looking south down University Street. The placement of the commemorative plaque bearing the "Brain Babies" and the inscription "Where shall wisdom be found and where is the place of understanding" is indicated as the rectangle at the lower right of the wall facing the viewer. (Fetherstonaugh, Durnford, Bolton, Chadwick, Architects, MNI Archives)

rugged concrete and heavy, fortress-like appearance, brutalism was the premier style for institutions in the 1970s, symbolizing endurance, functionality, and honesty. It was particularly popular among architects for university libraries, teaching buildings, and hospitals. Ellwood & Henderson's brutalist pavilion brought the growing Neuro complex up-to-date in 1978. Ironically, the heavy concrete image harmonized easily with the castle-like fortitude of Ross & Macdonald's 1934 scheme.

CONCLUSION

The MNI has been a steady and loyal architectural client for the past eighty-five years. Without exception, the institution hired top Montreal architects, all of whom had already done neighbouring buildings. One might conclude, in fact, that the most enduring influence on the architectural commissions of the MNI has been its immediate architectural context, despite the fact that at

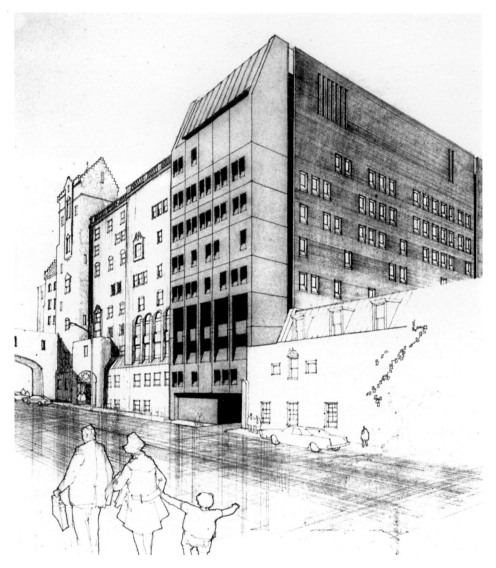

Figure T1.9: Perspective view of the Penfield Pavilion as it appears looking north up University Street. (MNI Archives)

the opening ceremony of the Neuro in 1934, Penfield named no fewer than four other institutions that had influenced the design of the new building. Ross & Macdonald's original scheme at the RVH had linked existing buildings and mimicked the Scottish baronial style of Henry Saxon Snell, the Maxwell brothers, and the firm's own work at the hospital. These ideas were retained in the as-built scheme of 1934, also by Ross & Macdonald, and echoed again in the post– Second World War extensions and renovations. So while the institution hired its medical staff from every corner of the earth and claimed a long list of worldly sites as inspiration, its own backyard was the architectural muse for a perfect little building.

Theme 2

Neurochemistry at the MNI

HANNA M. PAPPIUS

EARLY YEARS, 1934–1951

At the time of the opening of the MNI in 1934, biochemistry in general and that of the nervous system even more so was in its infancy. Neurochemistry, as a special discipline of science, did not exist. Nevertheless, a small laboratory of biological chemistry was established on the sixth floor of the new building, now the Rockefeller Pavilion, and there a neurologist at the RVH, Donald McEachern, supervised a clinical service for analysis of cerebrospinal fluid. McEachern subsequently became the neurologist-in-chief at the MNI, where he started research on acetylcholine metabolism and on the effect of epileptic seizures on the level of acetylcholine in the cerebrospinal fluid. With remarkable foresight, Wilder Penfield realized from the very beginning the importance of biochemical research to the understanding of neurological disorders, but it was not until 1944 that his vision of basic research in brain chemistry started to materialize, with the arrival of Kenneth Allan Caldwell Elliott.

Allan Elliott, also affectionately known to many as K.A.C., was born on 24 August 1903 in Kimberley, Union of South Africa. He matriculated with first-class honours in 1920 at St Andrews College in Grahamstown, and subsequently he attended Rhodes University College, where he studied physics and chemistry, again obtaining first-class honours in both his BSc and MSc. In October 1926, Elliott entered Selwyn College, Cambridge, as a graduate student, initially in organic chemistry under W.H. Mills, then in biochemistry under Sir Frederick Gowland "Hoppy" Hopkins, who greatly influenced him and for whom he cherished a life-long affection. These were the golden years of the Biochemical Institute on Tennis Court Road, Cambridge; Elliott lived at the hub of all that was most exciting in biological chemistry at the time. During this period he worked on biological oxidation-reduction systems, collaborating with such outstanding biochemists as M. Dixon, D. Keilin, and G. Bancroft, not to mention

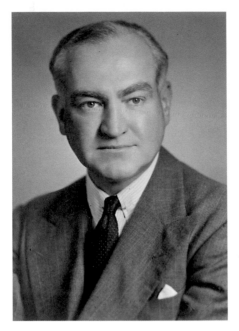

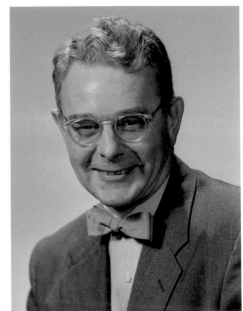

Figure T2.1: Donald McEachern, circa 1950.

Figure T2.2: K.A.C. Elliott, circa 1950.

his beloved "Hoppy." Elliott received the prestigious Beit Memorial Fellowship for Medical Research in 1929 and obtained his PhD in 1930. He continued his work on peroxidases in Munich, with the famous chemist Heinrich Wieland, returning briefly to Cambridge, where he was elected to the fellowship of Selwyn College. In 1933 he crossed the Atlantic to take up a research position at the Biochemical Research Foundation of the Franklin Institute in Philadelphia, and in 1943 he was appointed head of the Chemical Research Department of the Psychiatric Institute of the Pennsylvania Hospital and assistant professor of biochemistry at the University of Pennsylvania Medical School.

In the summer of 1944 Elliott received a telegram from Montreal asking him to come and talk with Wilder Penfield and Herbert Jasper. He was quickly convinced that the MNI really was a most unusual and inspiring place and in the fall of that year he joined its staff as acting neurochemist and assistant professor of neurology and biochemistry at McGill. He was named research neurochemist in 1945 and associate neurochemist in 1949. As he proudly re-counted to the end of his days, he was the first person anywhere officially to be called a neurochemist and, as everything at the MNI had a prefix "Neuro," his laboratory became the Neurochemistry Laboratory. Elliott continued his pioneering studies on brain metabolism at the MNI, while becoming an indispensable member of the institute team, engaging in collaborative research on a variety of clinical and basic problems, such as epilepsy with Penfield, acetylcholine metabolism with McEachern, and the effects of trauma and brain swelling with Jasper.

The methodology at the disposal of the neurochemist at that time was very limited, as compared to that available just a few decades later. Thus Elliott was able to revolutionize studies on brain metabolism by designing a simple humid chamber for preparation of cerebral cortex slices, in which approximately 100 per cent humidity was maintained. Uniform slices were cut using a Stadie-Riggs microtome, without wetting and without being allowed to dry out, before being rapidly weighed, and thus the results could be expressed in terms of the actual fresh weight of tissue. Oxygen utilization and the carbon dioxide and lactic acid production of the slices was measured in the Warburg apparatus, in which the volume of gas produced or absorbed over time was determined by calculation from changes in pressure.

With Nora Henderson, Marion Birmingham, and Jim Webb, K.A.C. investigated the effects of a variety of factors, such as different concentrations of potassium, glutamate, pH, oxygen tension, narcotics, and convulsants on aerobic and anaerobic metabolism of rat brain slices and homogenates. With Penfield, they demonstrated the absence of any fundamental defects in oxidative metabolism of human epileptogenic cortical tissue.

Head trauma and its consequence, brain swelling, were of particular concern at the time of war. Elliott and Jasper joined forces to get a better basic understanding of the processes involved in this serious complication of injury and sometimes of neurosurgery. They devised a method of determining brain tissue volume and applied it to measuring swelling and shrinkage induced experimentally. They carried out detailed studies on changes in local pH in the pia-arachnoid space and reactions of pial blood vessels to irrigation with buffered and unbuffered isotonic solutions.

Elliott's Solution

These studies led to the development of a solution, closely resembling spinal fluid, in fact often referred to as balanced artificial cerebrospinal fluid, and considered as most appropriate for use during lengthy neurosurgery. For decades "Elliott's solution" was used by neurosurgeons all over the world for irrigation of the brain during prolonged operations. In the MNI operating rooms, starting in 1947, it was used routinely, prepared daily by the clinical neurochemistry technicians.

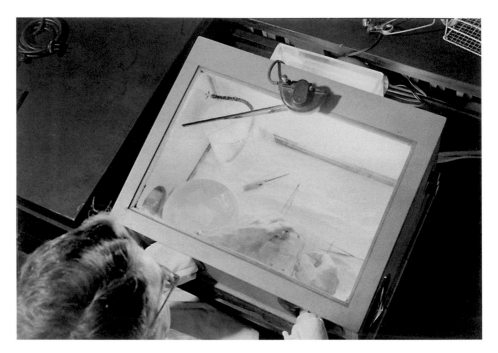

Figures T2.3 and T2.4: Elliott's humid chamber, circa 1948. Elliott and McEachern, in front of a drum on which contractions of leech muscle were recorded in the bio-assay for acetylcholine, 1949 (*opposite*).

Acetylcholine

McEachern received a five-year grant from the Rockefeller Foundation in 1945 for research on the neurochemistry of epilepsy and of psychotic states. This allowed him and Elliott to expand the studies on the acetylcholine (ACh) system, initiated earlier. Using the leech muscle bioassay, they demonstrated effects of anaesthetics and convulsants on brain content of ACh and on synthesis of ACh in brain slices. Among other effects, they reported that in the presence of calcium ions, in concentration similar to that in CSF, the synthesis of ACh was stimulated, while at higher concentrations it was inhibited. This was one of the earliest reports of the involvement of calcium in brain metabolism.

Under K.A.C. Elliott's direction, Roy Swank showed that with Nembutal anaesthesia ACh content of brain increases and falls as anaesthesia wears off. Hugh McLennan, using brain slices, studied factors affecting synthesis of ACh in great detail. He confirmed that high potassium accelerates the synthesis, but showed that, in the presence of low calcium, potassium inhibits it. He demonstrated that the carbon dioxide-bicarbonate buffer system is required for maximal synthesis and that any deviation from normal plasma concentration of

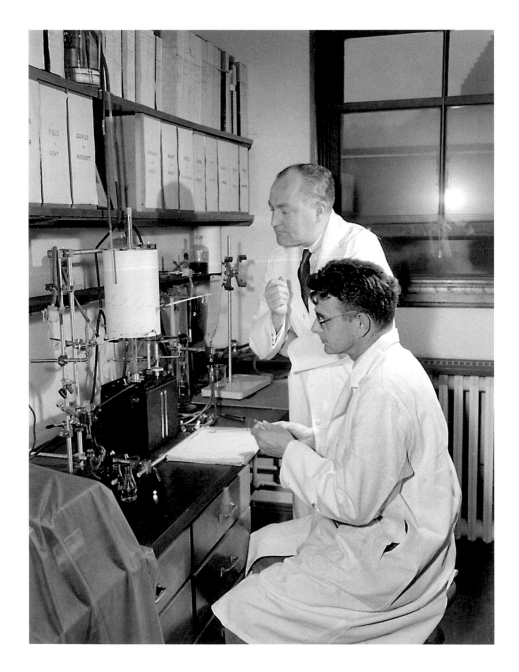

carbon dioxide, bicarbonate, or hydrogen ion depresses synthesis. Furthermore, he also found that synthesis of ACh was accelerated by very low concentrations of a variety of convulsant and anti-convulsant drugs. Elliott Brodkin showed that virtually all of the ACh found in the brain is present in a bound form, which is not physiologically active. Donald Tower, continuing the work started by McEachern, showed that CSF ACh content was increased by seizures. He then undertook a comprehensive survey of the whole acetylcholine system in various mammals, with special interest in normal and epileptogenic human brain tissue, measuring total ACh content, cholinesterase activity, and rates of production of free and bound ACh in tissue slices incubated in the presence of normal and high potassium. All components of the system showed decreased activity fairly regularly with ascending phylogenetic scale. Of particular interest was his finding that epileptogenic tissue tended to have an elevated cholinesterase activity and failed to produce bound ACh when incubated in vitro, and that the addition of glutamine or asparagine reversed these abnormalities. Similar results were obtained when seizures were induced experimentally. This raised the prospect of developing new therapy for epilepsy. Earlier work done in the laboratory had seemed to find a defect in the ACh system in the epileptogenic tissue, which could be corrected by glutamine, but Hania Pappius and Elliott reported in 1958 that these findings could not be repeated, and the great hope that glutamine would provide control of at least some types of seizures did not materialize.

Clinical Neurochemistry

Over the years, the small laboratory on the sixth floor for the determination of protein, sugar, chlorides, and Lange curves in the CSF expanded into the Ward Laboratory on the third floor and the clinical neurochemistry laboratory on the seventh floor, the last in the space that had been the famous MNI squash court. Lack of funds in the early years prevented expansion in the routine chemical analyses that could be offered to the clinicians. However, there was some space for research in neurological problems, such as lead absorption, vitamin B deficiency, hypothyroidism, chemical alterations in myasthenia gravis, and vitamin E in neuromuscular diseases. Most notably André Cipriani and Doris Brophy developed a new method of estimating CSF protein using a photoelectric colorimeter, which they published and became widely used. In 1942, in order to assist the interns and expedite the clinical work, the Ward Laboratory technician became responsible for doing all routine urinalyses and hematology tests. As a great innovation, in 1948, a full-time technician was engaged for all Ward Laboratory work, including drawing blood for Wasserman tests, thus saving the interns much valuable time and making for more speedy and efficient service. A photoelectric colorimeter was purchased for the Neurochemistry Laboratory, as were a flame photometer for sodium and potassium measurement and a ultraviolet light source for analysis of porphyrin content in urine. Gradually more tests were added to the list of tests that were routinely available. By

1953, procedures carried out by the laboratories per year reached an all-time high of 11,792. Of these, 5,967 were done in the Neurochemistry Laboratory and 5,825 in the Ward Laboratory, while 2,213 blood samples were drawn. These figures represented an average of 11 to 12 laboratory procedures carried out per patient. In addition, 4,350 litres of "Elliott's solution" were prepared for the operating rooms.

Donald McEachern was in charge of Clinical Neurochemistry until his death in 1952, except for one year (1944–45) when he was on leave of absence serving with the Royal Canadian Medical Army Corps and while K.A.C. Elliott temporarily took over. Doris Brophy was associated with neurochemistry at the institute from the opening of the original laboratory in 1935 and, as the head technician, contributed much to the development of a variety of technical procedures. She left the MNI in 1953.

THE DONNER LABORATORY OF EXPERIMENTAL NEUROCHEMISTRY

The Elliott Years, 1951–65

In 1951 Dr Penfield announced that, thanks to the generosity of Mr. William H. Donner and the Donner Canadian Foundation, the Donner Laboratory of Experimental Neurochemistry was being established on a separate scientific budget, according to the plaque at the entrance, "for as long as such work is carried on in the MNI." K.A.C. Elliott became its director, with the title of neurochemist, a position he held till 1965. He was also promoted to associate professor at that time.

In 1953, Hanna M. "Hania" Pappius joined the Donner Laboratory, as associate neurochemist and demonstrator in the Department of Experimental Neurology, and was promoted to lecturer a year later. At about the same time, Irving Heller, the up-and-coming neurologist, started his graduate training under Elliott's supervision, dividing his time between research and clinical responsibilities. Also in 1953, the seventh floor of the just-completed McConnell Wing became the home of the Department of Neurochemistry at the MNI. In the brand new laboratories work proceeded mostly on four main subjects: (1) energy metabolism of the brain, with emphasis on the role of electrolytes and phosphate derivatives, (2) the distribution of water in the brain and the nature of cerebral edema, (3) the role of neurophysiologically active substances, and (4) the metabolism of peripheral nerves.

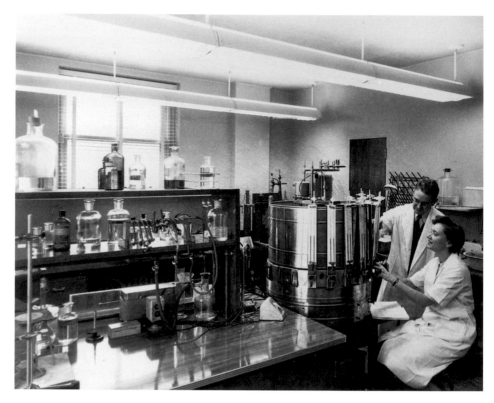

Figure T2.5: K.A.C. and Hania Pappius at the Warburg apparatus, 1953. (MNI Archives)

Sodium Pump

Investigations carried out under Elliott's direction by Pappius, Cross, Rosen-feld, Johnson, and Bilodeau were aimed at discovering the basic processes by which nervous tissue is maintained and exerts its functions and the manner in which they can be affected by metabolic and other factors. Substantial data were accumulated on the effects of different concentrations of ions, inhibitors, and drugs on the levels of adenosine triphosphate (ATP) and potassium in incubated rat-brain tissue slices. Both magnesium and, less strongly, calcium accelerated ATP hydrolysis by brain suspensions. Adenosine triphosphatase activity in the cerebral cortex was shown to be high enough to release all high-energy phosphate, which could be produced by esterification coupled with respiration. Of special interest was the finding that the ability to concentrate potassium in brain tissue in vitro was dependent specifically on sodium in the medium, but independent of the provision of high-energy phosphate, suggesting the action of a mechanism that extrudes sodium, a confirmation of the "sodium pump" theory. No difference between focal epileptogenic and normal human tissue was detected in magnesium- and calcium-activated triphosphatases, potassium and sodium contents, and the oxygen uptake rate.

Studies by Pappius and Elliott showed that rat cerebral cortex slices incubated for an hour under optimal aerobic conditions swelled by 30 to 40 per cent of their original volume. Using the distribution of "extracellular" markers to chemically delineate the extracellular space, it was possible to demonstrate that the swelling fluid accumulated there. Later studies with Igor Klatzo indicated that, in fact, the bulk of the swelling occurred in tissue damaged in the process of preparing the slices. By contrast, increase in the swelling in the presence of high concentration of potassium or glutamate occurred in the intracellular space. At the time, estimation of extracellular space in brain tissue by marker distribution was controversial, since the early electron micrographs showed close packing of all cellular elements and little, if any, extracellular space. Subsequently, Van Harreveld demonstrated occurrence of artifactual changes in the size of tissue compartments during fixation and dehydration for electron microscopy, supporting the validity of our methodology.

James Crossland, from the University of St Andrews, came for a few months in 1954 to clarify a discrepancy between his former work and that from Elliott's laboratory. Crossland and Pappius proved that the method of freezing the brain in situ with liquid air, used in Montreal, was valid and necessary for the determination of acetylcholine content of the brain under various physiological conditions. They demonstrated this further by showing an effect of insulin hypoglycemia on rat-brain acetylcholine level, which had been missed by others.

The GABA Story

Among Elliott's many achievements, the purification and chemical identification of a brain inhibitory substance, Factor I, as gamma-amino-butyric acid or GABA, was undoubtedly major. This was the beginning of the recognition of the importance of GABA and other amino acids as neurotransmitters. Up to that time it was recognized that the brain contained relatively large amounts of this amino acid, but the emphasis was on its metabolism and its potential contribution to cerebral energy metabolism. Its physiological function was totally unknown. Ernst Florey, an Austrian zoologist studying at the time in California, demonstrated that an extract of cattle brain had an inhibitory effect on the stretch receptor neuron in the abdomen of the crayfish. He called the unknown inhibitor Factor I. In 1954, on an invitation from K.A.C., Ernst and his wife and co-worker, Elizabeth, joined the Donner Laboratory to purify and identify Factor I. As a first step, Ernst and Hugh McLennan tested crude extracts on some

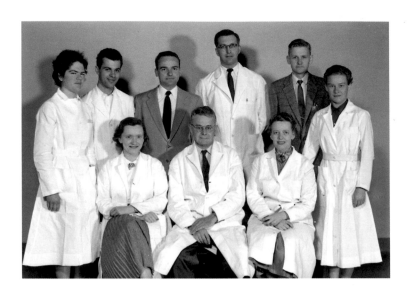

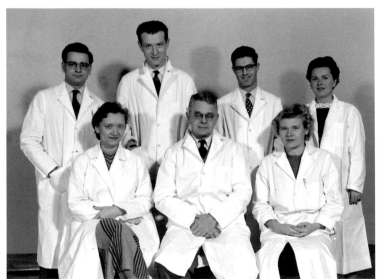

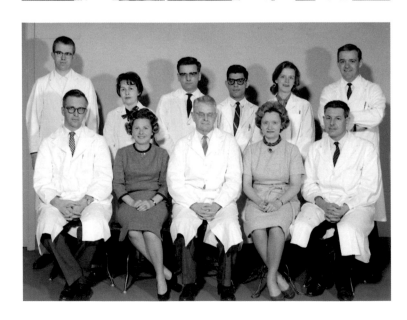

mammalian central and peripheral synapses and obtained evidence that Factor I had an inhibitory effect in these preparations, thus indicating its involvement also in mammalian synapses. The team then proceeded to develop a reliable and accurate bioassay to measure the amount of the inhibitor, using the crayfish stretch receptor. At that point Elliott induced Merck of Rahway, New Jersey, to delegate someone from their research team with appropriate experience to come and help in this project. Alva Bazemore arrived in Montreal and set about working up 100 pounds of beef brain, at first in big vats at the Merck plant on the outskirts of Montreal. As the isolation process progressed it became clear that the active substance was a stable, small amphoteric molecule. Many substances were tested in the bioassay for inhibitory activity, including all available amino acids, all without success. Then Elliott remembered that about five years earlier gamma-aminobutyric acid was shown to be present in brain. A supposedly pure sample of it was sent by Merck, but the material was found to be inactive. Bazemore was obliged to continue the rather tedious purification, finally obtaining pure active crystals, which were shown by infrared spectroscopy and chromatography to actually be gamma-aminobutyric acid. It was never explained what was in the obviously misnamed Merck sample, supposed to be GABA.

For the next six years GABA was the major research interest in the Donner Laboratory. Many studies followed, with numerous collaborators, on the identity of Factor I with GABA, its distribution and conditions affecting its brain content, and its failure to pass the blood-brain barrier when administered parenterally. Nico van Gelder contributed greatly to the understanding of bound, "occult," and free GABA, its equilibrium with glutamate, and the effect of anticonvulsants. Emilio Levin and Brenda Bollard developed precise chromatographic and enzymatic methods for measurement of GABA. Dick Lovell proved that in the brains of various species Factor I could be fully accounted for by their GABA content. Franz Hobbiger embarked on a comprehensive study of the pharmacological effects of GABA on intestinal smooth muscle and the respiratory and vascular systems.

Figure T2.6 (*Opposite*): Donner Laboratory. (*Top*) 1956: (*Sitting*) Hania Pappius, K.A.C., Mrs Budden. (*Standing*) Kathy Dickey, Michael Rosenfeld, Alva Bazemore, Irving Heller, Ernst Florey, Elizabeth Florey. (*Middle*) 1958: (*Sitting*) Hania Pappius, K.A.C., Dorothy Johnson. (*Standing*) Sigurd Hasse, Franz Hobbiger, Nico van Gelder, Ursula Feist. (*Bottom*) 1963: (*Sitting*) Irving Heller, Ursula Feist, K.A.C., Hania Pappius, Leon Wolfe. (*Standing*) Richard Lovell, Hanna Szylinger, Sigurd Hesse, Tariq Khan, Ania Kurnicki, Sandy Lowden.

Elliott went on to study amino acid alterations in epilepsy, the interrelation between glucose and free amino acids in the brain, and the effects of convulsions on the release of amino acids from proteins, all serving to establish the importance of amino acids as neurotransmitters or regulators of neuronal excitability.

Irving Heller initially compared the deoxyribonucleic acid content, cell densities, and metabolism of normal brain grey and white matter and human brain tumours to estimate metabolic rates in different cell types. Interestingly, he concluded that metabolic activity of the cerebral cortex is due mainly to neurons, despite the preponderance of glial elements, while the small neurons of the cerebellar cortex are less active than the glial cells. Subsequently, Heller's research concentrated on the metabolism of peripheral nerves with particular reference to the role of thiamine. Irving Heller spent a sabbatical year in 1971–72 with the renowned neurochemist Henry McIlwain, at the Institute of Psychiatry, Maudsley Hospital, London, studying advanced neurochemical techniques. Irving Heller and Hania Pappius shared supervision of the Clinical Neurochemistry Laboratory until the mid-1970s, when Heller left basic research to devote himself totally to his first love, clinical neurology.

In 1959, while still at the MNI, Elliott was appointed chairman of the Department of Biochemistry at McGill, a position he held for almost a decade. He continued as Gilman Cheney Professor of Biochemistry until 1971 and was made professor emeritus in 1973. On his retirement from McGill in 1971, Elliott joined the Canadian University Service Overseas and spent two years in Enugu, Nigeria, teaching biochemistry at the newly established medical school, to which he returned for two more periods during a third year.

Allan Elliott received a ScD from Cambridge University and was elected to fellowship of the Royal Society of Canada. He was chief editor of the *Canadian Journal of Biochemistry and Physiology*. With I.H. Page and J.H. Quastel, in 1955, he edited *Neurochemistry*, the first textbook in the field. He was a founding member of both the International and the American Societies for Neurochemistry. For many years he served on the Medical Advisory Board of the Multiple Sclerosis Society of Canada. In 1964 he travelled to the Chinese Medical College at Peking as the first Norman Bethune Exchange Professor. Throughout his life Allan Elliott was actively involved in organizations devoted to peace, democracy, and helping the disadvantaged and oppressed. In his later years he wrote sensitive essays expressing in a unique and refreshing manner his strong sense of awe at the vast complexity of the universe and of life processes and the role and origin of consciousness.

As he proclaimed on numerous occasions, K.A.C. loved life. Never one to live only for work, he loved music and dance, children's stories, and intelligent con-

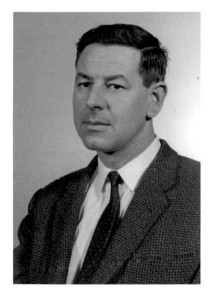 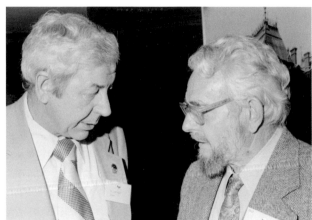

Figures T2.7 and T2.8: Leon Wolfe, 1961 (*left*). Leon Wolf and K.A.C. Elliott at the opening of the Penfield Pavilion, 1978 (*right*).

servation. In his youth he hiked, rode a motorbike, and climbed mountains, played rugby and tennis. To the very end of his life he sailed, fished, and skied cross-country. Elliott was honoured by the establishment in 1979 of the annual K.A.C. Elliott Lectureship at the MNI, to which he maintained a deep and intelligent loyalty to the end of his days. While he lived, he took enormous and infectious delight in these lectures, annually announcing his pleasure that they were not yet the Elliott Memorial Lectures. K.A.C. will be remembered not only for his scientific excellence and his mastery of scientific writing, but also for his integrity and fairness, his complete loyalty to the people and the causes he espoused, and the encouragement and support he gave to those around him, each according to his or her needs. Kenneth Allan Caldwell Elliott died in Montreal on 28 April 1986.

The Wolfe Years, 1965–90

Leon Wolfe was born on 25 March 1926 in Auckland, New Zealand. He obtained his BSc and MSc in 1947 and 1949 respectively, from Canterbury University College, University of New Zealand, in Christchurch, where he was a University of New Zealand and then a Royal Society of New Zealand Scholar. He went to England as an 1851 Exhibition Scholar and studied insect physiology in Cambridge under Sir Vincent Wigglesworth, obtaining his PhD (Cantab.) in 1952. After a stint as associate entomologist in the Science Service Laboratory in

London, Ontario, during which he studied the biology of blackflies, he entered medicine at the University of Western Ontario, graduating with an MD with Honours in 1958. He interned at the RVH and as a medical research fellow of the National Research Council of Canada, he trained for eighteen months under the eminent neurochemist Henry McIlwain, at the Maudsley Hospital, London, England. Wolfe returned to Montreal in 1960 as assistant professor in the Department of Neurology and Neurosurgery at McGill and associate neurochemist at the MNI. Wolfe was the director of the Donner Laboratory of Experimental Neurochemistry at the MNI and a neurochemist at the MNH from 1965 to 1990. He was promoted to professor in the Department of Neurology and Neurosurgery in 1970, becoming a Killam Professor at the MNI in 1992 and emeritus professor in 1995. Throughout this time he was a Medical Research Council of Canada career investigator.

Leon Wolfe was elected to the Royal Society of Canada. He was a visiting professor at universities in Bologna, Strasbourg, Rehovot, San Diego, and Helsinki, among others. As an invited lecturer and speaker at international meetings, too numerous to list, he discussed brain gangliosides and gangliosidoses, aspects of the prostaglandin system in physiology and pathophysiology, glycoprotein and glycolipid storage disorders, biochemical studies of ceroid lipofuscinoses (Batten's disease), age pigments in relation to Alzheimer's disease, and dolichols and their relationship to lysosomal membrane turnover, to name just some of his preoccupations. Complicated subject matter and difficult and outstanding biochemistry were always presented with aplomb.

Leon Wolfe had a joint appointment in the Department of Biochemistry. At different times he was an associate member of the McGill Centre for Studies on Aging and the McGill Nutrition and Food Science Centre, as well as a consultant on metabolic neurological diseases at both the Montreal Children's Hospital and the MNH. Throughout his career he served on a variety of university, departmental, and MNI committees and boards. He taught biochemistry regularly to medical students and in the Faculty of Science, also lecturing occasionally on a variety of subjects in many departments. He supervised an impressive number of graduate students and post-doctoral fellows. He was the deputy chief editor of the *Journal of Neurochemistry*, the premier journal in the field (1973–79), and chairman of the Publications Committee of the International Society for Neurochemistry (1979–83). He served on the editorial boards of the *Journal of Neurochemistry* (1969–73), *Prostaglandins* (1972–80), the *Canadian Journal of Neurological Sciences* (1973–81), *Neurochemical Pathology* (1982–93), and *Archives of Gerontology and Geriatrics* (1989–95). He was a sought-after referee for papers submitted to more than thirty national and international journals in biochemistry, neurochemistry, neuroscience, lipid research, neurology, neuropathology, clinical investigation, and paediatrics.

Leon Wolfe had several major research interests and he made significant contributions in a number of fields. His scientific achievements were recognized and respected worldwide. Some of his most important work is summarized below.

Gangliosides

Gangliosides are a class of acidic glycolipids with great structural complexity, which occur mainly in the grey matter of the brain. They were first isolated in 1925 and Wolfe's in-depth studies on this subject in the 1960s, mainly with Sandy Lowden, were pioneering. For their experiments they extracted gangliosides from rat, ox, cat, and human cerebral cortex, finding little difference between the different mammals. Wolfe and Lowden then developed techniques for isolation and identification of the complex chemical structure of these substances. Subsequently, the Wolfe team demonstrated that regions of the central nervous system rich in neurons contained the greatest amounts of gangliosides, while they were scarcely detectable in the corpus callosum and not at all in the optic nerve. Furthermore, chronic hypoxia and severe hypoglycemia, which lead to loss of cerebral cortical neurons, also resulted in greatly reduced ganglioside content of the cerebral cortex. These findings confirmed the neuronal location of the gangliosides. Separation of homogenized cerebral cortex into subcellular fractions showed that gangliosides occurred predominantly in membrane fractions, while none were found in clean preparations of nuclei, mitochondria, and myelin. Further studies indicated that gangliosides do not appear to occur in synaptic vesicles, but rather in the nerve-ending ghosts and associated membranes, suggesting that gangliosides are very likely concentrated mainly in dendrites and synaptic membranes. This hypothesis was supported by work with David Derry, who showed that gangliosides occurred in much greater amounts in clean isolated neurons and in the neuropil teased from immediately around the neuron cell body and dendrites then in isolated clumps of glial cells.

Studies with Matt Spence on the ganglioside content of rat cerebral hemispheres during development showed that considerable amounts of gangliosides were present at birth, and the adult brain contained a little more than twice the amount found in the newborn. The increase occurred in the first sixteen days of life and was somewhat diminished during myelination. These findings clearly indicated that gangliosides were not involved with myelination and were interpreted as indicating that increase of brain gangliosides during development was associated with expansion of the dendritic field.

Eicosanoids

Wolfe stumbled across prostaglandins in 1964 when, with Flavio Coceani, they detected, in perfusates of cat cerebellum and in brain extracts, the presence of an unknown substance that induced contraction of the "slow type" in the isolated rat stomach fundus. They established that they were dealing with water- and lipid-soluble acidic material that behaved in solvent partition systems like prostaglandins, chemically characterized in 1963 by Bergstrom and his co-workers at the Karolinska Institute, Sweden. Further support for this identification was obtained when they demonstrated that the type of contraction induced by crystalline prostaglandin E_1 (PGE$_1$), supplied by Bergstrom, was identical to that produced by their partially purified cerebellar perfusates.

Within a few years knowledge on the prostaglandins rapidly expanded worldwide, and the search was on for their physiological role and mechanism of action. Leon Wolfe was in his element. With Coceani, they chose the rat stomach for bioassay of a great variety of arachidonic acid metabolites and by-products, including prostaglandins. The fact that it had both cholinergic and adrenergic innervation and that the two networks could be stimulated independently was of particular interest. They showed that both the crystalline PGE$_1$ and a purified preparation of ox brain prostaglandins initiated contraction by a direct action on the smooth muscle membrane. Drugs that inhibited sympathetic fibres or receptors potentiated the action of prostaglandins, whereas those that stimulated sympathetic receptors were inhibitory. The presence of oxygen was absolutely necessary for initiation of the prostaglandin contraction.

In 1966, a chemist, Cecil Pace-Asciak, joined the Wolfe team, just as they demonstrated that the prostaglandin-like compounds released from the superfused cat cerebellum in vivo contained mostly prostaglandin F$_2$alpha. Experiments with labelled arachidonic acid indicated that direct conversion of the precursor to brain prostaglandins was very limited and that their formation in cerebral tissue arose almost entirely from endogenous substances. Further studies showed that prostaglandins of both E and F types were released spontaneously in vitro. Cholinergic, but not adrenergic nerve stimulation increased this release significantly and the increase was dependent on the rate of stimulation. Chromatographic characterization and quantification of the individual prostaglandins showed that PGE$_2$ and PGF$_2$alpha were the major prostaglandins formed and released during nerve stimulation. On the basis of these findings

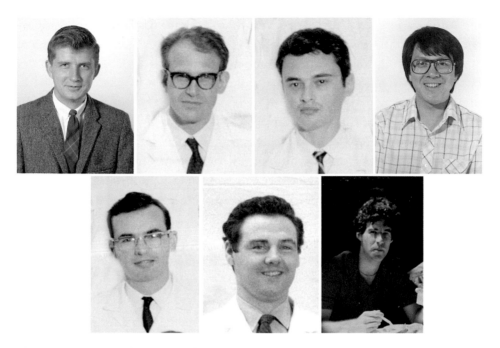

Figure T2.9: Some fellows and collaborators of L.S. Wolfe. (*Top row*) M. Spence,
F. Coceani, C. Pace-Asciak, N.M.K. Ng Ying Kin. (*Bottom row*) J. Callahan, J. Clarke,
L. Pellerin.

and some of their other data, Wolfe and his collaborators postulated that acetylcholine accelerates prostaglandin formation from precursors bound to membrane phospholipids.

To discover and determine the structure of the individual components of
the complex eicosanoid system, the bioassay was replaced by involved and
time-consuming but precise procedures. The new methodology consisted of
infra-red and nuclear magnetic resonance spectroscopy, mass spectroscopy of
derivatives, and gas liquid chromatography. Subsequently, the Wolfe team
contributed to all aspects of the rapidly exploding field of prostaglandins.

Pace-Asciak set up all the required methodology and made modifications
to increase the sensitivity to allow measurements in blood and CSF. Pace-
Asciak and Wolfe identified and chemically characterized a novel derivative
of prostanoic acid. During enzymatic conversion of arachidonic acid into
PGE_2, they identified and characterized three compounds derived from ex-
ogenous triatiated arachidonic acid and one derived from an endogenous,
unlabelled source.

Using guinea pig and rat cerebral cortex slices and homogenates, Wolfe and
Marion identified thromboxane B_2 as a compound accumulating during short

incubations. To their surprise the amounts of thromboxane B2 were consider-ably higher than those of PGE2 and PGF2alpha. Noradrenalin was shown to stimulate thromboxane formation. The discovery of the formation of this de-rivative of prostaglandin endoperoxides in nervous tissue implied the existence of another terminal pathway of prostaglandin metabolism and was a signifi-cant achievement of the MNI group.

Leon was always ready to apply his expertise to any project that might con-tribute to solving the riddle of the basic function of prostaglandins in the brain. As a first step, PGF2alpha was measured in human CSF obtained at routine pneumoencephalography. Normal levels were low, but measurable (50–100 pico.gms/ml). Considerable increases were found in patients with epilepsy, meningitis, and following cerebrovascular accidents and surgical trauma, with PGF2alpha, not PGE2, the dominant prostaglandin. However, there was little correlation with neurological symptoms.

The studies on synthesis and metabolism of prostaglandins in vivo and in vitro continued with Marion and Pappius. They showed that when the rat whole-brain hemispheres were frozen in liquid nitrogen immediately on re-moval, very low levels of PGF2alpha were found and PGE2 was undetectable, indicating that in vivo the prostaglandin content must be exceptionally small. In incubated slices, formation of both prostaglandins increased at an almost linear rate for one hour. Prostaglandins that were formed during the incubation diffused readily into the medium. Careful analysis of the data suggested exis-tence of specific binding sites for the prostaglandins, as well as non-specific sol-ubilization in tissue lipids. Catecholamines and adrenochrome greatly activated formation of PGF2alpha in slices and homogenates, probably through non-enzymatic reduction of endoperoxides. Indomethacin and ketanserin were potent inhibitors of the biosynthesis. In experiments in which labelled arachi-donic acid was added to the incubation medium, the prostaglandin biosynthe-sis in slices was shown to be derived from an intracellular pool that forms immediately after the death of the animal. PGF2alpha catabolism was very lim-ited, and PGE2 was converted to PGF2alpha. The biosynthetic capacity of brain tissue in vitro appeared to be orders of magnitude more than that in normal brain in situ. The labelling of rat brain lipids in vivo with ^{3}H-arachidonic acid and their subsequent analysis at different times post-mortem indicated that the released arachidonic acid originated from two specific phospholipids. An interesting finding, that following convulsions, free arachidonic acid and PGF2alpha in rat cerebral hemispheres increased but level of thromboxane B2 was not affected, suggested that there was relation in vivo between increased appearance of free arachidonic acid and the production of PGF2alpha, but not of thromboxane B2. This was in contrast to results in vitro, where production of both substances occurred and was stimulated by catecholamines.

In the late 1980s, Wolfe and Pellerin studied in detail the metabolism of prostaglandin D2 by human and rat cerebral cortex. PGD2 was discovered much later than PGF2alpha and PGE2. In the rat it was found to be quantitatively the main prostaglandin formed from endogenously released arachidonic acid, while only small amounts were found in the incubated human cerebral cortex. The difference turned out to be the presence in the human of an active enzyme, 11-ketoreductase, which further metabolized PGD2, but was missing in the rat. They concluded that PGD2 must be considered along with other eicosanoids in pathophysiological situations in the brain. At about the same time, in one of his many reviews, Wolfe stated that eicosanoids were definitely formed and metabolized in brain tissue and can have potent actions, but the biochemical and physiological processes they effect in vivo still remain difficult to define.

In the meantime, during a 1969–70 sabbatical leave in Strasburg, Wolfe developed a method for isolation of plasma membrane fraction from the brain in quantities sufficient to allow studies on its composition and metabolism. At the time this was of interest, as evidence was accumulating that the multi-enzyme system, called prostaglandin synthetase, required for biosynthesis of prostaglandins, was tightly bound to membrane elements. Arachidonic acid, the precursor of prostaglandin endoperoxides, had to be released from a complex lipid to start the whole process.

On his return to Montreal, Wolfe expanded his studies to the synthesis of the membrane-bound glycoproteins, present in the preparations of brain plasma and synaptic membranes. With Breckenridge and Ng Ying Kin, in elegant studies using a variety of sophisticated physico-chemical techniques, they first established the structure of brain dolichols (long-chain polyisoprenoid alcohols). They then demonstrated that the synthesis of the mannose core of the glycoproteins is a two-step process, involving first formation of the mannosyl-phosphonyl-dolicole, followed by a transfer of the sugar to the glycoprotein. Until then it was thought that the sugars were attached directly to the protein.

Throughout much of his life, among Wolfe's principal preoccupations was the identification of materials accumulating in the brain in inherited neurological diseases, with the view of establishing their underlying causes. In this he collaborated with his MNI colleagues Fred Andermann, George Karpati, Eva Andermann, and Stirling Carpenter, as well as other clinicians, providing the ability to isolate and characterize the complex molecules involved.

Gangliosidosis

In preparation for studies of human material, Wolfe and Callahan improved
the basic chemical chromatographic methodology to separate the individual
ganglioside types in the brain, which could then be degraded into individual
sugars and thus further characterized. In the first study of GM1-gangliosidosis
during life, following cerebral biopsy, they demonstrated, in a three-year-old
patient with progressive neurological deterioration that began at ten months
of age, a large increase in GM1-ganglioside in the cerebral cortex, and a marked
deficiency of the enzyme beta-galactosidase in the patient's brain, leukocytes,
and cultured fibroblasts. The patient excreted elevated amounts of highly
under-sulfated keratin sulfates in the urine. Abnormally low levels of beta-
galactosidase were also found in the leukocytes of both parents. In liver samples
obtained at autopsy in other cases of GM1-gangliosidosis, Wolfe and Callahan
showed an accumulation of keratin sulfates and were able to isolate and characterize them, again by methods they developed at the MNI. They concluded
that the presence of three biochemical criteria enable the unambiguous and
specific diagnosis of GM1-gangliosidosis: (1) the accumulation in the nervous
system of GM1-ganglioside, (2) the deficiency of beta-galactosidase, and (3) the
accumulation to varying degrees in the viscera, but not in the brain, of highly
water soluble under-sulfated glycosaminoglycans of the keratin sulfate type and
their excessive excretion in the urine. It also became clear that GM1-gangliosi-
dosis was an inborn error of metabolism quite distinct from Tay-Sachs disease,
in which GM_2-ganglioside accumulates. In further studies in patients with
GM1-gangliosidosis, the structure of oligosaccharides accumulating in the liver
was determined, and oligosaccharides and glycopeptides excreted in the urine
were characterized.

Ceramide Trihexosidosis

Fabry's disease is characterized by accumulation of ceramide trihexoside (CTH)
(galactosyl-galactosyl-glucosyl ceramide) in the serum and a number of tissues.
In 1967 Brady and co-workers showed this to be associated with a defect in the
catabolism of CTH, and in 1970 Kint showed this to be the result of a deficiency
of alpha-galactosidase. This was difficult to reconcile with the generally held
view that the linkages in the oligosaccharide portion of CTH were all of the
beta-stereo configuration. Wolfe and Clarke extracted and purified CTH from
pooled human kidney tissue and from the kidney of a patient who died from
Fabry's disease. Using nuclear magnetic resonance spectrometry and the measurement of optical rotations, they were able to demonstrate that the terminal
galactosidic linkage of the CTH molecule did in fact have the alpha-stereo con-

figuration. This finding was confirmed by enzymatic evidence that this linkage was susceptible to hydrolysis by alpha-galactosidase, but completely resistant to the action of beta-galactosidase. The results also showed that the CTH from normal tissue and from the Fabry's disease patient were indistinguishable from each other. In two patients with renal disease, but lacking the skin lesions typical of Fabry's disease, Clarke and Wolfe demonstrated the excretion of excessive quantities of CTH and low leucocyte alpha-galactosidase, thus confirming the diagnosis of Fabry's disease. In another patient with Fabry's disease who underwent renal transplantation, their data did not support the hypothesis that enzyme replacement by transplantation was effective in correcting the basic metabolic defect of the disease.

Neuronal Ceroid-Lipofucsinoses

Neuronal ceroid-lipofucsinoses (NLD) are a group of inherited metabolic disorders, also referred to as Batten disease. Although clinically described more than 100 years ago, the basic biochemical defect involved remained unknown. Studies in the Wolfe Laboratory on the chemical nature of the storage materials found in the urinary sediment of patients with NLD showed that they consisted of a lipid-soluble fraction and an auto-fluorescent insoluble residue. The insoluble materials were shown to have properties similar to retinoid-like structures, possibly complexed to protein or peptides. In the lipid-soluble extracts they identified and quantified greatly increased amounts of dolichols (long-chain polyisoprenoid alcohols) as compared to normal. They subsequently also demonstrated a very significant increase of dolichols in the cerebral cortex of such patients. While the accumulation of dolichols in the urinary sediment of NLD patients was the first biochemical marker of Batten disease, which helped clinicians to diagnose these patients, Wolfe's subsequent search for the biochemical pathogenic mechanism of this group of diseases eluded him and remains unexplained to this day.

Leonhard Scott Wolfe died on 3 December 2001 after a lengthy illness. Thus ended an amazing career of an outstanding neurochemist and medical scientist, who, for four decades, served the Montreal Neurological Institute and Hospital and McGill University with great distinction.

The Goad Unit, 1953–1995

I was born on 26 July 1925 in Łąkocin, Poland. In July 1940 I was fortunate to find myself in Montreal, as a war refugee. In 1942, on an Allied Nations Students Bursary and a University Bursary, I entered McGill, and in 1946 I obtained a BSc, with honours in biochemistry. From 1946 to 1953 I did graduate work

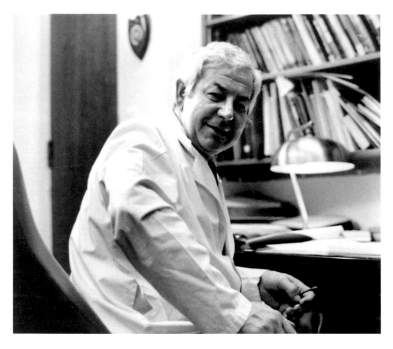

Figure T2.10: Leon Wolfe, 1978. (MNI Archives)

under the supervision of Dr Orville F. Denstedt in the Department of Biochemistry and received an MSc in 1948 and a PhD in 1953, both on the subject of metabolism of stored blood.

In early 1953, having just finished writing my PhD thesis, I received a message that a Dr Elliott at the MNI wished to see me. Without much enthusiasm, I made my way up University Street for what turned out to be a very short interview, as a result of which I started my work at the institute on 1 April of that year.

I remember wondering whether beginning a professional career on April Fool's Day was a good omen, never anticipating that I would be there for decades and that K.A.C. would become my mentor, a wonderful teacher and in the end a very loyal and trusted friend. His scientific method was impeccable, his thinking clear and logical, but above all he was a kind and understanding human being, who bore malice to no one and who refused to even suspect its presence in others. In the days when women's lib was unheard of, he understood the difficulties I had in combining a scientific career with raising a young family and, when necessary, made allowances for it. His support and recognition of my input into our joint work was most generous. When he decided to leave the MNI for the Department of Biochemistry and I opted to stay and on my own spread my wings, he did not begrudge me this choice. On the contrary, he extended every effort to ensure that I obtained the independence to which I aspired.

When Leon Wolfe became the director of the Donner Laboratory in 1965, I remained at the MNI officially as an independent researcher. In 1982, my laboratories were designated as the Goad Unit of the Donner Laboratory of Experimental Neurochemistry, in memory of Mr George Goad, former secretary-treasurer of the Donner Canadian Foundation, which at that time donated generously towards renovation and modernization of the Donner Labs. It was the beginning of nearly half a century of partnership with Leon, based on mutual respect and common goals. His enthusiasm for science in general and his global view of it, his deep knowledge and understanding of the brain and its workings, and his ready willingness to share his ideas made him an exciting colleague. He read widely, loved music and art, played the piano, was a potter, collected stamps, and played bridge, all with boundless energy. Life in his orbit was never dull and was a privilege. Progressing slowly up the academic ladder, in 1979 I was promoted to full professor in the Department of Neurology and Neurosurgery at McGill. During his sabbatical absences in 1969–70 and 1979–80 I substituted for Leon in the Donner Labs.

In 1969, Robert Katzman, then the Saul Korey Professor of Neurology at the Albert Einstein College of Medicine and later chair of the Department of Neurosciences at the University of California, San Diego School of Medicine, asked me to co-author a book with him on water and electrolytes in the brain, subjects of interest to both of us at the time. Later in his career, Bob became world-renowned for his work on Alzheimer's disease. *Brain Electrolytes and Fluid Metabolism* by Katzman and Pappius was published in 1973 and remains a classic in its field. Peter Gloor wrote in the 1972–73 MNI Annual Report, "This monumental work represents undoubtedly the most up-to-date and best documented treatise on this problem." In 1976, with enthusiastic support of Bill Feindel, I organized the Third International Workshop on the Dynamic Aspects of Cerebral Edema in Montreal. Participants from nine countries attended. With Bill, I co-edited its proceedings. In the intervening years, I lectured and participated in numerous workshops, symposia, and meetings. Among the most memorable was the Symposium on Biology of Neuroglia organized by the eminent Argentinian neuroscientist Eduardo De Robertis, held in conjunction with the Tenth Latin American Congress of Neurosurgery in Buenos Aires in 1963, followed by lectures at the University of Sao Paulo, the

Neurological Institutes in Montevideo and Santiago de Chile, and a paper at the Pan-American Congress of Neurology in Lima, with a little detour to Cusco and Machu Pichu.

In 1977, after an exciting sabbatical leave with Louis Sokoloff at the Laboratory of Cerebral Metabolism, National Institute of Mental Health in Bethesda, I refocused my research from edema to the study of the functional consequences of cerebral trauma. In 1986, I co-chaired with Leon Wolfe the Local Organizing Committee for the Annual Meeting of the American Society for Neurochemistry. I served on my share of university and institute committees, including the Research Ethics Committees of the Department of Neurology and Neurosurgery and the Allan Memorial Institute (Psychiatry), and the MNI Animal Care Committee, which I have chaired for many years. I served as a member of the Editorial Board of several journals, including the *Journal of Neurochemistry* and the *Journal of Cerebral Blood Flow and Metabolism*, and reviewed papers for a number of other international scientific publications. I closed my lab in 1995 and retired, receiving a post-retirement professorial appointment, which allowed me for many more years to continue to chair the MNI Animal Care Committee. In 2004, as a last service to an old friend and valued colleague, I organized the MNI Symposium to honour L.S. Wolfe. In 2005, at the same time as Bill Feindel and Don Baxter, I received the cherished MNI Life Achievement Award, and in 2009, I was made professor emerita at McGill. My extra-curricular professional activities were centred on the Polish Institute of Arts and Sciences in Canada and its McGill-affiliated Polish Library.

Cerebral Edema
When I originally joined K.A.C. Elliott, we studied, among other things, water and electrolyte distribution in brain tissue in vitro. On the basis of our results, I concluded that cortical slices were not an appropriate model for the condition most often encountered clinically and subsequently named vasogenic edema by Igor Klatzo. At that point I began a series of studies designed to chemically characterize various types of cerebral edema occurring in vivo. Because the subject was of special interest to clinicians, most of my early collaborators were neurosurgery and neurology fellows, who at the time were obliged to spend a year doing research.

It should be remembered that in the 1950s there were no definitive and rigid criteria for establishing that cerebral edema is present, and a variety of its models were used without considering that the resultant changes in volume of the brain were not necessarily caused by the same mechanism in every case. Determination of water content was not part of earlier reported investigations. By

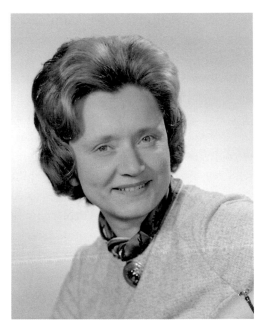
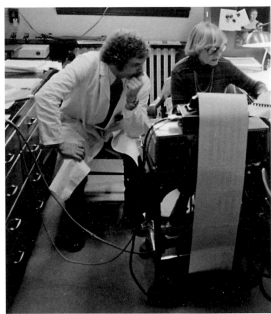

Figures T2.11 and T2.12: Hania Pappius, 1963 (*left*). Hania Pappius and Michael McHugh calculating results of deoxyglucose experiments, 1978 (*right*). (MNI Archives)

measuring water, potassium, and sodium contents, separately in grey and white matter, it was possible for us to define three different types of brain edema.

With D.R. Gulati, using focal freezing lesions on the exposed dura over the occipital region of one hemisphere in cats, we demonstrated that in trauma-induced edema, the fluid accumulated almost exclusively in the white matter, and with time spreading from the traumatized area. Decreased level of potassium was due to dilution by low potassium fluid, presumably derived from blood, but there was no net loss of this electrolyte, as determined in terms of dry weight of the tissue. With Lloyd Dayes we showed unequivocally that infusion of hypertonic solutions reduced brain volume, but that brain decompression was due to removal of water from normal tissue, rather than from the edematous tissue.

In contrast, studies with John Dossetor and J.H. Oh at the Renal Research Laboratory of the RVH indicated that osmotically induced water shifts associated with renal dialysis in dogs affected white and grey matter equally, while the sodium to potassium ratio remained unchanged.

At the time it was generally accepted that brain anoxia was always associated with cerebral edema. However, our efforts with John Norris to produce experimental anoxic edema were unsuccessful. Cats subjected to periods of hypoxia with and without severe hypercapnea developed symptoms of neurological damage and grossly abnormal EEGs, but the dry weight and electrolyte content of their brain tissues remained invariably within normal limits. On the other hand, when focal cerebral ischemia was produced in dogs by clipping the right middle cerebral artery, with time, vasogenic edema developed. In these experiments initially carried out by John Norris and continued by Shobu Shibata, with collaboration of the incomparable Charlie Hodge of the MNI Photography Department, serial fluorescent angiography was used to document the areas of ischemia and its persistence. Between twenty-four and forty-eight hours after the clip was applied, gross areas of infarction were evident macroscopically, and analysis of dry weight and electrolyte content indicated the presence of vasogenic cerebral edema. These results indicated that deprivation of oxygen with or without increase in carbon dioxide did not produce cerebral edema per se. Edema found as a consequence of ischemia was always associated with necrotic changes in the tissue.

Dexamethasone

Much effort was spent with Bill McCann on trying to establish to what extent steroids, the therapy of choice in neurosurgery and head trauma, control vasogenic edema. Freezing lesion in cats was used to induce edema, and dexamethasone (0.25 mgms/kg/day) was the steroid tested. Earlier results of sampling edematous tissue gave a measure of the degree of edema, but not its extent. The difference in weight between the traumatized and the control hemispheres was a somewhat insensitive measure, but the only available measure of the weight of the edema fluid. On the basis of our previous studies, which indicated that edema fluid in traumatized brain is derived from the blood, we attempted to tag the serum proteins by injecting I^{131} albumin (ISA) into the circulation, before the lesion was made, and comparing the amount of the marker in the two hemispheres with time after lesioning. This method did prove to be a more sensitive and less variable measure of the total edema fluid than comparing the hemisphere weights, but the two parameters had different time courses. Initially post-lesion the difference in ISA content followed closely the difference in weight of the two hemispheres. However, after the first twenty-four hours, the content of the marker remained unchanged, while the weight of the edema fluid continued to increase. We had to conclude that ISA uptake cannot be used as a quantative method for estimation of the amount of extravasated edema fluid, since the metabolic breakdown of the albumin, known to occur in the brain, after some time appears to balance its influx.

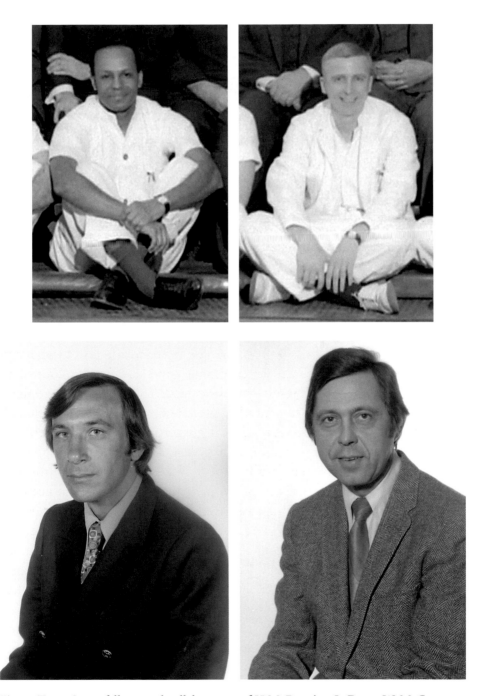

Figure T2.13: Some fellows and collaborators of H.M. Pappius: L. Dayes, W. McCann, C. Dila, and R. Hansebout. Dila and Hansebout were later appointed to the staff of the MNI Department of Neurosurgery. (MNI Archives)

On some of these animals, before the lesion, and forty-eight hours later, at the point of peak edema, McCann carried out EEG studies, which were then graded blindly by Christian Vera. Our results showed that dexamethasone had little or no effect at twenty-four hours post-lesion, but 48 hours after the lesion was made, it significantly diminished the edema, estimated both as an increase in weight and in ISA uptake in the traumatized hemisphere, suggesting that the drug did not prevent its formation. Dexamethasone strikingly improved the EEG abnormality present forty-eight hours after the lesion in untreated animals. However, no correlation could be demonstrated between the degree of edema and the extent of EEG abnormality, and between the effects of dexamethasone on the two parameters, suggesting that clinically beneficial effects of steroid therapy could not be fully explained by effects on cerebral edema. Similar conclusions were drawn from collaborative experiments with Neil Schaul, a fellow in the Department of Neurophysiology, who used more sophisticated EEG techniques and a larger group of animals. These studies indicated that in cats moderate cerebral edema did not result in EEG abnormalities, and delta waves occurred only in cases without a wide craniotomy, when severe edema led to secondary disturbances in midline structures.

Spinal Cord Trauma
A series of experimental studies on traumatized spinal cord and the action of steroids were carried out with Robert Hansebout, Marcial Lewin, Eugene Kuchner, and David Mercer. Standardized spinal cord injury was produced in cats by impact, and the neurological condition of the animals was rated daily according to the Tarlov system. Edema secondary to this injury was demonstrable on the second day after the lesion, spreading in both directions from the damaged segment, and became maximal between the third and sixth day. Dexamethasone had no significant effect on the spread or the degree of edema. On the other hand, animals pretreated with dexamethasone or given the steroid starting five hours after the lesion was made, showed significant clinical improvement. Further, a generalized decrease in potassium content of the spinal cord, not related to edema, which occurred in untreated animals starting on the third day after the lesion, was prevented in dexamethasone-treated animals. In fact, six days after lesioning, there was a highly significant correlation between the net potassium content of cord tissue and the functional state of the animal. These results also suggested that beneficial effects of dexamethasone on the functional state of animals were not mediated by its effects on edema. Rather, they were compatible with a direct action of steroids on the maintenance of the structural integrity of the spinal cord.

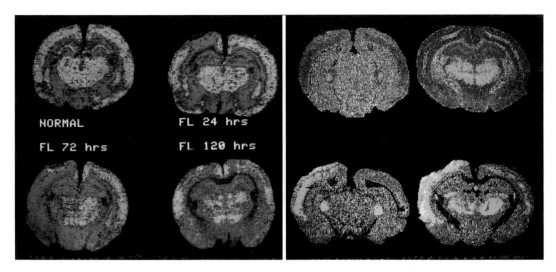

Figure T2.14: (*Left*) [¹⁴C]deoxyglucose colour-coded autoradiographs at selected anatomical locations in rat brain. (*Top row*) normal and one day after a freezing lesion. (*Bottom row*) three days and five days after lesioning. Note obvious decrease of glucose utilization at one and three days post-lesion, with return towards normal at five days. (*Right*) [¹²⁵I] HEAT colour-coded autoradiographs at selected anatomical locations in rat brain. (*Top row*) normal. (*Bottom row*) three days following a freezing lesion. Note obviously greater density of cortical areas of the lesioned (*left*) hemisphere as compared to unlesioned, indicating increased binding of a specific adrenergic receptor blocker. (H.M. Pappius and L.S. Wolfe, "Effect of Drugs on Local Cerebral Glucose Utilization in Traumatized Brain: Mechanism of Action of Steroids Revisited," in *Recent Progress in the Study and Therapy of Brain Edema,* ed. K.G. Go and A. Baethmann, 11–26 [New York: Plenum, 1984]); S. Dyve, Y-J. Yang, M. McHugh, A. Gjedde, and H.M. Pappius, "Effect of Injury on the Bi-Affinity alpha1-Adrenoreceptor Binding in Rat Brain *In Vivo,*" *Synapse* 19 [1995]: 88–96)

Experiments of Carl Dila showed that administration of fluid and pitressin in rats induced a condition within twenty-four to forty-eight hours that could be considered as an experimental model of the syndrome of inappropriate secretion of antidiuretic hormone. As the hyponatremia and hypo-osmolarity developed in the serum, the changes in muscle consisted of a decrease in sodium content and an increase in water content, equivalent to 12 per cent swelling. There was no loss of potassium from the muscle. In contrast, in brain the decrease in sodium was smaller; the water content increased only slightly, but there was a significant net loss of potassium. These studies suggest that neurological dysfunction associated with this syndrome is unlikely to be due to cerebral edema, but may be related to the decreased potassium content of brain tissue.

Finally, a study with Alan Yates, from the Department of Pathology, showed that cerebral edema measured chemically does not correlate well with edema as assessed by histological means. Dry weight, sodium, and potassium change progressively after death, so that post-mortem sampling is of little value.

Cerebral Function in Injured Brain

After years of concentrating on cerebral edema, tacitly assumed to be the underlying cause of the neurological abnormalities in conditions in which it occurs, my studies became focused on other mechanisms by which injury to the brain may result in malfunction. Until then the lack of a good method for assessing cerebral function in animals was a major obstacle to the study of functional disturbances in traumatized brain. This difficulty was overcome when Lou Sokoloff and his associates at the Laboratory of Cerebral Metabolism, National Institute of Mental Health in Bethesda, developed the deoxyglucose technique for measurement of local cerebral glucose utilization (LCGU) and validated the use of this method for mapping of cerebral functional activity in animals. Applying this approach in our studies, Hanna Szylinger, Michael McHugh, Ralph Dadoun, and I found that injury to the brain profoundly affected LCGU. With time after induction of a small, superficial focal freezing or heat lesion in the rat, significant depression of LCGU developed. This depression was most prominent throughout all of the cortical areas of the lesioned hemisphere (three days post-lesion 42 per cent of normal). Corresponding results in other regions were: contralateral cortical areas 86 per cent of normal, ipsilateral and contralateral subcortical structures 74 and 84 per cent of normal, respectively. Brain stem structures were not affected. In white matter bilaterally, LCGU depression reached its peak (61 and 64 per cent of normal, respectively) at twenty-four hours. LCGU returned to normal within five days in all affected areas. The observed changes, especially prominent in cortical tissue, were interpreted as representing a manifestation of cerebral dysfunction. Two further studies provided support for such an interpretation. In parallel experiments, using the [^{14}C]iodoantipyrine method, no corresponding changes in local cerebral blood flow were observed in traumatized brain. Further, a collaborative study with Marek Buczek and David Lust of the Laboratory of Experimental Neurological Surgery at the Case Western Reserve University in Cleveland, Ohio, showed that four energy-related metabolites, adenosine triphosphate, phosphocreatine, glucose, and lactate, were significantly increased in the lesioned hemisphere, with the most prominent effects observed in the cortical areas that exhibited the greatest depression in LCGU. Both the normal blood flow and the enriched metabolic profile were consistent with the hypothesis that decreased glucose use in the traumatized brain was caused by diminished need, due to inhibited activity, rather than by decreased supply of energy. This interpretation was also supported by our finding, with David Archer, that in the lesioned brain, reduction of cerebral metabolism by pentobarbital and isoflurane was limited by the metabolic depression that had already occurred as a result of injury. Since spatial distribution and time course of the observed changes in the LCGU did not parallel those of the development of cerebral edema, they could be regarded as independent of the edematous process.

Widespread depression of LCGU, which developed with time after the lesion in untreated animals, was significantly diminished by dexamethasone administered starting before or up to twenty-four hours after the lesion was made. Indomethacin and ibuprofen, inhibitors of the prostaglandin synthetase complex, were even more effective. The drugs induced most striking changes in cortical areas of the traumatized hemisphere, where the depression was most profound. However, the mechanisms of action of the steroid and the two non-steroidal anti-inflammatory drugs were not the same. Experiments with Leon Wolfe showed that indomethacin prevented the formation of prostaglandins in the traumatized brain by more than 90 per cent, while dexamethasone had no such effect. These results suggested that some components of arachidonic acid metabolism must be involved in functional disturbances resulting from trauma, while steroid action was mediated independently from the prostaglandin cascade.

Cortical Amines in Injured Brain

Both prostaglandins and steroids were known to influence neurotransmitter action and/or metabolism and, in the rat, both serotonergic and noradrenergic innervations are widely distributed to all parts of cerebral cortex – areas most affected in our model of traumatized brain. Furthermore, others have described changes in serotonin and catecholamine metabolism with cold injury and head trauma. We therefore considered the possibility that perturbations in these two neurotransmitter systems may have been underlying the LCGU changes we demonstrated in injured brain. Accordingly, in our model of trauma we investigated the effects of p-chloro-phenyl-alanine (PCPA), an inhibitor of serotonin synthesis, of ketanserin, a serotonin (5-HT2) receptor blocker, and of alpha-methyl-p-tyrosine (AMPT), an inhibitor of catecholamine synthesis. PCPA- and ketanserin-treated animals showed a very obvious amelioration of the depletion in LCGU. AMPT was even more effective, with nearly normal LCGU obtained in the traumatized brain. These results indicated that both neurotransmitter systems did in fact play a role in the functional cortical depression that develops in the injured brain. By contrast, in experiments with David Archer, two dihydropyridine calcium channel blockers failed to modify the depression in cortical LCGU induced by injury, suggesting that calcium does not mediate effects of neurotransmitters in the traumatized brain.

Tony Hakim joined the Donner Laboratory in 1978 to study, among other things, with my group, the effects of thiamine, vitamin B12, and folate deficiencies on local cerebral glucose utilization. He demonstrated that the primary metabolic consequence of thiamine deficiency was a widespread reduction in cerebral glucose utilization. Furthermore, with decreasing cerebral thiamine concentration, glucose utilization declined more rapidly in many of the structures that in humans develop histological lesions. With exposure of adult rats to nitrous oxide, as a model of B12 deficiency, LCGU was selectively diminished in cortical, auditory, and limbic structures. Folate deficiency had no effect on glucose utilization.

In the continuation of our search for mechanisms that may play a role in neurological disturbances resulting from brain injury, we expanded our investigations of cortical monoamines. Cortical serotonin metabolism was found to be increased throughout the lesioned hemisphere, and its complete inhibition with p-chlorophenylalanine ameliorated the decrease of LCGU. Cortical norepinephrine metabolism was bilaterally increased in focally injured brain, while experiments with Masaru Inoue showed that prazosin, a selective α_1-noradrenergic receptor ligand also normalized the LCGU. Furthermore, studies with Yu-Jia Yang, Albert Gjedde, and Suzan Dyve demonstrated that in vivo binding of ^{125}I-HEAT, another selective alpha$_1$-noradrenergic receptor blocker, was increased specifically in cortical areas of the lesioned hemisphere, but not in the subcortical structures, at the time of the greatest depression in LCGU. The major conclusion from these numerous studies was that the depressed functional state of a lesioned brain, as assessed by metabolic mapping with the deoxyglucose method, can be ameliorated by both inhibition of serotonin synthesis and blockage of the alpha$_1$-noradrenergic receptors.

Correlations

Studies with Colle and Holmes, of the Center for Research in Behavioral Neurobiology at Concordia University in Montreal, demonstrated that somatosensory deficits were significantly correlated with the extent of depression of glucose utilization in the cortical areas of the lesioned hemisphere in our model of trauma. Rats showed asymmetries in somatosensory responsiveness, decreases in running wheel activity, and difficulty with limb coordination. It was concluded that, as postulated, the observed behavioural changes were a manifestation of widespread functional depression, as reflected by decreased cortical glucose utilization throughout the lesioned hemisphere.

The final series of our experiments were designed to determine whether, in animals with focal brain lesions, behavioural deficits were correlated with time-course of cortical hypometabolism and of changes in serotonin metabolism and in alpha$_1$-noradrenergic receptor binding, and whether drugs known to modify the metabolic depression had any effect on behavioural status. We used the Morris water maze task, in which latency to find a submerged platform is considered a test of spatial memory. Progressive impairment of acquisition of the Morris task, of the unilateral increase of binding of HEAT and of hypometabolism mainly in cortical areas only, all showed a very similar time course, already demonstrable four hours post-lesion, reaching a maximum at day three and returning towards normal on days five to ten (50, 200, and 60 percent change, respectively). The drugs shown previously to modify the depression in LCGU, a non-steroidal anti-inflammatory drug, an inhibitor of serotonin synthesis, a specific serotonin receptor antagonist, and an alpha1-noradrenergic receptor blocker, also modified the binding of HEAT and the behavioural deficits. All groups of animals treated with these drugs showed subtle but statistically highly significant improvements in latency to locate the platform in the Morris test.

Good correlation between spatial memory deficits, changes in serotonin metabolism, and the alpha1-noradrenergic receptor binding and depression of cortical metabolism support the hypothesis that post-injury cortical hypometabolism is a reflection of cortical functional depression in which both the serotonergic and noradrenergic neurotransmitter systems play a role, compatible with their known inhibitory effects in the cortex and their postulated involvement in cortical information processing.

Clinical Neurochemistry

For about thirty-five years, starting in 1953, I was responsible for technical supervision of the Ward Laboratory on the third floor of the Rockefeller Pavilion, opposite the elevators, and the Clinical Neurochemistry on the seventh floor for chemical analysis of blood, cerebrospinal fluid, and urine. Irving Heller was in charge of the reports from the clinical point of view and maintained contacts with the clinicians and other MNI departments. For me, initially, this involved careful review of all aspects of the work and preparation of a new manual for both laboratories, in which revised directions for all procedures and technician duties were concisely presented. In addition to standard routine analyses, the Clinical Neurochemistry personnel continued to prepare Elliott's solution for the MNI operating rooms and, following a special request from the clinical services, a solution of Nupercaine in Elliott's, for use throughout the institute. These services were discontinued when, in 1968, Abbot Laboratories began producing Elliott's solution commercially.

In 1963, with the acquisition of a Technicon Auto Analyser, the seventh-floor laboratory was reorganized and completely renovated. This resulted in a major change in the scope of the services provided by the Neurochemistry Laboratory and, over time, a major increase in the amount of work performed there. Simultaneously, the workload in the Ward Laboratory also increased as new tests became available in RVH laboratories for which blood samples from MNI patients had to be drawn.

Thus in 1982–83 the Ward Lab technicians processed 23,891 hematology, 2,336 urinalysis, and 14,316 other tests, and 14,316 blood samples were procured for analysis in outside laboratories. In the Neurochemistry Laboratory 28,031 biochemical tests were performed. As more new biochemical tests were being developed and automation took over more and more of the routine hospital laboratory testing, the relatively small volume made our operation economically non-sustainable, and by the late 1980s the work was slowly transferred to RVH.

For most of the time when Irving Heller and I jointly administered the MNI Clinical Neurochemistry Laboratories, their personnel consisted of Margot Lienard-Boisjoly, Estelle Rossin-Arthiat, and Mitty Solomon, with occasional help from Hanna Szylinger. They were a devoted and dependable team. Estelle Rossin-Arthiat was the original organizer of the now traditional MNI Spring Fling.

CONCLUSION

It is important to recognize the contribution of the many animals that were and continue to be used in a vast number of studies on the brain, and that they cannot be replaced, if progress is to be achieved in our understanding of this very complicated organ. In this context it is interesting to read in the first MNI annual report (1934–35) that "the quarters for animals are planned carefully so that any type of animal can be made comfortable and each room has an outdoor runway on the roof exposed to the sun." Thus, concern for the welfare of experimental animals is a MNI tradition going back to the Penfield era. Over the years the standards for animal care and welfare have steadily evolved globally. Our Animal Care Facility, staffed by a dedicated and experienced team of ani-

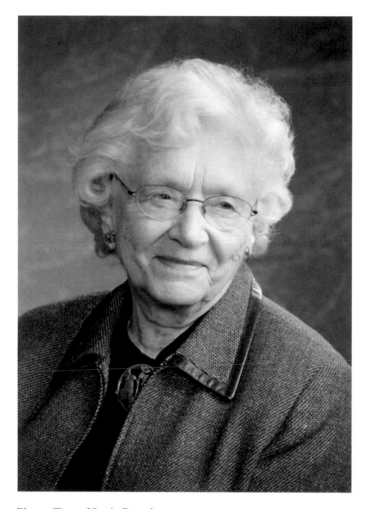

Figure T2.15: Hania Pappius, 2010.

mal care professionals, under the outstanding leadership of Janette Green since 1974, has enabled the MNI to meet and exceed these standards and consistently receive the Canadian Council of Animal Care Animal Practice Certificate. The appreciation of the MNI community was expressed by bestowing on the facility personnel of the MNI 2007 Outstanding Team Award.

The closing of the Donner Laboratory of Experimental Neurochemistry was not synonymous with the end to this science at the MNI. With modern advances in technology and their creative application to the development of new techniques, many a current researcher at the MNI is in fact a neurochemist, even if calling herself or himself something else.

Table T2.1
Elliott collaborators and students at the MNI

Alva Bazemore	Irving Heller	Hanna Pappius
Paula Berger-Strassberg	Nora Henderson	Wilder Penfield
Fernand Bilodeau	Franz Hobbiger	Al Pope
Marion Birmingham	Herbert Jasper	Mike Rosenfeld
Brenda Bollard	Dorothy Johnson	Karl Stern
Elliott Brodkin	Tariq Khan	Roy Swank
Jean Cross	Emilio Levin	Donald Tower
Jim Crossland	Dick Lovell	Nico van Gelder
Francis DeFeudis	Donald McEachern	Jim Web
Elizabeth Florey	Hugh McLennan	Leon Wolfe
Ernst Florey	R.L. Noble	

Table T2.2
Wolfe collaborators and students

Eva Andermann	Reynold Gold	Cecil Pace-Asciak
Fred Andermann	Roy Gravel	Jorma Palo
Vasu Appanna	Ronald Guttman	Hanna Pappius
Massimo Avoli	Matti Haltia	Sharon Parnes
Roy Baker	Webb Haymaker	Luc Pellerin
Violaine Bégin	Irving Heller	Arthur Perlin
Samuel Bercovic	Charles Hodge	Ronald Pokrupa
Richard Branan	Given Ivy	Lina Puglisi
Carol Breckenridge	Herbert Jasper	L.-Felipe Quesney
John Callahan	Stephen Jozeph	Klara Rostworowski
Stirling Carpenter	George Just	Charles Scriver
Joe Clark	Paige Kaplan	Robert Senior
Flavio Coceani	George Karpati	Roy Siktrom
John Crawhall	Robert Kinch	Ping-Ping Skelton
Audrey Cybulsky	Igor Klatzo	Maria Spatz
David Derry	Juergen Knaack	Mathew Spence
Robert Desnick	Ania Kurnicki	Antonio Suarez-Sanz
Christian Drapeau	Franc LeBlanc	Michel Vanasse
K.A.C. Elliott	A. Sandy Lowden	Gordon Watters
John Fawcett	Orval Mamer	John Wherrett
William Feindel	Jean Marion	Carl Witkop
Lindsey Foote	David Meek	Lucas Yamamoto
Peter Gillett	Jean Marie Mossard	Benjamin Zifkin
Uwe Goelert	N.M.K. Ng Ying Kin	

Table T2.3
Pappius collaborators and students

David Archer	Charlie Hodge	John W. Norris
Paula Berger	Masaru Inoue	J.H. Oh
Marek Buczek	Claudine Isaacs	Luc Pellerin
Stirling Carpenter	Dorothy Johnson	Ron Pokrupa
Lois Colle	Massako Kadekaro	Stanley Rapoport
James Crossland	M.A. Kallai	Mike Rosenfeld
Ralph Dadoun	Robert Katzman	Klara Rostworowski
Lloyd Dayes	Igor Klatzo	Ginette Sabourin
Jean-Claude Delhaye	Eugene Kuchner	Helen Sayaki
Catherine Dickey	Isabella Latawiec	Neil Schaul
Mirko Diksic	Marcial G. Lewin	Shobu Shibata
Carl J. Dila	David Lust	Louis Sokoloff
John Dossetor	Peter Madras	Maria Spatz
Suzan Dyve	Jean Marion	Hanna Szylinger
Victor Dzau	W.P. McCann	Chris Thomson
K.A.C. Elliott	Michael McHugh	Henry Tutt
Cesare Fieschi	David Mercer	Christian Vera
Albert Gjedde	Linda Michel	Yu-Jia Yang
D.R. Gulati	Bogumir Mrsulja	Alan Yates
Antoine Hakim	Beverly Murphy	Leon Wolfe
Robert R. Hansebout	Zoltan Nagy	

SELECT BIBLIOGRAPHY

Only salient publications are included. Complete reprint collections of papers by Elliott (144), Wolfe (218), and Pappius (104) can be found at the MNI Library.

K.A.C. Elliott

Bazemore, A.W., K.A.C. Elliott, and E. Florey. "Isolation of Factor I." *Journal of Neurochemistry* 1 (1957): 334–9.

Elliott, K.A.C. "An Unorthodox Career." *Bulletin of the Canadian Biochemical Society* 17 (1980): 14–16.

Elliott, K.A.C., and H.H. Jasper. "Physiological Salt Solutions for Brain Surgery: Studies of Local pH and Pial Vessel Reactions to Buffered and Unbuffered Isotonic Solutions." *Journal of Neurosurgery* 6 (1949): 140–52.

Elliott, K.A.C., I.H. Page, and J.H. Quastel, eds. *Neurochemistry: The Chemical Dynamics of Brain and Nerve*. Springfield, IL: Charles C. Thomas, 1955.

Elliott, K.A.C., and W. Penfield. "Respiration and Glycolysis of Focal Epileptogenic Human Brain Tissue." *Journal of Neurophysiology* 11 (1948): 485–90.

Elliott, K.A.C., and N.M. van Gelder. "Occlusion and Metabolism of γ-Aminobutyric Acid by Brain Tissue." *Journal of Neurochemistry* 3 (1958): 28–40.

Pappius, H.M., and K.A.C. Elliott. "Water Distribution in Incubated Slices of Brain and Other Tissues" *Canadian Journal of Biochemistry and Physiology* 34 (1956): 1007–22.

Tower, D.B., and K.A.C. Elliott. "Experimental Production and Control of an Abnormality in Acetylcholine Metabolism Present in Epileptic Cortex." *Journal of Applied Physiology* 5 (1953): 375–91.

Leon Wolfe

Callahan, J.W., and L.S. Wolfe. "Isolation and Characterization of Keratin Sulfates from the Liver of a Patient with GM_1-Gangliosidosis Type I." *Biochimica et Biophysica Acta* 215 (1970): 527–43.

Clarke, J.T.R., L.S. Wolfe, and A.S. Perlin. "Evidence for a Terminal Alpha-D-Galactopyranosyl Residue in Galactosylgalactosylglucosyl-Ceramide from Human Kidney." *Journal of Biological Chemistry* 246 (1971): 5563–9.

Coceani, F., and L.S. Wolfe. "Prostaglandins in Brain and the Release of Prostaglandin-Like Compounds from the Cat Cerebellar Cortex." *Canadian Journal of Physiology and Pharmacology* 43 (1965): 445–50.

Lowden, J.A., and L.S. Wolfe. "Studies on Brain Gangliosides. III. Evidence for the Location of Gangliosides Specifically in Neurons." *Canadian Journal of Biochemistry* 42 (1964): 1587–94.

Ng Ying Kin, N.M., and L.S. Wolfe. "Presence of Abnormal Amounts of Dolichols in the Urinary Sediment of Batten Disease Patients." *Pediatric Research* 16 (1982): 530–2.

Ng Ying Kin, N.M., L.S. Wolfe, J. Palo, and M. Haltia. "High Levels of Brain Dolichols in Enuronal Ceroid-Lipofuscinosis and Senescence." *Journal of Neurochemistry* 40 (1983): 1465–73.

Pace-Asciak, C., and L.S. Wolfe. "Biosynthesis of Prostaglandin E2 and F2a from Tritium-Labelled aArachidonic Acid by Rat Stomach Homogenate." *Biochimica et Biophysica Acta* 218 (1970): 539–42.

Spence, M.W., and L.S. Wolfe. "Gangliosides in Developing Rat Brain: Isolation and Composition of Subcellular Membranes Enriched in Gangliosides." *Canadian Journal of Biochemistry* 45 (1967): 671–88.

Wolfe, L.S., and L. Pellerin. "Arachidonic Acid Metabolites in the Rat and

Human Brain: New Findings on the Metabolism of Prostaglandin D_2 and Lipoxygenase Products." *Annals of the New York Academy of Sciences* 559 (1989): 74–83.

Wolfe, L.S., K. Rostworowski, and J. Marion. "Endogenous Formation of the Prostaglandin Endoperixide Metabilite, Thromboxane B_2, by Brain Tissue." *Biochemical and Biophysical Research Communication* 70 (1976): 907–13.

Hanna Pappius

Katzman, R., and H.M. Pappius. *Brain Electrolytes and Fluid Metabolism.* Baltimore, MD: Williams and Wilkins, 1973.

Lewin, M.G., R.T. Hansebout, and H.M. Pappius. "Chemical Characteristics of Traumatic Spinal Cord Edema in Cats." *Journal of Neurosurgery* 40 (1974): 65–75.

Pappius, H.M. "Biochemical Aspects of Brain Swelling." *Scientia* 103 (1968): 161–73.

– "Brain Injury: New Insights into Neurotransmitter and Receptor Mechanisms." *Neurochemical Research* 16 (1991): 941–9.

Pappius, H.M. "Cortical Hypometabolism in Injured Brain: New Correlations with the Noradrenergic and Serotonergic Systems and with Behavioral Deficits." *Neurochemical Research* 20 (1995): 1311–21.

Pappius, H.M., and W. Feindel, eds. *Dynamics of Brain Edema: Proceedings of the 3rd International Workshop on Dynamic Aspects of Cerebral Edema, Montreal, Canada, June 25–29, 1976.* Heidelberg: Springer-Verlag, 1976.

Pappius, H.M., and W.P. McCann. "Effects of Steroids on Cerebral Edema in Cats." *Archives of Neurology* 20 (1969): 207–16.

Shibata, S., C.P. Hodge, and H.M. Pappius. "Effects of Experimental Ischemia on Cerebral Water and Electrolytes." *Journal of Neurosurgery* 41 (1974): 146–59.

Theme 3

Multiple Sclerosis: Care and Research at the MNI

JACK ANTEL AND WILLIAM SHEREMATA

THE ORIGINS

The investigation of multiple sclerosis and the care of afflicted patients have been concerns of the MNI since its earliest days. From his early studies with del Río-Hortega that led to the discovery of the oligodendrocyte, Wilder Penfield pioneered in the study of glial cells – oligodendrocytes, astrocytes, and microglia – which are implicated in the pathophysiology of MS.[1] At that time, since there was no specific therapy for MS, patients suspected of suffering from this condition were evaluated on the neurosurgical service of the MNI to exclude other, treatable disorders. Even in the early years, however, there were concerns about environmental factors triggering or contributing to the course of the disease, and as early as 1934 William Cone, Colin Russel, and Robert Harwood published a paper implicating lead as a possible cause of MS.[2] The MNI's neuropathology laboratory allowed investigations of such putative mechanisms.[3] The chemistry laboratory carried out CSF analyses, including the colloidal gold test, which is now recognized as reflecting immunoglobulin production in the CNS.

THE MULTIPLE SCLEROSIS SOCIETY

The formal organization of a Multiple Sclerosis Program at the MNI occurred in the late 1940s, in concert with the formation of an organized MS Society in Montreal and the recruitment of Roy Swank to head a five-year research program directed at the disease.[4] Wilder Penfield served as honorary medical consultant to the society and Colin Russel was chair of the Medical Advisory Committee. Donald McEachren soon succeeded Russel, who was in ill health. In 1947, the society approved a large annual grant of $10,000 for three years to the MNI. Of the initial $10,000, $5,000 was allocated for MS research and $5,000

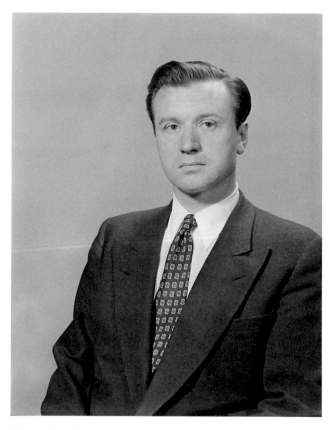

Figure T3.1: Bert Cosgrove circa 1954. (MNI Archives)

for clinical care, including physiotherapy and social service support. This was welcome and highlighted by Donald McEachren in his annual report as neurologist-in-chief: "With the support of the Colin Russel Chapter of the Multiple Sclerosis Society of Canada, a new Clinic for Physiotherapy has been opened in the Royal Victoria Hospital. The clinic has been furnished and redecorated by this group of keen supporters, and it is under the direction of Dr [Arthur] Young and Dr [Reuben] Rabinovitch."[5] The role of Social Services was an integral part of this comprehensive program, and received funding of its own towards its goals for MS patients, as reported by Elabel Davidson, head of the Department of Social Services: "Our survey of the paraplegic situation has also been used by the local multiple sclerosis unit in publicizing the incidence of this disease and the urgent need of support for medical research. It is our hope that social studies may be carried on concurrently with the medical research on multiple sclerosis so that we may know better how to help these patients."[6]

The useful role that a social worker could play within the program was recognized, as reported by Josephine Chiasson, the new head of Social Services: "The grant which the National Multiple Sclerosis Society has made to the Institute has made it possible for a social worker to participate in the clinical study of multiple sclerosis patients being carried on by our doctors and a dietician."[7] A further $6,000 grant was received from the province of Quebec in 1951 for "early detection of multiple sclerosis and predisposition."

ROY SWANK

Roy Swank first came to the MNI as a research fellow in the academic year 1939–40 and stayed until 1941, then returned to the institute in 1948 to direct a five-year research program into MS.[8] Swank's pending recruitment was met with much enthusiasm, as expressed by Donald McEachern: "We will soon welcome back Dr Roy Swank who will head an important new attack on the dread disease – multiple sclerosis. Plans have been laid to organize a new diagnostic and research clinic for multiple sclerosis and this will be opened in the early autumn. It will make available a wealth of clinical material, and will give to multiple sclerosis patients the newest and best that can be offered. Treatment facilities are already available in the daily Neurological Treatment Clinic, under Dr [Arthur] Young's direction, and this will serve as a testing ground for new techniques."[9] Upon his return to Montreal in September 1948, Swank's laboratory was in a space made available to him by William Cone in the already crowded neuropathology laboratory. Roy Swank's work derived from epidemiologic studies on the prevalence of MS, particularly in Norway, and its relation to dietary lipids.[10] Swank observed that the incidence of multiple sclerosis in Norway was very low along the coast and very high inland in the farming and dairy areas. He noted that "the fat intake, and in particular butter and animal fat in the diet, is very high inland and relatively low along the coast."[11] These observations led to a longitudinal study of the effects of a low fat diet on the clinical manifestation of MS, and the laboratory investigation of the effects of lipids on the circulation and on plasma proteins.[12] By 1953, Roy Swank could report, "This diet appears to lessen the severity of the disease by reducing the frequency and severity of the exacerbations. Its usefulness seems greatest early in the disease, before significant disability and a steady progression of symptoms have developed."[13] Roy Swank left the MNI after five years, for the University of Oregon.[14] The dietary approach continues to have adherents, with some recognition that it may modulate the immune response.

BERT COSGROVE AND THE MULTIPLE SCLEROSIS CLINIC

With the departure of Roy Swank, the MNI recruited J.B.R. "Bert" Cosgrove from the University of Manitoba to take over the MS program. Barry Arnason, then a medical student in Winnipeg, describes his first meeting with Cosgrove:

> A fond memory of him is imprinted in the tablets of my mind. There was a polio epidemic in Winnipeg in the summer of 1952 and I volunteered to try and help out at the infectious disease hospital. Mostly I ran errands and carried blood samples and the like and moved bodies from the iron lungs to the morgue. Burt was the neurologist who ran the show working 16 hours a day, deciding who had polio, who had western equine encephalitis that was also around, who had neither, who was next for one of the iron lungs, we had about 60 of them from all over the country, all filled, who needed a spinal tap and who didn't. I admired him greatly and I think it was during that dreadful time that my interest in neurology was kindled and my interest in immunology as well. The polio vaccine came out the next year.[15]

William Sheremata also recalls his first meeting with Bert Cosgrove, when he was recruited to the MNI in 1970, and his seven years of working with him in the MS Clinic: After my arrival in Montreal In the summer of 1971, I was introduced to J.B.R. Cosgrove. Although seemingly pleased to meet me, he did not express much interest in thoughts about the immunology of MS. He quietly pointed out that he had over 5,000 MS patients in his clinic and that his priority was to provide care for them. My help, he said, would be very much appreciated. Bert Cosgrove was a quiet man who did not deliberately set out to impress others. It was only by working with him that I began to appreciate his extraordinary knowledge of MS as a clinical disorder. Through him the important contributions of the great Douglas McAlpine at the Middlesex Hospital in London and Professor Brian Mathews at Oxford came into focus. Following McAlpine's death, Cosgrove was invited to edit *McAlpine Multiple Sclerosis*, the most influential text on the subject at the time, for a future edition. Bert asked me for assistance but, after I declined, he himself withdrew his candidacy for the task.

Cosgrove's awareness of the clinical nuances of multiple sclerosis was extraordinary. Unlike most neurologists at the time, who shared a nihilist attitude towards therapy, Cosgrove was interested in "treating" MS. He had learned from McAlpine's observations that oral steroids appeared to increase the rate of MS but that this was not the case for adrenocorticotropic hormone (ACTH). He pointed to salutary outcomes of the multicenter ACTH study published in 1970 as well as his own experience. Corsyntropin (Synacten; Sandoz), used in a clinical trial, he pointed out, stimulated an adrenal response that was only anabolic, unlike glucocorticoids that also induced a catabolic response. He felt this property of ACTH would enhance its salutary effect in acute exacerbations of MS. Bert Cosgrove was also interested in treating patients with the especially active forms of MS, "malignant MS," aggressively. He organized a committee to deal with this subject. It consisted of Barry Arnason (chairman of Neurology, University of Chicago), Kirk Osterland (new chairman of Immunology, McGill University), Cosgrove, and myself. The decision at the MNI was to institute an aggressive immunosuppressive protocol using azathioprine and prednisone over a period of two years, depending on achieving and maintaining a satisfactory clinical effect. This protocol was subsequently implemented for those patients who were still ambulatory after having at least three clinical exacerbations in their first year of illness. In 1971 we began to use high dose intravenous steroids for MS patients who were paraplegic as a result of spinal cord damage and swelling revealed by myelography. We extended this to patients with blind eyes and tumifactive swelling on an optic nerve shown by CT. Cosgrove thought that patients who appeared to have benefitted from a strict low animal fat diet more reflected their having less active forms of MS than response to the diet. This remains an important concern when assessing long term outcomes of more modern day clinical trials. From that point I was continuously astonished by his clinical prowess in the field. The occurrence of facial myokymia and paroxysmal symptoms in MS was revealed to me as not only interesting but unique to MS and helpful clinical signs in its diagnosis.[16] The availability of brain CT did not diminish Bert Cosgrove's emphasis on the clinical features of MS nor my appreciation of his expertise. Although I thought I knew the field of MS prior to my arrival at the MNI, I was quickly brought to my knees in admiration. The next several years in Montreal amounted to an extended clinical fellowship.

Cosgrove was impressed that psychological stress was a major problem related to onset and relapse of MS. He set up a study with the psychiatrist Lucien Gratton to evaluate the contribution of major life stressors in MS. The study was carried out, a data set generated, and the results analyzed. These revealed a correlation between onset and relapse of MS with such stressors. Serially studied, unselected MS patients in the Cosgrove-Gratton study were found to have suffered between 3 and 4 times as many major life stresses when compared with new referral of medical patients referred to psychiatry from medicine. However, Gratton abruptly returned to France in 1977 and no formal reports of the study data ensued. I presented a summary of the data that Cosgrove provided at a symposium of the International Neuropsychology Meeting in San Diego in 1978. Subsequent studies by Igor Grant, who was present at the symposium, and Mohr supported these findings.[17]

Bert Cosgrove also participated as a supervisor, with the Department of Immunology at the RVH, of the doctoral work in neuroimmunology conducted by Allan Sherwin that was directly relevant to understanding the immune response in the central nervous system in MS.[18] Such studies were identifying the presence of myelin directed antibodies in MS and in its animal model experimental allergic encephalomyelitis, led to an understanding of how antibodies present in the systemic circulation could access the central nervous system.[19]

Bert Cosgrove passed away on 11 May 1984. In his eulogy, Donald Baxter spoke for all who new Cosgrove: "Dr Cosgrove devoted virtually his entire professional career to this institution, and to the relief of the emotional and physical suffering of thousands of patients with chronic neurologic disease and in particular those with multiple sclerosis. His wise council is sorely missed by hundreds of patients. The residents and students have lost a teacher with unique experience and perspective in neurology, and his colleagues are the poorer without his friendship and steadying advice in times of difficulty."[20]

WILLIAM SHEREMATA

William Sheremata was recruited to McGill and the MNI in 1970, to advance the MS program. As he recalls, Preston Robb, the chief examiner at the Royal College of Physicians and Surgeons at the oral examinations in neurology held in Montreal in 1970, invited me to consider a position at McGill University. After further discussion and later after accepting his offer, he gave me his old laboratory on the sixth floor of the MNI which was located next to Wilder Penfield's' office. Dr Robb's laboratory was essentially in the same state as it had been in 1934 when the MNI opened. Soapstone sinks were still functional but other than countertops there was little else in the lab. It had served as the CSF laboratory for the MNI and RVH for many years under the supervision of Bert Cosgrove. Renovation of the laboratory was funded by a Medical Research Council establishment grant, supplemented the MNI. Research support was provided by the MRC, from the Multiple Sclerosis Society of Canada, and from local support. In the 1970s the Montreal community began effective fundraising and as a result became the largest source of funding for the MS Society of

Canada. The Society then accepted a recommendation from Bert Cosgrove that MS Clinics should receive some financial support from the Society. As a result, the MS Society of Canada then established a policy to fund university based MS Clinics. Funding was limited to a clinic secretary and a nurse, as well as some operational expenses.

Cosgrove thought that the presence of antibody in the CSF was important, referring to the work of Murray Bornstein, who had been a fellow at the MNI at the time but acknowledged that more investigation was needed. Performance of CSF analyses continued in the laboratory during our research endeavors, although we began measuring CSF immunoglobulin and albumin concentrations, as at the Massachusetts General Hospital in Boston, in addition to continuing performing CSF electrophoresis. Data developed in the laboratory was used to obtain approval for use of specific IgG and albumin measurement for the diagnosis of multiple sclerosis and autoimmune disease of the nervous system. After Link and Mueller in Stockholm published their observations showing that oligoclonal bands (OCBs) were present in the CSF of MS patients, we blindly examined electrophoretic strips independently of the clinical diagnosis.[21] Although we were using the same technology as in Stockholm, we found that OCBs appeared more often in CSF from seizure and Parkinson's patients than in MS.[22] A decision was made not to pursue OCB measurement at that time.

The new tissue culture facilities were focused on cellular immunology. The addition of another experienced laboratory technician greatly improved our research capacity. This new facility enabled us to perform "lymphoblastic transformation" as well as the bioassay to measure macrophage migration inhibitory factor. In the interval between 1972 and 1977 the laboratory was productive and a number of papers were published in major journals.[23] We found a prominent immune response to myelin basic protein at the very onset of MS exacerbations, a novel idea at the time, with diminishing responses during recovery in untreated patients. Subsequently, working with Mario Moscarello in Toronto, we found that antibody to myelin basic protein was not present at the onset of relapses but appeared later in the relapse and during early convalescence. Antibody levels were greatest when the cellular immune response had abated. Working with the apoprotein of myelin proteolipid was a challenge because it is highly polarized. Despite this, we detected an antibody response, although it was found in only a few subjects, and its presence did not correlate with a diagnosis of MS nor in the presence of any particular nervous system disorder nor any stage of multiple sclerosis.

While multiple sclerosis was the central problem investigated by the l aboratory, other demyelinating disorders, including isolated optic neuritis, Guillain-Barre syndrome, and subacute sclerosing encephalomyelitis (SSPE) were also subjects for investigation. With Jeffery Allen, a fellow in pediatric neurology, we performed, and published, the first analysis of CSF lymphocyte subsets in MS. Despite our achievements, our failure to measure RNA expression was a serious limitation but we did not have the resources to proceed in that direction.

The formal criteria for diagnosis of multiple sclerosis to be used for natural history and clinical trial purposes were initially defined in the mid-1960s by the Schumacher committee and required documentation of multiple sites of involvement of the CNS. An important clinical contribution to the MNI program was made by neuro-ophthalmologist Trevor Kirkham, who evaluated large numbers of patients. When para-clinical evidence of multi-focal lesions was incorporated into the diagnostic criteria in the early 1980s, physiologic evoked responses were added to the testing regimen at the MNI. The commitment of the MNI to a brain-imaging program resulted in access to magnetic resonance (MR) based imaging in 1984. MR-derived imaging criteria were subsequently incorporated into the diagnostic criteria.

The above MS directed clinical, laboratory, and imaging programs provided the infrastructure and environment to foster subsequent efforts in the MS field at the MNI. Donald Baxter, who became director in 1984, recruited Gordon Francis to succeed Bert Cosgrove at the MS clinic. Yves Lapierre joined Francis and subsequently became director of the MS clinic. Donald Baxter committed to the development of an MNI immunology program that soon included Jack Antel, Neil Cashman, Trevor Owens, V. Wee Yong, Mark Freedman, and, in early 2000s, Amit Bar-Or. Paul Giacomini also later joined the MS group. The infrastructure and resources of the Brain Imaging Centre allowed the subsequent cutting-edge application of magnetic resonance spectroscopy to MS by Douglas Arnold and Paul Matthews, of magnetic transfer imaging by Bruce Pike, and of quantitative analytic methods by Alan Evans and Douglas Arnold.

During the 1970s and 1980s, ongoing work at the Center for Neuroscience at the Montreal General Hospital and at McGill University contributed to the MS effort. Mike Rasminsky did some of the early neurophysiology of conduction by demyelinated axons. Albert Aguayo, Garth Bray, and their team utilized peripheral nerve allografts to demonstrate the potential for regeneration in the CNS, if a favourable micro-environment could be provided.

William Howard Feindel and the Origins of Neurosurgery in Saskatchewan

MARTHA RIESBERRY

DEVELOPING A DEPARTMENT

In 1955 the University of Saskatchewan created a new medical school to replace its two-year pre-medical program.[1] Dean W. Macleod recruited specialists of the highest calibre for the new medical school and to staff University Hospital. They came from many of the world's best academic and clinical centres – Queen Square, Johns Hopkins University, the Mayo Clinic, and the MNI – for the unique opportunities offered by a new medical school and teaching hospital.[2] William Feindel was given the responsibility of planning and developing the new Division of Neurosurgery. He had three goals for the department: provide a modern neurosurgical unit staffed and equipped for treating patients with major neurosurgical conditions, establish a program of clinical and laboratory research, and provide a stimulating environment for undergraduate and post-graduate teaching in neurosurgery.[3] Feindel was given generous funding from the university to purchase equipment and to hire the needed personnel.[4]

The neurosurgical ward at the UH included laboratory space and a classroom, but it had no intensive care unit or observation area. In 1957, three single-bed patient rooms were converted into a six-bed neurosurgical ICU – the first neurosurgical ICU in Canada – where patients could be observed from the nursing station.[5] The operating suite resembled those at the MNI and included an induction room, a viewing gallery, and eight X-ray viewing boxes installed on the wall, allowing the surgeon to view serial angiograms.[6] The first neurosurgical procedure at the UH was a twelve-hour excision of a 15 cm supra- and infra-tentorial meningioma performed by William Feindel under induced hypothermia and hypotension. The patient recovered and returned to his home with a new pair of shoes, a gift from the nursing staff.[7] Besides resecting brain tumours, Feindel clipped aneurysms and performed chemopallidectomies for Parkinson's disease. He also resected spinal cord tumours and herniated discs, and performed spinal cordotomies for the treatment of metastatic cancer pain.[8] William Feindel and Joseph Stratford pursued work they began at the MNI "on hypothermia during craniotomy for vascular lesions previously considered inoperable and continued experimental work on that subject – a suitable topic for the cold prairie winters."[9]

William Feindel performed epilepsy surgery, under local anaesthesia, as he had learned at the MNI, and wore the hooded facemask found useful in the prevention of infection during long cases, when a large area of cortex was exposed. He performed cortical stimulation to identify and thus preserve eloquent brain areas, and performed electrocorticography to locate the epileptic focus. This was accomplished using a closed-circuit television system set up between the viewing gallery and the operating room; a cable transmitted the electrico-cortical recording to an EEG machine in the gallery, and a television camera affixed above the EEG machine videotaped the electrographic recording. The recording was transmitted in real time to a television monitor in the operating room, where it could be easily seen by the neurosurgeon.[10] Having the EEG machine in the gallery reduced the interference from other operating room equipment and therefore improved the quality of the tracing. This was the first time that closed-circuit television was used in this way in Canada.

There were other firsts for Feindel in Saskatoon, such as his initial encounter with assisted ventilation:

> This was being introduced in 1955 by Dr Dobkin who had come from the MNI to the University Hospital at Saskatoon and was a great innovator in the use of new anesthetic drugs. An unnerving experience occurred when I was operating on a patient with a cerebellar tumor. I had been working near the floor of the fourth ventricle where vital functions such as breathing, heart rate and blood pressure were controlled by compact nerve centers. I asked Dobkin in the midst of the procedure if the patient's breathing was satisfactory. He replied, "The patient hasn't been breathing on his own for several hours." I did not realize that the new medication that Dobkin was using blocked the patient's own breathing rhythm so it could be controlled by the automatic respirator.[11]

The activities of the Division of Neurosurgery expanded quickly under Feindel's leadership. Although Joseph Stratford and Leslie Ivan had joined the department in 1956, by 1958 the department was serving the whole of Saskatchewan, with many referrals transferred urgently by air ambulance. The neurosurgical service became so busy that William Feindel recommended the addition of further clinical staff.[12] Feindel also encouraged the Division of Neurosurgery's cooperation with other services, and general surgery residents began rotating through neurosurgery for four months as part of their training. In 1955 Robert Murray, an ophthalmologist trained at Johns Hopkins University, brought a Zeiss binocular surgical microscope to the UH. William Feindel used this microscope for a number of neurosurgical procedures from 1955 on, making him one of the first micro-neurosurgeons.[13] Feindel did not report his microsurgical experience, as he preferred to use his magnifying loupes for most cases. Nonetheless, "he used the microscope for vascular and tumor cases in which magnification and lighting were critical" and acquired a microscope for the Cone Research Laboratory and operating room on his return to Montreal in 1959.[14]

Millie Erb-Weishoff was originally from Saskatchewan and had been an assistant director of nursing at the MNI. She was placed in charge of the neurosurgical operating room nursing staff and of the organization and preparation of its equipment at UH.[15] Ruth MacDonald, also from the MNI, joined her. As was the case at the Neuro, if a microscope drape or surgical hood mask could not be ordered, the nurses made them by hand.[16] Monica Tremblay was the head nurse on the ward. She had completed the postgraduate diploma course in neurosurgical nursing at the MNI.

TARDY ULNAR PALSY

William Feindel and Joseph Stratford presented three cases of decompression at the ulnar nerve at the elbow, without transposition, at the 28th meeting of the Royal College of Physicians and Surgeons of Canada in 1957, a procedure that was adopted worldwide. Doing so they introduced the term *cubital tunnel* and *cubital tunnel syndrome* as a cause for tardy ulnar palsy and described the functional anatomy of the cubital tunnel and how it is affected by flexion and extension of the elbow.[17]

THE SASKATOON SCANNER

William Feindel's major accomplishment in Saskatoon was the development of a clinically useful automatic radioisotope scanner, providing images of the brain in three axes, which he developed with Harold Johns, William Reid, Sylvia Fedoruk, and Joseph Stratford.[18] A second generation of this scanner was developed at the MNI upon Feindel's return, where it remained operational for fifteen years.

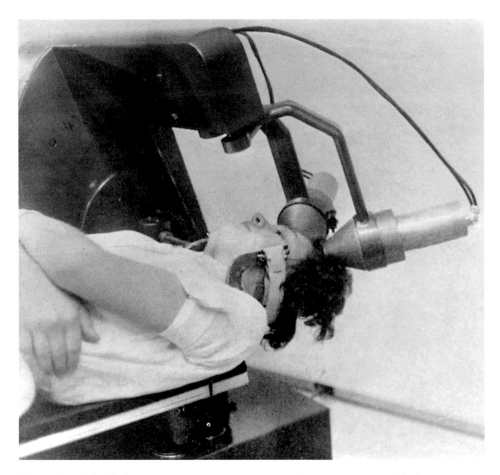

Figure T4.1: The Saskatoon contour automatic neuroisotope scanner with the twin radiation detectors mounted on a gantry. (MNI Archives)

William Feindel later recalled the development and function of the "Saskatoon Scanner":

The first use in Canada of radioactive tracers for the detection of tumours and strokes occurred curiously at the MNI "Satellite" on the prairie at University Hospital, Saskatoon. Drs Harold Johns and Bill Reid at the Saskatoon Cancer Clinic produced a prototype radioisotope scanner in 1956, with the assistance of physicist Sylvia Fedoruk and from a scan pattern proposed by neurosurgeon Bill Feindel. This first scanner had a novel contour scanning mechanism to avoid the "foreshortening" of the rectilinear scanner introduced by Sweet and Brownell in 1953. The Saskatoon device was designed so that both halves of the head would be scanned simultaneously, the parasagittal regions would be included, and the ends of the detectors would follow closely the contour of the skull, maintaining a fairly constant distance and geometry. The two detectors consisted of one-inch thick and one-inch diameter thallium-activated sodium iodide crystals coupled to photomultipliers and mounted in one-inch thick lead shields. Mounted on "bucket-handles," they scanned the head in a series of eight parasagittal arcs, starting at the nose, each describing 180°, and separated in coronal section by approximately 7.5°. The patient wore a rubber bathing cap in order to present a smooth surface to the detectors and allow fixation of the head in a cushioned clamp. The data were visualized by printing dots in proportion to the measured count rate and oblique dashes in proportion to the left/right difference in count rate between the two detectors. The scan took 30 minutes. Using I-131 labeled human serum albumin, the device showed considerable promise, with excellent correlation compared to other radiological procedures in 90 per cent of 115 cases studied with no false positives. An updated version was used from 1960 to 1975 at the MNI.[19]

CEREBRAL BLOOD FLOW STUDIES

Feindel, with the continued collaboration of Sylvia Fedoruk, devised an apparatus and technique to measure the carotid-jugular circulation time in pathological states in which the circulation time was delayed – as in cases of carotid occlusion or elevated intracranial pressure – or accelerated, as in arteriovenous malformations.[20]

TEACHING ACTIVITIES

A neurosurgical residency-training program was approved in 1955 and quickly expanded to include a second resident. William Feindel's teaching responsibilities included daily resident rounds and six hours a week of formal teaching.[21] Undergraduate teaching included didactic lectures to medical students, the teaching of surgical skills to second- and third-year students, and fourth-year bedside teaching.[22] Multidisciplinary teaching rounds with neurosurgical, neurological, and psychiatry residents were also instituted. Teaching was not limited to medical students and residents. Feindel also taught operating room nurses to improve their neurosurgical nursing skills. Neuropathology was added to the curriculum with the coming of Jerzy Olszewski in 1957; and a neurological sciences club met weekly with participants from anatomy, neurology, neurosurgery, pathology, and psychiatry starting in 1958. William Feindel also participated in public education, and he gave a radio lecture on *How Your Brain Works* in December 1955. This, Feindel recalled, was "oriented toward basic anatomical and physiological facts presented in a somewhat popular way.[23] Feindel also taught engineering students, encouraged further education in medical engineering, and gave joint lectures with the Colleges of Medicine and Engineering.[24]

Wilder Penfield visited Saskatoon on two occasions during Feindel's tenure. The first time was during the Canadian Neurological Society meeting in 1957, the second in 1959, to attend the University of Saskatchewan's Jubilee celebrations.[25] Penfield's Jubilee visit stemmed from Feindel's interdisciplinary activities and resulted in a small book, *Memory, Learning and Language: The Physical Basis of Mind*, edited by Feindel and published in 1960.[26]

The death of William Cone brought Feindel back to Montreal in 1959 as the first William Cone Professor of Neurosurgery at McGill University and the MNI.[27] Joseph Stratford succeeded Feindel as chief of the Department of Neurosurgery[28] Stratford later returned to Montreal to become neurosurgeon-in-chief and director of the Division of Neurosurgery at the Montreal General Hospital,[29] leaving behind a solid foundation for the future.[30]

Appendix 1

Japanese Chapter of the MNI
1955–1984

Japanese Chapter of the Montreal Neurological Institute, 1955–84

Name	Primay appointment	Year
Keiichi Amano	Neurosurgery	1970–71
Norio Arita	Cone Laboratory	1979–81
Mitsuru Ebe	Neurophysiology	1965–66
Kiyotaka Fujii	Cone Laboratory	1978
Yoshiya Iwama	Donner Laboratory	1956–57
Masahiro Izawa	Cone Laboratory	1982–83
Itsuki Jibiki	Neurophysiology	1982–83
Amami Kato	Cone Laboratory	1982–84
Hiroko Kato	Cone Laboratory	1970–71
Kazuo Kinoshita	Neurosurgery	1964–65
Michihiro Kirikae	Cone Laboratory	1984–86
Katsutoshi Kitamura	Neurosurgery	1957–58
Shin Kitamura	Cone Laboratory	1983–84
Keitaro Kobatake	Cone Laboratory	1981–83
Hiroshi Matsuda	Cone Laboratory	1984–85
Masayuki Matsunaga	Cone Laboratory	1978–81
Shigeaki Matuoka	Neurophysiology	1962–63
Mineo Motomiya	Cone Laboratory	1977–79
Yoku Nakagawa	Cone Laboratory	1975–77
Kirofumi Nakai	Cone Laboratory	1984–86
Shouzou Nakazawa	EEG	1966
Hideaki Nukui	Cone Laboratory	1977–79
Kazukiro Sako	Cone Laboratory	1981–83
Takashi Shibasaki	Cone Laboratory	1979–81

Name	Primay appointment	Year
Shobu Shibata	Neurochemistry	1970–71
Masato Shibuya	Cone Laboratory	1981–81
Hiroyuki Shimizu	Cone Laboratory	1979–81
Toshikiyo Shohmori	Neurophysiology	1964–67
Tohru Soejima	Cone Laboratory	1975–77
Eiichi Takara	Cone Laboratory	1984–86
Yukitaka Ushio	Neurosurgery	1967–69
June Wada	Electrophysiology	1955–56
Kouzou Yajima	Cone Laboratory	1981
Shinjirou Yamamoto	Neurophysiology	1950–59

* Holmberg and the Japanese Chapter of the MNI were instrumental in the building of the Rasmussen Reading Room in the MNI's Fellows Library.

Appendix 2

Fellows Day Lecturers
1957–1984

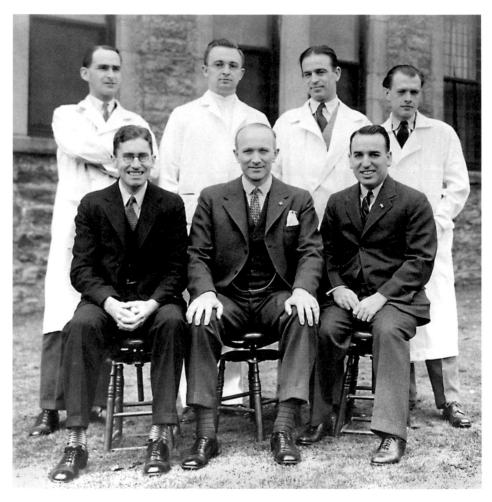

Figure A2: Standing are Kristian Kristiansen, Lyle Gage, Joseph Evans, Jerzy Chorobski, with Arthur Elvidge, Wilder Penfield and William Cone. (MNI Archives)

Fellows Day Lecturers, 1957–84

Year	Lecturer	Title
1957	Joseph P. Evans	Brain Injury: Present Concepts and Challenges
1958	Webb Haymaker	Kernicterus and Posticteric Encephalopathy
1959	Dorothy Russell	Reflections on Neuropathology
1960	Isadore Tarlov	Rigidity Due to Spinal Interneuron Destruction
1961	Guy Odom	Vascular Lesions of the Spinal Cord
1962	George Stavraky	Adaptation after Central Nervous System Damage
1963	Milton Shy	Newer Disorders of Muscle
1964	Kristian Kristiansen	Studies of the Vasomotor Control of the Cerebral Circulation
1965	Igor Klatzo	Experimental Studies on Blood-Brain Barrier and Brain Edema
1966	Robert H. Pudenz	Experiences in the Treatment of Trigeminal Neuralgia
1967	Arthur A. Ward Jr	Pathophysiology of Epilepsy
1968	Edwin Boldrey	Sensory Levels and Configuration Association with Painful Lesions Affecting the Spinal Roots and Peripheral Nerves in Man
1969	Kenneth M. Earle	Viral Encephalitis
1970	Donald Tower	Unknown
1971	C. Ajmone-Marsan	Unknown
1973	Claude Bertrand	Contributions to Stereotactic Neurosurgery and Its Applications to Neurological Diseases
1974	Sean Mullan	Unknown
1975	David Hubel	Unknown
1976	Keasley Welch	Dynamics of the Cerebral Spinal Fluid
1977	Herbert Jasper	Reflections on Forty Years of Epilepsy Research
1978	Phanor Perot	Somatosensory Evoked Potentials in Spinal Cord Injury
1979	Charles Branch Sr	Complications of Chymopapain Injection for the Treatment of Lumbar Disc Disease
1980	Henry Garretson	Arteriovenous Malformations
1983	Douglas Watt	Aerospace Medicine
1984	Blaine Nashold	The DREZ (Dorsal Root Entry Zone) Operation for Pain Relief

Appendix 3

Hughlings Jackson Lecturers
1935–1984

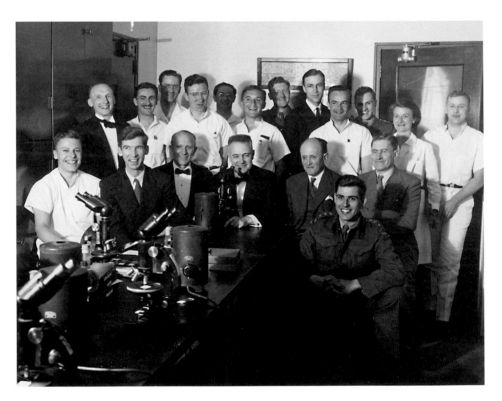

Figure A1: The 1944 Hughlings Jackson lecturer Percival Bailey, with the residents and staff of the MNI. (*Seated*) A.A. Ward, E.S. Lotspeich Jr, W. Penfield, P. Bailey, K. Stern, E.W. Peterson, A. Elvidge. (*Standing*): F.L. McNaughton, C.W. Hall, G. Morton, A.A. Moris, S. Spaner, C. Mushatt, D. Ross, J.P. Robb, unidentified, C. Bertrand, D. Bentley, T.S. Bennett. (MNI Archives)

Hughlings Jackson lecturers, 1935–84

Year	Lecturer	Lecture title
1935	Wilder G. Penfield	Epilepsy and Surgical Therapy
1936	MNI staff	Jackson's Teachings
1937	Karl S. Lashley	Factors Limiting Improvement after Central Nervous Lesions
1938	Detlev W. Bronk	Nerve Cells and Synapses in the Regulation of Organic Functions
1939	Walter B. Cannon	A Law of Denervation
1940	Charles H. Best	The Factors Affecting the Liberation of Insulin from the Pancreas
1941	Stephen W. Ranson	Experimental Studies of the Corpus Striatum
1942	Lord Adrian (1932)*	Sensory Areas of the Brain
1943	Philip Bard	Re-representation as a Principle of Central Nervous Organization
1944	Percival Bailey	The Cortical Organization of the Chimpanzee Brain
1945	Stanley Cobb	Some Problems on Neurocirculatory Asthenia
1946	Otto Loewi (1936)*	Problems Connected with the Effects of Nervous Impulse
1947	Sir Henry Dale (1936)*	Chemical Transmission and Central Synapse
1948	Derek Denny-Brown	Disorganization of Motor Function Resulting from Cerebral Lesions
1949	H. Cuthbert Bazett	Blood Temperature in Man and Its Control
1950	J. Godwin Greenfield	The Pathology of the Cerebellum and Related Motor Pathways
1951	J. Bertram Collip	The Endocrines in Relation to Neurology
1952	John C. Eccles (1963)*	Electrophysiology of the Neurons
1953	James C. White	Pain Conduction in Man: Studies on Its Transmission in Spinal Cord and Visceral Plexuses
1954	Théophile Alajouanine	On Some Aspects of Verbal Expression in Aphasia

Year	Lecturer	Lecture title
1955	Norman Dott	The Common Features of Brain Displacement by Tumour, by Hemorrhage, and by Violence
1956	Israel Weschler	On the Broadening Concepts of Neurology
1957	Herbert S. Gasser (1944)*	The Properties of Unmedullated Nerve Fibers with Afferent Function
1958	Donald O. Hebb	Intelligence, Brain Function, and Theory
1959	Herbert H. Jasper	Evolution of Concepts of Cerebral Localization since Hughlings Jackson
1960	Charles Symonds	Memory Disorder Following Brain Damage
1961	Wilder G. Penfield	The Brain's Record of Experience: Auditory and Visual
1962	Raymond D. Adams	Thiamine and the Human Nervous System
1963	Lord Russell Brain	Some Reflections on Brain and Mind
1964	Murray Barr	Some Principles and Examples in the New Field of Human Cytogenetics
1965	Paul Bucy	The Delusion of the Obvious
1966	Roger Sperry (1981)*	Mental Unity and Surgical Disconnection of the Cerebral Hemispheres
1967	John Z. Young	Information Storage in the Nervous System
1968	K.A.C. Elliott	Neurochemistry: An Aspect of the Interdisciplinary Basis of Neurology
1969	Holger Hyden	Some Brain Protein Changes Reflecting Neural Plasticity at Learning
1970	H. Houston Merritt	Pathophysiology of Parkinson's Disease and the Response of Symptoms to Treatment of Levodopa
1971	Clinton N. Woolsey	The Cortical Motor Maps of Monkey and Dog after Section of the Medullary Pyramid
1972	A. Earl Walker	Man and His Temporal Lobes
1973	Theodore Rasmussen	Some Dynamic Aspects of Focal Epilepsy
1974	Walle H. Nauta	The Problem of the Frontal Lobe: An Interpretation Based on Neuroanatomical Findings
1975	Ragnar Granit (1967)*	The Functional Role of the Muscle Spindles: Facts and Hypotheses

Year	Lecturer	Lecture title
1976	Miller Fisher	Some Clinical Pathological Aspects of Cerebral Vascular Disease
1977	Norman Geschwind	Left Inattention: A Paradox Resolved
1978	Vernon Mountcastle	A New Paradigm for Cerebral Function
1979	Brenda Milner	On the Duality of the Brain
1980	Donald Tower	Prospects and Challenge for Neurology and the Neurosciences
1982	David H. Hubel (1981)*	The Eye, the Brain, and Perception
1984	David Kuhl	Emission Imaging: An Emerging View of the Functioning Brain

* Year awarded the Nobel Prize

Notes

CHAPTER ONE

1 W. Penfield, "The Importance of the Montreal Neurological Institute," in *Neurological Biographies and Addresses* (London: Oxford University Press, 1936), 43. One of the sentences in which the pictograms appear recommends rubbing a poultice of blackfish brain upon the head to prevent grey hair. It doesn't work.

2 Ibid., 42–3.

3 Wilder Penfield, *No Man Alone: A Neurosurgeon's Life* (Toronto: Little, Brown, 1977), 63–4.

4 P. Del Río-Hortega and W. Penfield, "Cerebral Cicatrix: The Reaction of Neuroglia and Microglia to Brain Wounds," *Bulletin of the Johns Hopkins Hospital* 41 (1927): 278–303; W. Penfield, "The Radical Treatment of Traumatic Epilepsy," *Canadian Medical Association Journal* 23 (1930): 1–9.

5 Penfield, *No Man Alone*, 72.

6 Ibid., 25. Later in life, Wilder received a letter from his father explaining that the "call of the wild" drew him to the solitude of the forest. Charles Samuel Penfield to Wilder Penfield, 23 January 1913, file P142, C/D 33-5, Wilder Penfield Archive, Osler Library of the History of Medicine, McGill University, Montreal (hereafter WPA).

7 Penfield, *No Man Alone*, 15.

8 Penfield, diary 4 August 1935, file 13, box 1, Jefferson Lewis Fonds, Osler Library of the History of Medicine, McGill University, Montreal (hereafter JLF); Penfield, *No Man Alone*, xii.

9 Penfield, *No Man Alone*, 3.

10 Penfield, diary 4 August 1935, file 13, box 1, JLF.

11 Wilder Penfield to Jean Jefferson Penfield, 2 August 1904, file D-C/D 33-1, WPA.

12 Wilder Penfield to Jean Jefferson Penfield, 11 December 1910, file D-C/D 33-2, WPA.

13 Penfield, *No Man Alone*, 22.

14 Ibid.

15 E. Newton Harvey, *Edwin Grant Conklin, 1863–1952: A Biographical Memoire* (Washington: National Academy of Sciences, 1958). Conklin was associated with many learned societies in science, philosophy, and religion. He was a supporter of Darwin's theory of evolution.

16 Welsh had spent several years working in Germany with Rudolf Virchow and Julius Cohnheim. Rudolf Virchow (1821–1902), the father of modern pathology, believed that understanding the causes of disease was through scientific experimentation and by study under the microscope. Julius Cohnheim (1839–1884), Virchow's assistant, also specialized in pathological anatomy.

17 Martin wrote a textbook on biology with Thomas Huxley: *A Course of Practical Instruction in Elementary Biology* (London: Macmillan, 1875).

18 Michael Bliss, *William Osler: A Life in Medicine* (Toronto: University of Toronto Press, 1999), 168–71.

19 When the Johns Hopkins Hospital opened in 1889, Osler was physician-in-chief and professor of medicine; Welch was named professor of pathology; Halsted was professor of surgery; and Kelly, professor of gynaecology and obstetrics. Osler sought out the best physicians for his staff, basing his organization on management he had witnessed in German hospitals. Medical education at Hopkins followed Osler's respected philosophy of close bedside care for his patients, combined with well-equipped laboratories that would advance medical research in conjunction with combating disease. Osler followed the European model of clinical study. Having laboratory facilities in the hospital was crucial to gaining knowledge about medical conditions and proposing a cure for diseases.

20 Harvey, *Edward Grant Conklin*, 61.

21 Ibid., 70.

22 Penfield, *No Man Alone*, 18.

23 Ibid.

24 Abraham Flexner, *Abraham Flexner: An Autobiography* (New York: Simon and Schuster, 1960), 77.

25 Abraham Flexner, *Medical Education in the United States and Canada: A Report to the Carnegie Foundation for the Advancement of Teaching*, Carnegie Bulletin number 4 (New York: Carnegie Foundation, 1910).

26 Ibid., 235.

27 John Grier Hibben (1861–1933) had been ordained a Presbyterian minister and was a philosophy scholar before he succeeded Woodrow Wilson as president of Princeton University.

28 John Grier Hibben to Jean Jefferson Penfield, 7 February 1912, file D-C/D 33-2, WPA.

29 W. Penfield to Jean Jefferson Penfield, 7 February 1912, file D-C/D 33-2, WPA. Hibben also gave Penfield a letter of introduction to Princeton alumnus John Finney, a reputable surgeon at Johns Hopkins who was elected the first president of the American College of Surgeons.

30 Penfield, diary 11 January 1911, file 5, box 1, JLF.

31 Penfield, diary 10 November 1913, file 8, box 1, JLF.

32 John Miller Turpin Finney was a "surgeon's surgeon." His career in medicine was at Johns Hopkins Hospital, where he was assistant to the chief surgeon, William Halsted, from the time the hospital opened in 1889. Finney came from a devout Presbyterian family, as did Penfield, and coincidently suffered from the same form of acute appendicitis as Penfield's father had. Finney had also been a keen sportsman, playing

football at Princeton and at Harvard when he was in medical school. John L. Cameron, "John Miller Turpin Finney: The First President of the American College of Surgeons," *Journal of the American College of Surgeons* 208, no. 3 (2009): 327–32.

33 W. Penfield to Jean Jefferson Penfield, [26] March 1913, file D-C/D 33-2, WPA.

34 W. Penfield to Jean Jefferson Penfield, 20 October 1913, file D-C/D 33-2, WPA.

35 Penfield, diary 6 September 1914, file 8, box 1, JLF.

36 Penfield, *No Man Alone*, 33.

37 Bliss, *William Osler*, 85–6. In 1876, Osler spent the stipend he received for attending smallpox cases at the Montreal General Hospital to purchase fifteen Hartnack microscopes from Paris for the course he developed on microscopy and histology; Harvey Cushing, *The Life of Sir William Osler*, 2 vols (Oxford: Clarendon, 1925), 1:132.

38 William Feindel, "Highlights of Neurosurgery in Canada," *JAMA* 200, no. 10 (1967): 853–9.

39 William Osler, *The Principles and Practice of Medicine Designed for the Use of Practitioners and Students of Medicine* (New York: D. Appleton, 1892).

40 Bliss, *William Osler*, 185.

41 Richard L. Golden, *A History of William Osler's "The Principles and Practice of Medicine,"* Osler Library Studies in the History of Medicine, no. 8 (Montreal: Osler Library of the History of Medicine, 2004).

42 Osler had been chair of the board of electors when they appointed Professor Sherrington to the Waynflete Chair of Physiology on 7 November 1913.

43 Cushing stayed for a month during the summer of 1901, assisting Sherrington with his research on the cortical stimulation of primates, and sketching details of his techniques. Sherrington later used Cushing's drawings of the anthropoid brain when he and A.S.F. Leyton reported the results of their studies. John F. Fulton, *Harvey Cushing: A Biography*, 2 vols (Springfield, IL: Charles C. Thomas, 1946), 1:199.

44 John C. Eccles and William C. Gibson, *Sherrington: His Life and Thought* (Berlin: Springer-Verlag, 1979), 25.

45 William Feindel, "The Physiologist and the Neurosurgeon: The Enduring Influence of Charles Sherrington on the Career of Wilder Penfield," *Brain* 130, no. 11 (2007): 2758–65. "During the 'Exercises' the animals were prepared and examined on a table with a heated chamber, with the physiological changes such as nerve and muscle reflex action or blood pressure recorded on a 'smoked drum' or kymograph. A sample of such an experimental result, showing the effect of pituitary extract on the carotid artery pressure, was obtained by Penfield working with his partner Emile Holman, another Rhodes Scholar in Sherrington's class" (2759).

46 Charles S. Sherrington, *Mammalian Physiology: A Course of Practical Exercises* (Oxford: Clarendon, 1919).

47 Ibid., vi.

48 Penfield, *No Man Alone*, 36.

49 Ibid., 37.

50 Wilder Penfield, "A Medical Student's Memories of the Regius Professor," *Bulletin of the International Association of Medical Museums, Sir William Osler Memorial* 9 (1927): 387.

51 Penfield, *No Man Alone*, 39.

52 W. Penfield to Jean Jefferson Penfield, 18 March 1918, file D-C/D 33-3, WPA.

53 Fulton, *Harvey Cushing*, 1:162.

54 Mark C. Preul and William Feindel, "*The Art Is Long and the Life Short*: The Letters of Wilder Penfield and Harvey Cushing," *Journal of Neurosurgery* 95 (2001): 148.

55 Penfield, *No Man Alone*, 40.

56 Wilder Penfield, "William Osler, the Man I Remember," *Proceedings of the Charaka Club* 12 (1985): 52–8.

57 Wilder Penfield, "Alterations of the Golgi Apparatus in Nerve Cells," *Brain* 43, no. 3 (1920): 290–305.

58 Wilder Penfield and H.C. Bazett, "A Study of the Sherrington Decerebrate Animal in the Chronic as Well as the Acute Condition," *Brain* 45, no. 2 (1922): 185–265.

59 John Eccles and William Feindel, "Wilder Graves Penfield (1891–1976)," *Biographical Memoirs of Fellows of the Royal Society* 24 (1978): 472–513; William Feindel, "To Praise an Absent Friend," in *Images of the Neuro* (Montreal: Montreal Neurological Institute, 2013): 208–14.

60 Wilder Penfield, "Sir Charles Sherrington, O.M., G.B.E., F.R.S.," *Nature* 169 (1952): 698.

61 Holmes had trained in Dublin, and later in Frankfurt for two years, doing graduate work in neurology under Ludwig Edinger, from whom he "acquired the techniques which provided the basis for his anatomical and pathological studies of the next decade." Ian McDonald, "Gordon Holmes and the Neurological Heritage," *Brain* 130 (2007): 289.

62 Ibid., 289–90.

63 Wilder Penfield, "Osteogenetic Dural Endothelioma: The True Nature of Hemicraniosis," *Journal of Neurology and Psychopathology* 4 (May 1923): 27–34.

64 W. Penfield to Jean Jefferson Penfield, 3 July 1921, file D-C/D 33-3, WPA.

65 W. Penfield to Jean Jefferson Penfield, 20 May 1923, file D-C/D 33-3, WPA.

66 Penfield, *No Man Alone*, 90, 91.

67 Cajal was an eccentric but extraordinarily gifted scientist. Raised in Catalonia and stubbornly his own person, he managed to escape delinquency through the care of his physician father, who noticed his artistic talent and brought him along to illustrate autopsies. This changed the wayward direction of Cajal's youth, encouraging him to pursue a medical degree and eventually work to perfect staining techniques using silver and gold salts to examine brain tissue through the microscope. His beautiful drawings of neurons accompanied his research papers. Since Spain did not have the scientific standing of other European countries such as Germany and France, Cajal's Spanish publications were unobserved by the rest of the world, but his contribution to neurology was recognized by the Nobel committee when he received the Nobel Prize in Physiology or Medicine in 1906, along with Camillo Golgi. Eccles, *Sherrington*, 90.

68 W. Penfield, "Oligodendroglia and Its Relation to Classical Neuroglia," *Brain* 47 (1924): 430–52.

69 P. del Río-Hortega and W.G. Penfield, "Cerebral Cicatrix: The Reaction of Neuroglia and Microglia to Brain Wounds," *Bulletin of Johns Hopkins Hospital* 41 (1927): 278–303.

70 W. Penfield to Jean Jefferson Penfield, 29 May 1927, file D-C/D 33-3, WPA.

71 Edward Archibald to W. Penfield, 8 June 1927, file A/M 11-1/2, WPA.

72 W. Penfield to Edward Archibald, 17 July 1927, file A/M 11-1/2, WPA.

73 Penfield, *No Man Alone*, 134.

CHAPTER TWO

1 Edward Archibald to W. Penfield, 9 August 1927, file A/M 11-1/2, WPA.

2 W. Penfield to Archibald, 17 July 1927, file A/M 11-1/2, WPA.

3 Johannes Orth (1847–1923) was assistant to the pathologist Rudolf Virchow and succeeded him as director of the Institute of Pathology in Berlin following Virchow's death in 1902.

4 W.B Spaulding, "Charles Martin (1868–1953): A Notable Dean of McGill University," *Annals RCPSC* 24 (1991): 29–31.

5 Joseph Hanaway, Richard L. Cruess, and James Darragh, *McGill Medicine: The Second Half Century, 1885–1936* (Montreal and Kingston: McGill-Queen's University Press, 2006), 2:92, 98, 100.

6 William Osler, *A Circular Letter to Friends in Montreal*, 29 July 1919, Osler Library Archives, McGill University, Montreal. Osler also sent copies of his proposal to Sir Vincent Meredith, president of the Royal Victoria Hospital; Mr Farquhar Robertson, president of the Montreal General Hospital; and Dr Alexander Blackadder, acting dean of medicine at McGill during General Birkett's absence overseas. M.A. Entin, J. Hanaway, and T. Nimeh, "The Principal and the Dean," *Canadian Bulletin of Medical History / Bulletin canadien d'histoire de la médicine* 20 (2003): 151–70.

7 William Osler to John D. Rockefeller Jr, 28 August 1919, file 1.1.427.6.55, Rockefeller Archive Center (hereafter RAC).

8 William Osler, *The Principles and Practice of Medicine: Designed for the Use of Practitioners and Students of Medicine* (New York: D. Appleton, 1892).

9 William Feindel, *Images of the Neuro* (Montreal: Montreal Neurological Institute, 2013), 23–4.

10 Jeffrey D. Brison, *Rockefeller, Carnegie, and Canada: American Philanthropy and the Arts and Letters in Canada* (Montreal and Kingston: McGill-Queen's University Press, 2005), 24.

11 Frederick Gates to William Osler, 4 March 1902, quoted in Feindel, *Images of the Neuro*, 23.

12 William Osler to Frederick Gates, 5 March 1902, RU417 History Folder 5, Confidential Papers, box 1, McGill University Faculty of Medicine file, RAC.

13 William Osler to Frederick Gates, 26 April 1907, Harvey Cushing 1907–21, 19, F[rederick] T G[ates], box 1, RAC.

14 Cushing commented about Olser, "He seemed to have been pursued by fires" (Cushing, *Life of Sir William Osler*, 2:87), referring also to the fire at Johns Hopkins in 1904,

after which Osler received support from the Rockefellers for the hospital. Despite the Rockefellers' limit on grants to institutions outside the United States, they still donated $825,000 between 1897 and 1923 to the Baptist-sponsored Acadia University in Nova Scotia. William Feindel, "Osler and the Medico-Chirurgical Neurologists: Horsley, Cushing, and Penfield," *Journal of Neurosurgery* 99 (2003): 188–99.

15 Raymond B. Fosdick, *The Story of the Rockefeller Foundation* (New York: Harper, 1962); Rockefeller Institute for Medical Research, *The Rockefeller Institute for Medical Research: History, Organization and Equipment* (New York: Rockefeller Institute for Medical Research, 1911).

16 William Osler to John D. Rockefeller Jr, 28 August 1919, "The History of the Relations between the Rockefeller Foundation and the McGill University Faculty of Medicine between 1919 and 1925," 1.1.427.6.55, RAC.

17 George E. Vincent, president of the Rockefeller Foundation, to John W. Scane, McGill University's registrar, 24 December 1919, Rockefeller Foundation: Medical Education and Clinical Medicine, General Correspondence, RG0002, container 0068, file 01299, 1918–1924, McGill University Archives (hereafter MUA).

18 Marianne P. Fedunkiw, *Rockefeller Foundation Funding and Medical Education in Toronto, Montreal, and Halifax* (Montreal and Kingston: McGill-Queen's University Press, 2005), 94.

19 McGill University Faculty of Medicine file, 1919–1925, RAC.

20 The Opening of the Biological Building of McGill University – 5 October 1922, Campus Events RG83 c.1, *The Inaugural Address, Sir Charles Sherrington*, 5–12, MUA; Harvey Cushing, *The Life of Sir William Osler* (Oxford: Clarendon, 1925).

21 Meakins had graduated from McGill Medical School in 1904, studied at Johns Hopkins University and the New York Presbyterian Hospital, and spent two years as an intern for Charles Martin at the Royal Victoria Hospital. He was appointed director of experimental medicine at McGill in 1912. After his work during the war with the McGill Surgical Unit, he became the Christison Professor of Therapeutics at the University of Edinburgh.

22 Michael Barfoot, Christopher Lawrence, and Steven Sturdy, "The Trojan Horse: The Biochemical Laboratory of the Royal Infirmary of Edinburgh, 1921–1939," *Research Reports from the Rockefeller Archive Center*, Spring (1999): 19–21.

23 Ibid., 21.

24 Peter T. Macklem, "History of the Meakins-Christie Laboratories," in *Physiological Basis of Respiratory Disease*, ed. Qutayba Hamid, Joanne Shannon, and James Martin (Hamilton, ON: B.C. Decker, 2005), xvii.

25 Penfield, *No Man Alone*, 147.

26 Ibid.

27 Ibid., 148.

28 Ibid.

29 M.A. Entin, "Edward Archibald, Surgeon of the Royal Vic," Fontanus Monograph Series 16 (Montreal: McGill University Libraries, 2004), 74.

30 Penfield, *No Man Alone*, 153.

31 Ibid., 155.
32 W. Penfield to Edward Archibald, 16 September 1927, file A/M 11-1/2, WPA.
33 Penfield, *No Man Alone*, 63–4.
34 Ibid., 157.

CHAPTER THREE

1 M.A. Kennard, J.F. Fulton, and C.G. de Gutierrez-Mahoney, "Otfrid Foerster 1873–1941: An Appreciation," *Journal of Neurophysiology* 5 (1942): 1-17; Tze Ching Tan and P. McL. Black, "The Contributions of Otfrid Foerster (1873–1941) to Neurology and Neurosurgery," *Neurosurgery* 49, no. 5 (2001): 1231–5.

2 Klaus Joachim Zülch, *Otfrid Foerster: Physician and Naturalist (November 9, 1873–June 15, 1941)*, trans. A. Rosenauer and J.P. Evans (New York: Springer-Verlag, 1969), 3; K.J. Zülch, "Otfrid Foerster 1873–1941," *Surgical Neurology* 1 (1973): 313–16.

3 Fanya Kaplan, a member of a rival political faction, had shot Lenin in the neck in August 1918, and it was felt by some that his stroke was somehow related to that event. Although some believe that Foerster was in sympathy with this theory, Foerster himself does not mention it in his account of Lenin's last illness, and he is categorical in his conclusion: "Lenin's illness was arteriosclerosis." What Fanya Kaplan could not do with a Browning, nature did with a stroke. See O. Foerster, "Lenin's Last Illness," *Living Age*, 5 April 1924, 647–50; Robert Payne, *The Life and Death of Lenin* (Toronto: Grafton Books, 1987), 489. The cause of Lenin's death may have been neither the long-term effects of trauma to the carotid artery nor atherosclerotic stroke: it has been suggested that Lenin died from a ruptured cerebral aneurysm, and that "this finding was officially hidden … because of the prevailing theory at the time about the syphilitic origin of cerebral aneurysmsm." See J. Wronski, "Foerster's Activity and Neurosurgery in Wroclaw (Breslau)," *Zent bl Neurochir* 52 (1991): 153–63.

4 Upon his return to Breslau, Foerster joined Wernicke's clinic and helped in the preparation of *Atlas des Gehirns*, Wernicke's atlas of the human brain. See Kennard, Fulton, and de Gutierrez-Mahoney, "Otfrid Foerster," 2.

5 Pierre Marie and Jules Dejerine were about to be embroiled in a controversy that resounded loudly in French medical circles, regarding the role of Broca's area. Also, Dejerine was Babinski's rival for Charcot's chair at the University of Paris, which was awarded to Dejerine.

6 Kennard, Fulton, and de Gutierrez-Mahoney, "Otfrid Foerster," 1–2. In Switzerland, Foerster devoted himself to the rehabilitation of brain-damaged patients, then a sadly neglected field. So successful was Foerster at rehabilitating his patients that Wernicke would exclaim, "I have an assistant who makes the lame walk and the blind see." See Carlos Guillermo de Gutiérrez-Mahoney, "Otfrid Foerster: 1873–1941," *Archives of Neurology and Psychiatry* 46 (1941): 914.

7 De Gutiérrez-Mahoney, "Otfrid Foerster," 914. Only much later, in 1934, did Foerster enjoy the support of the Rockefeller Foundation, which financed an institute of brain research in Breslau, with Foerster its director. It was in such settings that Foerster

made his great contribution to the surgical treatment of epilepsy. Foerster's institute was destroyed without a trace – save for a few faded photographs – during the Second World War.

8 Kennard, Fulton, and de Gutierrez-Mahoney, "Otfrid Foerster," 4.

9 Wilder Penfield, "The Mechanism of Cicatricial Contraction of the Brain," *Brain* 50, nos 3–4 (1927): 499–517; Wilder Penfield and Richard C. Buckley, "Punctures of the Brain: The Factors Concerned in Gliosis and in Cicatricial Contraction," *Archives of Neurology and Psychiatry* 20, no. 1 (1928): 1–13.

10 Penfield, *No Man Alone*, 164.

11 Del Río-Hortega and Penfield, "Cerebral Cicatrix," 278–303.

12 Wilder Penfield, "Meningocerebral Adhesions: A Histological Study of the Results of Cerebral Incision and Cranioplasty," *Surgery, Gynecology and Obstetrics* 39 (1924): 803–10; Del Río-Ortega and Penfield, "Cerebral Cicatrix," 298–9; Penfield, "Mechanism of Cicatricial Contraction," 499–517.

13 Penfield, "Mechanism of Cicatricial Contraction," 514–15.

14 Otfrid Foerster, "Encephalographiesche Erfahrungen," *Zestchr. f. d. ges. Neurolog Psychiat* 94 (1925): 512–84; O. Foerster and W. Penfield, "Der narbenzug am und im gehirn bei traumatischer epilepsie in seine bedeutung fur das zustandekommen der anfalle und fur therapeutische bekampfung derselben," *Zestchr. f. d. ges. Neurolog Psychiat* 125 (1930): 475–572; W. Penfield, "The Radical Treatment of Traumatic Epilepsy and Its Rationale," *Canadian Medical Association Journal* 23 (1930): 189–97; O. Foerster and W. Penfield, "The Structural Basis of Traumatic Epilepsy and Results of Radical Operation," *Brain* 53 (1930): 99–119.

15 Foerster and Penfield, "Structural Basis of Traumatic Epilepsy," 99–102.

16 Wilder Penfield, "The Evidence for a Cerebral Vascular Mechanism in Epilepsy," *Annals of Internal Medicine* 7, no. 3 (1933): 303–10. A putative cortico-vascular mechanism in the onset of epileptic seizures was disproved by Joseph P. Evans in his doctoral dissertation, "A Study of Cerebral Cicatrix," in which he studied the effects of ischemia by applying a silver clip to the main branches of the middle cerebral artery. The period of post-occlusion observation lasted up to nine months, and the purpose of the experiment was to try to produce elements of Penfield's meningocerebral cicatrix. Penfield had stressed that connective tissue fibers within the cicatrix pulled it towards the meninges, and, at the same time, applied traction on the arteries encased within the scar. As these were anastomosed with the cortical arteries of the surrounding cortex, Penfield hypothesized that traction produced hypoxemia and thus contributed to the onset of seizures. Evans, however, was forced to concede that this was not the case. After observing that the central core of the infarcted tissue became a cystic cavity, and that the periphery of this cavity was rich in chromic inflammatory cells and gliosis, he observed "the almost complete absence of connective tissue elements from the cyst wall and … the absence of connective tissue infiltration into the adjacent tissue." Further, there was no infiltration of new blood vessels; and the dilatation of the ipsilateral ventricle did not result from traction." Rather, Evans states, "It is well to emphasize that atrophy alone may cause a shift of the ventricular system when little or no scar tissue is present." Thus,

rather than supporting Penfield's hypothesis, Evans's results constituted a major challenge to it. See Joseph P. Evans, "A Study of Cerebral Cicatrix" (PhD diss., McGill University, 1937), 74–5; J.N. Petersen and J.P. Evans, "The Anatomical End Result of Cerebral Arterial Occlusion: An Experimental and Clinical Correlation," *Transactions of the American Neurological Association* 63 (1937): 88–93.

17 Otfrid Foerster, "Die pathogenese des epileptischen Krampfanfalles," *Deutsche Zeitschrift für Nervenheilkunde* 94, no. 1 (1926): 15–53; Foerster and Penfield, "Structural Basis of Traumatic Epilepsy," 99–119.

18 J. Wro ski, "Foerster's Activity and Neurosurgery in Wrocław (Breslau)," *Zentralbl Neurochir* 52, no. 4 (1991), 154–63; N. Piotrowska and P. Winkler, "Otfrid Foerster, the Great Neurologist and Neurosurgeon from Breslau (Wrocław): His Influence on Early Neurosurgeons and Legacy to Present-Day Neurosurgery," *Journal of Neurosurgery* 107, no. 2 (2007): 451–6.

19 P. Bucy, "Neurosurgery in Darkness," *Surgical Neurology* 9, no. 6 (1978): 360.

20 P.C. Bucy, "Otfrid Foerster 1873–1941," *Surgical Neurology* 1 (1973): 316.

21 De Gutiérrez-Mahoney, "Otfrid Foerster," 916.

22 Bucy, "Neurosurgery in Darkness," 360.

23 Zülch, "Otfrid Foerster," 313–16.

24 O. Foerster and H. Altenburger, "Elektrobiologische Vorgänge an der menschlichen Hirnrinde," *Deutsche Zeitschrift für Nervenheilkunde* 135, nos 5–6 (1935): 277–88.

25 O. Foerster and W. Penfield, "Der Narbenzug am und in Gherin bei traumatischer Elilepsie in seiner Bedeutung fur das Zustandekommen der Angalle und fur die therapeurische Bekampgung derselbe," *Zeitschfift fur die gesamte Neurologie und Psychiatrie* 125 (1930): 475–572.

26 Zülch, *Otfrid Foerster,* 9.

27 Penfield, "Treatment of Traumatic Epilepsy," 189. Oskar Vogt had studied with Dejerine in Paris, and his wife, Cécile Mugnier, had studied with Dejerine's rival, Pierre Marie. Fortunately, this rivalry did not affect their scientific work or their family life. Their daughter, Marguerite, immigrated to America after the war and worked with Max Delbrück and Renato Delbucco, both Nobel laureates.

Oscar and Cécile Vogt were interested in correlating cortical function to the organization of the nerve cells within its layers, and produced one of the first human cytoarchitectomic maps. See Susan Forsburg, "Remembering Marguerite Vogt," *Women in Biology: The Internet Launch Pages,* last modified 2011, http://www-bcf. usc.edu/~forsburg/women/vogt.html.

28 I. Klatzo, *Cécile and Oskar Vogt: The Visionaries of Modern Neuroscience,* Acta Neurochirurgica Supplements, 80 (New York: Springer-Verlag Wein, 2002), 21.

29 Foerster and Penfield, "Structural Basis of Traumatic Epilepsy," 99–119; W. Penfield, "The Radical Treatment of Traumatic Epilepsy and Its Rationale," *Canadian Medical Association Journal* 23, no. 2 (1930): 189–97.

30 H.C., "Obituary, Professor O. Foerster," *British Medical Journal* 2 (1941): 634..

31 Kennard, Fulton, and de Gutierrez-Mahoney, "Otfrid Foerster 1873–1941," 1–17.

32 R. Brain, "Professor O. Foerster," *British Medical Journal* 2 (1941): 634.

CHAPTER FOUR

1   W. Penfield, "An Address on the Field of Neurosurgery," *Canadian Medical Association Journal* 19 (1928): 654–65.

2   L. Meakins and W.E. Gallie, "Edward William Archibald," *Canadian Medical Association Journal* 54 (1946): 194–7.

3   Joseph Hanaway, Richard Cruess, and James Darragh, *McGill Medicine* (Montreal and Kingston: McGill-Queen's University Press, 2006), 2:122–9.

4   M.A. Entin, "Edward Archibald, Surgeon of the Royal Vic," Fontanus Monograph Series 16 (Montreal: McGill University Libraries, 2004), 2.

5   C.K. Russel and V. Horsley, "Note on Apparent Re-representation in the Cerebral Cortex of the Type of Sensory Representation as It Exists in the Spinal Cord," *Brain* 29 (1906): 137–52.

6   Hanaway, Cruess, and Darragh, *McGill Medicine*, 2:122–9.

7   C.K. Russel, "Tumour of the Temporo-Sphenoidal Lobe and 'Dreamy States,'" *McGill Journal* 38 (1909): 3–7; W. Feindel, "Temporal Lobe Seizures," *Handbook of Clinical Neurology*, ed. O. Magnus and A.M. Lorentz de Haas (Amsterdam: North-Holland Publishing, 1974), 17:87–106.

8   E. Archibald, *Surgical Affections and Wounds of the Brain*, in *American Practice of Surgery*, ed. J.D. Bryant and A.H. Buck (New York: William Wood, 1908), 5:3–369; H. Cushing, *Surgery of the Head*, in *Surgery, Its Principles and Practice*, ed. W.W. Keen (Philadelphia: W.B. Saunders, 1920), 3:17–276.

9   "Dear Archibald, I wrote you last week acknowledging the big monograph, which I appreciated very much; so far as my chirurgical knowledge went it seemed first class, and I must say I was gratified to see a McGill man entrusted with so important a section. I knew your brother Sam would hold the position, it is a splendid one in every way. I hope to see you over this summer. With kind regards, Sincerely yours, [Signed] W Osler." See folder 3, box 36, Edward William Archibald Fonds, Osler Library of the History of Medicine, McGill University.

10 E. Archibald, "Puncture of the Corpus Callosum," *Canadian Medical Association Journal* 3 (1913): 451–6.

11 E. Archibald, "A Brief Survey of Some Experiences in the Surgery of the Present War," *Canadian Medical Association Journal* 6 (1916): 775–95; Archibald, "Gunshot Wounds of the Brain," *Canadian Medical Association Journal* 10 (1920): 778–9.

12 Hanaway, Cruess, and Darragh, *McGill Medicine*, 2:123.

13 File A/M 1-1/11, WPA. Penfield was tempted by an offer to consolidate neurology and neurosurgery at the University of Pennsylvania upon the retirement of Charles Frazier, the distinguished neurosurgeon. Penfield finally decided to "throw in [his] lot with McGill," and Francis Grant succeeded Frazier. See Penfield, *No Man Alone*, 284–310.

14 Ibid.

15 Ibid.

16 File A/M 11-1/3, WPA.

17 Archibald contracted pulmonary tuberculosis in 1901 and spent a year at the Trudeau Sanatorium in Saranac Lake, New York.

18 File C/SW 12, WPA.

19 Here Penfield does not do full justice to Archibald's treatise, which extended far be-
    yond head injury to cover the whole of neurosurgery as practised at the time.
    Archibald's section occupies 377 pages of volume 5 in Bryant and Buck's multivolume
    textbook of surgery. Beside head injury, Archibald discusses pathologies of neuro-
    surgical interest, such as meningiomas, gliomas, acoustic neuromas, and pituitary
    macroadenomas, to list only the tumours covered in his section. Archibald illustrates
    his text with excellent photographs of whole brain specimens from the Royal Victo-
    ria Hospital Museum. There are dramatic illustrations of infectious diseases affect-
    ing the skull and brain, and most notably of syphilitic involvement of the skull.
    Common neurosurgical conditions affecting children are also treated. A similar trea-
    tise on neurosurgery in Lewis's textbook of surgery, by Harvey Cushing himself, was
    published a year later. To many scholars, Archibald's book is more practical and bet-
    ter illustrated than Cushing's.

20 Montreal Neurological Institute, *Annual Report* (hereafter MNI, *MNI AR*), 1946–47
    (Montreal: McGill University, 1947), 9. Emphasis added.

21 Royal Victoria Hospital, *Thirty-Sixth Annual Report for the Year Ended 31st December
    1929* (hereafter RVH, *AR 1929*) (Montreal: Royal Victoria Hospital, 1930), 96–7.

22 Ibid.

23 Ibid.

24 File A/N 18-1/2, WPA.

25 William Feindel, like many others, benefited from Madeleine Ottman's generosity, as
    he later recalled: "When [I] first arrived at the Neuro as a Fellow in the 1940's [I] was
    surprised to see sophisticated Zeiss microscopes in [my] study cubicle on the sixth
    floor. More Zeiss microscopes, [I] saw, were available in the pathology laboratory. [I]
    was intrigued by the little plaque with the name Madeleine Ottman on each micro-
    scope. She was [related to someone] who had been operated on several years earlier
    by Dr Penfield … She was the first person who gave Dr Penfield a donation for his
    research without being asked. When she died three or four years later, she left $50,000
    to the Neuro, so Dr Penfield bought microscopes for the pathology lab."

26 W. Penfield and W.V. Cone, "Neuroglia and Microglia (The Metallic Methods)," in
    Handbook of Microscopical Technique, ed. C.E. McClung, 359–88 (New York: Paul B.
    Hoeber, 1929).

27 "Jones, Ottiwell Wood Jr," in *The Society of Neurological Surgeons* (Winston-Salem,
    NC: Wake Forest University Press, 2001), 486.

28 Ibid.

29 "Jones"; H. Rosegay, "A History of Neurological Surgery at the University of Califor-
    nia, San Francisco 1912–1995," UCSF Department of Neurological Surgery, 2012,
    http://neurosurgery.ucsf.edu/index.php/about_us_history.html.

30 File C/SW 7-1b, WPA.

31 L.J. Rubenstein, "Dorothy Stuart Russell 27 June 1895–19 October 1983," *Journal of
    Neuropathology* 142 (1984): iii–v; J.F. Geddes, "A Portrait of "The Lady": A Life of
    Dorothy Russell," *Journal of the Royal Society of Medicine* 90 (1997): 455–61; Geddes,
    "Why Do We Remember Dorothy Russell?," *Neuropathology and Applied Neurobi-
    ology* 24 (1998): 268–70; Queen Mary, University of London, "Professor Dorothy

Russell, LHMC Alumna, Pathology Institute Director," *Women at Queen Mary Online: A Virtual Exhibition*, http://www.women.qmul.ac.uk/virtual/women/atoz/russell.htm.

32 D.S. Russell, "Intravital Staining of Microglia with Trypan Blue," *American Journal of Pathology* 5 (1929): 451–8.

33 D.S. Russell, *Observations on the Pathology of Hydrocephalus* (London: Her Majesty's Stationery Office, the Medical Research Council, 1949); D.S. Russell and L.J. Rubenstein, *Pathology of Tumours of the Nervous System* (London: Edward Arnold, 1959).

34 J.P. Evans, "Exciting Beginnings," *Canadian Medical Association Journal* 116 (1977): 1367; RVH, *AR 1928*, ix, 85.

35 Evans, "Exciting Beginnings."

36 Ibid.

37 J.P. Evans, "A Study of the Effects of Cerebral Wounds and Cerebral Excisions: With a Review of the Literature of Post-Traumatic Epilepsy" (master's thesis, McGill University, 1930); Evans was also awarded a PhD in 1937. See Evans, "Study of Cerebral Cicatrix."

38 K. Kristiensen, "Arne Torkildsen (1899–1968)," *Journal of Neurological Science* 7 (1968): 605–9.

39 A. Torkildsen, "The Gross Anatomy of the Lateral Ventricles," *Journal of Anatomy* 68 (1934): 480–91.

40 Leonardo's nomenclature reflects the medieval cell doctrine, according to which, what we refer to as neurological and cognitive functions were located within the ventricles, which were considered "cells." The lateral ventricles were considered as one cell and referred to as the anterior cell, which received input from the five common senses – sight, smell, audition, taste, and touch. These sensory impressions were transferred to the second cell – our third ventricle – for analysis. The impressions felt to warrant it were committed to memory within the third cell, our fourth ventricle. See Ritchie Calder, *Leonardo & the Age of the Eye* (London: Heinemann, 1970), 181.

41 Torkildsen, "Gross Anatomy of the Lateral Ventricles."

42 A. Torkildsen and W. Penfield, "Ventriculographic Interpretations," *Archives of Neurology and Psychiatry* 30 (1933): 1011–21; A. Torkildsen, "A New Palliative Operation in Cases of Inoperable Occlusion of the Sylvian Aqueduct," *Acta chirurgica Scandinavica* 82 (1939): 117; W. Penfield, "The Torkildsen Procedure for Inoperable Occlusion of the Sylvian Aqueduct," *Canadian Medical Association Journal* 47 (1942): 62–3.

43 I.M. Tarlov, "The Structure and Functional Relationship of the Cerebrospinal Nerve Root" (master's thesis, McGill University, 1932); Tarlov, "Structure of the Nerve Root: I. Nature of the Junction between the Central and the Peripheral Nervous System," *Archives of Neurology and Psychiatry* 37, no. 3 (1937): 555–83; Tarlov, "Structure of the Nerve Root: II. Differentiation of Sensory from Motor Roots; Observations on Identification of Function in Roots of Mixed Cranial Nerves," *Archives of Neurology and Psychiatry* 37, no. 6 (1937): 1338–5; Tarlov, "Structure of the Filum Terminale," *Archives of Neurology and Psychiatry* 40, no. 1 (1938): 1–17; Tarlov, "Cysts, Perineurial, of the Sacral Roots: Another Cause, Removable, of Sciatic Pain," *Journal of the American Medical Association* 138, no. 10 (1948): 740–4.

44 Penfield thought that MCC caused a mechanical, reflex vasoconstriction, that rendered the surrounding cortex ischemic and epileptogenic. Thus, Gage proposed interrupting the sympathetic neural supply to the cerebral vasculature by severing the greater petrosal nerve and observing its effects on an animal's susceptibility to experimental epilepsy. See E.L. Gage, "The Effects of Vasomotor Nerve Section on Experimental Epilepsy" (master's thesis, McGill University, 1931), 5–7.

45 W. Penfield and L. Gage, "Cerebral Localization of Epileptic Manifestations," *Archives of Neurology and Psychiatry* 30, no. 4 (1933): 709–27.

46 W. Penfield and E. Boldrey, "Somatic Motor and Sensory Representations in the Cerebral Cortex of Man Studied by Electrical Stimulation," *Brain* 60 (1937): 389–43; W. Penfield and T. Rasmussen, *The Cerebral Cortex of Man* (New York: Macmillan, 1950).

47 Penfield and Gage, "Cerebral Localization of Epileptic Manifestations," 727.

48 RVH, *AR 1929*, 96–7; RVH, *AR 1930*, 88–9.

49 RVH, *AR 1931*, 88–91.

50 For details concerning Thomas Hoen's stay in Montreal, see D. Goulet, *Histoire de la Neurochirurgie au Québec* (Montreal: Carte Blanche, 2014), 69–76.

51 The ebullient Joseph Ransohoff, a major figure in American neurosurgery, succeeded Hoen in this position. Hoen is reputed to have had "meticulous technique, a steady hand, sure judgment and good instincts." B.S. Ray, "The Development of Neurosurgery in New York City," *Bulletin of the New York Academy of Medicine* 55 (1979): 932. Hoen returned to the MNI periodically as an invited speaker.

52 C. Russel and D.W. Stavraky, "The Syndrome of the Posterior Inferior Cerebellar Artery (with Two Illustrative Cases)," *Canadian Medical Association Journal* 30 (1934): 358–64.

53 C.G. Drake and G.W. Stavraky, "An Extension of the 'Law of Denervation' to Afferent Neurons," *Journal of Neurophysiology* 11 (1948): 229–38.

54 RVH, *AR 1932*, 81–2.

55 W.T. Grant and W.V. Cone, "Graduated Jugular Compression in the Lumbar Manometric Test for Spinal Subarachnoid Block," *Archives of Neurology and Psychiatry* 32 (1934): 1194–1201; H.M. Keith, "Experimentally Produced Convulsions Effect on Thujone Convulsions on Insulin and of Variations in Water Content of Brain," *Archives of Neurology and Psychiatry* 33 (1935): 353–9; H. Keith and G. Stavraky, "Experimental Convulsions Induced by Administration of Thujone: A Pharmacologic Study of the Influence of the Autonomic Nervous System on These Convulsions," *Archives of Neurology and Psychiatry* 34 (1935): 1022–40; W. Penfield, "Wilbur Sprong 1902–1934," *Neurological Biographies and Addresses*, 159.

56 W. Sprong, "Disappearance of Blood from Cerebrospinal Fluid in Traumatic Subarachnoid Hemorrhage: Ineffectiveness of Repeated Lumbar Punctures," *Journal of Surgery, Gynecology and Obstetrics* 58 (1934): 705–10.

57 W. Sprong, "Santiago Ramón y Cajal 1852–1934," *Neurological Biographies and Addresses*, 151–8.

58 Penfield, "Wilbur Sprong 1902–1934."

59 Ibid., 159.

60 RVH, *AR 1933*, 13–14, 17. The creation of the Montreal Neurological Institute would

not have been possible without the dedication of Sir Arthur Curie, who convinced the Board of Directors of the Royal Victoria Hospital of its necessity, obtained support for its hospital function from the province and the city, and raised the necessary funds from generous donors, to match funds from the Rockefeller Foundation. See W. Penfield, *The Difficult Art of Giving: The Epic of Alan Gregg* (Boston: Little, Brown, 1967); and Penfield, *No Man Alone*.

61 Frazier wrote a chapter on the surgery of cranial and peripheral nerves in Bryant and Buck's multi-volume treatise on surgery, which followed Edward Archibald's massive chapter on cranial neurosurgery. C.H. Frazier, "Surgery of the Cranial Nerves," in *American Practice of Surgery*, vol. 5, ed. J.D. Bryant and A.H. Buck, 370–418 (New York: William Wood, 1908).

62 W. Cone, C. Russel, and R.U. Harwood, "Lead as a Possible Cause of Multiple Sclerosis," *Archives of Neurology and Psychiatry* 31 (1934): 236–63; A.H. Gordon, "Dr F.H. MacKay: An Appreciation," *Canadian Medical Association Journal* 48 (1948): 393–4; O.R. Hyndman and W. Penfield, "Agenesis of the Corpus Callosum: Its Recognition by Ventriculography," *Archives of Neurology and Psychiatry* 37 (1937): 1251–70; Hyndman later joined Ralph Stuck, a fellow house officer, in the Department of Neurosurgery at the University of Colorado: G. Vander Ark, K. Lillehei, H. Fieger, H. McClintock, and J. Ogsbury, "Cyber Museum Featured Exhibit: The History of Neurosurgery in Colorado," Cyber Museum of Neurosurgery, http://www.neurosurgery.org/cybermuseum/coloradohistory/index.html.

63 RVH, *AR 1933*, 84–6.

64 W. Penfield, "Needle Pulling Forceps," *Journal of the American Medical Association* 91 (1928): 1187; Penfield, "Further Modification of Del Río-Hortega's Method of Staining Oligodendroglia," *American Journal of Pathology* 6 (1930): 445–7.

65 W. Penfield, "The Operative Treatment of Spontaneous Intracranial Haemorrhage," *Canadian Medical Association Journal* 28 (1933): 369–72.

66 W. Penfield and W. Cone, "Spina Bifida and Cranium Bifidum Results of Plastic Repair of Meningocele and Myelomeningocele by a New Method," *Journal of the American Medical Association* 98 (1932): 454–60.

67 W. Penfield and A. Young, "Nature of Von Recklinghausen's Disease and the Tumours Associated with It," *Archives of Neurology and Psychiatry* 23 (1930): 320–44; W. Penfield, "Tumors of the Sheaths of the Nervous System," *Archives of Neurology and Psychiatry* 27 (1932): 1298–1309; Penfield, "Tumors of the Sheaths of the Nervous System," in *Cytology and Cellular Pathology of the Nervous System*, ed. W. Penfield, 955–990 (New York, P.B. Hoeber, 1932); Penfield, "Classification of Brain Tumors and Its Practical Application," *British Medical Journal* 1 (1931): 337–42; Penfield, "The Classification of Gliomas and Neuroglia Cell Types," *Archives of Neurology and Psychiatry* 26 (1031): 745–53; A. Elvidge, W. Penfield, and W. Cone, "The Gliomas of the Central Nervous System: A Study of Two Hundred and Ten Cases," *Proceedings of the Association for Research in Nervous and Mental Diseases* 16 (1935): 107–81.

68 Penfield, "Classification of Brain Tumors and Its Practical Application."

69 K.H. Welch, "A Morphological Study of Human Glioblastoma Multiforme Transplanted to Guinea Pigs" (master's thesis, McGill University, 1947); H.D. Garretson,

"The Growth Characteristics of Glioblastoma Multiforme in the Anterior Chamber of the Guinea Pig Eye" (master's thesis, McGill University, 1968).

70 W. Penfield, ed., *Cytology and Cellular Pathology of the Nervous System* (New York: Paul B. Hoeber, 1932).

71 W. Penfield, "Diencephalic Autonomic Epilepsy," *Archives of Neurology and Psychiatry* 22 (1929): 358–74; Penfield, "The Influence of the Diencephalon and Hypophesis upon General Autonomic Function," *Canadian Medical Association Journal* 30 (1934): 589–98.

72 File C/SW 7-1b, WPA.

CHAPTER FIVE

1 R. Leblanc, "Fedor Krause: Pioneer Seizure Surgeon," *Epilepsia* 31 (1990): 616; W. Feindel, R. Leblanc, and A.N. de Almeida, "Epilepsy Surgery: Historical Highlights 1909–2009," *Epilepsia* 50, supplement 3 (2009): 131–51.

2 W. Penfield, "Epilepsy and Surgical Therapy," *Archives of Neurology and Psychiatry* 36 (1936): 449–84.

3 Penfield describes the care taken before a decision was made to ligate an artery putatively involved in the genesis of a patient's intra-operative seizure: "After the convulsion was over, however, it was observed that there were anaemic spots … over the cortex. … It seemed likely that this artery supplied in a general way the area of anemic spots. After consultation with Dr Russel, Dr Cobb, Dr Geyelin and Dr Spielmeyer. It was concluded that this artery could be ligated without fear of permanent paralysis or aphasia. Dr Cone was more fearful of aphasia. The artery was ligated in two points and the intervening artery removed. It was then found that the patient could not speak." The patient eventually recovered during his convalescence in hospital. (MNI Archives.)

4 Ibid.; W. Penfield and T. Erickson, *Epilepsy and Cerebral Localization: A Study of the Mechanism, Treatment and Prevention of Epileptic Seizures (with Special Chapters by Herbert H. Jasper and M.R. Harrower-Erickson)* (Springfield, IL: Charles C. Thomas, 1941).

5 See Penfield's draft of his Hughlings Jackson lecture in chapter 7.

6 O. Foerster and W. Spielmeyer, "Die Pathogenese des epileptischen Krampfanfalles," *Deutsche Zeitschrift für Nervenheilkunde* 94, no. 1 (1926): 15. Cited in W. Penfield, "The Evidence for a Cerebral Vascular Mechanism in Epilepsy," *Annals of Internal Medicine* 7 (1933): 301–10.

7 W. Penfield, "The Mechanism of Cicatricial Contraction in the Brain," *Brain* 50 (1927): 499–517; Penfield, "The Radical Treatment of Traumatic Epilepsy and Its Rationale," *Canadian Medical Association Journal* 23 (1930): 189–97.

8 Penfield, "Radical Treatment of Traumatic Epilepsy and Its Rationale," 196.

9 Penfield, "Mechanism of Cicatricial Contraction in the Brain," 1927; del Río-Hortega and Penfield, "Cerebral Cicatrix," 278–303; W. Penfield and R.C. Buckley, "Punctures of the Brain: Factors Concerned in Gliosis and in Cicatricial Contraction," *Archives of Neurology & Psychiatry* 20 (1928): 1–13.

10 W. Penfield, "Intracerebral Vascular Nerves," *Archives of Neurology and Psychiatry* 27 (1932): 30–40.

11 Ibid.

12 Ibid.

13 Ibid., 15.

14 Penfield met Cobb when they were both students at Johns Hopkins, he as a medical student, Cobb as Adolf Meyer's graduate student. Cobb went on to Harvard, where he did a surgical internship with Harvey Cushing and later was instrumental in the introduction of Dilantin for the treatment of epilepsy. Cobb and Penfield remained life-long friends, and when Cobb died, Penfield gave his eulogy at Harvard Chapel. W. Penfield, "Hail and Fairwell," *Archives of Neurology* 19 (1968): 233–4.

15 J. Chorobski, "Part 1: A Vasodilator Nervous Pathway to the Cerebral Vessels from the Central Nervous system. Part 2: On the Occurrence of Afferent Nerve Fibers in the Internal Carotid Plexus" (master's thesis, McGill University, 1932); S. Cobb and J.E. Finesinger, "Cerebral Circulation XIX: The Vagal Pathway of the Vasodilator Impulses," *Archives of Neurology and Psychiatry* 28 (1932): 1234–56; J. Chorobski and W. Penfield, "Cerebral Vasodilator Nerves and Their Pathway from the Medulla Oblongata with Observations on the Pial and Intracerebral Vascular Plexus," *Archives of Neurology and Psychiatry* 28 (1932): 1257–89.

16 Cobb and Finesinger, "Cerebral Circulation XIX."

17 File C/D 13, WPA.

18 Cobb and Finesigner, "Cerebral Circulation XIX"; Chorobski and Penfield, "Cerebral Vasodilator Nerves and Their Pathway from the Medulla Oblongata."

19 File C/SW 7, WPA.

20 Chorobski, "Vasodilator Nervous Pathway."

21 W. Penfield, "The Evidence for a Cerebral Vascular Mechanism in Epilepsy," *Annals of Internal Medicine* 7 (1933): 301–10.

22 Ibid.

23 Florey was elevated to the peerage and received the Nobel Prize in Medicine or Physiology in 1945, with Sir Ernst Boris Chain and Sir Alexander Fleming, for his role in the synthesis of penicillin.

24 H.W. Florey, "Microscopical Observations on the Circulation of the Blood in the Cerebral Cortex," *Brain* 48 (1925): 43–64.

25 Ray, "Development of Neurosurgery in New York City," 931–2.

26 M. Riser, P. Mériel, and J. Planques, "Les spasmes vasculaires en neurologie. Etude clinique et expérimentale," *Encéphale* 26 (1931): 501–28.

27 F.A. Echlin, "Cerebral Ischaemia and Its Relation to Epilepsy" (master's thesis, McGill University, 1939).

28 Ibid.; F.A. Echlin, "Vasospasm and Focal Cerebral Ischemia: An Experimental Study," *Archives of Neurology and Psychiatry* 47 (1942): 36.

29 Ray, "Development of Neurosurgery"; Echlin and Hoen took turns caring for Geoffrey Jefferson during his convalescence from a serious heart attack suffered while in New York City. It would be Jefferson's last contact with the MNI.

30 F.A. Echlin, "Spasm of Basilar and Vertebral Arteries Caused by Experimental Subarachnoid Hemorrhage," *Journal of Neurosurgery* 23 (1965): 1–11.

31 F.A. Echlin, "Experimental Vasospasm, Acute and Chronic, Due to Blood in the Subarachnoid Space," *Journal of Neurosurgery* 35 (1971): 646–56.

32 Mississippi Conference on Subarachnoid Hemorrhage and Cerebrovascular Spasm, *Subarachnoid Hemorrhage and Cerebrovascular Spasm*, ed. Robert R. Smith and James T. Robertson (Springfield, IL: Charles C. Thomas, 1975).

33 W. Penfield, R.A. Lende, and T. Rasmussen, "Manipulation Hemiplegia: An Untoward Complication in the Surgery of Focal Epilepsy," *Journal of Neurosurgery* 18 (1961): 771.

34 R.A. Lende, "Local Spasm in Cerebral Arteries" (master's thesis, McGill University, 1956).

35 R.A. Lende, "Local Spasm in Cerebral Arteries," *Journal of Neurosurgery* 17 (1960): 90–103.

36 Lende had been preceded in Colorado by MNI fellows Ralph Stuck and Olan Hyndman, who had taken positions at the Denver General Hospital in 1939 and 1943, respectively; and by Maitland Baldwin and Keasley Welch, who had succeeded each other as chair of the Department of Neurosurgery at the University of Colorado. See Vander Ark et al., "Cyber Museum Featured Exhibit."

37 R.A. Lende and C.N. Woolsey, "Sensory and Motor Localization in Cerebral Cortex of Porcupine (Erethizon dorsatum)," *Journal of Neurophysiology* 19 (1956): 544–63.

38 "Perot, Phanor L. Jr," in *The Society of Neurological Surgeons* (Winston-Salem, NC: Wake Forest University Press, 2001), 300.

39 S.N. Chou, "Richard A. Lende Winter Neurosurgery Conference," *Surgical Neurology* 39 (1993): 243–6.

40 "Odom, Guy Leary," in *The Society of Neurological Surgeons* (Winston-Salem, NC: Wake Forest University Press, 2001), 292.

41 J. Kapp, S.J. Mahaley Jr, and G.L. Odom, "Cerebral Arterial Spasm. Parts 1–3," *Journal of Neurosurgery* 29 (1968): 331–56.

42 E.W. Peterson, B.S. Kent, and W.V. Cone, "Intracranial Pressure in the Human at Altitude," *Archives of Neurology and Psychiatry* 52 (1944): 520–5.

43 Henneman was interested mainly in the neurons and interneurons of the spinal cord. He is chiefly remembered for Henneman's law, which relates the function of spinal neurons to their size.

44 E.W. Peterson, J. Valberg, and D.S. Whittingham, "Electrically Induced Thrombosis of the Cavernous Sinus in the Treatment of Carotid Cavernous Fistula," in International Congress of Neurological Surgery, *Abstracts of Papers, Scientific Exhibits and Motion Pictures*, ed. Charles G. Drake and Roger Duvoisin (Amsterdam: Excerpta Medica Foundation, 1969).

45 E.W. Peterson, J. Metuzale, and D.H. Johnson, "The Relief of Cerebral Vasospasm by Topically Applied Ethylene Diamine Tetra-Acetic Acid (EDTA)," *Excerpta Medica, International Congress Series* 193 (1969): 72; E.W. Peterson, R. Searle, F. Mandy and R. Leblanc, "A Chronic Experimental Model for the Production of Subarachnoid Haemorrhage," *British Journal of Surgery* 60 (1973): 316–17.

46 E.W. Peterson, R. Searle, F. Mandy, and R. Leblanc, "Reversal of Cerebral Vasospasm," *Lancet* 301, no. 7818 (1973): 1513; E.W. Peterson, R. Searle, F. Mandy, and R. Leblanc, "The Reversal of Experimental Vasospasm by Dibutiryl-3'-5'-Adenosine Monophos-

phate," *Journal of Neurosurgery* 39 (1973): 730–34; E.W. Peterson, R. Leblanc, and F. Lebel, "Cyclic Adenosine Monophosphate Antagonism of Prostaglandin Induced Vasospasm," *Surgical Neurology* 4 (1975): 490–6.

47 E.W. Peterson and R. Leblanc, "A Theory of the Mechanism of Cerebral Vasospasm and Its Reversal: The Role of Calcium and Cyclic-AMP," *Canadian Journal of Neurological Sciences* 3 (1976): 223–6.

48 R. Leblanc, "Calcium Antagonism in Cerebral Vasospasm" (master's thesis, McGill University, 1984); Feindel, Yamamoto, and Leon Wolfe, the director of the Donner Laboratory of Experimental Neurochemistry, had studied the role of prostaglandins in the genesis and treatment of cerebral vasospasm in the early 1970s. See Y.L. Yamamoto, W. Feindel, L.S. Wolfe, H. Katoh, and C.P. Hodge, "Effects of Prostaglandins on Cerebral Blood Flow," *European Neurology* 6 (1971–2): 144–52; Y. Yamamoto, W. Feindel, L.S. Wolfe, H. Katoh, and C.P. Hodge, "Experimental Vasoconstriction of Cerebral Arteries by Prostaglandins," *Journal of Neurosurgery* 37 (1972): 385–97.

49 R. Leblanc, W. Feindel, Y.L. Yamamoto, J.G. Milton, and M.M. Frojmovic, "Reversal of Acute Cerebral Vasospasm by the Calcium Antagonist Verapamil," *Canadian Journal of Neurological Science* 11 (1984): 42–7; R. Leblanc, W. Feindel, Y.L. Yamamoto, J.G. Milton, M.M. Frojmovic, and C.P. Hodge, "The Effects of Calcium Antagonism on the Epicerebral Circulation in Early Vasospasm," *Stroke* 15 (1984): 1017–20.

50 F. Espinosa, B. Weir, and D. Boisvert, "Chronic Cerebral Vasospasm after Large Subarachnoid Hemorrhage in Monkeys," *Journal of Neurosurgery* 57 (1982): 224–32.

51 B. Weir, *Aneurysms Affecting the Nervous System* (Baltimore, MD: Williams and Wilkins, 1987).

52 B. Weir and S. Mullan, "The University of Chicago Neurosurgical Program," *Neurosurgery* 39 (1996): 376–9; Bryce Weir has written that, "as was usual for Dr Penfield's trainees during that era, he [Rasmussen] went from being a junior staff man at the Montreal Neurological Institute to become the Professor of Neurological Surgery elsewhere." See B. Weir, "Theodore Rasmussen 1910–2001," *Canadian Journal of Neurological Science* 29 (2002): 289–90.

53 S. Mullan and W. Penfield, "Illusions of Comparative Interpretation and Emotion Production by Epileptic Discharge and by Electrical Stimulation in the Temporal Cortex," *Archives of Neurology and Psychiatry* 81 (1959): 269–84.

54 Weir and Mullan, "University of Chicago Neurosurgical Program." Sean Mullan is perhaps best remembered for his innovative work on the induced thrombosis of cerebral aneurysms and of carotid-cavernous fistulas, an interest that he shared with another MNI fellow, Eric Peterson. Henry Garretson at the MNI also attempted to produce thrombosis of cerebral aneurysms in 1964, using a stereotactic device that was, as Gilles Bertrand has written, "essentially a ball joint that could be screwed into a burr hole, but which incorporated a graduation in the anteroposterior and lateral direction for the probe support." S. Mullan, "Experiences with Surgical Thrombosis of Intracranial Berry Aneurysms and Carotid Cavernous Fistulas," *Journal of Neurosurgery* 41 (1974): 657–70; Mullan, "Treatment of Carotid-Cavernous Fistulas by Cavernous Sinus Occlusion," *Journal of Neurosurgery* 50 (1979): 131–44; G. Bertrand, "Stereotactic Surgery at McGill: The Early Years," *Neurosurgery* 54 (2004): 1244–52.

CHAPTER SIX

1   The donors are recognized by a plaque in the vestibule of the institute, which reads, "McGill University acknowledges with gratitude generous donations toward the erection and maintenance of this building." On it are listed the Rockefeller Foundation, the Province of Quebec, the City of Montreal, Sir Herbert Holt, J.W. McConnell, Walter Stewart, and anonymous benefactors. Two were Lewis Reford and his wife, and their names are noted on the Foundation Plaque at its entrance. Lewis Reford had studied neurosurgery with Harvey Cushing at Johns Hopkins. Reford returned to Montreal in 1911 and was appointed to the Royal Victoria Hospital. He served overseas in the Royal Canadian Army Medical Corps at the No. 3 Canadian General Hospital (McGill) from 1915 to 1919. Reford's interest in neurosurgery was life-long. He advised Edward Archibald on Penfield's recruitment. After his death on 31 May 1919, Mrs Reford established the Lewis L. Reford Fellowship, given annually to a neurosurgeon in training, as well as a Fellows Fund, its income to be used for the needs of the Fellows Society. William Feindel was awarded the first Reford Fellowship in 1951.

2   Montreal Neurological Institute, *Neurological Biographies and Addresses*, 42. *La Nature* was first created in white marble by the French sculptor Louis-Ernest Barrias in 1889 for the Faculty of Medicine at Bordeaux. A second version by Barrias in polychrome marble and onyx, also dated 1899, was commissioned by the Conservatoire national des arts et métiers. It became part of the Louvre collection and is now at the Musée d'Orsay. A copy was made for the staircase of the old Faculty of Medicine of the University of Paris, now renamed the University of Paris V René Descartes.

3   As William Feindel recalled, Penfield had prevailed upon Sir Arthur Currie, principal of McGill University, to provide him with a letter to the Canadian Legation in Paris to request the permission of the French authorities to make a copy of the statue. In this he was aided by Walter Wells Bosworth, an American architect in Paris, who also secured the services of Adolphe Galli, reputed to make the best copies of sculpture in Paris. *Nature* was expertly carved from "a bloc of marble of great beauty" at a cost of fifty thousand old francs – the franc was then based on the gold standard – borne by four generous friends of the institute, Mr and Mrs A.A. Hodgson and Dr and Mrs Lewis Reford. The statue arrived in Montreal in the summer of 1934. Barnet Phillips, the reception hall's architect, suggested Belgian black marble for the base, to match the dark border of the flooring and the black Belgian colour of the lining of the room. See file D-C/D 33-4, WPA.

4   Montreal Neurological Institute, *Neurological Biographies*, 42–5.

5   The Hughlings Jackson Amphitheatre has been converted into offices and storage areas. It was replaced by the Jeanne Timmins Auditorium when the Webster Pavilion was built in 1985.

6   File A/N 24-2, WPA.

7   MNI, *MNI AR*, 1936, 6.

8   Ibid.

9   N. Petersen, *MNI AR*, 1934, 6–7; H.S. Hayden, "A New Technique for Surgical Photography in the Operating Room," *Photographic Journal* 76 (1936): 205–9.

10 P. Robb, *The Development of Neurology at McGill* (Montreal: Preston Robb, 1989), 49.

11 Montreal Neurological Institute, *Neurological Biographies*.

12 Ibid., 37.

13 Ibid., 29.

14 Ibid., 29.

15 Cushing, a great bibliophile, did not linger at the institute after the opening ceremonies. He "'escaped' with William Francis [the Osler librarian] to the medical faculty's building down the hill, to see the Osler Library." See P. Robb, *Development of Neurology,* 48.

16 Ibid., 39.

17 Ibid., 39.

18 D. Goulet, *Histoire de la neurologie au Québec* (Outremont: Carte Blanche, 2011), 91–2.

19 Ibid., 93.

20 A. Bellerose and R. Amyot, "Metastatic Epidural Abscess of the Spinal Marrow," *Canadian Medical Association Journal* 27 (1932): 629–31.

21 MNI, *MNI AR*, 1934–35, 18–29; MNI, *MNI AR*, 1936, 22–3.

22 Goulet, *Histoire de la neurologie*, 105–6.

23 MNI, *MNI AR*, 1934–35, 18–29; MNI, *MNI AR*, 1936, 22–3.

24 Goulet, *Histoire de la neurologie*, 87.

25 Ibid., 100.

26 Montreal Neurological Institute, *Neurological Biographies and Addresses*, 54.

CHAPTER SEVEN

1 "André J. Cipriani (1908–1956)." http://media.cns-snc.ca/history/pioneers/cipriani/cipriani.html.

2 E.B. Boldrey, "Architectonic Subdivision of the Mammalian Cerebral Cortex Including a Report of the Electrical Stimulation on One Hundred and Five Human Cerebral Corticices" (master's thesis, McGill University, 1936).

3 W. Penfield and E.B. Boldrey, "Somatic Motor and Sensory Representation in the Cerebral Cortex of Man as Studied by Electrical Stimulation," *Brain* 60 (1937): 389–443. Edwin Boldrey joined the faculty of the University of California School of Medicine in San Francisco in 1940 and ascended the academic ladder to full professorship and chair of the Department of Neurological Surgery.

4 MNI, *MNI AR*, 1934–35, 5.

5 MNI, *MNI AR*, 1936, 6.

6 A. Elvidge, W. Penfield, and W. Cone, "The Gliomas of the Central Nervous System: A Study of Two Hundred and Ten Verified Cases," *Association for Research in Nervous and Mental Diseases* 16 (1937): 107–81.

7 Ibid.; G. Roussy, J. L'Hermitte, and L. Corniel, "Essai de classification des tumeurs cérébrales," *Annales d'Anatomie Pathologique et d' Anatomie Normale Médico- Chirurgicale* 1 (1924): 333–78; J. Globus and I. Strauss, "Spongioblastoma Multiforme: A Primary Malignant Form of Brain Neoplasm: Its Clinical and Atomic Features," *Archives of Neurology and Psychiatry* 14 (1925): 139–91.

8   G.E. Tremble and W. Penfield, "Operative Exposure of the Facial Canal with Removal of a Tumor of the Greater Superficial Petrosal Nerve," *Archives of Otolaryngology* 23 (1936): 573–9.

9   W. Penfield, "A Technique for Demonstrating the Perivascular Nerves of the Pia Mater and Central Nervous System," *American Journal of Pathology* 11 (1935): 1007–10; W. Penfield and N.C. Norcross, "Subdural Traction and Post-traumatic Headache: Stuy of Pathology and Therapeusis," *Archives of Neurology and Psychiatry* 36 (1936): 75–94.

10 W. Penfield, "Epilepsy and Surgical Therapy," *Archives of Neurology and Psychiatry* 36 (1936): 449–84.

11 A.J. Kilgour and H.W. Williams, "Walter Spielmeyer," *American Journal of Psychiatry* 92 (1935): 255–7.

12 J.P. Evans, "A Study of the Sensory Defects Resulting from Excision of Cerebral Substance in Humans," *Proceedings of the Association for Research in Nervous and Mental Disease* 15 (1934): 331–70.

13 Penfield and Rasmussen, *Cerebral Cortex of Man*.

14 A. Anderson and W. Haymaker, "Elaboration of Hormones by Pituitary Cells Growing in Vitro," *Proceedings of the Society for Experimental Biology and Medicine* 33 (1935): 313–16; W. Haymaker and A. Anderson, "Homiografting of Rat Pituitary Grown in Vitro," *Journal of Pathology and Bacteriology* 42 (1936): 339–410.

15 W. Haymaker and J. Sanchez-Perez, "Río-Hortega's Double Silver Impregnation Technique Adapted to the Staining of Tissue Cultures," *Science* 82 (1935): 355–6.

16 W. Penfield, "Oligodendroglia and Its Relation to Classical Neuroglia," *Brain* 47 (1924): 430–52; del Río-Hortega and Penfield, "Cerebral Cicatrix," 278–303; J.M. Sanchez-Perez, "Hortega's Silver Stains in Neuropathology," *Technical Methods and Bulletin of International Association of Medical Museums* 15 (1936): 78–83.

17 M. Marcé, "Note sur l'action toxique de l'essence d'absinthe," *Comptes rendus hebdomadaires des séances de l'académie des sciences* 58 (1864): 628–9; H.M. Keith, "Experimentally Produced Convulsions: Effect on Thujone Convulsions of Insulin and of Variations in Water Content of Brain," *Archives of Neurology and Psychiatry* 33 (1935): 353–9; H.M. Keith and G. Stavraky, "Experimental Convulsions Induced by Administration of Thujone: A Pharmacological Study of the Influence of the Autonomic Nervous System on These Convulsions," *Archives of Neurology and Psychiatry* 34 (1935): 1022–40; G.W. Stavraky, "Response of Cerebral Blood Vessels to Electric Stimulation of the Thalamus and Hypothalamic Regions," *Archives of Neurology and Psychiatry* 35 (1936): 1002–5; A.S. Gill and D.K. Binder, "Wilder Penfield, Pío del Río-Hortega, and the Discovery of Oligodendroglia," *Neurosurgery* 60 (2007): 940–8.

18 Lord Tweedsmuir was born John Buchan. He was an author of adventure novels, most notably of *The Thirty-Nine Steps*, which was made into a film by Alfred Hitchcock, in 1935. See MNI, *MNI AR*, 1936, 10.

19 J. Lewis, *Something Hidden: A Biography of Wilder Penfield* (Toronto: Doubleday Canada, 1981), 163–4.

20 W/U 34, WPA.

21 W. Penfield to F.M.R. Walshe, 22 March 1935, file C/D 20, WPA.

22 P. Robb, *The Development of Neurology at McGill* (Montreal: Montreal Neurological Institute, 1989), 50, 59, 60.

CHAPTER EIGHT

 1 M. Preul, W. Feindel, T.F. Dagy, J. Stratford, and G. Bertrand, "Arthur Roland Elvidge (1899–1985): Contributions to the Diagnosis of Brain Tumors and Cerebrovascular Disease," *Journal of Neurosurgery* 88 (1998): 162–71.

 2 W. Penfield to S. Cobb, 28 August 1935, file C/D 14-4, WPA.

 3 A. Egas Moniz, "L'encéphalographie arterielle, son importance dans la localisationes tumeurs cerebrales," *Revue Neurologique* 2 (1927): 72–90.

 4 P. Robb, *The Development of Neurology at McGill* (Montreal: Montreal Neurological Institute, 1989), 58.

 5 Although well known in Europe, cerebral angiography was largely unknown in North America at the time. Preul et al., "Arthur Roland Elvidge (1899–1985)."

 6 A.R. Elvidge, "The Cerebral Vessels Studied by Angiography," *Proceedings of the Association for Research in Nervous and Mental Disease* 18 (1938): 110–49.

 7 MNI, *MNI AR*, 1936, 11.

 8 H.R. Geyelin and W. Penfield, "Cerebral Calcification Epilepsy: Endarteritis Calcificans Cerebri," *Archives of Neurology and Psychiatry* 21 (1929): 1020–43.

 9 W. Penfield and A. Ward, "Calcifying Epileptogenic Lesions," *Archives of Neurology and Psychiatry* 60 (1948): 20–36.

10 R. Leblanc, D. Melancon, D. Wilkinson, and T. Kirkham, "Hereditary Neurocutaneous Angiomatosis: Report of Four Cases," *Journal of Neurosurgery* 85 (1996): 1135–42.

11 Elvidge, "Cerebral Vessels Studied by Angiography," 120.

12 Preul et al., "Arthur Roland Elvidge (1899–1985)."

13 C-109, MNI Archives.

14 A.R. Elvidge and W. Feindel, "Surgical Treatment of Aneurysm of the Anterior Cerebral and of the Anterior Communicating Arteries Diagnosed by Angiography and Electroencephalography," *Journal of Neurosurgery* 7 (1950): 13–32.

15 Ibid., 28.

16 J.H. Boucoud, "Dr Elvidge Remembered," in *Nursing Highlights 1934 to 1990, Montreal Neurological Institute & Hospital. A Narrative of the Reflections, Revelations, Anticipations and Dreams of Nursing at the Montreal Neurological Institute*, ed. E. Barrowman, M. Cavanaugh, L. Dalicandro, M. Everett, P. Robb, and C.E. Robertson (Montreal: Montreal Neurological Institute, 1992), 64–5; Preul et al., "Arthur Roland Elvidge (1899–1985)."

17 Preul et al., "Arthur Roland Elvidge (1899–1985)."

18 Ibid.

19 S.H. Knowles, "The Healer," in Baxter, *Francis L. McNaughton*, 5–6.

20 W. Feindel, "The Healer," in Baxter, *Francis L. McNaughton*, 5.

21 F.L. McNaughton, "The Use of Ergotamine Tartrate in Migraine," *Canadian Medical Association Journal* 33 (1935): 664–5.

22 F.L. McNaughton, "The Innervation of the Intracranial Blood Vessels and Dural Si-
    nuses," *Proceedings of the Association for Research in Nervous and Mental Diseases* 18
    (1938): 178–200; McNaughton, "The Distribution of Sensory Nerves to the Dura
    Mater and Cerebral Vessels" (master's thesis, McGill University, 1941); W. Feindel, W.
    Penfield, and F.L. McNaughton, "The Tentorial Nerves and Localization of Intracra-
    nial Pain in Man," *Neurology* 10 (1960): 555–63; D. Lloyd-Smith and F.L. McNaughton,
    "Methysergide (Sansert) in the Prevention of Migraine: A Clinical Trial," *Canadian
    Medical Association Journal* 89 (1963): 1221–3.

23 P. Robb, "The Neurologist," in Baxter, *Francis L. McNaughton*, 2–3.

24 Ibid.

25 B.H. Smith and F.L. McNaughton, "Mysoline, a New Anticonvulsant Drug: Its Value
    in Refractory Cases of Epilepsy," *Canadian Medical Association Journal* 68 (1953): 464–
    7; J.A. Aguilar, H.K. Martin, and F.L. McNaughton, "Aminoglutethimide in the Treat-
    ment of Epilepsy," *Canadian Medical Association Journal*, 84 (1961): 374–6.

26 F. McNaughton, "Observations on Diagnosis and Medical Treatment," in *Epilepsy and
    the Functional Anatomy of the Human Brain*, ed. W. Penfield and H.H. Jasper, 540–68
    (Boston: Little, Brown, 1954).

27 MacLeod, "The Humanitarian."

28 M. Avoli, "Herbert H. Jasper and the Basic Mechanisms of the Epilepsies," in *Jasper's
    Basic Mechanisms of the Epilepsies [Internet]*. 4th ed., ed. J.L. Noebels et al. (Bethesda,
    MD: National Center for Biotechnology Information, 2012).

29 L. Lapicque, "Recherches quantitatives sur l'excitation électrique des nerfs traitée
    comme une polarisation," *Journal de physiologie et de pathologie générale* 9 (1907):
    620–35; H.H. Jasper and A.M. Monnier, "Transmission of Excitation between Excised
    Nonmyelinated Nerves," *Journal of Cellular Physiology* 11 (1938): 259–77.

30 H.H. Jasper, "Some Highlights of 70 Years in Neuroscience Research," in *The History
    of Neuroscience in Autobiography*, ed. L.R. Squire (Washington, DC: Society for Neu-
    roscience, 1996), 1:326.

31 Avoli, "Herbert H. Jasper and the Basic Mechanisms of the Epilepsies"; H.H. Jasper
    and L. Carmichael, "Electrical Potentials from the Intact Human Brain," *Science* 81
    (1935): 51–3.

32 O. Foerster and H. Altenburger, "Elektrobiologische Vorgänge an der menschlichen
    Hirnrinde," *Deutsche Zeitschrift für Nervenheilkunde* 135 (1935): 277–88.

33 W. Penfield, "Herbert Jasper," in "Recent Contributions to Neurophysiology: Inter-
    national Symposium in Neurosciences in Honor of Herbert H. Jasper," ed. J.P.
    Cordeau and P. Gloor, supplement, *Electroencephalography and Clinical Neurophysi-
    ology* 31 (1972): 10.

34 Avoli, "Herbert H. Jasper and the Basic Mechanisms of the Epilepsies."

35 W. Feindel, "Herbert Henri Jasper 1906–1999: An Appreciation," *Canadian Journal of
    Neurological Sciences* 26 (1999): 224–9.

36 Jasper, "Some Highlights," 332–3.

37 MNI, *AR, 1938–1939*, 17–18; T. Erickson, "Neurogenic Hyperthermia" (master's thesis,
    McGill University, 1934); Erickson, "The Nature and the Spread of the Epileptic Dis-
    charge" (PhD diss., McGill University, 1937).

38 H.H. Jasper and H.L. Andrews, "Electroencephalography," *Archives of Neurology and Psychiatry* 39 (1938): 96–115; H.H. Jasper and W. Hawke, "Electroencephalography," *Archives of Neurology and Psychiatry* 39 (1938): 885–901; H.H. Jasper and I.C. Nichols, "Electrical Signs of Cortical Function in Epilepsy and Allied Disorders," *American Journal of Psychiatry* 94 (1938): 835–51.

39 Penfield and Erickson, *Epilepsy and Cerebral Localization* (Springfield: Thomas, 1941).

40 W. Penfield and H.H. Jasper, *Epilepsy and the Functional Anatomy of the Human Brain* (Boston: Little, Brown, 1954)

41 Avoli, "Herbert H. Jasper and the Basic Mechanisms of the Epilepsies."

42 H.H. Jasper and C. Ajmone-Marsan, "Thalamocortical Integrating Mechanisms," *Research Publication of the Association for Research in Nervous and Mental Diseases* 30 (1952): 493–512; H.H. Jasper and C. Ajmone-Marsan, *A Stereotaxic Atlas of the Diencephalon of the Cat* (Ottawa: National Research Council of Canada, 1954); H.H. Jasper, R. Naquet, and E.V. King, "Thalamocortical Recruiting Responses in Sensory Receiving Areas in the Cat," *Electroencephalography and Clinical Neurophysiology* 7 (1955): 99–114; H.H. Jasper, "History of the Early Development of Electroencephalography and Clinical Neurophysiology at the Montreal Neurological Institute: The First 25 Years, 1939–1964," *Canadian Journal of Neurological Sciences* 18 (1991): 533–48.

43 P. Gloor, "Electrophysiological Studies of the Amygdala in the Cat" (PhD diss., McGill University, 1957); Gloor, "Amygdala," in *Handbook of Physiology: II. Neurophysiology*, ed. J. Field, H.W. Magoun, and E.V. Hall, 1395–1420 (Washington: American Physiological Society, 1960); Gloor, *The Temporal Lobe and Limbic System* (New York: Oxford University Press, 1999).

44 Jasper, "Some Highlights," 341.

45 H.H. Jasper and G. Bertrand, "Recording from Microelectrodes in Stereotaxic Surgery for Parkinson's Disease," *Journal of Neurosurgery* 24 (1966): 219–21.

46 H.H. Jasper, R.T. Khan, and K.A.C. Elliott, "Amino Acids Released from the Cerebral Cortex in Relation to Its State of Activation," *Science* 147 (1965): 1448–9; G.C. Celesia and H.H. Jasper, "Acetylcholine Released from Cerebral Cortex in Relation to State of Activation," *Neurology* 16 (1966): 1053–63.

47 H.H. Jasper, A.A. Ward, and A. Pope, *Basic Mechanisms of the Epilepsies* (Boston: Little, Brown, 1969).

CHAPTER NINE

1 G. Odom and K. Stern, "Morphologic Alterations of the Neuron Due to Tumour Invasion," *Archives of Pathology* 39 (1945): 221–5; K. Stern and K.A.C. Elliott, "Experimental Observations on the So-Called Senile Changes of Intracellular Neuro-Fibrilis," *American Journal of Psychiatry* 106 (1949): 190–4; K. Stern, "Thalamo-Frontal Projection in Man," *Journal of Anatomy* 76 (1951): 302–7.

2 K. Stern, *The Pillar of Fire* (New York: Harcourt, Brace, 1951).

3 D. Avery, "Wartime Medical Cooperation across the Pacific: Wilder Penfield and the Anglo-American Medical Missions to the Soviet Union and China, 1943–1944," *Pacific Science* 54 (2000): 289–98.

4   S.P. Humphreys, "Study of the Vascular and Cytological Changes in the Cerebral Cicatrix" (MSc thesis, McGill University, 1939); W. Penfield, "Epilepsy and the Cerebral Lesions of Birth and Infancy," *Canadian Medical Association Journal* 41 (1939): 527–34; Penfield, "The Epilepsies: With a Note on Radical Therapy," *New England Journal of Medicine* 221 (1939): 209–18; W. Penfield and S. Humphreys, "Epilpetogenic Lesions of the Brain: A Histologic Study," *Archives of Neurology and Psychiatry* 43 (1940): 240–61; W. Penfield and A.W. Keith, "Focal Epileptic Lesions of Birth and Infancy with a Report of Eight Cases," *American Journal of Diseases of Children* 59 (1940): 718–38.

5   Chart no. 4203, MNI Archives.

6   W.V. Cone, M-109, MNI Archives.

7   Neuropathology report S-295-38, MNI Archives.

8   Jason Karamchandani, personal communication, 10 December 2014.

9   W. Penfield, M-109, MNI Archives.

10 Penfield and Humphreys, "Epilpetogenic Lesions of the Brain" 256.

11 Penfield, "The Epilepsies: With a Note on Radical Therapy," *New England Journal of Medicine* 221 (1939): 217.

12 S. Love and D. Lewis, *Greenfield's Neuropathology*, 8th ed. (London: Hodder Arnold, 2008), 391–5.

13 Ibid.; D. Ellison, *Neuropathology a Reference Text of CNS Pathology*, (Edinburgh: Mosby, 2013): 84–8.

14 W. Penfield, "The Circulation of the Epileptic Brain," *Proceedings of the Association for Research in Nervous and Mental Disease* 28 (1937): 605–37.

15 Ibid.

16 W. Penfield, M-109, MNI Archives.

17 N.C. Norcross, "Studies in Cerebral Circulation" (MSc thesis, McGill University, 1936); W.M. Nichols, "Changes in the Circulation of the Brain and Spinal Cord Associated with Nervous Activity" (MSc thesis, McGill university 1938); F.A. Echlin, "Cerebral Ischemia and Its Relation to Epilepsy" (MSc thesis, McGill University, 1939); Erickson, "Nature and Spread of the Epileptic Discharge"; S.P. Humphreys, "Study of the Vascular and Cytological Changes in the Cerebral Cicatrix" (MSc thesis, McGill University, 1939).

18 K. von Santha and A. Cipriani, "Focal Alterations in Subcortical Circulation Resulting from Stimulation of the Cerebral Cortex," *Association for Research in Nervous and Mental Disease* 18 (1938): 346–62.

19 W. Penfield, K. von Santha, and A. Cipriani, "Cerebral Blood Flow during Induced Epileptiform Seizures in Animals and Man," *Journal of Neurophysiology* 2 (1939): 257–67.

20 Erickson, "Nature and the Spread of the Epileptic Discharge"; T. Erickson, "The Spread of the Epileptic Discharge: An Experimental Study of the After Discharge Induced by Electrical Stimulation of the Cerebral Cortex," *Archives of Neurology and Psychiatry* 43 (1940): 429–52.

21 Erickson, "Nature and the Spread of the Epileptic Discharge," 47.

22 Ibid., 52, 54.

23 Ibid., 132.

24 W.P. Van Wagonen and R.Y. Herren, "Surgical Division of Commissural Pathways in

the Corpus Callosum: Relation to Spread of an Epileptic Attack," *Archives of Neurology and Psychiatry* 44 (1940): 740–59; D.H. Wilson, C. Culver, M. Waddington, and M. Gazzaniga, "Disconnection of the Cerebral Hemispheres: An Alternative to Hemispherectomy for the Control of Intractable Seizures," *Neurology* 25 (1975): 1149–53.

25 O.R. Hyndman and W. Penfield, "Agenesis of the Corpus Callosum: Its Recognition by Ventriculography," *Archives of Neurology and Psychiatry* 37 (1937): 1251–70.

26 W. Penfield and E. Boldrey, "Cortical Spread of Epileptic Discharge and the Conditioning of Effect of Habitual Seizures," *American Journal of Psychiatry* 96 (1939): 280.

27 W. Penfield, "Engrams in the Human Brain Mechanisms of Memory," *Proceedings of the Royal Society of Medicine* 61 (1968): 831–40; G.V. Goddard, "Development of Epileptic Seizures through Brain Stimulation at Low Intensity," *Nature* 214 (1967): 1020–1; G.V. Goddard and R.M. Douglas, "Does the Engram of Kindling Model the Engram of Normal Long Term Memory," *Canadian Journal of Neurological Sciences* 2 (1975): 385–94.

    Penfield published a disappointing chapter on the conditioned reflex, "Consciousness, Memory and Man's Conditioned Reflex," in which he mentions Pavlov and the conditioned reflex but once, in a short paragraph lost within the chapter's thirty pages. His "Engrams in the Human Brain Mechanisms of Memory" is also wanting, although he does seem to ascribe a role to conditioned reflexes in the acquisition of sensorimotor skills, and for engrams in recording "the permanent impression left behind by psychical experience in the brain's cellular network." See W. Penfield, "Consciousness, Memory and Man's Conditioned Reflex," in *On the Biology of Learning*, ed. K.H. Pribram (New York: Harcourt, Brace, 1969), 158; Penfield, "Engrams."

28 A.E. Childe and W. Penfield, "Anatomic and Pneumographical Studies of the Temporal Horn with a Further Note of Pneumographic Analysis of the Cerebral Ventricles," *Archives of Neurology, Neurosurgery and Psychiatry* 37 (1937): 1021–34.

29 J. Kershman, "The Medulloblast and the Medulloblastoma: A Study of Human Embryos," *Archives of Neurology and Psychiatry* 40 (1938): 937–67; Kershman, "Genesis of Microglia in the Human Brain," *Archives of Neurology and Psychiatry* 41 (1939): 24–50.

30 Kershman, "Genesis of Microglia."

31 W. Penfield, T.C. Erickson, and I. Tarlov, "Relation of Intracranial Tumours and Symptomatic Epilepsy," *Archives of Neurology and Psychology* 44 (1940): 300–17.

32 W. Penfield and D. McEachern, "Intracranial Tumours," *Oxford Medicine* 6 (1938): 137–224.

33 W. Penfield and E. Boldrey, "Somatic Motor and Sensory Representation in the Cerebral Cortex of Man as Studied by Electrical Stimulation," *Brain* 60 (1937): 389–443.

34 W. Penfield, "The Cerebral Cortex in Man, I. The Cerebral Cortex and Consciousness," *Archives of Neurology, Neurosurgery and Psychiatry* 40 (1938): 417–42.

35 W. Penfield, *Mystery of the Mind: A Critical Study of Consciousness and the Human Brain* (Princeton: Princeton University Press, 1975).

CHAPTER TEN

1 MNI, *MNI AR*, 1939–40, 3.
2 T. Copp, "The Development of Neuropsychiatry in the Canadian Army (Overseas),"
   in *Canadian Health Care and the State*, ed. David Naylor (Montreal and Kingston:
   McGill-Queen's University Press, 1992), 80.
3 H. Elliott, "Lieut.-Col. O.W. Stewart," *Canadian Medical Association Journal* 63 (1950):
   524; MNI, *MNI AR*, 1950–51, 48.
4 MNI, *MNI AR*, 1936; J. Cameron, "Captain W. Martin Nichols: 'Doc Nic' Camp Medical Officer at Stalag Luft 1 RAMC," in *World War II – Prisoners of War – Stalag Luft
   I: A Collection of Stories, Photos, Art and Information on Stalag Luft I*, http://www.
   merkki.com/nicholsmartin.htm.
5 Copp, "Development of Neuropsychiatry," 67.
6 F.L. McNaughton, "Colin Russel: Pioneer of Canadian Neurology," *Canadian Medical
   Association Journal* 77 (1957): 719–23; C.K. Russel and V. Horsley, "Note on Apparent
   Re-representation in the Cerebral Cortex of the Type of Sensory Representation as It
   Exists in the Spinal Cord," *Brain* 29 (1906): 137–52.
7 C.K. Russel, "Tumour of the Temporo-Sphenoidal Lobe and 'Dreamy States,'" *McGill
   Journal* 38 (1909): 3–7. The "dreamy state" accompanying some aspects of temporal
   lobe epilepsy originating from mesial temporal lobe structures presents a variable
   picture of confusion, a feeling of unreality, feelings of déjà vu, automatic, stereotyp-
   ical movements, and other complex phenomena for which the patient has partial or
   no memory. See W. Feindel, "Temporal Lobe Seizures," in *Handbook of Clinical Neurology*, ed. O. Magnus and A.M. Lorentz de Haas (Amsterdam: North-Holland Publishing, 1974), 17:87–106.
8 Anonymous, "The Canadian Neurosurgical Centre, Hackwood Park, Basingstoke,"
   British Journal of Surgery 32 (1945): 525–30. It had been planned that Penfield would
   replace Cone in England later, but as preparations for his departure moved apace, a
   small shadow was seen on his chest X-ray. Despite Penfield's efforts to have it over-
   looked, this small shadow precluded him from active service. Penfield did visit Basingstoke, but in civilian garb. Unable to be in uniform, Penfield felt out of place and
   did not return.
9 Canadian military nurses of either sex are referred to as "nursing sisters." "Canadian
   Army Medical Corps Nursing Sisters," Historica Canada, http://www.thecanadia-
   nencyclopedia.ca/en/article/canadian-army-medical-corps-nursing-sisters/.
10 MNI, *MNI AR*, 1940–41, 9.
11 Ibid., 10.
12 Anonymous, "Canadian Neurosurgical Centre," 526.
13 W. Penfield, *Military Neurosurgery* (Ottawa: Government Distribution Office, Government Printing Bureau, 1941), 40–2.
14 O.W. Stewart, C.K. Russel, and W.V. Cone, "Injury to the Central Nervous System by
   Blast: Observations on a Pheasant," *Lancet* 237 (1941): 172–4.

15 E.H. Botterell, E.A. Carmichael, and W.V. Cone, "Sulphanilamide and Salphapyridine in Experimental Cerebral Wounds," *Journal of Neurology and Psychiatry* 4 (1941): 163–74.

16 Botterell's devotion to injured troops led him to create the first North American centre devoted to the rehabilitation of patients afflicted with a spinal cord injury. See "History," Surgery, University of Toronto, Division of Neurosurgery, last modified 19 January 2015, http://neurosurgery.utoronto.ca/about/history.htm.

17 McNaughton, "Colin Russel," 722.

18 MNI, *MNI AR*, 1939–40.

19 See Veterans Affairs Canada, "Royal Red Cross Class 2 (ARRC)," Veterans Affairs Canada, last modified 9 December 2014, http://www.veterans.gc.ca/eng/remembrance/medals-decorations/orders-decorations/arrc. See also Helen Kendall, interviewed in "World War One Continues: Nursing-Sisters," *Cape Breton's Magazine* 34 (1983): 6; Manuscript Group 12.275, Helen Kendall Fonds, Beaton Institute, Cape Breton University; R. Carpenter, "The First Ice Hockey Champions," Legends of Australian Ice, http://icelegendsaustralia.com/1stIceChampions-hockey-intro.html#.

20 L.M. Stewart, "Off to War," in Barrowman et al., *Nursing Highlights*, 36–8.

21 M. Bashow and E.B. Sparling, "Freda," in ibid., 38–9.

22 Ibid., 44.

23 Ibid., 39.

24 Ibid., 40–1.

25 Ibid., 42.

26 W. Stewart to W. Penfield, 23 April 1945, file C/G 45 (O), WPA.

27 The touching story of Freda Bossy is told by her *consoeurs* M. Bashow and Eva Sparling, in Barrowman et al., *Nursing Highlights*, 38–45.

CHAPTER ELEVEN

1 MNI, *MNI AR*, 1940–41, 7.

2 Ibid., 9.

3 Ibid., 7.

4 MNI, *MNI AR*, 1939–40, 14.

5 MNI, *MNI AR*, 1941–42, 2.

6 MNI, *MNI AR*, 1940–41, 7–9; MNI, *MNI AR*, 1944–45, 25.

7 H.H. Jasper, A. Cipriani, E.S. Lotspeich, T.S. Bennett, Thorn, Clinton, Chapman, and Mitchell, "Experimental Investigations on the Effects of Acceleration in Animals," in MNI, *MNI AR*, 1942–43, 19; D. McEachren, B.D.B. Layton, and E.G. Burr, "Canadian Army Night Vision Training and Testing Unit," *War Medicine* 5 (1944): 83; E.W. Peterson, M. Bornstein, and H.H. Jasper, "The Effect of Morphine Sulphate and Sulphathiozole on Altitude Tolerance," in MNI, *MNI AR*, 1944–45, 25; E.W. Peterson, B.S. Kent, and W.V. Cone, "Intracranial Pressure in the Human Subject at Altitude," *Archives of Neurology and Psychiatry* 52 (1944): 520–5; H.H. Jasper, E.W. Peterson, and M.B. Bornstein, "Cerebrospinal Fluid Pressure under Conditions Existing at High Altitudes: A Critical Review," *Archives of Neurology and Psychiatry* 52 (1944): 400–8.

8   MNI, *MNI AR*, 1940–41, 7; M.R. Harrower-Erickson, "Psychological Factors in Avia-
     tion Medicine," *Canadian Medical Association Journal* 44 (1941): 348–52.

9   H.H. Jasper and A. Vineberg, "Estimation of the Depth of Skin Burns," in MRI, *RR,
     1942–43*, 19.

10 P.O. Lehman, D. McEachern, and G. Morton, "Seasickness and Other Forms of Mo-
     tion Sickness," *War Medicine* 2 (1942): 410–28; W. Penfield, D. McEachern, W. Mc-
     Nall, O.W. Stewart, W.S. Fields, B.A. Campbell, G. Morton, A. Cipriani, and H.H.
     Jasper, "Experimental Investigation of Motion Sickness," in MRI *AR, 1942–1943*, 19; G.
     Morton, A. Cipriani, and D. McEachern, "Mechanism of Motion Sickness," *Archives
     of Neurology and Psychiatry* 57 (1947): 58–70.

11 B.P. Babkin and M.B. Bornstein, "The Effects of Swinging and Binaural Galvanic
     Stimulation on Gastric Motility in the Dog," *Revue Canadienne de Biologie* 2 (1943):
     336–49.

12 F.C. MacIntosh, "Boris Petrovich Babkin 1877–1950," *Revue canadienne de biologie* 10
     (1951): 3–7; I. deDurgh Daly, S.A. Komarov, and E.G. Young, "Boris Petrovitch Babkin.
     1877–1950," *Obituary Notices of Fellows of the Royal Society* 8 (1952): 12–23; I.T. Beck,
     "The Life, Achievements and Legacy of a Great Canadian Investigator: Professor Boris
     Petrovich Babkin (1877–1950)," *Canadian Journal of Gastroenterology* 20 (2006): 579–
     88.

13 A.R. Elvidge, "Head Injuries," *Canadian Medical Association Journal* 38 (1938): 26–33;
     Elvidge, "The Post-traumatic Convulsive and Allied States," in *Injuries of the Skull,
     Brain and Spinal Cord*, ed. S. Brock, 233–73 (Baltimore, MD: Williams and Wilkins,
     1940); P.O. Lehmann and A. Elvidge, "Posttraumatic Headache and Dizziness," *Cana-
     dian Medical Association Journal* 47 (1942): 197–201; W. Penfield and W.V. Cone, "El-
     ementary Principles of the Treatment of Head Injuries," *Canadian Medical Association
     Journal* 48 (1943): 99–104; F.L. McNaughton and W.D. Ross, "Head Injury: A Study of
     Patients with Chronic Post-traumatic Complaints," *Archives of Neurology and Psy-
     chiatry* 52 (1944): 255–69; H.H. Jasper, J. Kershman, and A. Elvidge, "Electroen-
     cephalographic Studies of Injury to the Head," *Archives of Neurology and Psychiatry*
     44 (1940): 328–48; H.H. Jasper and W. Penfield, "Electroencephalograms in Post-trau-
     matic Epilepsy," *American Journal of Psychiatry* 100 (1943): 365–77; W. Penfield, "Post-
     traumatic Epilepsy," *American Journal of Psychiatry* 100 (1944): 750–51; H.H. Jasper
     and M.B. Bornstein, "Analysis of Changes in the Electrical Activity of the Brain Pro-
     duced by Experimental Trauma," in MNI, *MNI AR*, 1944–45, 25; H.H., Jasper J. Ker-
     shman, and A. Elvidge, "Electroencephalography in Head Injury," *Research in Nervous
     and Mental Diseases* 24 (1945): 388–420; M.B. Bornstein, "Presence and Action of
     Acetylcholine in Experimental Brain Trauma," *Journal of Neurophysiology* 9 (1946):
     349–66.

14 R. Pudenz, "The Repair of Cranial Defects with Tantalum," *Journal of the American
     Medical Association* 121 (1943): 478–81.

15 Y.C. Chao, S. Humphreys, and W. Penfield, "A New Method of Preventing Adhesions:
     The Use of Amnioplastin after Craniotomy," *British Medical Journal* 1 (1940): 517–19;
     R. Pudenz and G. Odom, "Meningocerebral Adhesions," *Surgery* 12 (1942): 318–44.

16 K.A.C. Elliott, H.H. Jasper, and J. Meyer, "The Physio-Pathological Nature of Brain

Swelling and Oedema Following Traumatic Injury or Exposure," in MNI, *MNI AR*, 1944–45, 25; M. Prados, B. Strowger, and W.H. Feindel, "Studies on Cerebral Edema; Reaction of the Brain to Air Exposure; Pathologic Changes," *Archives of Neurology and Psychiatry* 54 (1945): 163–74; M. Prados, B. Strowger, and W.H. Feindel, "Studies on Cerebral Edema; Reaction of the Brain to Exposure to Air; Physiologic Changes," *Archives of Neurology and Psychiatry* 54 (1945): 290–300; H.H. Jasper and K.A.C. Elliott, "The Effect of Various Kinds of Irrigation Fluids on the Local pH Pial Vessels, Functional Stage and Subsequent Condition of the Cerebral Cortex Exposed at Operation," in MNI, *MNI AR*, 1944–45, 25.

17   R. Amyot, "Méningites purulentes traitées et guéries par le Sulfapyridine," *Union médicale du Canada* 70 (1941): 604; E.F. Hurteau, "The Intracranial Use of Sulphonamides: Experimental Study of the Histology and Rate of Absorption," *Canadian Medical Association Journal* 44 (1941): 352–5; E.F. Hurteau, "The Intracranial Use of Sulfadiazine: Experimental Study of the Histology and Rate of Absorption," *Canadian Medical Association Journal* 45 (1942): 15–17; A. Elvidge, "Effect of Sulphonamide Injection on the Reticuloendothelial System," in MRI, *RR, 1942–43*, 19; W.V. Cone, H.H. Jasper, R. Pudenz, and T.S. Bennett, "Effect of Local Application, Intrathecal Injection and Intravenous Injection of Sulphonamides upon Cerebral Function," in MNI, *MNI AR*, 1942–43, 19; H.H. Jasper, W.V. Cone, R. Pudenz, and T.S. Bennet, "The Electroencephalograms of Monkeys Following the Application of Microcrystalline Sulfonamides to the Brain," *Surgery, Genecology & Obstetrics* 76 (1943): 599–611; C. Corona, "Experimental and Clinical Studies of Aseptic Meningitis," in MNI, *MNI AR, 1944–45*, 26.

18   W.V. Cone and W.H. Bridgers, "A Combined Tidal Irrigator and Cystometer for Management of the Paralyzed Bladder," *Surgery, Genecology & Obstetrics* 75 (1942): 61–6; W.V. Cone, "Fusion of Vertebrae Following Removal of the Intervertebral Disc in Monkeys," in MNI, *MNI AR*, 1942–43, 19; D. McEachern and W.V, Cone, "Clinical Points on Ruptured Intervertebral Discs: Low Back Pain and Sciatica," *Canadian Medical Association Journal* 49 (1943): 33–5.

19   H.H. Jasper and J.P. Robb, "Clinical and Experimental Studies of Changes in Electrical Skin Resistance in Peripheral Nerve Lesions," MNI, *RR 1944–45*, 31; H.H. Jasper, R. Notman, and J. Meyer, "Electromyography in Peripheral Nerve Lesions with Histological Controls," in MNI, *RR, 1944–45*, 45.

20   C. Bertrand and Hurtz, "Methods of Nerve Suture," in MNI, *MNI AR*, 1942–43, 19; P.O. Lehmam, "Wound Reactions to Different Suture Materials," in ibid., 19.

21   H. Elliott, "The McGill Hammer," *Canadian Medical Association Journal* 42 (1940): 575.

22   "History of the Chairs," Department of Pathology, Anatomy, and Cell Biology, Sidney Kimmel Medical College, Thomas Jefferson University, http://www.jefferson.edu/university/jmc/departments/pathology/history.html; V.H. Moon, *Shock and Related Capillary Phenomena* (New York: Oxford University Press, 1938).

23   J. Scudder, "Studies in Blood Preservation: The Stability of Plasma Proteins," *Annals of Surgery* 112 (1940): 502–19. Scudder's collaborator at Columbia was Charles Drew,

a McGill graduate and surgeon who had a determining influence on Clarence Green, the first African-American neurosurgeon. Greene did his neurosurgery training at the MNI with Penfield and Cone.

24 W. Stetten, "The Blood Plasma for Great Britain Project," *Bulletin of the New York Academy of Medicine* 17 (1941): 27–38.

25 C.H. Shelden, R. Pudenz, J.S. Restarski, and W.M. Craig, "The Lucite Calvarium: A Method for Direct Observation of the Brain. I. The Surgical and Lucite Processing Techniques," *Journal of Neurosurgery* 1 (1944): 67–75; R. Pudenz and C.H. Shelden, "The Lucite Calvarium: A Method for Direct Observation of the Brain. II. Cranial Trauma and Brain Movement," *Journal of Neurosurgery* 3 (1946): 487–505. MNI, *MNI AR*, 1943–44, 32.

26 J.F. Fulton, *Harvey Cushing: A Biography* (Springfield: Charles Thomas, 1946)

27 MNI, *MNI AR*, 1944–45, 31–2.

28 W. Penfield, "Bilateral Frontal Gyrectomy and Postoperative Intelligence," *Research Publication of the Association for Research in Nervous and Mental Disease* 27 (1948): 519–34; D.E. Cameron and M.D. Prados, "Bilateral Frontal Gyrectomy: Psychiatric Results," *Research Publication of the Association for Research in Nervous and Mental Disease* 27 (1948): 534–7.

29 Erickson, "Neurogenic Hyperthermia"; Erickson, "Nature and the Spread of the Epileptic Discharge"; Erickson, "Spread of the Epileptic Discharge."

30 W. Penfield and T.C. Erickson, *Epilepsy and Cerebral Localization* (Oxford: Charles C. Thomas, 1941).

31 "Erickson, Theodore Charles," in *The Society of Neurological Surgeons* (Winston-Salem, NC: Wake Forest University Press, 2001), 455.

32 H. Cushing, *The Life of Sir William Osler*, 2 vols (Oxford: Oxford University Press, 1925).

33 MNI, *MNI AR*, 1939–1949, 17.

34 W. Penfield, "The Passing of Harvey Cushing," *Yale Journal of Biology and Medicine* 12 (1940): 325–6.

35 M.C. Preul and W. Feindel, "Origins of Wilder Penfield's Surgical Technique: The Role of the 'Cushing Ritual' and Influences from the European Experience," *Journal of Neurosurgery* 75 (1991): 816.

CHAPTER TWELVE

1 D. McEachern, MNI, *MNI AR*, 1941–42, 10–11.

2 MNI, *MNI AR*, 1942–43, 16–18.

3 MNI, *MNI AR*, 1941–42, 12.

4 MNI, *MNI AR*, 1942–43, 11.

5 The same was true of the nursing staff, although some left for personal reasons rather than military service, as Eileen Flanagan, director of nursing, reported: "As the War goes on, the difficulties in maintaining a stable nursing staff increase. During 1941 we have lost twenty members of the staff: eight have been married; two have joined

the R.C.A.M.C. [Royal Canadian Army Medical Corps]; two the Naval Nursing Service; two the Air Force Nursing Service and one the Victorian Order of Nurses." See MNI, *MNI AR*, 1941–42, 22.

6 A shadow was seen on Dr Penfield's chest X-ray, WPA.

7 MNI, *MNI AR*, 1941–42, 7.

8 Ibid., 11.

9 Ibid.

10 W. Penfield, MNI, *MNI AR*, 1943–44, 16.

11 Elizabeth McRea-Welch to Norma Isaacs, 27 August 1978, MNI Archives.

12 It is now in the OR head nurse's office and is reproduced here as figure 12.1.

13 William Feindel first worked as a research assistant with Miguel Prados, and later studied the effects of steroids on cerebral edema. MNI, *MNI AR*, 1943–44, 24.

14 Welch to Isaacs, 27 August 1978.

15 Peter Lehmann holds the distinction of having been the first Canadian-born senior resident of the institute, and of having performed the first thalamotomy for Parkinson's disease at the University of British Columbia in 1960. See C.R. Honey and S.P. Ravikant, "Surgery for Parkinson's Disease," *British Columbia Medical Journal* 43 (2001): 210–13. Claude Bertrand, the first French-Canadian fellow at the MNI, graduated in medicine from the Université de Montréal in 1940 and was awarded a Rhodes Scholarship upon his graduation, but took up residency at Oxford only after the war, in 1946. Bertrand was thus at Oxford with another MNI fellow, William Feindel, and both studied in Wilfrid Le Gros Clark's laboratory. Feindel would eventually become the third director of the MNI. Bertrand established the first Department of Neurosurgery at Hôpital Notre-Dame in 1947, the Université de Montréal's major teaching hospital. Feindel's dissertation was entitled "A Study of Neural Patterns by the Aid of Intravital Methylene Blue"; Bertrand's was "Diffusion and Absorption within the Brain."

16 MNI, *MNI AR*, 1941–42, 15; MNI, *MNI AR*, 1943–44, 9–11.

17 "Part of the early history of nursing was the romance and flirtation between the fellows and nurses which blossomed everywhere. Many long-standing marriages began here: those of Faith Lyman Feindel, Suzanne Langevin Power, Pat Murray McRea, Elizabeth McRea Welch, Rita Edward Lehmann, Vetha Merritt Paine (the operating room was apparently a hot-bed of Romance!) Goldie Jasper, Mary Buell Jacob, Arlene Croft Tower plus many, many more." See E.S. Vindicaire, "Romance and Marriage," in Barrowman et al., *Nursing Highlights 1934 to 1990*, 246.

18 W. Penfield, "The British-American-Canadian Surgical Mission to the U.S.S.R," *Canadian Medical Association Journal* 49 (1943): 455–61; Penfield, "Medicine in Free China," *British Medical Journal* 1 (1944): 821–2; D. Avery, "Wartime Medical Cooperation across the Pacific: Wilder Penfield and the Anglo-American Medical Missions to the Soviet Union and China, 1943–1944," *Pacific Science* 54 (2000): 289–98.

19 Avery, "Wartime Medical Cooperation."

20 Ibid.

21 Ibid., 292.

22 MNI, *MNI AR*, 1942–43, 8–9.

23 Avery, "Wartime Medical Cooperation," 293.

24 Twenty years after meeting with Chiang Kai-shek, it was now Mao who was "to China, what George Washington was to the United States of America, an unvanquished general and the first head of the new nation." NP-7, WPA.

25 J. Norman Petersen's early career showed great promise. From McGill's medical school and the Royal Victoria Hospital, he travelled to Boston and Philadelphia, to the National Hospital at Queen Square, London, and to la Salpêtrière in Paris. Petersen then studied under some of the famous Continental neurologists, including Spielmeyer in Germany, Brouwer in Holland, and Guillain in Paris. As William Feindel recalled, "All recognized Petersen's scholarly, gentle temperament. His devotion to the Institute was unmatched, as evidenced by his meticulous preparation of the annual reports during the Institute's first ten years. Norman Peterson had suffered from gout from an early age. Despite his progressing physical incapacity, which compelled him to use crutches and later a wheelchair, he continued actively teaching neurology. His lectures reflected his intellectual brilliance, good judgment and great experience, combined with a spiritual equanimity. In spite of a very painful and crippling illness, his loyalty to his colleagues and patients endeared him to his many friends. I came to know Dr Petersen in the latter part of his illness, when Petersen was confined to the bedroom and living room on the eighth floor of the Institute, and I occupied the room next door. I found Petersen to be gracious, open to enlightened conversation – sometimes peppered with pithy and astute comments about some of the characters at the Institute – despite his evident physical immobility and discomfort. Petersen's last Annual Report was written on his sickbed in the Residents' Suite at the Institute. He died 'in harness' as he wished it, beloved by all, first of the Institute's attending staff to go. Had this incongruous disease not struck him down, he would have undoubtedly become one of the leading figures in Canadian neurology, a continuing strength at the Institute. The tragedy of his untimely death reverberated through the halls of the Institute for many months." W. Feindel, reminiscence, M-109, MNI Archives.

26 MNI, *MNI AR*, 1944–45, 19.

27 Ibid., 14.

28 Ibid., 9–10.

29 C.M. Rémillard, B.G. Zifkin, A. Sherwin, and W. Feindel, "George A. Savoy, Visionary Benefactor of Canadians with Epilepsy, and the History of the Savoy Foundation for Epilepsy," *Canadian Journal of Neurological Science* 23 (1996): 80–2.

30 MNI, *MNI AR*, 1944–45, 37–8.

31 Of great significance to the institute was the recruitment of K.A.C. Elliot as neurochemist. His coming, however, was not without cost, as the space allocated for the fellows' squash court was reassigned to accommodate his laboratory.

32 MNI, *MNI AR*, 1944–45, 29.

33 Ibid., 7.

CHAPTER THIRTEEN

1 The exact quotation is "The significance of the building lies in the things which it houses … Within the shell should lie a living mollusk, a collective creature that is expected from time to time to form a pearl of great value." W. Penfield, "The Significance of the Montreal Neurological Institute," *Neurological Biographies and Addresses* (London: Oxford University Press, 1936), 52.

2 W.M. Nichols, "Changes in the Circulation of the Brain and Spinal Cord Associated with Nervous Activity" (master's thesis, McGill University, 1938).

3 C/G 40, WPA.

4 A/N 11 4/2, WPA.

5 Cameron, "Captain W. Martin Nichols."

6 C/G 41, WPA.

7 Nichols was president of the Society of British Neurological Surgeons from 1972 to 1974.

8 J. Bidzinski, "Jerzy Choróbski," *Surgical Neurology* 26 (1986): 425–7.

9 De Martel, like Chorobski's father, had also lost a son in the Great War and could not bear to see the Germans enter Paris for a second time in a generation. He committed suicide as they marched into Paris. Following his sojourn in the French capital, Chorobski returned to Poland, to the Neurological Clinic at the University of Warsaw.

10 J. Choróbski, "1. A Vasodilator Nervous Pathway to the Cerebral Vessels from the Central Nervous System. 2. On the Occurrence of Afferent Nerve Fibers in the Internal Carotid Plexus" (PhD diss., McGill University, 1932); J. Choróbski and W. Penfield, "Cerebral Vasodilator Nerves and Their Pathway from the Medulla Oblongata," *Archives of Neurology and Psychiatry* 28 (1932): 1257–69.

11 J. Choróbski and L. Davis, "Cyst Formation of the Skull," *Surgery, Gynecology & Obstetrics* 58 (1934): 12–31.

12 J. Subczynski, *In the Shadow of Satan* (Marco Island, FL: Keller Publishing, 2006).

13 J. Bidzinski, "Jerzy Choróbski," *Surgical Neurology* 26 (1986): 426

14 Ibid. Chorobski's experience was not unique among MNI fellows. Anatole Dekaban, a fellow at the institute from 1949 to 1951, was similarly involved with the Polish resistance. Unlike Chorobski, Dekaban was able to escape Communist rule when he fled Poland in 1947. See the Anatole S. and Pamela D. Dekaban Fund at http://dekaban.engin.umich.edu/fund/.

15 P.C. Bucy, "Editor's Comment," in *Modern Neurosurgical Giants*, ed. P.C. Bucy (New York: Elsivier, 1986), 60.

16 Bidzinski, "Jerzy Choróbski."

17 Ibid.

18 A.E. Carmichael, "E.A. Carmichael Editor 1938–1948," *Journal of Neurology, Neurosurgery and Psychiatry* 44 (1981): 859–60.

19 C/D 13, WPA.

20 A listing and discussion of Jerzy Chorobski's most important papers can be found in Bidzinski, "Jerzy Choróbski."

21 C/D 13, WPA

22 Ibid.

23 Ibid.

24 Ibid.

25 M. Hiller, "Wilgress, Leilun Dana," *Canadian Encyclopedia* (Edmonton: Hurtig Publishers, 1986): 3:1944.

26 C/D 13, WPA.

27 Ibid.

28 C.M. Fisher, *Memoirs of a Neurologist* (Rutland VT: Academy Books, 1992), 1:85–129.

29 Fisher comments on the effects of war on the previously thriving metropolis's now deserted streets: "It was downtown Toronto on a Sunday afternoon." Ibid., 87.

30 Ibid.

31 Ibid., 96.

32 Ibid.

33 Ibid., 120.

34 Ibid.

35 Ibid., 128–9.

36 E.D. McKenzie, "Mystery Man of Stalag XVII-B," We Pledge Allegiance: True War Stories, http://www.wepledgeallegiance.com/MysteryMan.htm.

37 P. Robb, "Dr Reuben Rabinovitch: An Appreciation," *Canadian Medical Association Journal* 93 (1965): 941–2.

38 A. Sicard, "Thierry de Martel, seigneur de la chirurgie et homme d'honneur," *Histoire des Sciences médicales* 26 (1992): 99–104; R. Rabinovitch, "Clovis Vincent, Neurosurgeon and Patriot," *Journal of Neurosurgery* 2 (1945): 530–4; Robb, "Dr Reuben Rabinovitch," 32–4.

39 Rabinovitch, "Clovis Vincent."

40 M. Seldin, *A Letter: Dr Reuben Rabinovitch 1908–1967* (Montreal: Montreal Neurological Institute, 1967), 11–13.

41 Ibid.

42 Ibid.

43 Ibid.

44 This is an extract from a letter to the editor of the *Montreal Star*. The letter was reprinted in the *Canadian Jewish Review*. See H. MacLennan, "Hugh MacLennan, Noted Canadian Author, Pays Tribute to the Late Dr Rabinovitch," *Canadian Jewish Review*, 22 October 1965. It was also published in H. MacLennan, *A Letter: Dr Reuben Rabinovitch 1908–1967* (Montreal: Montreal Neurological Institute, 1967), 10. Hugh MacLennan, a Montreal author and McGill English professor, wrote *The Watch That Ends the Night* about life and love on the night shift of a big city hospital. See H. MacLennan, *The Watch That Ends the Night* (Montreal and Kingston: McGill-Queen's University Press, 2009).

CHAPTER FOURTEEN

1 F. Andermann, "In Celebration of a Life Well Lived: Dr James Preston Robb April 4, 1914 – September 25, 2004," *Epilepsia* 46 (2005) 603–4; P. Robb, *The Development of Neurology at McGill University* (Montreal: Montreal Neurological Institute, 1989), 123–5.

2 F. Andermann, "In Celebration of a Life Well Lived: Dr James Preston Robb April 4, 1914 – September 25, 2004," *NeuroImage*, December 2004, 4–8.

3 Ibid.

4 P. Robb, *NINDS Monograph No. 1. Public Health Service Publication No. 1357* (Washington, DC: US Government Printing Office, 1965).

5 Robb was a visiting professor at the University of Nairobi in his retirement from the MNI.

6 W. Penfield, MNI, *MNI AR*, 1947–48, 5.

7 F. McNaughton, ibid., 28, 30; W.V. Cone, MNI, *MNI AR*, 1948–49, 26.

8 Anonymous, "Clarence Sumner Greene," *Journal of the National Medical Association* 50 (1958): 139–40; J.B. Barber Jr, "The Howard Division of Neurosurgery," *Journal of the National Medical Association* 59 (1967): 477–9; S. McLelland 3rd and K.S. Harris, "Clarence Sumner Greene Sr: The First African-American Neurosurgeon," *Neurosurgery* 59 (2006): 1325–7; S. McLelland 3rd, "The Montreal Neurological Institute: Training of the First African-American Neurosurgeons," *Journal of the National Medical Association* 99 (2007): 1071–3.

9 J.B. Barber, "Post-MNI ('58–'61) Activities: Second Letter," in *McGill Neurosurgical Reunion Round Robin* (Montreal: Montreal Neurological Institute and Hospital, 1995), 1.

10 Charles Drew was an African-American graduate of McGill Medical School who did his surgical residency at Freedmen's Hospital before moving on to Columbia Presbyterian Hospital. While at Columbia he worked with John Scudder on the storing of blood plasma. He later returned to Freedmen's Hospital as head of the Department of Surgery. Cone's role in Drew's career warrants further exploration. See "The Charles R. Drew Papers: Biographical Information," Profiles in Science, National Library of Medicine, http://profiles.nlm.nih.gov/ps/retrieve/Narrative/BG/p-nid/336; "Charles Drew," Biography.com, http://www.biography.com/people/charles-drew-9279094.

11 J.B. Barber, "Post-MNI ('58–'61) Activities: Second Letter," in *McGill Neurosurgical Reunion Round Robin* (Montreal: Montreal Neurological Institute and Hospital, 1995), 4.

12 Ibid.

13 H.M. Pappius and L.A. Dayes, "Hypertonic Urea: Its Effect on the Distribution of Water and Electrolytes in Normal and Edematous Brain Tissues," *Archives of Neurology* 3 (1965): 395–402.

14 From 1947 to 1967, three of the first four African-American neurosurgeons in the United States were trained at the MNI. However, despite the changing climate for visible minorities, by 1968 there were only twelve African-American neurosurgeons practising in the United States. Barber, "Post-MNI ('58–'61) Activities."

15 S. Yamada, "George Austin, MD," *Neurological Research* 23 (2001): 1–4; McLelland 3rd, "Montreal Neurological Institute."

16 MNI, *MNI AR*, 1946–47, 8.

17 Ibid.

18 Ibid., 9; emphasis added.

19 MNI, *MNI AR*, 1948–49, 5; emphasis added.

20 W.V. Cone, MNI, *MNI AR*, 1945–46, 13; emphasis added. Cone was also appreciative of another who would one day lead the MNI: "Finally, now that the laboratory activities are returning to normalcy, I would like to acknowledge indebtedness to Dr William Feindel, who in his last year in Medicine at McGill carried, in addition to his scholastic work, the duties of neuropathological fellow last year." Ibid., 22.

21 MNI, *MNI AR*, 1946–47, 29.

22 Ibid., 31, 38–9; MNI, *MNI AR*, 1947–48, 29, 30; H.H. Jasper and J. Droogleever-Fortuyn, "Thalamocortical System and the Electrical Activity of the Brain," *Federation Proceedings* 7 (1948): 61–2; H. Jasper, J. Hunter, and R. Knighton, "Experimental Studies of Thalamo-Cortical Systems," *Transactions of the American Neurological Association* 73 (1948): 210–12; J. Droogleever-Fortuyn, "Experimental Studies on Thalamo-Cortical Mechanisms," *Clinical Neurophysiology* 3 (1951): 394–400; J.S. Meyer and J. Hunter, "Behavior Deficits Following Diencephalic Lesions," *Neurology* 2 (1952): 112–30.

23 W. Penfield and K. Kristiansen, "Seizure Onset and the Localization of Epileptic Discharge," *Transactions of the American Neurological Association* 73 (1948): 73–80; K. Kristiansen and G. Courtois, "Rhythmic Electrical Activity from Isolated Cerebral Cortex," *Electroencephalography and Clinical Neurophysiology* 1 (1949): 265–71.

24 B.R. Kaada, K.H. Pribram, and J.A. Epstein, "Respiratory and Vascular Responses in Monkeys from Temporal Pole, Insula, Orbital Surface and Cingulate Gyrus: A Preliminary Report," *Journal of Neurophysiology* 12 (1949): 347–56; B.R. Kaada and H.H. Jasper, "Respiratory Responses to Stimulation of Temporal Pole, Insula, and Hippocampal and Limbic Gyri in Man," *Archives of Neurology and Psychiatry* 68 (1952): 609–19.

25 W. Penfield and H. Steelman, "The Treatment of Focal Epilepsy by Cortical Excision," *Annals of Surgery* 126 (1947): 740–62; W. Penfield and H. Flanigin, "Surgical Therapy of Temporal Lobe Seizures," *Archives of Neurology and Psychiatry* 64 (1950): 491–500.

26 J. Hunter and H.H. Jasper, "A Method of Analysis of Seizure Pattern and Electroencephalogram: A Cinematographic Technique," *Electroencephalography and Clinical Neurophysiology* 1 (1949): 113–14.

27 W. Penfield, "Obituary: Pio del Río-Hortega," *Archives of Neurology and Psychiatry* 54 (1945): 413–16; M. Prados and W. Gibson, "Pio del Río-Hortega 1882–1945," *Journal of Neurosurgery* 3 (1946): 275–84.

28 MNI, *MNI AR*, 1946–47, 30.

29 Ibid., 18, 26; W.V. Gibson, "The Diagnostic Problem in Poliomyelitis," *Canadian Medical Association Journal* 57 (1947): 531–6.

30 "Dr William C. Gibson: A Tribute from Green College, UBC," Green College, http://www.greencollege.ubc.ca/database/rte/files/William%20C%20Gibson%20Biography.pdf.

31 W. Penfield, "Ferrier Lecture: Some Observations on the Cerebral Cortex of Man," *Proceedings of the Royal Society of London. Series B, Biological Sciences* 134 (1947): 329–47.

32 W. Penfield and T. Rasmussen, *The Cerebral Cortex of Man: A Clinical Study of Localization of Function* (New York: MacMillan, 1950).

33 W. Penfield, "Neurology in Canada and the Osler Centennial," *Canadian Medical Association Journal* 61 (1949): 69–73.

34 W. Penfield and H.H. Jasper, "Highest Level Seizures," *Proceedings of the Association for Research in Nervous and Mental Disease* 26 (1947): 252–71; W. Penfield, "Epileptic Manifestations of Cortical and Supracortical Discharge," *Electroencephalography and Clinical Neurophysiology* 1 (1949): 3–10; H.H. Jasper, "Diffuse Projection Systems: The Integrative Action of the Thalamic Reticular System," *Electroencephalography and Clinical Neurophysiology* 1 (1949): 405–20.

35 Penfield, "Epileptic Manifestations of Cortical and Supracortical Discharge," 3.

36 MNI, *MNI AR*, 1947–48, 34; MNI, *MNI AR*, 1948–49, 32.

37 B. Babkin, "Origin of the Theory of Conditioned Reflexes: Sechenov, Hughlings Jackson, Pavlov," *Archives of Neurology and Psychiatry* 60 (1948): 520.

38 Ibid., 521.

39 Ibid.

40 *The Mystery of the Mind* is Penfield's final word on the brain-mind-soul question, but it is not his clearest expression on it, which instead can be found in his "Brain Mechanisms Related to Consciousness." See W. Penfield, "Brain Mechanisms Related to Consciousness: Epilepsy Points the Way," *Japanese Journal of Brain Physiology* 106 (1969): 1–18.

CHAPTER FIFTEEN

1 Penfield and Rasmussen, *Cerebral Cortex of Man*.

2 W. Penfield, "Some Observations on the Cerebral Cortex of Man," *Proceedings of the Royal Socisty of London B: Biological Sciences* 134 (1947): 329–47.

3 Ibid., vii.

4 Ibid., ix.

5 The homunculus, in its various guises, and the correlation of its grotesque shapes to the cortical areas that they represent, has been the subject of recent interest: G.S. Gandhoke, P. Nakaji, A. Abla, W. Feindel, R.F. Spetzler, and M.C. Preul, "The Homunculus: A Life, in and out of Realism," *Journal of Neurosurgery* 115 (2011): A425–A426; W. Feindel, "Little Man in the Cerebral Machine," 24 September 2011, MNI Archives; W. Feindel, "Homunculus," Neuro Critical Care Society, Montreal, 11 October 2011; Z. Ward, "The Changing Face of Penfield's Homunculus," *Osler Library Newsletter* 119 (2013): 13–14.

6 "Donald B. Tower," in *Neuroscience in Autobiography,* ed. L.R. Squire (New York: Academic, 2001), 3:433; emphasis added. http://www.sfn.org/~/media/SfN/Documents/TheHistoryofNeuroscience/Volume%203/c13.ashx.

7 Penfield and Rasmussen, *Cerebral Cortex of Man*, 13.

8 Ibid., 25, 56: emphasis added.

9 T. Rasmussen and W. Penfield, "Further Studies of the Sensory and Motor Cerebral Cortex of Man," *Federation Proceedings* 6 (1947): 452–60; W. Penfield, "A Second Somatic Sensory Area in the Cerebral Cortex of Man," *Transactions of the American Neurological Association* 74 (1949): 184–6; W. Penfield and T. Rasmussen, "Vocalization and Arrest of Speech," *Archives of Neurology and Psychiatry* 61 (1949): 21–7.

10 M. Critchley, "Sir Francis Walshe (1886–1973)," *Journal of the Neurological Sciences* 19 (1973): 255–6.

11 Ibid.

12 F.M.R. Walshe to W. Penfield, 25 April 1943, file C/G 20, WPA.

13 Penfield, "Some Observations on the Cerebral Cortex of Man."

14 F.M.R. Walshe to W. Penfield, 6 August 1946, file C/G 20, WPA.

15 File C/G 20, WPA.

16 "Donald B. Tower," 433–4.

17 Penfield and Rasmussen, *Cerebral Cortex of Man*, 90, 106.

18 Boldrey, "Architectonic Subdivision of the Mammalian Cerebral Cortex"; W. Penfield and E. Boldrey, "Somatic Motor and Sensory Representation in the Cerebral Cortex of Man as Studied by Electrical Stimulation," *Brain* 60 (1937): 389–443.

19 C. Vogt and O. Vogt, "Die vergleiohend-arkitektonische und die vergleichend-reizphysiologische Felderung der Grosshirnrinde unter besonderer Beriicksichtigunj der Menschlichen," *NatUrwissenschaften* 14 (1926): 1191.

20 Boldrey, "Architectonic Subdivision," 173–4.

21 R.M. Brickner, "A Human Cortical Area Producing Repetitive Phenomena When Stimulated," *Journal of Neurophysiology* 3 (1940): 128–30.

22 W. Penfield and K. Welch, "The Supplementary Motor Area in the Cerebral Cortex of Man," *Transactions of the American Neurological Association* 74 (1949): 179–84; W. Penfield and K. Welch, "The Supplementary Motor Area of the Cerebral Cortex of Man," *Archives of Neurology and Psychiatry* 66 (1951): 289–317. While at the MNI, Keasley Welch wrote a far-sighted MSc thesis on tumour-mediated neo-vascularization in transplanted glioblatomas, a subject that did not reach the mainstream of oncological research for another fifty years. During his first day on the neurosurgical service, Welch was taught how to gown and glove "the Neuro way" – a complicated affair designed to minimize the risk of infection – by the operating room supervisor, Elizabeth MacRae, whom he later married. After serving in the United States Army Medical Corps, Welch took a position at the University of Colorado, one of four former MNI fellows to do so – Maitland Baldwin, Richard Lende, and Milton Shy were the other three. After sixteen years at Colorado, Welch was appointed chief of neurosurgery at Brigham and Women's and Children's Hospital of Harvard University, where he stayed until retirement. See K.M. Welch, "A Morphological Study of Human Glioblastoma Multiforme Transplanted to Guinea Pigs" (master's thesis, McGill University, 1947).

23 Penfield and Welsh, "Supplementary Motor Area," 180; emphasis added.

24 W. Penfield, "Observations on Cerebral Localization of Function," *Comptes Rendus, IV Congres Neurologique International*, vol. 3, lecture 1 (1949): 427.

25 P. Robb, "A Study of the Effects of Cortical Excision on Speech in Patients with Previous Cerebral Injuries" (master's thesis, McGill University, 1946); J.P. Robb, "Effects of Cortical Excision and Stimulation of the Frontal Lobe on Speech," *Association for Research in Nervous and Mental Disease* 27 (1947): 587–609.

26 L. Roberts, "A Study of Certain Alterations in Speech during Stimulation of Specific Cortical Regions" (master's thesis, McGill University, 1949).

27 Ibid.; L. Roberts, "Localization of Speech in the Cerebral Cortex," *Transactions of the American Neurological Association* 56 (1951): 43–50.

28 J. Dejerine, "Sur un cas de cécité verbale avec agraphie, suivi d'autopsie," *Comptes rendus hebdomadaires des séances et mémoires de la société de biologie* 3, no. 9 (1891): 197–201.

29 Roberts, "Study of Certain Alterations," 28–9.

30 Roberts, "Localization of Speech," 46.

31 Ibid., 185.

32 W. Penfield and L. Roberts, *Speech and Brain Mechanisms* (Princeton, NJ: Princeton University Press, 1959).

33 J. Dejerine and A. Dejerine-Klumpke, *Anatomie des centres nerveux* (Paris: Ruff, 1901), 2:247–8; P. Marie and C. Foix, "Les aphasies de guerre," *Neurologie* 24 (1917): 53–87; A.R. Luria, *Traumatic Aphasia* (The Hague: Mouton, 1970).

34 *Speech and Brain Mechanisms* was Lamar Roberts's last publication from the MNI. A graduate of Duke University, Roberts had come to the institute as an intern in neurosurgery in 1948 and completed his residency in 1952, whereupon he was called to San Diego for military service in the United States Navy. Roberts returned to the MNI in 1954 as a staff neurosurgeon, where he continued his work on language, and on epileptogenic conditioned responses with Herbert Jasper and Frank Morrell. Lamar Roberts left the institute in 1958 to become the inaugural head of the Division of Neurosurgery at the University of Florida, Gainesville. Albert Rhoton succeeded him in 1972. See F. Morrell, L. Roberts, and H.H. Jasper, "Effect of Focal Epileptogenic Lesions and Their Ablation upon Conditioned Electrical Responses of the Brain in the Monkey," *Electroencephalography and Clinical Neurology* 8 (1956): 217–36; MNI, *MNI AR*, 1958–59, 11.

35 Dejerine, *Anatomie des centres nerveux*, figs 248, 247; Penfield and Roberts, *Speech and Brain Mechanisms*, fig. X-4, 201.

36 A-L. Foville, *Traité complet de l'anatomie, de la physiologie et de la pathologie du système nerveux cérébro-spinal* (Paris: Fortin, Masson, 1844); Dejerine, *Anatomie des centres nerveux*, 247–52.

37 Dejerine, *Anatomie des centres nerveux*, trans. R. Leblanc, 247; capitalization and emphasis in original.

38 Penfield and Roberts, *Speech and Brain Mechanisms*, 136.

39 Dejerine, *Anatomie des centres nerveux*, 248.

40 Ibid.

41 Penfield and Roberts, *Speech and Brain Mechanisms*, 188.

42 T. Rasmussen and B. Milner, "Clinical and Surgical Studies of the Cerebral Speech Areas in Man," in *Cerebral Localization*, ed. K.J. Zulch, O. Creutzfeldt, and G.C. Galbraith, 238–57 (Berlin: Springer-Verlag, 1975).

43 S. Finger, "Francis Schiller (1909–2003)," *Journal of the History of the Neurosciences* 13 (2004): 353–7.

44 F. Schiller, "Aphasia Studied in Patients with Missile Wounds," *Journal of Neurology, Neurosurgery and Psychiatry* 10 (1947): 183–97.

45 Roberts, "Study of Certain Alterations," 13, 34.

46 Roberts, "Alterations in Speech," 34.

47 F. Schiller, *Paul Broca: Founder of French Anthropology, Explorer of the Brain* (Oakland: University of California Press, 1979).

48 F. Schiller, "Consciousness Reconsidered," *Archives of Neurology and Psychiatry* 67 (1952): 199–227.

49 "Symposium on Brain and Mind," *Archives of Neurology and Psychiatry* 67 (1952): 135–227.

50 S. Cobb, "On the Nature and Locus of Mind," *Archives of Neurology and Psychiatry* 67 (1952): 172.

51 Schiller, "Aphasia Studied in Patients."

52 W. Penfield, "Memory Mechanisms," *Archives of Neurology and Psychiatry* 67 (1952): 196.

CHAPTER SIXTEEN

1 W. Penfield and H. Erickson, *Epilepsy and Cerebral Localization* (Baltimore, MD: Charles C. Thomas, 1941).

2 Ibid., 301.

3 H.H. Jasper and J. Kershman, "Electroencephalographic Classification of the Epilepsies," *Archives of Neurology and Psychiatry* 45 (1941): 939–40.

4 Harry Steelman earned his medical degree from Duke University in 1943 and trained in neurosurgery at the MNI from 1944 to 1947. Steelman then relocated to the Walter Reed Army Medical Center in Washington DC, where he served as chief of neurological surgery during the Korean War. After his discharge from the Army, Steelman moved to Phoenix, Arizona, where he pursued his interest in the surgical treatment of epilepsy, in collaboration with John Green, the founder of the Barrow Neurological Institute. See W. Penfield and H. Steelman, "The Treatment of Focal Epilepsy by Cortical Excision," *Annals of Surgery* 126 (1947): 740–61.

5 Ibid., 760. Emphasis added.

6 Ibid., 762.

7 W. Penfield and A. Ward, "Calcifying Epileptogenic Lesions, Hemangioma Calcificans: Report of a Case," *Archives of Neurology and Psychiatry* 60 (1948): 20–36.

8 Herman Flanigin came to the MNI in 1946 to complete a residency in neurosurgery. He also worked with Herbert Jasper to further enhance his understanding of epilepsy before returning to Oklahoma City in 1950, where he performed the first temporal lobectomy for the treatment of epilepsy. See W. Penfield and H. Flanigin, "Surgical Therapy of Temporal Lobe Seizures," *Archives of Neurology and Psychiatry* 64 (1950): 491–500.

9 Penfield and Flanigin, "Surgical Therapy of Temporal Lobe Seizures," 497; emphasis added.

10 "This type of experience in a number of patients through the years ... plus increasing confidence in the cortical EEG, has led to the gradual development of our present plan of cortical excision." T. Rasmussen, "Cortical Excision for Medically Refractory Focal Epilepsy," in *Epilepsy Proceedings of the Hans Berger Centenary Symposium*, ed. P. Harris and C. Mawdsley (Edinburgh: Churchill Livingston, 1974), 229.

11 M. Baldwin, "Functional Representation in the Temporal Lobe of Man" (master's thesis, McGill University, 1952).

12 Ibid., 8–9.

13 Ibid., 98–101.

14 W. Penfield and M. Baldwin, "Temporal Lobe Seizures and the Technique of Subtotal Temporal Lobectomy," *Annals of Surgery* 136 (1952): 629.

15 W. Feindel and W. Penfield, "Localization of Discharrge in Temporal Lobe Automatism," *Archives of Neurology and Psychiatry* 72 (1954): 605–30.

16 Penfield and Baldwin, "Temporal Lobe Seizures," 632.

17 K.M. Earle, M. Baldwin, and W. Penfield, "Incisural Sclerosis and Temporal Lobe Seizures Produced by Hippocampal Herniation at Birth," *Archives of Neurology and Psychiatry* 69 (1953): 27–42.

18 Penfield and Baldwin, "Temporal Lobe Seizures," 634. It has been said that everything has been written but not everything has been read. This is certainly the case for incisural sclerosis, as it was first described by Chaslin in 1889, and rediscovered by Spielmeyer in 1930. See P. Chaslin, "Note sur l'anatomie pathologique de l'épilepsie essentielle: la sclérose névroglique." *Comptes rendus hebdomadaires des séances et mémoires de la société de biologie* 1 (1889): 169–71; W. Spielmeyer, "Anatomic Substratum of the Convulsive State," *Archives of Neurology and Psychiatry* 23 (1930): 869–75.

19 W. Feindel, W. Penfield, and H.H. Jasper, "Localization of Epileptic Discharge in Temporal Lobe Automatism," *Transactions of the American Neurological Association* 77 (1952): 14–17; W. Feindel and W. Penfield, "Localization of Discharge in Temporal Lobe Automatism," *Archives of Neurology and Psychiatry* 72 (1954): 605–30; W. Feindel and P. Gloor, "Comparison of Electroencephalographic Effects of Stimulation of Amygdala and Brainstem Reticular Formation in Cats," *Electroencephalography and Clinical Neurophysiology* 6 (1954): 389–402; H.H. Jasper and T. Rasmussen, "Studies of Clinical and Electrical Responses to Deep Temporal Stimulation in Man with Some Consideration of Functional Anatomy," *Proceedings of the Association for Research in Nervous and Mental Disease* 36 (1956): 316–34.

20 Jasper and Kershman, "Electroencephalographic Classification," 939–40.

21 Jasper and Rasmussen, "Studies of Clinical and Electrical Responses."

22 P. Gloor, A. Olivier, L.F. Quesney, F Andermann and S. Horowitz, "The Role of the Limbic System in Experiential Phenomena of Temporal Lobe Epilepsy," *Annals of Neurology* 12 (1982): 129–44.

23 W. Penfield, MNI, *MNI AR*, 1949–50, 5.

24 Ibid., 8; emphasis added.

25 Ibid., 8–9.

26 Ibid., 5.

27 Ibid., 6.
28 Ibid.
29 MNI, *MNI AR*, 1948–49, 44.
30 MNI, *MNI AR*, 1949–50, 6–7; emphasis added.
31 Ibid., 32–3.
32 B.P. Babkin, "I.V. Pavlov, 1849–1949," *Canadian Medical Association Journal* 34 (1936): 438–9.
33 F.C. MacIntosh, "Boris Petrovich Babkin 1877–1950," *Revue Canadienne de Biologie* 10 (1951): 3–7; I. deDurgh Daly, S.A. Komarov, and E.G. Young, "Boris Petrovitch Babkin, 1877–1950," *Obituary Notices of Fellows of the Royal Society* 8 (1952): 12–23.

CHAPTER SEVENTEEN

1 MNI, *MNI AR*, 1950–51, 6–7.
2 "These nominations only make official the friendly relations that we have entertained with Neurology in Quebec over many years, and more recently with its neurosurgery. They constitute an acknowledgment of the excellent work accomplished by our colleagues in the Provincial capital." Trans. R. Leblanc. See MNI, *AR, 1950–51,* 6.
3 MNI, *MNI AR*, 1949–50, 10.
4 F. McNaughton to W. Penfield, 10 November 1943, Francis Lothian McNaughton Fonds, Osler Library of the History of Medicine, McGill University.
5 P. Robb, MNI, *MNI AR*, 1974–75, 28; D. Goulet, *Histoire de la Neurologie au Québec* (Montreal: Carte Blanche, 2011), 319–20.
6 J.B. Martin, MNI, *MNI AR*, 1977–78, 28; Goulet, *Histoire.*
7 A. Delmas and G. Bertrand, "La Veine retro-rolandique," *Comptes rendus de l'Association d'anatomie* 37 (1950): 1–7; A. Delmas, B. Pertuiset, and G. Bertrand, "Veins of the Temporal Lobe," *Revue d'otoneuroophtalmolgie* 23 (1951): 224–30.
8 G. Bertrand, "Dynamic Factors in the Evolution of Syringomyelia and Syringobulbia," *Clinical Neurosurgery* 20 (1973): 322–33.
9 G. Bertrand, "Stereotactic Surgery at McGill: The Early Years," *Neurosurgery* 54 (2001): 1244–52; H.H. Jasper and G. Bertrand, "Recording from Microelectrodes in Stereotaxic Surgery for Parkinson's Disease," *Journal of Neurosurgery* 24 (1966): 219–21; H.H. Jasper and G. Bertrand, "Stereotaxic Microelectrode Studies of Single Thalamic Cells and Fibers in Patients with Dyskinesia," *Transactions of the American Neurological Association* 89 (1964): 79–82; H.H. Jasper and G. Bertrand, "Thalamic Units Involved in Somatic Sensation and Voluntary and Involuntary Movements in Man," in *The Thalamus*, ed. D.F. Purpura and M.D. Yahr, 365–90 (New York: Columbia University Press, 1966).
10 C.J. Thompson and G. Bertrand, "A Computer Program to Aid the Neurosurgeon to Locate Probes Used during Stereotactic Surgery of Deep Cerebral Structures," *Computer Methods and Programs in Biomedicine* 2 (1972): 265–76.
11 Francis LeBlanc left the institute to become professor of clinical neurosciences in the Faculty of Medicine at the University of Calgary, where he specialized in spinal

surgery. LeBlanc later returned to the MNI for a short stay, to treat one of the attending neurosurgeons for a lumbar disc herniation. The University of Calgary established the Frank LeBlanc Chair in Spinal Cord Research in 2009.

12 A. Olivier, W.W. Boling, and T. Taniverdi, *Techniques in Epilepsy Surgery: The MNI Approach* (Cambridge: Cambridge University Press, 2012).

13 J.C. Thomas and E.M. Davidson, *Social Problems of the Epileptic Patient: Report of a Medical Social Study / Problèmes sociaux de l'épileptique. Compte rendu d'une étude médicosociale* (Montreal: Montreal Neurological Institute, 1949): 62.

14 G. Jefferson, "The Mind of Mechanical Man," *British Medical Journal*, 25 June 1949, 1105–10.

CHAPTER EIGHTEEN

1 W. Penfield, MNI, *MNI AR*, 1951–52, 4.

2 Ibid., 28.

3 H.H. Jasper and C. Ajmone-Marsan produced a widely used stereotaxic atlas of the cat. Jerzy Olszewski produced two atlases, one of the *Macaca mulatta*, and the other, with Donald Baxter, of man. Olszewski and Baxter's atlas has achieved classic status and remains in print. See H.H. Jasper and C. Ajmone-Marsan, *Stereotaxic Atlas of the Diencephalon of the Cat* (Ottawa: National Research Council of Canada, 1954); J. Olszewski, *The Thalamus of the Macaca Mulatta: An Atlas for Use with the Stereotaxic Instrument* (Basel: S. Karger, 1952); J. Olszewski and D. Baxter, *Cytoarchitecture of the Human Brain Stem* (Basel: S. Karger, 1954).

4 D.H. Hubel, in *The History of Neuroscience in Autobiography,* ed. L.R. Squire (Washington, DC: Society for Neuroscience, 1996), 1:299. http://www.sfn.org/~/media/sfn/documents/autobiographies/c9.ashx.

5 Ibid., 300.

6 Ibid.

7 Ibid.

8 W. Penfield, MNI, *MNI AR*, 1952–53, 8.

9 Ibid., 10.

10 J.C. Eccles, "Hypotheses Relating to the Brain-Mind Problem," *Nature* 168 (1951): 53–7.

11 MNI, *MNI AR*, 1951–52, 6.

12 B. McArdle, "Myopathy Due to a Defect in Muscle Glycogen Breakdown," *Clinical Science* 10 (1951): 13–33.

13 MNI, *MNI AR*, 1952–53, 5.

14 Ibid., 5.

15 E. Flanagan, "The Parts of Pisces," in *Fair Shake: The Autobiographical Essays by McGill Women,* ed. M. Gillett and K.A. Sibbald, 40–53 (Montreal: Eden, 1984), 42.

16 Ibid., 44.

17 Ibid., 45.

18 Ibid., 45–6.

19 As impressed as she might have been for this unexpected beneficence, it is clear that

the night belonged to another unexpected guest, as Flanagan recounts: "Mrs Dorothy Killam … had flown from the Bahamas for the occasion and, to the delight of the guests, she was wearing her famous diamonds. These were a great part of her estate and contributed to her munificent bequest to the Institute." Ibid., 46.

20 Ibid., 46–7.

21 E. Desjardins, E.C. Flanagan, and S. Giroux, *Heritage: History of the Nursing Profession in Quebec from the Augustinians and Jeanne Mance to Medicare* (Montreal: Association of Nurses of the Province of Québec, 1971).

22 G.J. Wherrett, *The Miracle of the Empty Beds: A History of Tuberculosis in Canada* (Toronto: University of Toronto Press, 1977).

23 Flanagan, "Parts of Pisces," 48.

24 MNI, *MNI AR*, 1951–52, 5–6.

25 W. Cone and S.E. Barrera, "The Brain and the Cerebrospinal Fluid in Acute Aseptic Cerebral Embolism: An Experimental and Pathologic Study," *Archives of Neurology and Psychiatry* 25 (1931): 546.

26 Evans, "Study of Cerebral Cicatrix."

27 Fisher, *Memoirs of a Neurologist*.

28 Ibid., 61.

29 Ibid.

30 Personal communication, Eric Peterson to Richard Leblanc, 1976.

31 M. Fisher, "Occlusion of the Internal Carotid Artery," *Archives of Neurology and Psychiatry* 65 (1951): 347.

32 C.M. Fisher, "Concerning Strokes," *Canadian Medical Association Journal* 69 (1952): 257–68; Fisher, "Occlusion of the Carotid Arteries," *Archives of Neurology and Psychiatry* 72 (1954): 187–204.

33 Fisher, "Occlusion of the Carotid Arteries."

34 C.M. Fisher, "Observations of the Fundus Oculi in Transient Monocular Blindness," *Neurology* 9 (1959): 333–47.

35 M. Fisher, "Occlusion of the Internal Carotid Artery," *Archives of Neurology and Psychiatry* 65 (1951): 377.

36 C.M. Fisher, "Occlusion of the Carotid Arteries," *Archives of Neurology and Psychiatry* 72 (1954): 203. Miller Fisher's papers on carotid occlusion largely eclipsed Arthur Elvidge's correlation of hemiplegia with occlusion of the internal carotid and middle cerebral arteries as demonstrated by angiography, published in December 1951. A.R. Elvidge and A. Werner, "Hemiplegia and Thrombosis of the Internal Carotid System," *Archives of Neurology and Psychiatry* 66 (1951): 752–82.

37 Fisher, *Memoirs of a Neurologist*, 58–61.

CHAPTER NINETEEN

1 Ibid.

2 R.L. Maitland, "National Institute of Neurological Diseases and Blindness: Development and Growth (1960–1968)," in *The Nervous System*, ed. R.O. Brady and D.B. Tower (New York: Raven, 1975), 1:xxxiii–xlvi; D.B. Tower, "The Impact of the NINCDS on the

Neurosciences: An Essay Written for the Centennial of the NIH," *Journal of Neuroscience* 7 (1987): 1601–6.

3   E. Goldensohn, "George Milton Shy 1919–1967," *Archives of Neurology* 18 (1968): 453–4.

4   G.M. Shy, S. Brendle, R. Rabinovitch, and D. McEachern, "The Effects of Cortisone in Certain Neuromuscular Disorders," *Journal of the American Medical Association* 144 (1950): 1353–8.

5   G.M. Shy and G.A. Drager, "A Neurological Syndrome Associated with Orthostatic Hypotension: A Clinical-Pathological Study," *Archives of Neurology* 12 (1960): 511–27.

6   F.H. O'Brien and A.S Dekaban, "Maitland Baldwin Sept. 29, 1918–Feb. 9, 1970," *Neurology* 21 (1971): 872.

7   C. Ajmone-Marsan, "Clinical Neurophysiology and Epilepsy in the Early Years of the NINDB Intramural Program," in *Mind, Brain, Body, and Behavior*, ed. I.G. Farreras, C. Hannaway, and V.A. Harden (Amsterdam: IOS, 2004), 155.

8   M. Baldwin, P. Bailey, C. Ajmone-Marsan, I. Klatzo, and D. Tower, *Temporal Lobe Epilepsy: A Colloquium Sponsored by the National Institute of Neurological Diseases and Blindness, National Institute of Health, Bethesda, Maryland, in Cooperation with the International League against Epilepsy* (Springfield, IL: Charles C. Thomas, 1958).

9   Paul Mclean was one of the most original thinkers in the neurosciences of the last century. He is most remembered for his intriguing *Triune Brain in Evolution: Role in Paleocerebral Functions* (New York: Plenum, 1990).

10 Cosimo Ajmone-Marsan to William Feindel, 28 March 1986, MNI Archives.

11 Cosimo Ajmone-Marsan served as president of the American Epilepsy Society in 1973 and as editor-in-chief of the IBRO Symposia Monograph Series from 1978 to 1984. Among his distinctions is the Award for Ambassador of Epilepsy in recognition of outstanding contributions. Ajmone-Marsan left the NIH in 1979 for the University of Miami School of Medicine, where he remained, as head of the Electroencephalography Laboratory in the Department of Neurology, until his retirement in 1997. See Ajmone-Marsan, *Mind, Brain, Body, and Behavior*, 151–68.

12 Ibid.

13 J.M. Van Buren, "The Cortical Representation of the Feeding Reflex" (master's thesis, McGill University, 1950).

14 G.A. Ojeman, "In Memoriam Arthur Allen Ward, Jr, MD, 1916–1997," *Epilepsia* 39 (1998): 560–4; G.U. Mehta, J.D. Heiss, J.K. Park, A.R. Asthagiri, and R.R. Lonser, "Neurological Surgery at the National Institutes of Health," *World Neurosurgery* 74 (2010): 49–59.

15 C.L. Li, "Anatomical Study of Fiber Connections of the Temporal Pole in the Cat" (master's thesis, McGill University, 1950).

16 H.H. Jasper, MNI, *MNI AR*, 1953–54, 36–7.

17 C-L. Li, "Microelectrode Studies of the Electrical Activity of the Cerebral Cortex" (PhD diss., McGill University, 1954).

18 Z.M. Rap, "In Memory of Professor Igor Klatzo (1916–2007)," *Folia Neuropathologica* 45 (2007): 153–4.

19 I. Klatzo, "Cecile and Oskar Vogt: The Visionaries of Modern Neuroscience," *Acta Neurochirurgica Supplement (Book 80)* (New York: Springer Wein, 2002).

20 I. Klatzo, "A Study of Glioblastoma Multiforme by the Golgi Method," *American Journal of Pathology* 28 (1952): 357–67; Klatzo, "A Study of Glia by the Golgi Method," *Laboratory Investigation* 1 (1952): 345–50.

21 I. Klatzo, "Presidential Address: Neuropathological Aspects of Brain Edema," *Journal of Neuropathology and Experimental Neurology* 26 (1967): 1–14; I. Klatzo, D.C. Gajdusek, and V. Zigas, "Pathology of Kuru," *Laboratory Investigation* 8 (1959): 799–847.

22 Klatzo, "Cecile and Oskar Vogt."

23 D.B. Tower, "The Role of Acetylcholine in Neural Activity with Particular Reference to Craniocerebral Trauma and Epilepsy" (master's thesis, McGill University, 1948); Tower, "A Study of the Acetylcholine System in the Cerebral Cortex of Various Mammals and in the Human Epileptogenic Focus and of Certain Factors which Affect Its Activity" (PhD diss., McGill University, 1951).

24 "Tower," *History of Neuroscience in Autobiography*, 430.

25 Ibid, 434.

26 Ibid.

27 Ibid.

CHAPTER TWENTY

1 Montreal Neurological Institute, *Prospect and Retrospect in Neurology: 2nd Foundation Volume Published for the Staff, to Commemorate the Opening of the McConnell Wing and the 2nd Foundation of the Montreal Neurological Institute of McGill University* (Boston: Little Brown, 1955).

2 Ibid., 23.

3 Ibid., viii–x.

4 W. Feindel, "Children of the Brain: A Cerebral Christmas Card," *NeuroImage* (December 1987): 1–3.

5 Ibid.

6 M. Filer Spence-Sales, "The Advance of Neurology," in Barrowman et al., *Nursing Highlights,* 162–5.

7 File A/N 33, WPA.

8 Although not mentioned by Filer, the parallel with Gauguin's *D'où venons-nous? Que sommes-nous? Où allons-nous?* is obvious. Wilder Penfield had a more prosaic view of the mural, describing it as "an artistic fantasy that moves through history from barbaric trepanation and the mystery of Aesculapius to the science of the future." See W. Penfield, *Prospects and Retrospect in Neurology* (Boston: Little, Brown and Company, 1955), x.

9 John Kershman died suddenly, at the age of forty-four, in 1951. As Penfield recalled, "He was an indefatigable worker who had achieved true distinction as clinician and electroencephalographer and who gave promise of greater things. Kindness, understanding, and humor came and went with Jack Kershman." Donald McEachern also

passed away in 1951, at the age of forty-seven. "Each of these two gifted men," wrote Francis McNaughton, "created for himself a unique position in the life of the Institute which no one else can hope to fill. Their work, their scientific achievements, their personalities, are built into the very walls of this place, and their influence upon us continues in a thousand ways." MNI, *MNI AR*, 1951–52, 5, 20.

10 File A/N 33, WPA. In this, Filer is in good company: Goya painted the Duchess of Alba in a pose highly reminiscent of Filer's patient, in a state of deshabille (*La maja desnuda*) and more chastely covered (*La maja vestida*).

11 J.N. Walton, *Brain's Diseases of the Nervous System* (Oxford: Oxford University Press, 1969).

12 W. Penfield and H.H. Jasper, *Epilepsy and the Functional Anatomy of the Human Brain* (Boston: Little, Brown, 1954).

13 W.R. Amberson, "Epilepsy and the Functional Anatomy of the Human Brain," *Science* 119 (1954): 645–6.

14 W. Penfield, "Epileptic Automatism and the Centrencephalic Integrating System," *Research Publication of the Association for Research in Nervous and Mental Diseases* 30 (1952): 513–28.

15 W. Penfield, "The Cerebral Cortex and Consciousness: The Harvey Lecture, 1936," *Archives of Neurology and Psychiatry* 40 (1938): 441–2.

16 W. Penfield, "Epileptic Automatism and the Centrencephalic Integrating System," *Association for the Research in Nervous and Mental Disease* 30 (1952): 513.

17 Ibid., 513.

18 W. Penfield and H.H. Jasper, *Epilepsy and the Functional Anatomy of the Human Brain* (Boston: Little, Brown, 1954): 481–2.

19 F.M.R. Walshe, "The Brain-Stem and the 'Highest Level' of Function in the Nervous System: With Particular Reference to the 'Automatic Apparatus' of Carpenter (1950) and to the 'Centrencephalic Integrating System' of Penfield," *Brain* 80 (1957): 537.

20 W. Penfield, "Centrencephalic Integrating System," *Brain* 81 (1958): 232; emphasis in the original.

21 For letters between Penfield and Walshe, see file C/D 20, WPA.

CHAPTER TWENTY-ONE

1 W. Penfield, MNI, *MNI AR*, 1954–55, 6.

2 J. Hanbery and H.H. Jasper, "Independence of Diffuse Thalamo-Cortical Projection System Shown by Specific Nuclear Destructions," *Journal of Neurophysiology* 16 (1953): 252–71; J. Hanbery, C. Ajmone-Marsan, and M. Dilworth, "Pathways of Non-Specific Thalamo-Cortical Projection System," *Electroencephalography and Clinical Neurophysiology* 6 (1954): 103–18; B.S. Nashold, "Observations on the Thalamocortical Projections" (master's thesis, McGill University, 1954); B.S. Nashold, J. Hanbery, and J. Olszewski, "Observations on the Diffuse Thalamic Projections," *Electroencephalography and Clinical Neurophysiology* 7 (1955): 609–20.

3 I. Heller, "The Desoxyribonucleic Acid Content, Cell Densities and Metabolism of Normal Brain and Human Brain Tumours" (master's thesis, McGill University, 1954);

I. Heller and K.C.A. Elliott, "The Metabolism of Normal Brain and Human Gliomas in Relation to Cell Type and Density," *Canadian Journal of Biochemistry and Physiology* 33 (1955): 395–403.

4   MNI, *MNI AR*, 1954–55, 7.

5   Ibid., 21–2.

6   K.H. Pribram, "Hemispheric Specialization: Evolution or Revolution," *Annals of the New York Academy of Sciences* 299 (1977): 18.

7   K.H. Pribram, "What Makes Man Human," *James Arthur Lecture on the Evolution of the Human Brain* 39 (1970), American Museum of Natural History. http://digitallibrary.amnh.org/handle/2246/5998.

8   I. Tattersall, "Karl Pribram, the James Arthur Lectures, and What Makes Us Human," *Journal of Biomedical Discovery and Collaboration* 1 (2006): 15. doi: 10.1186/1747-5333-1-15,

9   The MNI contingent in Saskatoon eventually also included neurosurgeons Joseph Stratford and Kenneth Paine, neurologists Donald Baxter and Allan Bailey, neuroradiologist Sidney Traub, neuroanaesthetist Allen Dobkin, and neuropathologists Jerzy Olszewski and Bohdan Rozdilsky. Sidney Traub had studied meningiomas as a research fellow at the institute, and Bohdan Rozdilsky had just finished his MSc with Olszewski. See B. Rozdilsky, "Permeability of Cerebral Blood Vessels to Protein Molecules in Convulsive Zeizures" (master's thesis, McGill University, 1956).

10   Personal papers 1940–1989, box 9, Feindel Fonds.

11   W. Penfield, MNI, *MNI AR*, 1955–56, 9.

12   A. Gregg, "Medical Institute," in *Prospects and Retrospects in Neurology Second Foundation Volume* (Boston: Little, Brown and Comapnt, 1955), 20.

13   Ibid., 6.

14   Ibid.,10.

15   André Pasquet's contributions to neurosurgical anaesthesia were pioneering, and his insights into the management of patients operated upon with the aid of local anacsthesia are as valid today as they were when Penfield was operating. See C.R. Stephen and A. Pasquet, "Anesthesia for Neurosurgical Procedures: Analysis of 1,000 Cases," *Current Research in Anesthesiology and Analgesia* 28 (1949): 77–88.

16   A. Olivier, "Epilepsy Surgery at the MNI: From Archibald to the Creation of the Shirley and Mark Rayport Fellowship in Surgery of Epilepsy," *Epilepsia* 51, supplement 1 (2010): 97–100.

17   "Kindling: A Symposium on Basic Research in Neuroscience, Vancouver, May 16–17, 1975," ed. J.A. Wada, *Canadian Journal of Neurological Sciences* 2 (1975): 383–522.

18   F. Morrell, "Effect of Focal Epileptogenic Lesions on the Connecting Function of Brain" (master's thesis, McGill University, 1955).

19   J. Engel, "Frank Morrell (1926–1996)," *Epilepsia* 38 (1997): 261–2.

20   P. Gloor, "Electrophysiological Studies on the Connections of the Amygdaloid Nucleus of the Cat. I. The Neuronal Organization of the Amygdaloid Projection System," *Electroencephalography and Clinical Neurophysiology* 7 (1955): 223–42; Gloor, "Electrophysiological Studies on the Connections of the Amygdaloid Nucleus of the Cat. II. The Electrophysiological Properties of the Amygdaloid Projection System,"

Electroencephalography and Clinical Neurophysiology 7 (1955): 243–64; D.H. Ingvar, "Electrical Activity of Isolated Cortex in the Un-Anaesthetized Cat with Intact Brain Stem," *Acta Physiologica Scandinavia* 33 (1955): 151–68; Ingvar, "Extraneuronal Influence upon the Electrical Activity of Isolated Cortex Following Stimulation of the Reticular System," *Acta Physiologica Scandinavia* 33 (1955): 169–93; Ingvar, "Reproduction of the 3 per Second Spike and Wave EEG Pattern by Subcortical Electrical Stimulation in Cats," *Acta Physiologica Scandinavia* 33 (1955): 137–50; D.H. Ingvar and J. Hunter, "Influence of Visual Cortex upon Light Impulses in the Brain Stem of the Unanaesthetized Cat," *Acta Physiologica Scandinavia* 33 (1955): 194–218.

21 Israel Weschler, of Columbia University, gave the 1956 Hughlings Jackson Lecture, "On the Broadening Concepts of Neurology."

22 D.J. Beck and D. Russell, "Experiments on Thrombosis of the Superior Longitudinal Sinus," *Journal of Neurosurgery* 3 (1946): 337–47.

23 C.E. Gilkes, "An Account of the Life and Achievements of Miss Diana Beck, Neurosurgeon (1902–1956)," *Neurosurgery* 62 (2008): 738–42.

24 Sir Geoffrey Keynes was neither neurologist or neurosurgeon, nor neuroscientist or researcher, but a general surgeon from St Bartholomew's Hospital, London. Sir Geoffrey had gained fame for the treatment of myasthenia gravis by thymectomy. His topic was "The Thymus and Myasthenia Gravis and Thymectomy."

25 W. Penfield, "Glimpse of Neurophysiology in the Soviet Union," *Canadian Medical Association Journal* 73 (1955): 891-9

26 Ibid., 891–2. D.O. Hebb and W. Penfield, "Human Behavior after Extensive Bilateral Removal from the Frontal Lobes," *Archives of Neurology and Psycghiatry* 44 (1940): 421–38.

27 Penfield, "Glimpse of Neurophysiology in the Soviet Union," 896.

28 W. Penfield, MNI, *MNI AR*, 1956–57, 8.

29 Penfield, "Glimpse of Neurophysiology in the Soviet Union," 899.

30 A. Solzhenitsyn, *In the First Circle* (New York: Harper Perennial, 2009); G. Gorelik, "The Top-Secret Life of Lev Landau," *Scientific American* 277 (August 1997): 72–7.

31 W. Penfield and M.E. Faulk, "The Insula: Further Observations on Its Functions," *Brain* 78 (1955): 448, 268-9.

CHAPTER TWENTY-TWO

1 W. Penfield and J. Evans, "The Frontal Lobe in Man: A Clinical Study of Maximum Removals," *Brain* 58 (1935): 115–33.

2 A. Crompton, "From the Archives," *Brain* 129 (2006): 827; Penfield and Evans, "Frontal Lobe in Man," 117.

3 File C/SW 7-1b, WPA.

4 J.H. Harlow, "Recovery from the Passage of an Iron Bar through the Head (1868)," *Publications of the Massachusetts Medical Society* 2 (1868): 327–47, cited in C. Blakemore, *Mechanics of the Mind*. BBC Reith Lecture 1976 (Cambridge: Cambridge University Press, 1977), 11–27.

5   Penfield and Evans, "Frontal Lobe in Man," 131.

6   Ibid., 119.

7   Crompton, "From the Archives," 829.

8   E. Ring, "Dr Molly Harrower (November 26, 1982)," Oral History Project. George A. Smathers Library, University of Florida Digital Collections, http://ufdc.ufl.edu/UF00006059/00001/2j?search=harrower.

9   W. Pickren, "Profile: Molly Harrower," Psychology's Feminist Voices, http://www.feministvoices.com/molly-harrower/.

10 Ibid.

11 M.R. Harrower-Erickson, "Changes in Figure-Ground Perception in Patients with Cortical Lesions," *British Journal of Surgery* 30 (1939): 47–51.

12 M. Harrower-Erickson, MNI, *MNI AR*, 1940–1941, 16.

13 Ibid., 8; M.R. Harrower-Erickson, "The Contribution of the Rorschach Method to Wartime Psychological Problems," *Journal of Mental Science* 86 (1940): 366–77; Harrower Erickson, "Psychological Factors in Aviation Medicine," *Canadian Medical Association Journal* 44 (1941): 348–52; Harrower-Erickson, "Large Scale Investigation with the Rorschach Method," *Journal of Consulting Psychology* 7 (1943): 120–6.

14 "Peter M. Milner," Society for Neuroscience, http://www.sfn.org/~/media/SfN/Documents/TheHistoryofNeuroscience/Volume%208/PeterMilner.ashx.

15 Ring, "Dr Molly Harrower."

16 Pickren, "Profile of Molly Harrower."

17 R.F. Brown and P.M. Milner, "The Legacy of Donald O. Hebb: More Than the Hebb Synapse," *Nature Reviews Neuroscience* 4 (2003): 1013.

18 D.O. Hebb, *The Organization of Behavior: A Neuropsychological Theory* (New York: Wiley, 1949). Hebb's concept was proven by Holger Hyden in 1962, and, renamed "long-term potentiation," led to a Nobel Prize for Erick Kandel. Wilder Penfield gave an informative lecture to the Royal Society of Medicine on the search for elusive engrams of the brain in 1968, to which he referred as the neurological equivalent of the *Hunting of the Snark*. See H. Hyden and E. Egyhazi, "Nuclear RNA Changes in Nerve Cells during a Learning Experiment in Rats," *Proceedings of the National Academy of Sciences* 48 (1962): 1366–73; E.R. Kandel, *Search of Memory: The Emergence of a New Science of Mind* (New York: Norton, 2006), 284; W. Penfield, "Engrams in the Human Brain: Mechanisms of Memory," *Proceedings of the Royal Society of Medicine* 61 (1968): 831–40.

19 D.O. Hebb, "Intelligence in Man after Large Removals of Cerebral Tissue: Report of Four Left Frontal Lobe Cases," *Journal of General Psychology* 21 (1939): 73–87.

20 D.O. Hebb and W. Penfield, "Human Behavior after Extensive Bilateral Removal from the Frontal Lobes," *Archives of Neurology and Psychiatry* 44 (1940): 421–38.

21 Ibid., 435.

22 B. Milner, "Brenda Milner," *The History of Neuroscience in Autobiography Volume 2*, ed. L.S. Squire (Washington, DC: Society for Neuroscience, 1998), 282.

23 B. Milner, "Intellectual Effects of Temporal-Lobe Damage in Man" (PhD diss., McGill University, 1952).

24 Milner, "Brenda Milner," 283.

25 B. Milner, "Effects of Different Brain Lesions on Card Sorting," *Archives of Neurology* 9 (1963): 90–110.

26 Milner, "Brenda Milner."

27 M. Jones-Gotman and B. Milner, "Design Fluency: The Invention of Nonsense Drawings after Focal Cortical Lesions," *Neuropsychologia* 15 (1977): 653–74.

28 Kluver and Bucy, "'Psychic Blindness.'"

29 H.H. Jasper and J. Kershman, "Electroencephalographic Classification of the Epilepsies," *Archives of Neurology and Psychiatry* 45 (1941): 903–43; W. Feindel, W. Penfield, and H.H. Jasper, "Localization of Epileptic Discharge in Temporal Lobe Automatism," *Transactions of the American Neurological Association* 77 (1952): 14–17.

30 Milner, "Intellectual Effects of Temporal-Lobe Damage in Man," 47.

31 Milner, "Brenda Milner," 285.

32 Ibid.

33 W. Penfield and B. Milner, "Memory Deficit Produced by Bilateral Lesions in the Hippocampal Zone," *Archives of Neurology and Psychiatry* 79 (1958): 475–97; Milner, "Brenda Milner."

34 Milner, "Brenda Milner"; B. Milner, S. Corkin, and H.-L. Teuber, "Further Analysis of the Hippocampal Amnesic Syndrome: 14-Year Follow-up Study of H.M," *Neuropsychology* 6 (1968): 215–34; S. Corkin, *Permanent Present Tense: The Unforgettable Life of the Amnesic Patient, H.M.* (New York: Basic Books, 2013).

35 Milner, "Brenda Milner," 286; W.B. Scoville, R.H. Dunsmore, W.T. Liberson, C.E. Henry, and A. Pepe, "Observations on Medial Temporal Lobotomy and Uncotomy in the Treatment of Psychotic States: Preliminary Review of 19 Operative Cases Compared with 60 Frontal Lobotomy and Undercutting Cases," *Proceedings of the Association of Research in Nervous and Mental Disease* 31 (1953): 347–69; W.B. Scoville and B. Milner, "Loss of Recent Memory after Bilateral Hippocampal Lesions," *Journal of Neurology, Neurosurgery and Psychiatry* 20 (1957): 11–21.

36 Scoville and Milner, "Loss of Recent Memory"; Corkin, *Permanent Present Tense*, 55.

37 Milner, "Brenda Milner," 287; W.B. Scoville, "The Limbic Lobe in Man," *Journal of Neurosurgery* 11 (1954): 65.

38 Milner, "Brenda Milner."

39 Ibid., 287.

40 S. Corkin, "Acquisition of Motor Skill after Bilateral Medial Temporal-Lobe Excision," *Neuropsychology* 6 (1968): 255–65.

41 Milner, "Brenda Milner," 287, 289.

42 S. Corkin, D.G. Amaral, R.G. González, K.A. Johnson, and B.T. Hyman, "H.M.'s Medial Temporal Lobe Lesion: Findings from Magnetic Resonance Imaging," *Journal of Neuroscience* 17 (1997): 3964–79.

43 W. Penfield and G. Mathieson, "Memory: Autopsy Findings and Comments on the Role of Hippocampus in Experiential Recall," *Archives of Neurology* 31 (1974): 153.

44 W. Penfield, "The Interpretive Cortex," *Science* 129 (1959): 1719.

45 W. Penfield and G. Mathieson, "Memory: Autopsy Findings," 152.

46 Ibid., 154.

47 B. Milner, "Wilder Penfield: His Legacy to Neurology; Memory Mechanisms," *Canadian Medical Association Journal* 116 (1977): 1376.

48 A.R. Luria, *The Working Brain* (Basic Books, 1973), 15, 46.

49 Milner, "Brenda Milner." 293.

50 J. Emde Boas, "Juhn A. Wada and the Sodium Amytal Test: The First (and Last?) 50 Years," *Journal of the History of the Neurosciences* 8 (1999): 286–92.

51 Electroconvulsive therapy for the treatment of psychiatric illness was instituted on the presumption that schizophrenia and epilepsy were mutually exclusive conditions, and that causing epileptic seizures in a controlled environment mitigated psychotic episodes.

52 J. Wada, "Clinical Experimental Observations of Carotid Artery Injections of Sodium Amytal," *Brain and Cognition* 33 (1997): 11–13; Wada, "Youthful Season Revisited," *Brain and Cognition* 33 (1997): 7–10; J. Wada and T. Rasmussen "Intracarotid Injection of Sodium Amytal for the Lateralization of Cerebral Speech Dominance: Experimental and Clinical Observations," *Journal of Neurosurgery* 17 (1960): 266–82.

53 MNI, *MNI AR*, 1956–57, 38.

54 Wada and Rasmussen, "Intracarotid Injection of Sodium Amytal."

55 Ibid. Juhn Wada subsequently obtained his Canadian citizenship and took a position at the University of British Columbia, where he has remained for the whole of his distinguished career.

56 C. Branch, B. Milner, and T. Rasmussen, "Intracarotid Sodium Amytal for the Lateralisation of Cerebral Speech Dominance," *Journal of Neurosurgery* 21 (1964): 399–405; T. Rasmussen and B. Milner, "The Role of Early Left-Brain Injury in Determining Lateralization of Cerebral Speech Function," *Annals of the New York Academy of Sciences* 299 (1977): 355–69. Charles L. Branch Sr graduated from Vanderbilt University Medical School in 1953. He began his neurosurgical training at the University of Chicago but completed it at the MNI. Branch remained on the faculty of the MNI until 1968, when he took a position at the University of Texas in San Antonio. See C. Branch, "Microelectrode Study of Betz Cells in the Unanesthetized Cat" (master's thesis, McGill University, 1958).

57 B. Milner, "Hemispheric Specialization and Interaction," in *The Neurosciences: Third Study Program*, ed. F.O. Schmitt and F.G. Worden (Cambridge, MA: MIT Press, 1974), 3–4, 75–89.

58 B. Milner, "Sparing of Language Functions after Early Unilateral Brain Damage," *Neurosciences Research Program Bulletin* 12 (1974): 213–17; Rasmussen and Milner, "Role of Early Left-Brain Injury," 362–5; J. Dejerine, *Anatomie des centres nerveux* (Paris: Ruff, 1901), 247–8.

59 B. Milner, "Amobarbital Memory Testing: Some Personal Reflections," *Brain and Cognition* 33 (1997): 14–17; Milner, "Brenda Milner."

60 B. Milner, C. Branch, and T. Rasmussen, "Study of Short-Term Memory after Intracarotid Injection of Sodium Amytal," *Transactions of the American Neurological Association* 87 (1962): 224–6; Milner, "Amobarbital Memory Testing"; Milner, "Brenda Milner."

CHAPTER TWENTY-THREE

1 MNI, *MNI AR*, 1956–57, 22–3.

2 Ibid., 12.

3 See Appendix 2.

4 G. Bertrand, "Stereotactic Surgery at McGill: The Early Years," *Neurosurgery* 54 (2004): 1244–52.

5 L. Roberts, "Functional Plasticity in Cortical Speech Areas and Integration of Speech," *Archives of Neurology and Psychiatry* 79 (1958): 275–83.

6 V.P. Bersnev, N.L. Ryabukha, A.V. Vereshchako, and V.N. Musikhin, "The Saint Petersburg Academy of Postgraduate Education: To the 75th Anniversary of Its Faculty of Neurosurgery," Russian Neurosurgery, http://www.neuro.neva.ru/en/Articles_2010 _1/polenov.files/001.files/bersnev.shtml.

7 T. Rasmusen, MNI, *MNI AR*, 1957–58, 11; B.L. Lichterman, "Wilder Penfield and Soviet Neuroscience," *Ninth Annual Meeting of the International Society for the History of the Neurosciences (ISHN)*, Session 8, Special Lecture, Montreal, Quebec, Canada, 28 June 2004; A.-L. Christensen, E. Golgberg, and D. Bougakov, *Luria's Legacy in the 21st Century* (Oxford: Oxford University Press, 2009), 106.

8 H.H. Jasper and J. Majkowski, "Discussion: Pavlovian Conference on Higher Nervous Activity," *Annals of the New York Academy of Sciences* 92 (1961): 970–3.

9 M.J. Mossakowski, "The Activity of the Succinic Dehydrogenase in Glial Tumors," *Journal of Neuropathology and Experimental Neurology* 21 (1962): 137–46; M.J. Mossakowski, G. Mathieson, and J.M. Cummings, "A Parkinsonian Syndrome in the Course of Subacute Encephalitis," *Neurology* 11 (1961): 461–9; Mossakowski, Mathieson, and Cummings, "The Relationship of Metachromatic Leucodystrophy and Amaurotic Idiocy," *Brain* 84 (1961): 585–604.

10 MNI, *MNI AR*, 1958–59, 24; J.P. Cordeau, J. Gybels, H.H. Jasper, and L.J. Poirier, "Microelectrode Studies of Unit Discharge in the Sensorimotor Cortex," *Neurology* 10 (1960): 591–600.

11 MNI, *MNI AR*, 1957–58, 36.

12 Ibid., 9; J. Klingler and P. Gloor, "The Connections of the Amygdala and of the Anterior Temporal Cortex in the Human Brain," *Journal of Comparative Neurology* 115 (1960): 333–69.

13 B.C. Pevehouse, "A Study of Cerebral Edema Induced by Hypothermal Injury" (master's thesis, McGill University, 1961). Theodore Rasmusen became Pevehouse's thesis advisor after William Cone's death.

14 K.A.C. Elliott, A. Bazemore, and E. Florey, "Factor I and γ-Aminobutyric Acid," *Nature* 178 (1956): 1052–3.

15 G. Bertrand, "Studies on Cortical Localization in the Monkey: The Supplementary Motor Area" (master's thesis, McGill University, 1953); Bertrand, "Spinal Efferent Pathways from the Supplementary Motor Area," *Brain* 79 (1956): 461–73.

16 A.R. Elvidge, and A. Martinez-Coll, "Long-term Follow-up of 106 Cases of Astrocytoma, 1928-1939," *Journal of Neurosurgery* 13 (1956): 230–43; A.R. Elvidge, "Astrocy-

toma of the Brain and Spinal Cord: A Review of 176 Cases, 1940–1949," *Journal of Neurosurgery* 13 (1956): 413–43.

17 Gloor, "Electrophysiological Studies of the Amygdala in the Cat"; P. Gloor, "The Pattern of Conduction of Amygdaloid Seizure Discharge," *Archives of Neurology and Psychiatry* 77 (1957): 247–58.

18 R.A. Lende and C.N. Woolsey, "Sensory and Motor Localization in Cerebral Cortex of Porcupine," *Journal of Neurophysiology* 19 (1956): 544–63.

19 T. Rasmussen, J. Olszewski, and D. Lloyd-Smith, "Focal Seizures Due to Chronic Localized Encephalitis," *Neurology* 8 (1958): 435–45; T. Rasmussen and W. McCann, "Clinical Studies of Patients with Focal Epilepsy Due to 'Chronic Encephalitis,'" *Transactions of the American Neurological Association* 93 (1968): 89–94.

20 M.J. Aguilar and T. Rasmussen, "The Role of Encephalitis in Progression of Epilepsy," *Archive of Neurology* 2 (1960): 663–76; Y. Robitaille, "Neuropathologic Aspects of Chronic Encephalitis," in *Chronic Encephalitis and Epilepsy Rasmussen's Syndrome*, ed. F. Andermann, 79–110 (Boston: Butterworth-Heinemann, 1992).

21 M.J. Aguilar, "The Role of Chronic Encephalitis in the Pathogenesis of Epilepsy" (master's thesis, McGill University, 1958).

22 F. Andermann, "Chronic Encephalitis and Rasmussen's Syndrome," in Andermann, *Chronic Encephalitis*, viii–ix; Robitaille, "Neuropathologic Aspects of Chronic Encephalitis," 79–110; A. Grenier, J. Antel, and C.K. Osterland, "Immunologic Studies in Chronic Encephalitis of Rasmussen," in Andermann, *Chronic Encephalitis*, 125–34; D.M. Asher and D.C. Gajdusek, "Virologic Studies in Chronic Encephalitis," in Andermann, *Chronic Encephalitis*, 147–58.

23 A. Olivier, "Corticectomy for the Treatment of Seizures Due to Chronic Encephalitis," in Andermann, *Chronic Encephalitis*, 205–12; J.-G. Villemure, F. Andermann, and T. Rasmussen, "Hemispherectomy for the Treatment of Epilepsy Due to Chronic Encephalitis," in Andermann, *Chronic Encephalitis*, 235–41.

24 D.H. Ingvar and U. Sodrberg, "A New Method for Measuring Cerebral Blood Flow in Relation to the Electroencephalogram," *Electroencephalography and Clinical Neurophysiology* 8 (1956): 403–12.

25 B.B. Boycott and J.Z. Young, "A Memory System in Octopus Vulgaris Lamarck," *Proceedings of the Royal Society of London B Biological Sciences* 143 (1955): 449–80; J.Z. Young, "What Squids and Octopuses Tell Us about Brains and Memories," *James Arthur Lecture on the Evolution of the Human Brain* 46 (1976), American Museum of Natural History. http://digitallibrary.amnh.org/handle/2246/6004.

26 H.S. Gasser, "Properties of Dorsal Root Unmedullated Fibers on the Two Sides of the Ganglion," *General Physiology* 38 (1955): 709–28.

27 D.O. Hebb, "Intelligence, Brain Function and Theory of Mind," *Brain* 82 (1959): 260–75.

28 MNI, *MNI AR*, 1956–57, 49–51.

29 "Evans, Joseph P.," in *The Society of Neurological Surgeons* (Winston-Salem, NC: Wake Forest University Press, 2001), 456.

CHAPTER TWENTY-FOUR

1 Lewis, *Something Hidden*, 256–7.
2 F. Feindel, "Reminiscences of a Scrub Nurse," in Barrowman et al., *Nursing Highlights 1934–1990*, 92–6.
3 E. Flanagan, "The Peter Pan Statue and Its Acquisition: 1952–1959," in Barrowman et al. *Nursing Highlights 1934–1990*, 165–7.

CHAPTER TWENTY-FIVE

1 MNI, *AR, 1958–59*, 6–7. Why had he done it? We always strive to find rational answers for irrational acts. Perhaps Eileen Flanagan was correct: "Dr Penfield never recovered from the shock of Dr Cone's death – never understood that it was his alienation from Dr Cone which made him so unhappy. It was that he announced his resignation from the Institute at a meeting in the amphitheatre without telling Dr Cone [illegible] his partner in the original undertaking. Dr Cone felt he had been betrayed – that was the real reason, not that he would not be offered the Directorship." See file C/D 33–3, WPA.
2 MNI, *AR, 1958–59*, 8–9.
3 Ibid., 23.
4 R.L. Rovit, P. Gloor, and L.R. Henderson Jr, "Temporal Lobe Epilepsy: A Study Using Multiple Basal Electrodes. 1. Description of Method," *Neurochirurgia* 3 (1960): 6–19; R.L. Rovit and P. Gloor, "Temporal Lobe Epilepsy: A Study Using Multiple Basal Electrodes. II. Clinical EEG Findings," *Neurochirurgia* 3 (1960): 19–34; R.L. Rovit, P. Gloor, and T. Rasmussen, "Sphenoidal Electrodes in the Electrographic Study of Patients with Temporal Lobe Epilepsy: An Evaluation," *Journal of Neurosurgery* 18 (1961): 151–8.
5 R.L. Rovit, "The Electroencephalographic Effects of Intracarotid Injections of Sodium Amytal in Patients with Epilepsy" (master's thesis, McGill University, 1961). Richard Lee Rovit held a number of academic positions following his departure from the MNI in 1960. He was appointed associate professor of surgery (neurosurgery) at the Jefferson Medical College in Philadelphia in 1961, chairman of the Department of Neurological Surgery at St Vincent's Hospital and Medical Center in New York, and professor of clinical neurological surgery at New York University School of Medicine from 1966 to 1993. In 1994 he became professor of neurological surgery at New York Medical College, Valhalla, New York. "Rovit, Richard Lee," in *The Society of Neurological Surgeons* (Winston-Salem, NC: Wake Forest University press, 2001), 317.
6 MNI, *AR, 1958–59*, 9, 32.
7 G. Schaltenbrand and P. Bailey, *Introduction to Stereotaxis with an Atlas of the Human Brain* (Stuttgart: Thieme, 1959).
8 G. Bertrand, J. Blundell, and R. Musella, "Electrical Exploration of the Internal Capsule and Neighboring Structures during Stereotaxic Procedures," *Journal of Neurosurgery* 22 (1965): 333–43; G. Bertrand, "Stereotactic Surgery at McGill: The Early Years," *Neurosurgery* 54 (2004): 1244–52.

9 L.S. Stepien, J.P. Cordeau, and T. Rasmusen, "The Effect of Temporal Lobe and Hippocampal Lesions on Auditory and Visual Recent Memory," *Brain* 83 (1960): 470–89.

10 H.H. Jasper and P. Gloor,(MNI, *AR, 1959–60,* 40; G.D. Smirnov, "Georgii Donatovich Smirnov," *Neurophysiology* 5 (1973): 502–3.

11 MNI, *AR, 1959–60,* 9.

12 MNI, *AR, 1958–59,* 10, 35; H.H. Jasper, G. Arfel-Capdevielle, and T. Rasmussen, "Evaluation of EEG and Cortical Electrographic Studies for Prognosis of Seizures Following Surgical Excision of Epileptogenic Lesions," *Epilepsia* 2 (1961): 130–7.

13 D. Sullivan, "Dr A. Maxwell House Brought Health Care to Remote Places," *Globe and Mail,* 18 November 2013.

14 F.B. Maroun, J.C. Jacob, and W.D. Heneghan, *Diastematomyelia* (St Louis, MO: Warren H. Green, 1976).

15 P.N. Tandon and R. Ramamurthi, *Textbook of Neurosurgery,* 3 vols., 3rd ed. (New Delhi: Jaypee Brothers Medical Publishers, 2012).

16 S. Carpenter and G. Karpati, *Pathology of Skeletal Muscle* (Oxford: Oxford University Press, 2001).

17 MNI, *AR, 1959–60,* 19.

18 P. Gloor, C.L. Vera, and L. Sperti, "Electrophysiological Studies of Hippocampal Neurons. I. Configuration and Laminar Analysis of the 'Resting' Potential Gradient, of the Main-Transient Response to Perforant Path, Fimbrial and Mossy Fiber Volleys and of 'Spontaneous' Activity," *Electroencephalography and Clinical Neurophysiology* 15 (1963): 353–78; P. Gloor, L. Sperti, and C.L. Vera, "Electrophysiological Studies of Hippocampal Neurons. II. Secondary Postsynaptic Events and Single Cell Unit Discharges," *Electroencephalography and Clinical Neurophysiology* 15 (1963): 379–402; P. Gloor, C.L. Vera, and L. Sperti, "Electrophysiological Studies of Hippocampal Neurons. III. Responses of Hippocampal Neurons to Repetitive Perforant Path Volleys," *Electroencephalography and Clinical Neurophysiology* 17 (1964): 353–70; P. Gloor, L. Sperti, and C.L. Vera, "A Consideration of Feedback Mechanisms in the Genesis and Maintenance of Hippocampal Seizure Activity," *Epilepsia* 5 (1964): 213–38.

19 W. Maani, "History of Neurosurgery in Jordan," Slideshare, http://www.slideshare.net/WalidMaani/history-of-neurosurgery-in-jordan.

20 G. Jefferson, "Sir Hugh Cairns 1896–1952," *British Medical Journal* 2 (1952): 233–5.

21 P. H. Schurr, *So That Was Life: Biography of Sir Geoffrey Jefferson* (London: Royal Society of Medicine, 1997)

22 MNI, *AR, 1959–60,* 5.

23 Ibid., 8.

24 Ibid., 6.

25 See Appendix 4.

26 T. Rasmussen, "Montreal Neurological Institute, McGill University, Quarter-Century Founding Celebration," *World Neurology* 1 (1960): 113–27. All quotes are from this article, unless otherwise indicated.

27 J. Chorobski and T. Bacia, "On the Coexistence of Epileptic Seizures and Abnormal Involuntary Movements," *Journal of Neurology, Neurosurgery and Psychiatry* 24 (1961): 151–7.

28 Ibid., 119.

29 Ibid., 120.

30 Ibid., 122.

31 I.J. Lebish, D.G. Simons, H. Yagoda, H. Janssen, and W. Haymaker, "Observations on Mice Exposed to Cosmic Radiation in the Stratosphere: A Longevity and Pathological Study of 85 Mice," *Military Medicine* 124 (1959): 835–47.

32 T. Rasmussen, "Montreal Neurological Institute, McGill University, Quarter-Century Founding Celebration," *World Neurology* 1 (1960): 122.

33 Ibid., 121.

34 H.H. Jasper, "Evolution of Conceptions of Cerebral Localization since Hughlings Jackson," *World Neurology* 1 (1960): 97–109.

35 Ibid., 101.

36 Ibid., 102. Emphasis added.

37 W. Penfield, "The Cerebral Cortex of Man. I. The Cerebral Cortex and Consciousness," *Archives of Neurology and Psychiatry* 40 (1938): 417–42; Penfield, "Epileptic Automatisms and the Centrencephalic Integrating System," *Association for Research in Nervous and Mental Disease* 30 (1952): 513–28.

38 Jasper, "Evolution of Conceptions of Cerebral Localization," 107; Penfield, "Epileptic Automatisms."

39 Cone's contributions to the treatment of hydrocephalus have been largely forgotten, since he committed none of his ideas to paper. Ira Jackson's is the only record of Cone's activities in this field. Jackson's address is reproduced here in some detail, as the journal in which it appeared, *World Neurology*, was short lived in its original form, and surviving copies are difficult to access.

40 T. Rasmussen, "Montreal Neurological Institute, McGill University, Quarter-Century Founding Celebration," *World Neurology* 1 (1960): 124.

41 Ibid.

42 Ibid., 125.

43 Ibid., 116–17.

CHAPTER TWENTY-SIX

1 Willaim Feindel reminiscence, MNI Archives.

2 T.B. Rasmussen, "Experimental Ligation of the Cerebral Arteries of the Dog" (master's thesis, University of Minnesota, 1938).

3 T.B. Rasmussen and H. Freedman, "Treatment of Causalgia: An Analysis of 100 Cases," *Journal of Neurosurgery* 3 (1946): 165–73.

4 Penfield and Rasmussen, *Cerebral Cortex of Man.*

5 B. Weir, "Theodore Rasmussen, 1910–2002," *Canadian Journal of Neurological Sciences* 29 (2002): 289–90.

6 Harvey and Rasmussen were prescient in their use of electroencephalography to assess the effects of ischemia, since intra-operative EEG later became commonplace during carotid endarterectomy to alert the surgeon that the period of carotid clamping was approaching the limits of tolerance. Similarly, the temporary occlusion of an intracranial artery would gain its place in the neurosurgical armamentarium

when neurosurgeons, emboldened by their success in the microsurgical clipping of cerebral aneurysms, began operating on larger, more complex aneurysms by temporarily occluding the parent artery during their dissection. See J. Harvey and T. Rasmussen, "Electroencephalographic Changes Associated with Experimental Temporary Focal Cerebral Anemia," *Electroencephalography and Clinical Neurophysiology* 3 (1051): 341–51.

7   R. Lende, "Local Spasm in Cerebral Arteries" (master's thesis, McGill University, 1956); Lende, "Local Spasm in Cerebral Arteries," *Journal of Neurosurgery* 17 (1960): 90–103; W. Penfield, R.A. Lende, and T. Rasmussen, "Manipulation Hemiplegia: An Untoward Complication in the Surgery of Focal Epilepsy," *Journal of Neurosurgery* 18 (1961): 760–76.

8   P. Robb, MNI, *MNI AR*, 1960–61, 26.

9   Ibid., 6.

10 MNI, *MNI AR*, 1961–62, 25

11 Ibid., 25

12 "Bertha Cameron," in Barrowman et al., *Nursing Highlights 1934–1990*, 117–18.

13 J. MacMillan Walker, "The Director as a Person," inBarrowman et al., *Nursing Highlights 1934–1990*, 118–19.

14 MNI, *MNI AR*, 1961–62, 25–6.

15 M. Pigeon, "Health Care in Québec in the Second Half of the 20th Century," McCord Museum, http://www.mccord-museum.qc.ca/scripts/explore.php?Lang=1&elementid=110__true&tableid=11&tablename=theme&contentlong.

16 MNI, *MNI AR*, 1961–62, 25–6.

17 MNI, *MNI AR*, 1960–61, 20.

18 Ibid., 22.

19 H.A. Pappius and D.R. Gulati, "Water and Electrolyte Content of Cerebral Tissues in Experimentally Induced Edema," *Acta Neuropathologica* 2 (1963): 451–60; T. Rasmussen and and D.R. Gulati, "Cortisone in the Treatment of Postoperative Cerebral Edema," *Journal of Neurosurgery* 19 (1962): 535–44.

20 See Appendix 2.

21 W.H. Feindel and S. Fedoruk, "Measurement of Brain Circulation Time by Radio-Active Iodinated Albumin," *Canadian Journal of Surgery* 3 (1960): 312–18; W. Feindel, R.L. Rovit, and L. Stephens-Newsham, "Localization of Intracranial Vascular Lesions by Radioactive Isotopes and an Automatic Contour Brain Scanner," *Journal of Neurosurgery* 18 (1961): 811–21; W. Feindel. "Detection of Intracranial Lesions by Contour Brain Scanning with Radioisotopes," *Postgraduate Medicine* 31 (1962): 15–23.

22 W.K. Welch, "A Morphological Study of Human Glioblastoma Multiforme Transplanted to Guinea Pigs" (master's thesis, McGill University, 1947).

23 H.D. Garretson, "The Growth Characteristics of Glioblastoma Multiforme in the Anterior Chamber of the Guinea Pig Eye" (PhD diss., McGill University, 1968), 138.

24 G. Stent, "Prematurity and Uniqueness in Scientific Discovery," *Scientific American*, December 1972, 84–93.

25 MNI, *MNI AR*, 1960–61, 23; MNI, *MNI AR*, 1962–63, 39.

26 A.L. Sherwin, M.R. Richter, J.B.R. Cosgrove, and B. Rose, "Myelin Binding Antibodies in Experimental 'Allergic' Encephalomyelitis," *Science* 134 (1961): 1370–2.

27 F.O. Schmitt, "Molecular and Ultrastructural Correlates of Function in Neurons, Neuronal Nets, and the Brain," *Naturwissenschaften* 53 (1966): 71–9.

28 J.D. Robertson, "The Occurrence of a Subunit Pattern in the Unit Membranes of Club Endings in Mauthner Cell Synapses in Goldfish Brain," *Journal of Cell Biology* 19 (1963): 201–21.

29 D.K.C. MacDonald, *Near Zero: An Introduction to Low Temperature Physics* (New York: Anchor Books, 1961).

30 D. Sheer, *Electrical Stimulation of the Brain: An Inter-disciplinary Survey of Neurobehavioral Integrative Systems* (Austin: University of Texas Press, 1961), 203–31, 277–87, 519–33, 533–53, 557–62.

31 W. Penfield, "A Surgeon's Chance Encounters with Mechanisms Related to Consciousness," *Journal of the Royal College of Surgeons of Edinburgh* 5 (1960): 173–90; Penfield, "Activation of the Record of Human Experience," *Journal of the Royal College of Surgeons of England* 29 (1961) 77–84.

32 P. Perot and W. Penfield, "Hallucinations of Past Experience and Experiential Responses to Stimulation of Temporal Cortex," *Transactions of the American Neurological Association* 85 (1960): 80–4.

33 W. Penfield and P. Perot, "The Brain's Record of Auditory and Visual Experience: A Final Summary and Discussion," *Brain* 86 (1963): 595–696.

34 W. Penfield, "The Permanent Record of the Stream of Consciousness: Proceedings of the 14th International of Psychology, Montreal, 1954," *Annual Volume of Physiology and Experimental Medical Sciences* 1 (1955): 24–7; Penfield, "The Role of the Temporal Cortex in Certain Psychical Phenomena: Maudsley Lecture," *Journal of Mental Science* 101 (1955): 451–65; Penfield, "Some Mechanisms of Consciousness Discovered during Electrical Stimulation of the Brain," *Proceedings of the National Academy of Sciences* 44 (1958): 51–66; Penfield, "The Role of the Temporal Cortex in Recall of Past Experience and Interpretation of the Present," *Ciba Foundation Symposium on the Neurological Basis of Behavior* (London: Churchill, 1958), 149–74; S. Mullan and W. Penfield, "Illusions of Comparative Interpretation and Emotion Production by Epileptic Discharge and by Electrical Stimulation in the Temporal Cortex," *Archives of Neurology and Psychiatry* 81 (1959): 269–84; Penfield, "Interpretive Cortex."

CHAPTER TWENTY-SEVEN

1 MNI, *MNI AR*, 1962–63, 20.

2 MNI, *MNI AR*, 1963–64, 19.

3 Ibid., 19–20.

4 I. Heller, "Biochemical Studies of Peripheral Nerve Metabolism with Particular Reference to the Role of Thiamine" (PhD diss., McGill University, 1962).

5 A.L. Sherwin, M. Richter, J.B.R. Cosgrove, and B. Rose, "Myelin-Binding Antibodies in Experimental Allergie Encephalomyelitis," *Science* 134 (1961): 1370; A.L. Sherwin, "Immunochemical Studies of the Nervous System" (PhD diss., McGill University, 1965).

6   A.H. Eisen, G. Karpati, T. Laszlo, F. Andermann, J.P. Robb, and H.L. Bacal, "Immunologic Deficiency in Ataxia Telangiectasia," *New England Journal of Medicine* 272 (1965): 18–22.

7   Allan Morton freely acknowledged the photographic talent of Charles Hodge and his assistants, Garneau and Kalaby, and the graphic artistry of Eleanor Sweezey in the realization of the figures illustrating his thesis. See A. Morton, "The Hypothalamic Magnocellular Nuclei in Man" (master's thesis, McGill University, 1961).

8   P. Perot, "Mesencephalic-Thalamic Relations in the Mechanism of the Experimental Wave and Spike Complex in the Cat" (PhD diss., McGill University, 1963); B. Weir, "The Reticular Formation in Petit Mal Epilepsy" (master's thesis, McGill University, 1963); R. Hansebout, "The Effects of Intracarotid Methotrexate on the Rhesus Monkey" (master's thesis, McGill University, 1964); W.M. Nichols, "Changes in the Circulation of the Brain and Spinal Cord Associated with Nervous Activity" (master's thesis, McGill University, 1938).

9   P. Perot, B. Weir, and T. Rasmussen, "Tuberous Sclerosis: Surgical Therapy for Seizures," *Archives of Neurology* 15 (1966): 498–506; B. Weir and A. Elvidge, "Oligodendrogliomas: An Analysis of 63 Cases," *Journal of Neurosurgery* 29 (1968): 500–5.

10 B. Milner, MNI, *MNI AR*, 1962–63, 44.

11 Ibid.

12 L. Taylor, "Backwardness in Reading and Brain Dysfunction" (master's thesis, McGill University, 1961); MNI, *MNI AR*, 1962–1963, 44.

13 D. Kimura, "Visual and Auditory Perception after Temporal-Lobe Damage" (PhD diss., McGill University, 1961); Kimura, "Some Effects of Temporal-Lobe Damage on Auditory Perception," *Canadian Journal of Psychology* 15 (1961): 156–65; Kimura, "Cerebral Dominance and the Perception of Verbal Stimuli," *Canadian Journal of Psychology* 15 (1961): 166–71.

14 D. Kimura, "Perception of Unfamiliar Stimuli after Right Temporal Lobe Damage," *Archives of Neurology* 8 (1963): 264–71; Kimura, "Speech Lateralization in Young Children as Determined by an Auditory Test," *Journal of Comparative and Physiological Psychology* 56 (1963): 899–902.

15 MNI, *MNI AR*, 1962–63, 44; M. Studdert-Kennedy and D.P. Shankweiler, "Hemispheric Specialization for Speech Perception," *Journal of the Acoustical Society of America* 48 (1970): 579–94.

16 S.H. Corkin, "Somesthetic Function after Focal Cerebral Damage in Man" (PhD diss., McGill University, 1964).

17 Corkin, *Permanent Present Tense.*

18 Milner, Corkin, and Teuber, "Further Analysis of the Hippocampal Amnesic Syndrome."

19 P.M. Corsi, "Human Memory and the Medial Temporal Region of the Brain" (PhD diss., McGill University, 1972).

20 B. Milner, P. Corsi, and G. Leonard, "Frontal-Lobe Contribution to Recency Judgments," *Neuropsychologia* 29 (1991): 601–18.

21 L.B. Taylor, "Localisation of Cerebral Lesions by Psychological Testing," *Clinical Neurosurgery* 16 (1969): 269–87.

22 D.L. McRea, C. Branch, and B. Milner, "The Occipital Horns and Cerebral Dominance," *Neurology* 18 (1968): 95–8.

23 N. Geschwind and W. Levitsky, "Human Brain: Left-Right Asymmetries in Temporal Speech Region," *Science* 161 (1968): 186–7.

24 G. Ratcliff, C. Dila, L.Taylor, and B. Milner, "The Morphological Asymmetry of the Hemispheres and Cerebral Dominance for Speech: Possible Relationship," *Brain and Language* 11 (1980): 87–98.

25 Ibid., 88.

26 MNI, *MNI AR,* 1967–68, 52; MNI, *MNI AR,* 1969–70, 55; B. Milner, L. Taylor, and R. Sperry, "Lateralized Suppression of Dichotically Presented Digits after Commissural Section in Man," *Science* 161 (1968): 184–6; B. Milner, L. Taylor, and M. Jones-Gotman, "Lessons from Cerebral Commissurotomy: Auditory Attention, Haptic Memory, and Visual Images in Verbal Associative-Learning," in *Brain Circuits and the Functions of the Mind: Essays in Honor of Roger W. Sperry*, ed. C. Trevarthen, 293–303 (Cambridge: Cambridge University Press, 1990).

27 A.B. Rothballer, "Studies on the Adrenaline-Sensitive Component of the Reticular Activating System" (master's thesis, McGill University, 1955). Professor George W. Stavraky of the University of Western Ontario gave the 1962 Annual Fellows' Lecture, "Adaptation after Central Nervous System Damage." Milton Shy, of the University of Pennsylvania, gave the 1963 lecture, "Newer Disorders of Muscle." Professor Alf Brodal, from the University of Oslo, gave the neuroanatomy lecture, "The Vestibular Nuclei and Their Connections."

28 R. Brain, "Some Reflections on Brain and Mind," *Brain* 86 (1963): 381–402.

29 "The Nobel Prize in Physics 1962," Nobelprize.org, http://www.nobelprize.org/nobel_prizes/physics/laureates/1962/.

30 G. Gorelik, "The Top-Secret Life of Lev Landau," *Scientific American*, August 1997, 72–7.

31 Kapitsa was awarded the 1978 Nobel Prize for his work in low-temperature physics.

32 A. Solzhenitsyn, *In The First Circle* (New York: Harper Perennial, 2009).

33 Taken from a diary by Wilder Penfield. The names cited are Evgeny Mikhailovich Lifshitz, Mstislav Vsevolodovitch Keldych, Boris Yegorov, and Propper Graschenko.

34 W. Penfield, Diary, February 1962, Moscow – Consultation.

35 Ibid.

36 Smirnov had studied mechanisms of attention with Herbert Jasper at the MNI and had been an organizer of the International Colloquium in Moscow that led to the founding of the International Brain Research Organization. See MNI, *MNI AR*, 1958–59, 9; MNI, *MNI AR*, 1959–60, 40.

37 Penfield, *Mystery of the Mind*, 67–72.

38 G.D. Smirnov to Wilder Penfield, 9 December 1970.

CHAPTER TWENTY-EIGHT

1 "Comrade Norman Bethune, a member of the Communist Party of Canada, was around fifty when he was sent by the Communist Parties of Canada and the United

States to China; he made light of travelling thousands of miles to help us in our War of Resistance Against Japan. He arrived in Yenan in the spring of last year, went to work in the Wutai Mountains, and to our great sorrow died a martyr at his post. What kind of spirit is this that makes a foreigner selflessly adopt the cause of the Chinese people's liberation as his own? It is the spirit of internationalism, the spirit of communism, from which every Chinese Communist must learn." Mao Tse-tung, "In Memory of Norman Bethune," *Selected Works of Mao Tse-tung*, https://www.marxists. org/reference/archive/mao/selected-works/volume-2/mswv2_25.htm#bm1.

2 Bethune Secretariat, "Bethune: His Time and Legacy," news release, 16–18 November 1979.

3 Ibid.

4 L. Hannant, ed., *The Politics of Passion: Norman Bethune's Writing and Art* (Toronto: University of Toronto Press, 1968), 71–117.

5 W. MacLeod, "The Humanitarian," in *Francis L. McNaughton 1906–1986*, ed. D. Baxter (Montreal: Montreal Neurological Institute, 1986), 9–11.

6 W. Penfield, "Oriental Renaissance in Education and Medicine," *Science* 141 (1963): 1158.

7 W. Feindel, MNI, *MNI AR*, 1978–79, 40–1.

8 Penfield, "Oriental Renaissance in Education," 1154.

9 Penfield does not name the "Chinese graduate student," nor does he question why a research fellow could write to Mao, let alone why Mao would be interested in intervening on Penfield's behalf. See Wilder Penfield to Norman Robertson, 15 November 1961, file C/SW 12, WPA. The only Chinese national at the institute at the time was Chen I. Tsay, who appears in the staff photograph of the academic year 1955–56 as an assistant resident in neurosurgery. The following year he is listed both as a resident in neurosurgery and as a fellow in electroencephalography. See MNI, *MNI AR*, 1955–56, 19; MNI, *MNI AR*, 1956–57, 17–18, 31.

10 File C/SW 12, WPA.

11 J.W. Lella, "Osler and Bethune: 'Sons of the Manse' and Their 'Angelical Conjunction of Medicine and Divinity,'" *Osler Library Newsletter* 119 (2013): 2–5.

12 *Heart of Spain*, Internet Movie Database, http://www.imdb.com/title/tt0162986/.

13 Hazen Sise was an architect who participated in the creation of such beautiful and iconic structures as the Beaver Lake Pavilion on Mount Royal and the Salle Wilfrid-Pelletier at Montreal's Place des Arts, and the National Arts Centre in Ottawa. Sise had accompanied Bethune to Spain and was a founding member of the Norman Bethune Foundation, with Francis McNaughton and others. See McLoed, "Humanitarian."

14 File C/SW 12, WPA.

15 W. Penfield, "Oriental Renaissance in Education and Medicine: A Canadian Physician Sees a Sudden Renaissance of Western Learning on the Chinese Mainland," *Science* 141 (1963): 1153–61.

16 File C/SW 12, WPA.

17 K.A.C. Elliott, "Observations on Medical Science and Education in the People's Republic of China," *Canadian Medical Association Journal* 92 (1965): 73–6.

18 W. Feindel, MNI, *MNI AR*, 1978–79, 40; McLeod, "Humanitarian."

19 D.B. Tower and W. Feindel, "Impressions of Neurology and Neurosurgery in the People's Republic of China," *Annals of Neurology* 7 (1980): 395–405.

20 W. Feindel, MNI, *MNI AR*, 1979–80, 44–5.

21 Ibid., 40–1.

22 Ibid., 44–5; W. Feindel, MNI, *MNI AR*, 1980–81, 48.

CHAPTER TWENTY-NINE

1 MNI, *MNI AR*, 1963–64, 17–18, 36.

2 Ibid., 17–18.

3 Ibid., 7.

4 W. Penfield and P. Perot, "The Brain's Record of Auditory and Visual Experience: A Final Summary and Discussion," *Brain* 86 (1963): 595–696.

5 MNI, *MNI AR*, 1963–64, 36.

6 H.H. Jasper and G. Bertrand, "Stereotaxic Microelectrode Studies of Single Thalamic Cells and Fibres in Patients with Dyskinesia," *Transactions of the American Neurological Association* 89 (1964): 79–82; G. Bertrand and H.H. Jasper, "Microelectrode Recording of Unit Activity in the Human Thalamus," *Confinia Neurologica* 26 (1965): 205–8; G. Bertrand, J. Blundell, and R. Musella, "Electrical Exploration of the Internal Capsule and Neighbouring Structures during Stereotactic Procedures," *Journal of Neurosurgery* 22 (1965): 333–43; H.H. Jasper and G. Bertrand, "Recording from Microelectrodes in Stereotactic Surgery for Parkinson's Disease," *Journal of Neurosurgery* 24 (1966): 219–21; Jasper and Bertrand, "Thalamic Units Involved in Somatic Sensation and Voluntary and Involuntary Movements in Man," in *The Thalamus*, ed. D.P. Purpura and M.D. Yahr, 365–90 (New York: Columbia University Press); G. Bertrand, H.H. Jasper, and A. Wong, "Microelectrode Study of the Human Thalamus: Functional Organization in the Ventro-Basal Complex," *Confinia Neurologica* 29 (1966): 81–6. These and other achievements in neurophysiology were facilitated by the work of Eddy Puodziunas and his assistant, George Lootus, who built, maintained, and modified some of the apparatus used in stereotactic procedures.

7 W. Penfield and M.E. Faulk, "The Insula: Further Observations on Its Function," *Brain* 78 (1955): 445–70.

8 W.C. Kite Jr, "The Cortical Representation of Gastric Motor Function" (master's thesis, McGill University, 1949).

9 H. Silfvenius, P. Gloor, and T. Rasmussen, "Evaluation of Insular Ablation in Surgical Treatment of Temporal Lobe Epilepsy," *Epilepsia* 5 (1964): 307–20. There have been recent attempts to define an epileptic semiology specific to the insula, and a renewal, in some quarters, of resecting insular cortex using microsurgical techniques to avoid manipulation of the branches of the middle cerebral artery.

10 C. Drake, "Surgical Treatment of Ruptured Aneurysms of the Basilar Artery," *Journal of Neurosurgery Neurosurgery* 23 (1964): 457–73.

11 M.A. Falconer, E.A. Serafetinides, and J.A. Coesellis, "Etiology and Pathogenesis of Temporal Lobe Epilepsy," *Archives of Neurology* 10 (1964): 233–48.

12 V.G. Longo and D.A. Bovet, "Neuropharmacological Investigations of Hallucinogenic

Drugs: Laboratory Results versus Clinical Trials," *Acta Neurochirurgica* 12 (1964): 215–29.

13 M.L. Barr and E.G. Bertram, "A Morphological Distinction between Neurons of the Male and Female, and the Behaviour of the Nucleolar Satellite during Accelerated Nucleoprotein Synthesis," *Nature* 163 (1949): 676–7.

14 *À tout prendre*, Internet Movie Database, http://www.imdb.com/title/tt0057725/.

15 MNI, *MNI AR*, 1962–63, 7.

16 W. Feindel, R.L. Rovit, and L. Stephens-Newsham. "Localization of Intracranial Vascular Lesions by Radioactive Isotopes and an Automatic Contour Brain Scanner," *Journal of Neurosurgery* 18 (1961): 811–21.

17 The Cone Laboratory also benefited from the expert help of Nicholas Rumin and Robert Stolk in the technical design of the radioactive detection apparatus.

18 W. Feindel and M. Diksic, "Yazokazu Lucas Yamamoto, MD, PhD (1928–2003) Neurosurgeon, Nuclear Physician and Scientist," *NeuroImage*, February 2004, n.p.

19 S. Fedoruk and W. Feindel, "Measurement of Brain Circulation Time by Radioactive Iodinated Albumin," *Canadian Journal of Surgery* 3 (1960): 312–18.

20 Perot, "Mesencephalic-Thalamic Relations."

21 Penfield and Perot, "The Brain's Record of Auditory and Visual Experience."

22 W. Feindel and P. Perot, "Red Cerebral Veins: A Report on Arteriovenous Shunts in Tumors and Cerebral Scars," *Journal of Neurosurgery* 22 (1965): 315–25.

23 Ibid., 323.

24 Ibid., 322.

25 W. Feindel, Y.L. Yamamoto, and C.P. Hodge, "Red Cerebral Veins and the Cerebral Steal Syndrome: Evidence from Fluorescein Angiography and Microregional Blood Flow by Radioisotopes during Excision of an Angioma," *Journal of Neurosurgery* 35 (1971): 167.

26 W. Feindel, MNI, *MNI AR*, 1970–71, 57.

27 Garretson was appointed director of the Division of Neurological Surgery at the University of Louisville in 1971, where he continued to teach and to practise surgery until his retirement in 1997.

28 W. Feindel, H. Garretson, Y.L. Yamamoto, P. Perot, and N. Rumin, "Blood Flow Patterns in the Cerebral Vessels and Cortex in Man: Studies by Intracarotid Injection of Radioisotopes and Coomassie Blue Dye," *Journal of Neurosurgery* 23 (1965): 12–22; H. Garretson, P. Perot, Y.L. Yamamoto, and W. Feindel, "Intracarotid Coomassie Blue Dye as an Aid in the Surgery of Intracranial Vascular Lesions," *Journal of Neurosurgery* 26 (1967): 577–83.

29 Feindel et al., "Blood Flow Patterns," 19.

30 Ibid., 22–3.

31 Ibid.

32 R.L. de CH, Saunders, W. Feindel, and V.R. Carvalho, "X-ray Microscopy of the Blood Vessels of the Human Brain," *Medical and Biological Illustration* 15 (1965): 108–22, 234–46.

33 W. Feindel, "Charles Hodge, OC, FRPS, FBPA, FIMI (1924–2001) Neurophotographer Extraordinaire," *NeuroImage*, July 2001, 3–6.

34 Marcus Arts joined Charles Hodge in 1976 and became head of Neurophotography in 2001, when Charles Hodge entered the darkroom forever. Arts was joined by Susan Kaup, Helmut Bernhard, Jean-Paul Acco, Tony Rizzuto, and Anthony Revoy as he oversaw the expansion and modernization of Neurophotography into the Department of Neuro Media Services. See V. Svoboda, "Neuro Media Services and Radiology," *NeuroImage*, September 2013, n.p.

35 Charles Hodge was the first Canadian to be elected a fellow of the Biological Photographic Association, in 1958. He was awarded the first William Gordon Award for outstanding biophotography in 1969. The following year he was awarded the gold medal of the Royal Photographic Society of Great Britain, the only photographer in North America to have this distinction. Hodge was made Louis Schmidt Laureate for 1975, the highest honour of the Biological Photographic Association. He became an honorary fellow of the Royal Photographic Society of Great Britain in 1984, and an honorary fellow of the Institute of Medical Illustrators of Great Britain in 1990. In 1992 he was appointed to the Order of Canada. See Feindel, "Charles Hodge."

36 W. Feindel, Y.L. Yamamoto, and C.O. Hodge, "Intracarotid Fluorescein Angiography: A New Method for Examination of the Epicerebral Circulation in Man," *Canadian Medical Association Journal* 96 (1967): 1–7; W. Feindel, C.P. Hodge, and Y.L. Yamamoto, "Epicerebral Angiography by Fluorescein during Craniotomy," *Progress in Brain Research* 30 (1968): 471–7; C.P. Hodge, Y.L. Yamamoto, and W. Feindel, "Fluorescein Angiography of the Brain: The Photographic Procedure," *Journal of the Biological Photographic Association* 46 (1978): 67–79; J.E. Little and C.P. Hodge, "Quality Reproduction of Large Electroencephalograms," *Journal of the Biological Photographic Association* 46 (1978): 133–5; C.J. Thompson and C.P. Hodge, "A Digital Databack Timer," *Journal of the Biological Photographic Association* 46 (1978): 61–6.

37 Y.L. Yamamoto, K.M. Phillips, C.P. Hodge, and W. Feindel, "Microregional Blood Flow Changes in Experimental Cerebral Ischemia: Effects of Arterial Carbon Dioxide Studied by Fluorescein Angiography and Xenon 133 Clearance," *Journal of Neurosurgery* 35 (1971): 155–66; T. Soejima, Y.L. Yamamoto, E. Meyer, W. Feindel, and C.P. Hodge, "Protective Effects of Steroids on the Corticomicrocirculation Injured by Cold," *Journal of Neurosurgery* 51 (1979): 188–200; J.R. Little, Y.L. Yamamoto, W. Feindel, E. Meyer, and C.P. Hodge, "Superficial Temporal Artery to Middle Cerebral Artery Anastomosis: Intraoperative Evaluation by Fluorescein Angiography and Xenon-133 Clearance," *Journal of Neurosurgery* 50 (1979): 560–9; R. Leblanc, W. Feindel, Y.L. Yamamoto, J.G. Milton, M.M. Frojmovich, and C.P. Hodge, "The Effects of Calcium Antagonism on the Epicerebral Circulation in Early Vasospasm," *Stroke* 15 (1984): 1017–20.

38 J. Tyler, R. Leblanc, E. Meyer, A. Dagher, Y.l. Yamamoto, M. Diksic, and A. Hakim, "Hemodynamic and Metabolic Effects of Cerebral Arteriovenous Malformations," *Stroke* 20 (1989): 890–8; R. Leblanc and J.R. Little, "Hemodynamics of Cerebral Arteriovenous Malformations," *Clinical Neurosurgery* 36 (1989): 299–317.

CHAPTER THIRTY

1   MNI, *MNI AR*, 1963–64, 17.

2   File C/G 64 (H-I-J), WPA.

3   T. Rasmussen, MNI, *MNI AR*, 1964–65, 8.

4   File A/N 32-10, WPA.

5   H.H. Jasper, "On Leaving McGill for l'Université de Montreal," Memoirs, chapter 15: 1–3, William Feindel Fonds, Montreal Neurological Institute.

6   Ibid.

7   Ibid.

8   MNI, *MNI AR*, 1964–65, 19. Herbert Jasper's departure was not the only loss to the institute: Reuben Rabinovitch passed away suddenly, on 16 September 1965. As McNaughton noted, "He loved the Neurological Institute and served it well. He also gave his patients the most remarkable care and attention, and they were devoted to him … Rab will be missed by all." Anonymous, MNI, *MNI AR*, 1965–66, front matter. True to Rab's concern for the residents and fellows, Mr and Mrs Sydney Caplan, two close friends of Reuben Rabinovitch, made a generous donation in his honour, to be used for the acquisition of books and monographs for the Fellows Library. The passing of Dorothy Killam, "a good friend and a staunch supporter," was also noted (MNI, *MNI AR*, 1965–66, 7). Mrs Killam's husband had provided the funds necessary to establish the Laboratory for Research in Chronic Neurological Diseases at the institute, in 1948. Mrs Killam bequeathed a substantial sum as a general endowment and for the establishment of scholarships for advanced studies.

9   P. Gloor, C.L. Vera, and L. Sperti, "Electrophysiological Studies of Hippocampal Neurons. 3. Responses of Hippocampal Neurons to Repetitive Perforant Path Volleys," *Electroencephalography and Clinical Neurophysiology* 17 (1964): 353–70; P. Gloor, L. Sperti, and C.L. Vera, "A Consideration of Feedback Mechanisms in the Genesis and Maintenance of Hippocampal Seizure Activity," *Epilepsia* 5 (1964): 213–38; R. Caruthers, K. Mueller, and P. Gloor, "Interaction of Evoked Potentials of Neocortical and Hypothalamic Origin in the Amygdala," *Science* 144 (1964): 422–3.

10 P. Lampert and S. Carpenter, "Electron Microscopic Studies on the Vascular Permeability and the Mechanism of Demyelination in Experimental Allergic Encephalomyelitis," *Journal of Neuropathology and Experimental Neurology* 24 (1965): 11–24.

11 G. Mathgieson, MNI, *MNI AR*, 1966–67, 20, 45; S. Carpenter, "Proximal Axonal Enlargement in Motor Neuron Disease," *Neurology* 18 (1968): 841–51.

12 MNI, *MNI AR*, 1966–67, 22.

13 Carpenter and Karpati, *Pathology of Skeletal Muscle*.

14 M. Sinnreich and F. Andermann, "George Karpati (1934–2009)," *Canadian Journal of Neurological Sciences* 36 (2009): 282.

15 P. Webster, "George Karpati," *Lancet* 373 (2009): 1246.

16 E.E. Zubrzycka-Gaarn, D.E. Bulman, G. Karpati, A.H.M. Burghes, B. Belfall, H.J. Klamut, J. Talbot, R.S. Hodges, P.N. Ray, and R.G Worton, "The Duchenne Muscular

Dystrophy Gene Product Is Localized in Sarcolemma of Human Skeletal Muscle," *Nature* 333 (1988): 466–9.

17 Webster, "George Karpati."

18 Helmut Bernhard, personal communication, 2014.

19 MNI, *MNI AR*, 1960–61, 33; MNI, *MNI AR*, 1966–67, 37; R. Ethier, MNI, *MNI AR*, 1967–68, 37.

20 J.A. Simpson, "Myasthenia Gravis as an Autoimmune Disease: Clinical Aspects," *Annals of the New York Academy of Sciences* 135 (1966): 506–16.

21 D.A. Brewerton, F.D. Hart, A. Nicholls, M. Caffrey, D.C.O. James, and R.D. Sturrock, "Ankylosing Spondylitis and HL-A 27," *Lancet* 1 (1973): 904–7.

22 K. Krnjevic and A. Silver, "A Histochemical Study of Cholinergic Fibres in the Cerebral Cortex," *Journal of Anatomy* 99 (1965): 711–59.

23 P.C. Bucy, "The Delusion of the Obvious," *Perspectives in Biology and Medicine* 9 (1966): 358–68.

24 R.W. Sperry, "Mental Unity following Surgical Disconnection of the Cerebral Hemispheres," *Harvey Lectures* 62 (1966–7): 293–323.

25 R.M. Donaghy and G. Yasargil, "Microangeional Surgery and Its Techniques," *Progress in Brain Research* 30 (1968): 263–7.

26 MNI, *MNI AR*, 1967–68, 9.

27 P. Gloor, MNI, *MNI AR*, 1968–69, 22–3.

28 D.M. Derry and L.S. Wolfe, "Gangliosides in Isolated Neurons and Glial Cells," *Science* 158 (1967): 1450–52; G. Karpati and W.K. Engel, "Transformation of the Histochemical Profile of Skeletal Muscle by 'Foreign Innervation,'" *Nature* 215 (1967): 1509–10; R.J. Broughton, "Sleep Disorders: Disorders of Arousal?," *Science* 159 (1968): 1070–8; B. Milner, L. Taylor, and R.W. Sperry, "Lateralized Suppression of Dichotically Presented Digits after Commissural Section in Man," *Science* 161 (1968): 184–6; A.L. Sherwin, G. Karpati, and J.A. Buckle, "Imminohisto-Chemical Localization of Creatine Phosphokinase in Skeletal Muscle," *Proceedings of the National Academy of Sciences of the United States of America* 64 (1969): 171–5.

29 J.A. Buckle and A.L. Sherwin, "Organ Specificity of Creatine Phosphokinase Muscle Isoenzyme," *Immunochemistry* 6 (1969): 681–7; A.L. Sherwin, F.E. LeBlanc, and W.P. McCann, "Altered LDH Isoenzymes in Brain Tumors," *Archives of Neurology* 18 (1968): 311–15.

30 L.S. Wolfe, MNI, *MNI AR*, 1967–68, 39, 41; MNI, *MNI AR*, 1968–69, 42–4; P. Gloor, MNI, *MNI AR*, 1969–70, 25, 42.

31 A.A. Eisen and A.L. Sherwin, "Serum Creatine Phosphokinase Activity in Cerebral Infarction," *Neurology* 18 (1968): 263–8.

32 P. Gloor, J.T. Murphy, and J.J. Dreifuss, "Electrophysiological Studies of Amygdalo-Hypothalamic Connections," *Annals of the New York Academy of Sciences* 157 (1969): 629–41; F.E. LeBlanc and J.P. Cordeau, "Modulation of Pyramidal Tract Cell Activity by Ventrolateral Thalamic Regions: Its Possible Role in Tremorogenic Mechanisms," *Brain Research* 14 (1969): 255–70; G. Mathews, G. Bertrand, and R. Broughton, "Thalamic Somatosensory Evoked Potentials in Parkinsonian Patients: Correlation with Unit Responses and Thalamic Stimulation," *Electroencephalography and Clinical Neu-*

rophysiology 28 (1970): 98–9; J.J. Dreifuss, J.T. Murphy, and P. Gloor, "Contrasting Effects of Two Identified Amygdaloid Efferent Pathways on Single Hypothalamic Neurons," *Journal of Neurophysiology* 31 (1968): 237–48; J.T. Murphy and L.P. Renaud, "Inhibitory Interneurons in the Ventromedial Nucleus of the Hypothalamus," *Brain Research* 9 (1968): 385–9; A. Morton, "The Time Course of Retrograde Neuron Loss in the Hypothalamic Niagno-Cellular Nuclei of Man," *Brain* 93 (1970): 329–36.

33 P. Gloor, "Generalized Cortico-Reticular Epilepsies: Some Considerations on the Pathophysiology of Generalized Bilaterally Synchronous Spike and Wave Discharge," *Epilepsia* 9 (1968): 249–63; P. Gloor, O. Kalabay, and N. Giard, "The Electroencephalogram in Diffuse Encephalopathies: Electroencephalographic Correlates of Grey and White Matter Lesions," *Brain* 91 (1968): 779–802; P. Gloor, "Epileptogenic Action of Penicillin," *Annals of the New York Academy of Sciences* 166 (1969): 350–60.

34 P. Gloor, MNI, *MNI AR*, 1967–68, 44; MNI, *MNI AR*, 1968–69, 47; C.W. Needham and C.J. Dila, "Synchronizing and Desynchronizing Systems of the Old Brain," *Brain Research* 11 (1968): 285–93; C.J. Dila, "A Midbrain Projection to the Centre Median Nucleus of the Thalamus: A Neurophysiological Study," *Brain Research* 25 (1971): 63–74.

35 Carl Dila joined the Department of Neurosurgery at the institute at the end of his residency. Charles Needham left Montreal after his residency in neurosurgery and held academic positions at Yale, the University of California at Los Angeles, and the University of Arizona.

36 MNI, *MNI AR*, 1968–69, 34.

37 W. Penfield and H. Steelman, "The Treatment of Focal Epilepsy by Cortical Excision," *Annals of Surgery* 126 (1947): 740–62.

38 Stephen Nutik joined former MNI fellow Maurice Héon in the Department of Neurosurgery at the Université de Sherbrooke. Roger Broughton, Vital Montpetit, and Robert Nelson relocated to the University of Ottawa. Leo Renaud moved to the Montreal General Hospital before becoming head of Neurology at the University of Ottawa.

39 J.Z. Young, "The Organization of a Memory System," *Proceedings of the Royal Society of London B Biological Sciences* 163 (1965): 285–320; J.Z. Young, "Two Memory Stores in One Brain," *Endeavour* 24 (1965): 13–20.

40 H. Hyden and E. Egyhazi, "Nuclear RNA Changes in Nerve Cells during a Learning Experiment in Rats," *Proceedings of the National Academy of Sciences* 48 (1962): 1366–73; S.P.R Rose, "Holger Hyden and the Biochemistry of Memory," *Brain Research Bulletin* 50 (1999): 443. The Hebbian concept of the engram had by then entered the realm of quantum physics, with Neils Bohr commenting at the inauguration of the Institute of Genetics at the University of Cologne in 1962, "The fact that everything which has come into our consciousness is remembered points to its leaving permanent marks in the organism." See N. Bohr, "Light and Life Revisited, 1962," in *The Philosophical Writings of Neils Bohn* (Woodbridge, CT: Ox Bow, 1987), 3:28.

41 *Clinical Neurosurgery* 16 (1969): 234–50, 251–68, 269–87, 288–314, 328–55, 356–75.

42 W. Feindel, "Symposium on Recent Research on the Cerebral Microcirculation," *Journal of Neurosurgery* 35 (1971): 123–80.

43 MNI, *MNI AR*, 1968–69, 6.

44   Ibid., 26–7.

45   Ibid., 29.

46   W. Penfield, "Speech, Perception and the Uncommitted Cortex," in *Brain and Conscious Experience Study Week on Brain and Conscious Experience, September 28–October 4, 1964*, Pontificia Academia Scientiarum, ed. J.C. Eccles, 319–47 (New York: Springer Verlag, 1966); W. Penfield, "Conditioning the Uncommitted Cortex for Language Learning," *Brain* 88 (1965): 787–98.

47   Penfield, "Speech, Perception and the Uncommitted Cortex," 217–18. P. Teilhard de Chardin, *Le Phénomène humain* (Paris: Le Seuil, 1955). It is uncertain if Penfield read de Chardin. A review of *The Phenomenon of Man* (New York: Harper, 1959) was recommended to Penfield by Stanley Cobb in a letter dated 5 January 1961, WPA.

48   W. Penfield, "Speech, Perception and the Uncommitted Cortex," in Eccles, *Study Week on Brain and Conscious Experience*, 218.

49   Penfield, *Mystery of the Mind*.

50   P. Gloor, *Hans Berger, On the Electroencephalogram of Man: The Fourteen Original Reports on the Human Electroencephalogram* (Amsterdam: Elsevier Publishing, 1969).

51   P. Gloor, "The Work of Hans Berger," *Electroencephalography and Clinical Neurophysiology* 27 (1969): 649; P. Gloor, "Hanz Berger: Psychophysiology and the Discovery of the Human Electroencephalogram," in *Berger Centenary Symposium on Epilepsy*, ed. P. Harris and C. Mawdslwy, 353–73 (Churchill Livingston, 1974); P. Gloor, "Berger Lecture: Is Berger's Dream Coming True?," *Electroencephalography and Clinical Neurophysiology* 90 (1994): 253–66.

52   This conceptualization was also favoured by Pavlov, who felt that a conditioned reflex was constituted by a connection "between a point in the brain's subcortex, which supported instincts, and a point in its cortex, where associations were built." See M. Specter, "Drool Ivan Pavlov's Real Quest," *New Yorker*, 24 November 2014.

53   Gloor, "Work of Hans Berger," 649.

54   File W/U 416, WPA.

55   File W/U 418, WPA.

56   Hans Berger, "Psychophysiology and the Discovery of the Human Electroencephalogram," Hans Berger Centennial Symposium on Brain–Mind Relationships, 23 May 1973, Montreal Neurological Institute.

57   Penfield, *Mystery of the Mind*, ix.

CHAPTER THIRTY-ONE

1   T. Rasmussen, MNI, *MNI AR*, 1969–70, 7–8.

2   Ibid., 8.

3   Ibid., 10.

4   MNI, *MNI AR*, 1967–68, 44; MNI, *MNI AR*, 1968–69, 47.

5   "Douglas Skuce deserves special praise for having done an enormous amount of work, well beyond the call of duty, in bringing this project to fruition." See Pierre Gloor in MNI, *MNI AR*, 1969–70, 25–6.

6 John Ives, a graduate of Strathclyde University, Glasgow, replaced Ralph Jell, who left the MNI in November 1969 to take a position in the Department of Physiology at the University of Manitoba in Winnipeg. See MNI, *MNI AR*, 1969–70, 48.

7 Ibid., 25–6, 46.

8 P. Gloor, MNI, *MNI AR*, 1970–71, 49–50. The MNI's commitment to ever more powerful computer-assisted research was matched by the willingness of the Medical Research Council of Canada to join in this farsighted endeavour. This joint effort was highlighted by Christopher Thompson's annual report to the MNI staff in 1981: "In 1970, the Montreal Neurological Institute acquired its first PDP-12 computer from a Medical Research Council major equipment grant for projects in neurophysiology, stereotaxic surgery, and electromyography. I joined the staff at the same time as an MRC professional assistant and have been supported by MRC ever since. In 1972, Jean Gotman took over computer applications in neurophysiology and EEG, supported by a Killam scholarship and now by an MRC scholarship. The introduction of computed tomography in 1973 and of positron emission tomography in 1975 opened up a whole new spectrum of medical imaging applications. Dr Terence Peters in 1978 took over the X-ray applications of computers. In 1979 we moved into the Penfield wing with two PDP-11/60 computers, the larger system in the Research Computing Laboratory, the smaller in the EEG department. With these systems we have gone from one computer which could be used by only one person at a time to two that can serve many users at once. Time on the old computer was heavily booked for preparation of programs since changing needs require continuing program development. Developing new programs can now be done concurrently with all other tasks." See C. Thompson, MNI, *MNI AR*, 1980–81, 94.

9 MNI, *MNI AR*, 1969–70, 30; R. Hansebout, E.W. Peterson, T.R. Ringer, and N.D. Durie, "Experiences with Core Temperature Maintenance during the Course of Regional Profound Brain Hypothermia," *Medical Research Engineering* 9 (1970): 9–13; C. Romero-Sierra, A. Sierhuis, R. Hansebout, and M. Lewin, "A New Method for Localized Spinal-Cord Cooling," *Medical and Biological Engineering* 12 (1974): 188–93; J.D. Wells and R.R. Hansebout, "Local Hypothermia in Experimental Spinal Cord Trauma," *Surgical Neurology* 10 (1978): 200–4.

10 Governement du Québec, "Historical Background," Régie de l'assurance maladie du Québec, http://www.ramq.gouv.qc.ca/en/regie/Pages/historical-background.aspx.

11 MNI, *MNI AR*, 1970–71, 9–10.

12 C.J. Hackwell, MNI, *MNI AR*, 1973–74, 41–2.

13 C.J. Hackwell, "1970 to 1974," in *Nursing Highlights 1934–1990*, ed. E. Barrowman, M. Cavanaugh, L. Dalicandro, M. Everett, P. Robb, and C.E. Robertson, 219–21.

14 A.F. Sadikot, M.M. Chakravarty, C. Bertrand, V. V. Rymar, A. Al-Subaie, and D. Louis, "Creation of Computerized 3D MRI-Integrated Atlases of the Human Basal Ganglia and Thalamus," *Frontiers in Systems Neuroscience* 5 (2011): 71.

15 W. Feindel, MNI, *MNI AR*, 1971–72, 34; G. Bertrand, H.H. Jasper, and A. Wong, "Microelectrode Study of the Human Thalamus: Functional Organization in the Ventrobasal Complex," *Confinia Neurologica* 29 (1967): 81–6; G. Bertrand, H.H. Jasper, A.

Wong, and G. Matthews, "Microelectrode Recording during Stereotactic Surgery," *Clinical Neurosurgery* 16 (1969): 328–55; C.J. Thompson and G. Bertrand, "A Computer Program to Aid the Neurosurgeon to Locate Probes Used during Stereotaxic Surgery on Deep Cerebral Structures," *Computer Programs in Biomedicine* 2 (1972): 265–76; G. Bertrand, A. Oliver, and C.J. Thompson, "The Computerized Brain Atlas: Its Use in Stereotaxic Surgery," *Transactions of the American Neurological Association* 98 (1973): 233; G. Bertrand, A. Olivier, and C.J. Thompson, "Computerized Display of Stereotaxic Brain Maps and Probe Tracts," *Acta Neurochirurgica* 21 (1974): 235–43; T.L. Hardy, "Computer Display of the Electrophysiological Topography of the Diencephalon during Stereotaxic Surgery" (master's thesis, McGill University, 1975); C.J. Thompson, T. Hardy, and G. Bertand, "A System for Anatomical and Functional Mapping of the Human Thalamus," *Computers and Biomedical Research* 10 (1977): 9–24.

16   T.L. Hardy, G. Bertrand, and C.J. Thompson, "The Position and Organization of Motor Fibers in the Internal Capsule Found during Stereotactic Surgery," *Applied Neurophysiology* 42 (1979): 160–70; T.L. Hardy, G. Bertrand, and C.J. Thompson, "Thalamic Recordings during Stereotactic Surgery. I. Surgery Topography of Evoked and Nonevoked Rhythmic Cellular Activity," *Applied Neurophysiology* 42 (1979): 185–97; T.L. Hardy, G. Bertrand, and C.J. Thompson, "Thalamic Recordings during Stereotactic Surgery. II. Location of Quick-Adapting Touch-Evoked (Novelty) Cellular Responses," *Applied Neurophysiology* 42 (1979): 198–202; T.L. Hardy, G. Bertrand, and C.J. Thompson, "Organization and Topography of Sensory Responses in the Internal Capsule and Nucleus Ventralis Caudalis Found during Stereotactic Surgery," *Applied Neurophysiology* 42 (1980), 335–51; T.L. Hardy, G. Bertrand, and C.J. Thompson, "Position and Organization of Thalamic Cellular Activity during Diencephalic Recording. I. Pressure-Evoked Activity," *Applied Neurophysiology* 43 (1980): 18–27; T.L. Hardy, G. Bertrand, and C.J. Thompson, "Touch-Evoked Thalamic Cellular Activity: The Variable Position of the Anterior Border of Somesthetic SI Thalamus and Somatotopography," *Applied Neurophysiology* 44 (1981): 302–13.

17   A.F. Sadikot et al., "Creation of Computerized 3D MRI-Integrated Atlases."

18   J.C. Eccles, M. Ito, and J. Zentagothal, *The Cerebellum as a Neuronal Machine* (Berlin: Springer-Verlag, 1967).

19   MNI, *MNI AR*, 1969–70, 6.

20   Ibid.

21   Ibid., 46.

22   J.R. Ives, C.J. Thompson, and J.F. Woods, "Acquisition by Telemetry and Computer Analysis of 4-Channel, Long-Term EEG Recordings from Patient Subject to 'Petit Mal' Absence Attacks," American Electroencephalographic Society, 26th Annual Meeting, Houston, October 1972; J.R. Ives, C.J. Thompson, and J.F. Woods, "Technical Contribution: Acquisition by Telemetry and Computer Analysis of 4-Channel Term EEG Recordings from Patients Subject to 'Petit-Mal' Absence Attacks," *Electroencephalography and Clinical Neurophysiology* 34 (1973): 665–8. Stevens and her collaborators at the University of Oregon had previously devised a similar system. J.R. Stevens, H. Kodama ,B. Lonsbury and L. Mills"Ultradian Characteristics of Spon-

taneous Seizure Discharges Recorded by Radiotelemetry in Man," *Electroencephalography and Clinical Neurophysiology* 31 (1971): 313–25.

23 P. Gloor, MNI, *MNI AR*, 1981–82, 71.

CHAPTER THIRTY-TWO

1 MNI, *MNI AR*, 1971–72, 12. Rasmussen is quoting Allan Gregg, of the Rockefeller Institution, innaugural address at the opening of the McConnell Wing of the MNI. See A. Gregg, *Prospects and Retrospects in Neurology* (Boston: Little, Brown, 1955), 12.

2 Ibid.

3 W. Feindel, MNI, *MNI AR*, 1971–72, 15–16; MNI, *MNI AR*, 1970–71, 34, 57; MNI, *MNI AR*, 1972–73, 60. Some of the early work supported by the Webster Research Fund resulted in a number of influential publications: Y.L. Yamamoto, E.Meyer, and W. Feindel, "Multichannel Miniature Semiconductor Detector System with On-line Computer Analysis for Measurement of Miniregional Cerebral Blood Flow," *IEEE Transactions on Nuclear Science* n.s. 22 (1974): 383–87; Y.L Yamamoto, C.J. Thompson, E. Meyer, J.S. Robertson, and W. Feindel, "Dynamic Positron Emission Tomography for Study of Cerebral Hemodynamics in a Cross Section of the Head Using Positron-Emitting 68Ga-EDTA and 77Kr," *Journal of Computer Assisted Tomography* 1 (1977): 43–56; E. Meyer, "A Transform Method and Semiconductor Detector System Applied to Regional Cerebral Blood Flow Analysis" (PhD diss., McGill University, 1980).

4 MNI, *MNI AR*, 1972–73, 12.

5 MNI, *MNI AR*, 1973–74, 7.

6 MNI, *MNI AR*, 1972–73, 15.

7 MNI, *MNI AR*, 1971–72, 16.

8 MNI, *MNI AR*, 1973–74, 10.

9 MNI, *MNI AR*, 1974–75, 46.

10 Ibid., 46–7.

11 P. Murray, "Studies on the Comparison of Flow Patterns and Regional Cerebral Blood Flow before and after Cerebral Revascularization for Selective Middle Cerebral Artery Occlusion in the Dog" (master's thesis, McGill University, 1978)

12 S. Nutik, "Thermal Afferents to Posterior Hypothalamic Neurons" (PhD diss., McGill University, 1971).

13 MNI, *MNI AR*, 1972–73, 36.

14 F. Andermann, ed., "Krabbe's Globoid Cell Leukodystrophy. Galacterocerebroside 0-Galactosidase Deficiency: A Multidisciplinary Approach to the Study of Patients with Progressive Neurological Disease. Grand Rounds at the Montreal Neurological Institute and Hospital – Chairman Theodore B. Rasmussen, MD," *Canadian Medical Association Journal* 105 (1971): 505–11.

15 P. Gloor, O. Kalabay, and N. Giard, "The Electroencephalogram in Diffuse Encephalopathies: Electroencephalographic Correlates of Grey and White Matter Lesions," *Brain* 91 (1968): 779–802.

16 Eva Andermann completed her doctoral dissertation on focal epilepsy and related

disorders, and she was appointed assistant electroencephalographer. Dr Andermann became an internationally recognized neurogeneticist and expert in the management of the gravid epileptic patient, an area in which she was ably assisted by her graduate student Linda Dansky. See E. Andermann, "Focal Epilepsy and Related Disorders: Genetic, Metabolic and Prognostic Studies" (PhD diss., McGill University, 1972); L. Dansky, E. Andermann, F. Andermann, and A. Sherwin, "The Outcome of Pregnancy in Epileptic Women," *Canadian Journal of Neurological Sciences* 1 (1974): 264–5; L.V. Dansky, "Marriage and Reproduction in Epileptic Patients" (master's thesis, McGill University,1978); Dansky, "Outcome of Pregnancy in Epileptic Women: A Prospective Evaluation of Genetic and Environmental Risk Factors" (PhD diss., McGill University, 1989).

17   L. Wolfe, MNI, *MNI AR*, 1976–77, 51.

18   MNI, *MNI AR*, 1970–71, 45; MNI, *MNI AR*, 1971–72, 53.

19   The conditions studied included infantile myotonic dystrophy, juvenile Tay-Sachs disease, Sandhoff's disease, juvenile dystonic lipidosis, cerebromacular degeneration, Lafora's disease, Werdnig-Hoffmann disease, Duchenne disease, dermatomyositis, acid maltase deficiency, and the Guillain-Barré syndrome.

20   S. Carpenter, G. Karpati, F. Andermann, J.C. Jacob, and E. Andermann, "The Ultrastructural Characteristics of the Abnormal Cytosomes in Batten-Kufs' Disease," *Brain* 100 (1977): 137–6; L.S. Wolfe, N.M.K. Ng Ying Kin, R.R. Baker, S. Carpenter, and F. Andermann, "Identification of Retinoyl Complexes as the Autofluorescent Component of the Neuronal Storage Material in Batten's Disease," *Science* 195 (1977): 1360–2.

21   E. Andermann, C. Remillard, C. Goyer, L. Blitzer, F. Andermann, and A. Barbeau, "Genetic and Family Studies in Friedreich's Ataxia," *Canadian Journal of Neurological Sciences* 3 (1976): 287–301.

22   E. Andermann, F. Andermann, M. Joubert, G. Karpati, S. Carpenter, and D. Melancon. "Familial Agenesis of the Corpus Callosum with Anterior Horn Cell Disease: A Syndrome of Mental Retardation, Areflexia, and Paraparesis," *Transactions of the American Neurological Association* 97 (1972): 242–4; E. Andermann, F. Andermann, S. Carpenter, G. Karpati, A. Eisen, D. Mélançon, J. Bergeron, "Agenesis of the Corpus Callosum with Sensorimotor Neuronopathy: A New Autosomal Recessive Malformation Syndrome with High Frequency in Charlevoix County, Quebec," Fifth International Conference on Birth Defects, Montreal, August, 1977; E. Andermann, F. Andermann, D. Bergeron, P. Lanvin, R. Nagy, and J. Bergeron, "Familial Agenesis of the Corpus Callosum with Sensori-Motor Neuronopathy: Genetic and Epidemiological Studies of over 170 Patients," *Canadian Journal of Neurological Sciences* 6 (1979): 400; J.R. Nagy, "Familial Agenesis of the Corpus Callosum with Sensorimotor Neuronopathy: Genetic and Epidemiological Studies" (master's thesis, McGill University, 1982).

23   E. Andermann, MNI, *MNI AR*, 1976–77, 68.

24   M. Joubert, J.J. Eisenring, J.P. Robb, and F. Andermann, "Familial Agenesis of the Cerebellar Vermis: A Syndrome of Episodic Hyperpnea, Abnormal Eye Movements, Ataxia, and Retardation," *Neurology* 19 (1969): 813–25; E. Andermann, F. Andermann,

M. Joubert, D. Mélançon, G. Karpati, and S. Carpenter, "Three Familial Midline Malformation Syndromes of the Central Nervous System: Agenesis of the Corpus Callosum and Anterior Horn-Cell Disease; Agenesis of Cerebellar Vermis; and Atrophy of the Cerebellar Vermis," *Birth Defects Original Article Series* 11 (1975): 269–93.

25   E. Andermann, MNI, *MNI AR*, 1978–79, 73.

26   P. Gloor, MNI, *MNI AR*, 1975–76, 36–7.

27   G. Bertrand, H.H. Jasper, A. Wong, and G. Mathews, "Microelectrode Recording during Stereotaxic Surgery," *Clinical Neurosurgery* 16 (1969): 328–55.

28   MNI, *MNI AR*, 1973–74, 53.

29   J.R. Ives, C.J. Thompson, and J.F. Woods, "Technical Contribution: Acquisition by Telemetry and Computer Analysis of 4-Channel Term EEG Recordings from Patients Subject to 'Petit-Mal' Absence Attacks," *Electroencephalography and Clinical Neurophysiology* 34 (1973): 665–8; J. Gotman, D.R. Skuce, C.J. Thompson, P. Gloor, J.R. Yves, and W.F. Ray, "Clinical Applications of Spectral Analysis and Extraction of Features from Electroencephalograms with Slow Waves in Adult Patients," *Electroencephalography and Clinical Neurophysiology* 35 (1973): 225–35; J.R. Ives, C.J. Thompson, P. Gloor, A. Olivier, and J.F. Woods, "The On-line Computer Detection and Recording of Spontaneous Temporal Lobe Epileptic Seizures from Patients with Implanted Depth Electrodes via a Radio-Telemetry Link," *Electroencephalography and Clinical Neurophysiology* 37 (1974): 205; J. Ives and J.F. Woods, "4-Channel 24-Hour Cassette Recorder for Long-Term EEG Monitoring of Ambulatory Patients," *Electroencephalography and Clinical Neurophysiology* 39 (1975): 88–92; J. Gotman, P. Gloor, and W.F. Ray, "A Quantitative Comparison of Traditional Reading of the EEG and Interpretation of Computer-Extracted Features in Patients with Supratentorial Brain Lesions," *Electroencephalography and Clinical Neurophysiology* 38 (1975): 623–39; J.R. Ives, A. Wilkins, M. Jones, F. Andermann, and J. Woods, "Twenty-Seven Days in the Life of an Epileptic Patient," *Biotelemetry* 3 (1976): 177–80; J. Gotman and P. Gloor, "Automatic Recognition and Quantification of Interictal Epileptic Activity in the Human Scalp EEG," *Electroencephalography Clinical Neurophysiology* 41 (1976): 513–29; J.R. Ives, C.J. Thompson, and P. Gloor, "Seizure Monitoring: A New Tool in Electro-Encephalography," *Electroencephalography and Clinical Neurophysiology* 41 (1976): 422–7; J.R. Ives and P. Gloor, "Automatic Nocturnal Sleep Sampling: A Useful Method in Clinical Electroencephalography," *Electroencephalography and Clinical Neurophysiology* 43 (1977): 880–4.

30   H.H. Jasper and J. Kershman, "Electroencephalographic Classification of the Epilepsies," *Archives of Neurology & Psychiatry* 45 (1941): 930. R.R. Rovit, P. Gloor, and L.T. Henderson Jr, "Temporal Lobe Epilepsy: A Study Using Multiple Basal Electrodes. 1. Description of Method," *Neurochirurgia* 3 (1960): 6–19; R.R. Rovit and P. Gloor, "Temporal Lobe Epilepsy: A Study Using Multiple Basal Electrodes. II. Clinical EEG Findings," *Neurochirurgia* 3 (1960): 19–34; R.R. Rovit, P. Gloor, and T. Rasmussen, "Sphenoidal Electrodes in the Electrographic Study of Patients with Temporal Lobe Epilepsy: An Evaluation," *Journal of Neurosurgery* 18 (1961): 151–8; J.R. Ives, "EEG Monitoring of Ambulatory Epileptic Patients," supplemente, *Postgraduate Medical Journal* 52, no. 7 (1976): 86–91.

31 Quesney, a refined and considerate gentleman, died in the midst of a brilliant career in a motor vehicle accident in Spain in 2005, having taken an influential position at the University of Madrid. See L.F. Quesney, "Pathophysiology of Generalized Penicillin Epilepsy in the Cat: The Role of Cortical and Subcortial Structures" (PhD diss., McGill University, 1977).

32 P. Gloor, "Generalized Epilepsy with Bilateral Synchronous Spike and Wave Discharge: New Findings concerning Its Physiological Mechanisms," supplement, *Electroencephalography and Clinical Neurophysiology* 34 (1978): 245–9; L.F. Quesney and P. Gloor, "Generalized Penicillin Epilepsy in the Cat: Correlation between Electrophysiological Data and Distribution of 14C-Penicillin in the Brain," *Epilepsia* 19 (1978): 35–45; P. Gloor, L.F. Quesney, and H. Zumstein, "Pathophysiology of Generalized Penicillin Epilepsy in the Cat: The Role of Cortical and Subcortical Structures. II. Topical Application of Penicillin to the Cerebral Cortex and to Subcortical Structures," *Electroencephalography and Clinical Neurophysiology* 43 (1977): 79–94; L.F. Quesney, F. Andermann, S. Lal, and S. Prelevic, "Transient Abolition of Generalized Photosensitive Epileptic Discharge in Humans by Apomorphine, a Dopamine-Receptor Agonist," *Neurology* 30 (1980): 169–74; L.F. Quesney, F. Andermann, and P. Gloor, "Dopaminergic Mechanism in Generalized Photosensitive Epilepsy," *Neurology* 31 (1981): 1542–4; P. Gloor, A. Olivier, L.F. Quesney, F. Andermann, and S. Horowitz, "The Role of the Limbic System in Experiential Phenomena of Temporal Lobe Epilepsy," *Annals of Neurology* 12 (1982): 129–44; A. Olivier, P. Gloor, L.F. Quesney, and F. Andermann, "The Indications for and the Role of Depth Electrode Recording in Epilepsy," *Applied Neurophysiology* 46 (1983): 33–6; L.F. Quesney, "Pathophysiology of Generalized Photosensitive Epilepsy in the Cat," *Epilepsia* 25 (1984): 61–9; A. Olivier, P. Gloor, F. Andermann, and L.F. Quesney, "The Place of Stereotactic Depth Electrode Recording in Epilepsy," *Applied Neurophysiology* 48 (1985): 395–9; L.F. Quesney and P. Gloor, "Localization of Epileptic Foci," supplement, *Electroencephalography and Clinical Neurophysiology* 37 (1985): 165–200; J. Gotman, J.R. Ives, P. Gloor, L.F. Quesney, and P. Bergsma, "Monitoring at the Montreal Neurological Institute," supplement, *Electroencephalography and Clinical Neurophysiology* 37 (1985): 327–40; N. So, P. Gloor, L.F. Quesney, M. Jones-Gotman, A. Olivier, and F. Andermann, "Depth Electrode Investigations in Patients with Bitemporal Epileptiform Abnormalities," *Annals of Neurology* 25 (1989): 423–31.

33 J. Gotman, D.R. Skuce, C.J. Thompson, P. Gloor, J.R. Ives, and W.F. Ray, "Clinical Applications of Spectral Analysis and Extraction of Features from Electroencephalograms with Slow Waves in Adult Patients," *Electroencephalography and Clinical Neurophysiology* 35 (1973): 225–35; J. Gotman, "Computer Analysis of the Clinical EEG" (PhD diss., McGill University, 1976); J. Gotman, P. Gloor, and N. Schaul, "Comparison of Traditional Reading of the EEG and Automatic Recognition of Interictal Epileptic Activity," *Electroencephalography and Clinical Neurophysiology* 44 (1978): 48–60.

34 N.M. Van Gelder, A.L. Sherwin, and T. Rasmussen, "Amino Acid Content of Epileptogenic Human Brain: Focal versus Surrounding Regions," *Brain Research* 40 (1972): 385–93; N.M. Van Gelder, "Glutamate Dehydrogenase, Glutamic Acid Decarboxylase,

and GABA Amino Transferase in Epileptic Mouse Cortex," *Canadian Journal of Physiology and Pharmacology* 52 (1974): 952–9; A. Sherwin, L.F. Quesney, S. Gauthier, A. Olivier, Y. Robitaille, Y. McQuaid, C. Harvey, and N. van Gelder, "Enzyme Changes in Actively Spiking Areas of Human Epileptic Cerebral Cortex," *Neurology* 34 (1984): 927–33; Y. Robitaille and A. Sherwin, "High Affinity (3H) Beta-Alanine Uptake by Scar Margins of Ferric Chloride-Induced Epileptogenic Foci in Rat Isocortex," *Journal of Neuropathology and Experimental Neurology* 43 (1984): 376–83.

35 MNI, *MNI AR*, 1974–75, 56–8; P. Gloor and G. Testa, "Generalized Penicillin Epilepsy in the Cat: Effects of Intra-Carotid and Intra-Vertebral Pentylenetetrazol and Amobarbital Injections," *Electroencephalography and Clinical Neurophysiology* 36 (1974): 499–515; S. Prelevic, W.M. Burxham, and P. Gloor, "A Microelectrode Study of Amygdaloid Afferents: Temporal Neocortical Inputs," *Brain Research* 105 (1976): 437–57; L.-P. Quesney, "Pathophysiology of Generalized Penicillin Epilepsy in the Cat: The Role of Cortical and Subcortical Structures" (PhD diss., McGill University, 1977).

36 MNI, *MNI AR*, 1973–74, 60–1.

37 G. Mathieson, "Pathologic Aspects of Epilepsy with Special Reference to the Surgical Pathology of Focal Cerebral Seizures," in *Advances in Neurology*, vol. 8, *Neurosurgical Management of the Epilepsies*, ed. D.P. Purpura, J.K. Penry, and R.D. Walter, 107–38 (New York: Raven, 1975).

38 G. Mathieson, "Pathology of Temporal Lobe Foci," in *Advances in Neurology*, vol. 11, *Complex Partial Seizures*, ed. J.K. Penry and D.D. Daly, 163–85 (New York: Raven, 1975).

39 W. Penfield and B. Milner, "Memory Deficit Produced by Bilateral Lesions in the Hippocampal Zone," *Archives of Neurology and Psychiatry* 79 (1958): 475–97.

40 Ibid.

41 W. Penfield and G. Mathieson, "Memory: Autopsy Findings and Comments on the Role of Hippocampus in Experiential Recall," *Archives of Neurology* 31 (1974): 145–54.

42 G.M. Remillard, R. Ethier, and F. Andermann, "Temporal Lobe Epilepsy and Perinatal Occlusion of the Posterior Cerebral Artery: A Syndrome Analogous to Infantile Hemiplegia and a Demonstrable Etiology in Some Patients with Temporal Lobe Epilepsy," *Neurology* 24 (1974): 1001–9.

43 MNI, *MNI AR*, 1972–73, 15.

44 J. Ambrose, "Computerized X-ray Scanning of the Brain," *Journal of Neurosurgery* 40 (1974): 679–95.

45 MNI, *MNI AR*, 1973–74, 11, 48.

46 I.E. Leppik, C.J. Thompson, R. Ethier, and A.L. Sherwin, "Diatrizoate in Computed Cranial Tomography: A Quantitative Study," *Investigative Radiology* 12 (1977): 21–6.

CHAPTER THIRTY-THREE

1 MNI, *MNI AR*, 1973–74, 7–9.

2 W. Feindel, ibid., 9.

3 MNI, *MNI AR*, 1974–75, 5.

4 MNI, *MNI AR*, 1973–74, 12.

5 Ibid., 10.

6 Martin's appointment had been preceded by administrative changes in the governance of the institute and of the Department of Neurology and Neurosurgery. Since the founding of the Montreal Neurological Institute in 1934, the director of the institute was also chair of the Department of Neurology and Neurosurgery at McGill University. The two positions were separated in 1977. The departmental budget became the responsibility of the chair, who reported to the dean of medicine. The MNI budget, however, remained the responsibility of its director, who reported to the principal and the board of governors. Thus, the director of the MNI still remained responsible for its endowment funds, which he used for research, teaching, the recruitment of research staff, and for allocation of space and resources necessary to the institute's research activities. The chair of the Department of Neurology and Neurosurgery was freed of these responsibilities and could devote his time to undergraduate and postgraduate teaching at the McGill hospitals, among other responsibilities of the chair of a department at a major university. See MNI, *MNI AR*, 1978–79, 38; MNI, *MNI AR*, 1979–80, 48–9.

7 MNI, *MNI AR*, 1975–76, 55; MNI, *MNI AR*, 1976–77, 13, 76.

8 J. Olszewski and D. Baxter, *Cytoarchitecture of the Human Brainstem* (Philadelphia: J.B. Lippincott, 1954).

9 R. Ethier, D.G. King, D. Melancon, G. Bélanger, S. Taylor, and C. Thompson, "Development of High Resolution Computed Tomography of the Spinal Cord," *Journal of Computer Assisted Tomography* 3 (1979): 433–8.

10 MNI, *MNI AR*, 1974–75, 1; C.J. Hackwell and C. Robertson, "The Hackwell-Robertson Years," in Barrowman et al., *Nursing Highlights 1934 to 1990*, 219–37.

11 L. Weiskrantz, E.K. Warrington, M.D. Sanders, and J. Marshall, "Visual Capacity in the Hemianopic Field following a Restricted Occipital Ablation," *Brain* 97 (1974): 709–28; E.K. Warrington, "The Selective Impairment of Semantic Memory," *Quarterly Journal of Experimental Psychology* 27 (1975): 635–57.

12 MNI, *MNI AR*, 1973–74, 12.

13 R. Granit, "The Functional Role of the Muscle Spindles: Facts and Hypotheses," *Brain* 98 (1975): 531–56.

14 T. Rasmussen, "Postoperative Superficial Hemosiderosis of the Brain, Its Diagnosis, Treatment and Prevention," *Transactions of the American Neurological Association* 98 (1973): 133–7.

15 D.P. Purpura, J.K. Penry, and D.D. Daly, eds., *Advances in Neurology*, vol. 8, *Neurosurgical Management of the Epilepsies* (New York: Raven, 1975); J.K. Penry and D.D. Daly, eds., *Advances in Neurology*, vol. 11, *Complex Partial Seizures* (New York: Raven, 1975).

16 G. Vinken and P. Bruyn, "The Epilepsies," in *Handbook of Clinical Neurology Volume 15* (Amsterdam: North-Holland Publishing, 1974).

17 P. Gloor, "Temporal Lobe Epilepsy: Its Possible Contribution to the Understanding of the Functional Significance of the Amygdala and of Its Interaction with Neorcortical-Temporal Mechanisms," in *Symposium on the Neurobiology of the Amygdala, Bar Harbor, Maine, 1971*, ed. B.E. Eleftheriou, 423–57 (New York: Plenum, 1971).

18 P. Gloor, *The Temporal Lobe and Limbic System* (Oxford: Oxford University Press, 1999).

19 A.M. Pappius and W. Feindel, eds., *Dynamics of Brain Edema: Proceedings of the 3rd International Workshop on Dynamic Aspects of Cerebral Edema, Montreal, Canada, June 25–29, 1976* (Heidelberg: Springer-Verlag, 1976).

20 R. Katzman and H.M. Pappius, eds., *Brain Electrolytes and Fluid Metabolism* (Baltimore, MD: Williams and Wilkins, 1973).

21 R. Katzman, R. Clasen, I. Klatzo, J.S. Meyer, H.M. Pappius, and A.G. Waltz, "Brain Edema in Stroke," *Stroke* 8 (1977): 512–40.

22 H. Schneider, D. Janz, C. Gardner-Thorpe, H. Meinardi, and A.L. Sherwin, eds., *Clinical Pharmacology of Anti-Epileptic Drugs* (Berlin: Springer-Verlag, 1975).

23 W.G. Bradlev, D. Gardner-Medwin, and J.N. Walton, eds., *Recent Advances in Myology* (Amsterdam: Excerpta Medica, 1975), 51–5, 258–66, 274–84, 374–9.

24 M.K. Jones, "Imagery as a Mnemonic Aid after Left Temporal Lobectomy" (master's thesis, McGill University, 1971); Jones, "Reduced Visual Inventiveness after Focal Right Hemisphere Lesions in Man" (PhD diss., McGill University, 1975); M.K. Jones-Gotman and B. Milner, "Right Temporal-Lobe Contribution to Image-Mediated Verbal Learning," *Neuropsychologia* 16 (1978): 61–71; M.K. Jones-Gotman, "Incidental Learning of Image-Mediated or Pronounced Words after Right Temporal Lobectomy," *Cortex* 15 (1979): 187–97.

25 B. Milner, "Interhemispheric Differences in the Localization of Psychological Processes in Man," *British Medical Bulletin* 27 (1971): 272–7.

26 B. Milner, "Hemispheric Specialization: Scope and Limits," in *The Neurosciences: Third Study Program*, ed. F.O. Schmitt and F.G. Worden, 75–89 (Boston: MIT Press, 1974).

27 Michael Dogali pursued a career in neurosurgery in California, and Ilo Leppik took a position in the Department of Experimental and Clinical Pharmacology at the University of Minnesota College of Pharmacy. Kenneth Laxer later moved to California and pursued his interest in the care of epileptic patients. Jean-Guy Villemure would have a distinguished career in four major universities on two continents.

28 File J 13-1, WPA.

CHAPTER THIRTY-FOUR

1 A. Blum, "A Bedside Conversation with Wilder Penfield," *Canadian Medical Association Journal* 183 (2011): 745–6.

2 MNI, *MNI AR*, 1975–76, 38–9.

3 W. Feindel, "Wilder Penfield: His Legacy to Neurology," *Archives of Neurology* 116 (1977): 1365–77.

4 H.H. Jasper, "The Centrencephalic System," *Canadian Medical Association Journal* 116 (1977): 1371–2. The centrencephalic integrating system is undergoing a revival of sorts, especially as it relates to consciousness and epilepsy. See R. Llinas and D. Paré, "Of Dreaming and Wakefulness," *Neuroscience* 44 (1991): 521–35; R. Llinas and Urs Ribar,

"Consciousness and the Brain: The Thalamocortical Dialogue in Health and Disease," *Annals of the New York Academy of Sciences* 929 (2001): 166–75; A.D. Norden and H. Blumenfeld, "The Role of Subcortical Structures in Human Epilepsy," *Epilepsy and Behavior* 3 (2002): 219–31; L. Yu and H. Blumenfeld, "Theories of Impaired Consciousness in Epilepsy," *Annals of the New York Academy of Sciences* 1157 (2009): 48–60.

5 File 14, box 2, Francis Lothian McNaughton Fonds, Osler Library of the History of Medicine, McGill University.

CHAPTER THIRTY-FIVE

1 File E/K 78-9-15, WPA.

2 Although officially opened, the pavilion still needed completion of its inner structure, which took another year. See MNI, *MNI AR*, 1980–81, 43.

3 G. Scotti, R. Ethier, D. Melançon, K.Terbrugge, and S. Tchang, "Computed Tomography in the Evaluation of Intracranial Aneurysms and Subarachnoid Hemorrhage," *Radiology* 23 (1977): 85–90; G. Scotti, K. Terbrugge, D. Melançon, and G. Bélanger, "Evaluation of the Age of Subdural Hematomas by Computerized Tomography," *Journal of Neurosurgery* 47 (1977): 311–15; S. Tchang, G. Scotti, K. Terbrugge, D. Mélançon, G. Bélanger, C. Milner, and R. Ethier," Computerized Tomography as a Possible Aid to Histological Grading of Supratentorial Gliomas," *Journal of Neurosurgery* 46 (1977): 735–9; K. Terbrugge, G. Scotti, R. Ethier, D. Mélançon, S. Tchang, and C. Milner, "Computed Tomography in Intracranial Arteriovenous Malformations," *Radiology* 122 (1977): 703–5.

4 MNI, *MNI AR*, 1981–82, 81.

5 J.D. Wells and R.R. Hansebout, "Local Hypothermia in Experimental Spinal Cord Trauma," *Surgical Neurology* 10 (1978): 200–4.

6 MNI, *MNI AR*, 1977–78, 8–9.

7 R. Leblanc and M. Preul, "William H. Feindel (1918–2014)," *Journal of Neurosurgery* 122 (2015): 449–52.

8 See Bernard Becker Medical Library, "The H. Richard Tyler Collection of the American Academy of Neurology Library," https://becker.wustl.edu/resources/arb/rare-books/tyler-collection.

9 L.F. Kromer, A. Bjorklund, and U. Stenevi, "Intracephalic Implants: A Technique for Studying Neuronal Interactions," *Science* 204 (1979): 1117–19.

10 F.O. Schmitt, "Introduction," in G.M. Edelman and V.B. Mountcastle, *The Mindful Brain* (Cambridge, MA: MIT Press, 1978), 2; V.B. Mountcastle, "The Columnar Organization of the Neocortex," *Brain* 120 (1997): 701–22; V.B. Mountcastle, "An Organizing Principle for Cerebral Function," in Edelman and Mountcastle, *Mindful Brain*, 7–50.

11 I.P. Pavlov, "Conditioned Reflexes in Dogs after Destruction of Different Parts of the Cerebral Hemispheres," in *Lectures on Conditioned Reflexes: Twenty-Five Years of Objective Study of the Higher Nervous Activity (Behaviour) in Animals*, ed. W.H. Gantt,

G. Volborth, and W.B. Cannon, 97–8 (New York: International Publishers, 1928); emphasis in the original.

12   B. Milner, "Complementary Functional Specializations of the Human Cerebral Hemispheres," in *Nerve Cells, Transmitters and Behavior*, ed. R. Levi-Montalcini, 601–28 (Vatican City: Pontifical Academy of Sciences, 1980).

13   T. Rasmussen and B. Milner, "The Role of Early Left-Brain Injury in Determining Lateralization of Cerebral Speech Functions," *Annals of the New York Academy of Sciences* 299 (1977): 355–69.

14   MNI, *MNI AR,* 1974 75, 10.

15   W. Feindel, ed., "The First International Symposium on Positron Emission Tomography," *Journal of Computer Assisted Tomography* 2 (1978): 637–64.

16   C.J. Thompson, Y.L. Yamamoto, and E. Meyer, "Positome II: A High Efficiency PET Device for Dynamic Studies," *Journal of Computer Assisted Tomography* 2 (1978): 650–1; E. Meyer, "A Transform Method and Semiconductor Detector System Applied to Regional Cerebral Blood Flow Analysis" (PhD diss., McGill University, 1980).

17   Y.L. Yamamoto, C.J. Thompson, E. Meyer, and W. Feindel, "Positron Emission Tomography for Measurement of Regional Cerebral Blood Flow," *Advances in Neurology* 30 (1981): 41–53.

18   P.E. Roland, E. Meyer, Y.L. Yamamoto, and C.J. Thompson, "Dynamic Positron Emission Tomography as a Tool in Neuroscience: Functional Brain-Mapping in Normal Human Volunteers," supplement, *Journal of Cerebral Blood Flow and Metabolism* 1 (1981): S463–4; P.E. Roland, E. Meyer, T. Shibasaki, Y.L. Yamamoto, and C.J. Thompson, "Regional Cerebral Blood Flow Changes in Cortex and Basal Ganglia during Voluntary Movements in Normal Human Volunteers," *Journal of Neurophysiology* 48 (1982): 467–80.

19   R. Leblanc and E. Meyer, "Functional PET Scanning in the Treatment of AVMs," *Journal of Neurosurgery* 73 (1990): 615–19.

CHAPTER THIRTY-SIX

1   MNI, *MNI AR*, 1979–80, 5–56; MNI, *MNI AR*, 1981–82, 72–3.

2   Agapito Lorenzo initiated the electromyography laboratory at the institute in 1967, then left for the United States the following year, and the laboratory came under the direction of Andrew Eisen, who established its international reputation.

3   W. Feindel, MNI, *MNI AR*, 1982–83, 14.

4   Beyond his expertise in the neuropathology of epilepsy, Yves Robitaille was expert in the pathology related to Alzheimer's disease. With collaborators at the Douglas Hospital Research Centre he explored the role of cholinergic and somatostatinergic systems in Alzheimer's disease and other forms of dementia.

5   Joy Arpin trained in neurosurgery at the MNI and did a year of postgraduate training in neuroradiology at the Massachusetts General Hospital in Boston. Her principal interest at the institute was in the microsurgical treatment of vascular disease. John Wells, a graduate of Tulane University Medical School in Louisiana, had worked

with Robert Hansebout during his residency at the MNI. Wells later left the MNI to join Robert Hansebout at McMaster University. Antoine Hakim had an influential career at the MNI, especially in the imaging of cerebrovascular disease. Hakim relocated to the University of Ottawa in 1992 as professor and chair of neurology. David Thomas rendered great service to the institute before moving on to the University of Calgary.

6 MNI, *MNI AR*, 1982–83, 58.

7 R. Leblanc, R. Ethier, and J.R. Little, "Computerized Tomographic Findings in Arteriovenous Malformations of the Brain," *Journal of Neurosurgery* 51 (1979): 765–72; R. Leblanc and A. O'Gorman, "Neonatal Intracranial Hemorrhage: A Clinical and Serial Computerized Tomographic Study," *Journal of Neurosurgery* 53 (1980): 642–51; R. Leblanc, W. Feindel, and R. Ethier, "Epilepsy from Cerebral Arteriovenous Malformations," *Canadian Journal of Neurological Sciences* 8 (1981): 7–13; R. Leblanc, W. Feindel, T. Yamamoto, J.G. Milton, and M.M. Frojmovic, "Reversal of Acute Cerebral Casospasm by the Calcium Antagonist Verapamil," *Canadian Journal of Neurological Sciences* 11 (1984): 42–7; R. Leblanc, W. Feindel, T. Yamamoto, J.G. Milton, M.M. Frojmovic, and C.P. Hodge, "The Effects of Calcium Antagonism on the Epicerebral Circulation in Early Vasospasm," *Stroke* 15 (1984): 1017–20.

8 Richard Leblanc was appointed to the staff of the MNI in 1982. He and Donatella Tampieri, an interventional neuroradiologist, inaugurated the Vascular Neuro-interventional Group. He later became director of the Brain Tumour and Skull Base Surgery Programs at the MNI, while maintaining an interest in the surgical treatment of epilepsy associated with cortical migration disorders. He was made professor in the Department of Neurology and Neurosurgery at McGill University in 1998. See R. Leblanc, "Calcium Antagonism in Cerebral Vasospasm" (master's thesis, McGill University, 1984).

9 L. Friedman and B.E. Jones, "Study of Sleep-Wakefulness States by Computer Graphics and Cluster Analysis before and after Lesions of the Pontine Tegmentum in the Cat," *Electroencephalography and Clinical Neurophysiology* 57 (1984): 43–56.

10 A. Parent, L. Descarries, and A. Beaudet, "Organization of Ascending Serotonin Systems in the Adult Rat Brain: A Radioauto-graphic Study after Intraventricular Administration of H5-Hydroxytryptamine," *Neuroscience* 6 (1981): 115–38.

11 E. Hamel and A. Beaudet, "Electron Microscopic Autoradiographic Localization of Opioid Receptors in Rat Neostriatum," *Nature* 312 (1984): 155–7.

12 International Society for Cerebral Blood Flow & Metabolism, *Brain Bits* 40 (June 2014), http://iscbfm.org/PDFS/3a/3a882aa9-f6b4-496f-982e-69a6988c64c1.pdf.

13 A.M. Hakim, "The Cerebral Ischemic Penumbra," *Canadian Journal of Neurological Sciences* 14 (1987): 557–9.

14 R. Leblanc, J.L. Tyler, G. Mohr, E. Meyer, M. Doksic, L. Yamamoto, L. Taylor, S. Gauthier, and A. Hakim, "Hemodynamic and Metabolic Effects of Cerebral Revascularization," *Journal of Neurosurgery* 66 (1987): 529–35; R. Leblanc, Y.L. Yamamoto, J.L. Tyler, and A. Hakim, "Borderzone Ischemia," *Annals of Neurology* 22 (1987): 707–13. R. Leblanc, Y.L. Yamamoto, J.L. Tyler, and A. Hakim, "Hemodynamic and Metabolic

Effects of Extracranial Carotid Disease," *Canadian Journal of Neurological Sciences* 16 (1989): 51–7. R. Leblanc, "Physiological Studies in Cerebrovascular Disease," *Clinical Neurosurgery* 37 (1991): 289–311.

15 MNI, *MNI AR*, 1974–75, 11.

16 D. Guitton, M. Crommelinck, and A. Roucoux, "Stimulation of the Superior Colliculus in the Alert Cat. I. Eye Movements and Neck EMG Activity Evoked When the Head Is Restrained," *Experimental Brain Research* 39 (1980): 63–73; A. Roucoux, D. Guitton, and M. Crommelinck, "Stimulation of the Superior Colliculus in the Alert Cat. II. Eye and Head Movements Evoked When the Head Is Unrestrained," *Experimental Brain Research* 39 (1980): 75–85.

17 D.G. Tanji, S.P. Wise, R.W. Dykes, and E.G. Jones, "Cytoarchitecture and Thalamic Connectivity of Third Somatosensory Area of Cat Cerebral Cortex," *Journal of Neurophysiology* 41 (1978): 268–84; R.W. Dykes, "Parallel Processing of Somatosensory Information: A Theory," *Brain Research Reviews* 6 (1983), 47 115; R.W. Dykes, P. Landi y, R. Metherate, and T.P. Hicks, "Functional Role of GABA in Cat Primary Somatosensory Cortex: Shaping Receptive Fields of Cortical Neurons," *Journal of Neurophysiology* 52 (1984): 1066–93.

18 M. Avoli, "The Respective Roles of the Thalamus and Cortex in Feline Pencillin-Induced Generalized Epilepsy" (PhD. diss., McGill University, 1982).

19 R.S. McLachlan, P. Gloor, and M. Avoli, "Differential Participation of Some 'Specific' and 'Non-Specific' Thalamic Nuclei in Generalized Spike and Wave Discharges of Feline Generalized Penicillin Epilepsy," *Brain Research* 307 (1984): 277–87.

20 MNI, *MNI AR*, 1980–81, 89; M. Petrides and B. Milner, "Deficits on Subject-Ordered Tasks after Frontal- and Temporal-Lobe Lesions in Man," *Neuropsychologia* 20 (1982): 249–62.

21 MNI, *MNI AR*, 1982–83, 56; MNI, *MNI AR*, 1983–84, 85–6.

22 MNI, *MNI AR*, 1983–84, 108–9.

23 ALS Society of Quebec, "Dr Heather Durham Dedicates Life to Studying ALS," accessed October 16, 2014, http://sla-quebec.ca/news_detail.php?id=32.

24 P. Holland, G.A. Cates, B.S. Wenger, and B.L. Raney, "Myogenesis of Normal and Dystrophic Chick Embryonic Skeletal Muscle Cells in Vitro: Biosynthesis of Plasma Membrane Proteins," *Canadian Journal of Biochemistry* 58 (1980): 1156–64; P.C. Holland, S.D.J. Pena, and C.W. Guerin, "Developmental Regulation of Neuraminidase-Sensitive Lectin-Binding Glycoproteins during Myogenesis of Rat L-6 Myoblasts," *Biochemistry Journal* 218 (1984): 465–73.

25 S. Carpenter and G. Karpati, *Pathology of Skeletal Muscle* (Edinburgh: Churchill Livingstone, 1984).

26 D. Melançon, G. Bélanger, S. Taylor, and R. Ethier, "Percutaneous Spinal Cord Puncture," presented at the Montreal Neurological Institute, March 1978; D. Tampieri, D. Mélançon, and R. Ethier, "Spinal Cord Puncture: Diagnostic and Therapeutic Aspects," in *Imaging of Brain Metabolism Spine and Cord Interventional Neuroradiology Free Communications: XVth Congress of the European Society of Neuroradiology Würzburg, September 13th–17th, 1988*, 197–200 (Berlin: Springer, 1989).

27 Denis Mélançon, personal communication, 11 February 2015.

28 MNI, *MNI AR*, 1981–82, 96; M. Diksic, S. Farrokhzad, Y.L. Yamamoto, and W. Feindel, "Synthesis of 'No-Carrier Added' 1,3-bis-(2-chloroethyl)nitrosourea (BCNU)," *Journal of Nuclear Medicine* 23 (1982): 895–9; M. Diksic, S. Sako, W. Feindel, A. Kato, and Y.L. Yamamoto, "Pharmacokinetics of Positron-Labeled 1,3-bis(2-chloroethyl) Nitrosourea in Human Brain Tumors Using Positron Emission Tomography," *Cancer Research* 44 (1984): 3120–4.

29 A. Olivier and G. Bertrand, "Stereotaxic Device for Percutaneous Twist-Drill Insertion of Depth Electrodes and for Brain Biopsy," *Journal of Neurosurgery* 56 (1982): 307–8; A. Olivier and G. Bertrand, "A New Head Clamp for Stereotactic and Intracranial Procedures: Technical Note," *Applied Neurophysiology* 46 (1983): 272–5; T.M. Peters and A. Olivier, "C.T. Aided Stereotaxy for Depth Electrode Implantation and Biopsy," *Canadian Journal of Neurological Sciences* 10 (1983): 166–9; T.M. Peters, A. Olivier, and G. Bertrand, "The Role of Computed Tomographic and Digital Radiographic Techniques in Stereotactic Procedures for Electrode Implantation and Mapping, and Lesion Localization," *Applied Neurophysiology* 46 (1983): 200–5.

30 MNI, *MNI AR*, 1983–84, 57.

31 J. Ives, C.J. Thompson, and P. Gloor, "Seizure Monitoring: A New Tool in Electroencephalography," *Electroencephalography and Clinical Neurophysiology* 41 (1976): 422–7; J. Gotman, "A Computer System to Assist in the Evaluation of the EEGs of Epileptic Patients," *Behavioral Research Methods and Instrumentation* 13 (1981): 525–31; Gotman, "Automatic Recognition of Epileptic Seizures in the EEG," *Electroencephalography and Clinical Neurophysiology* 54 (1982): 530–40; J. Gotman, J.R. Ives, P. Gloor, L.F. Quesney, and P. Bergsma, "Monitoring at the Montreal Neurological Institute," supplement, *Electroencephalography and Clinical Neurophysiology* 37 (1985): 327–40; J. Gotman, J.R. Ives, and P. Gloor, "Automatic Recognition of Inter-ictal Epileptic Activity in Prolonged EEG Recordings," *Electroencephalography and Clinical Neurophysiology* 46 (1979): 510–20.

32 MNI, *MNI AR*, 1978–79, 60; P. Gloor, A. Olivier, L.F. Quesney, F. Andermann, and S. Horowitz, "The Role of the Limbic System in Experiential Phenomena of Temporal Lobe Epilepsy," *Annals of Neurology* 12 (1982): 129–44.

33 MNI, *MNI AR*, 1980–81, 72.

34 Ibid., 69–70.

35 F. Morrell, T. Rasmussen, L. de Toledo-Morrell, L.F. Quesney, and P. Gloor, "Frontal Lobe Epilepsy of Neoplastic Etiology: Incidence of Secondary Epileptogenesis," *Epilepsia* 25 (1984): 654–5.

36 F. Morrell, T. Rasmussen, P. Gloor, and L. de Toledo-Morrell, "Secondary Epileptogenic Foci in Patients with Verified Temporal Lobe Tumors," *Electroencephalography and Clinical Neurophysiology* 54 (1983): 26; F. Morrell, T. Rasmussen, L. de Toledo-Morrell, L.F. Quesney, and P. Gloor, "Frontal Lobe Epilepsy of Neoplastic Etiology: Incidence of Secondary Epileptogenesis," *Epilepsia* 25 (1984): 654–5; F. Morrell, "Secondary Epileptogenesis in Man," *Archives of Neurology* 42 (1985): 318–35.

37 The original Norfolk and Norwich University Hospital was the site of the 1868 meeting of the British Association for the Advancement of Science attended by Broca and

Hughlings Jackson, who both addressed the topic of aphasia. See M.P. Lorch, "The Merest Logomachy: The 1868 Norwich Discussion of Aphasia by Hughlings Jackson and Broca," *Brain* 131 (2008): 1658–70.

38 T.B. Rasmussen, "Wilder Penfield: His Legacy to Neurology. Surgical Treatment of Epilepsy," *Canadian Medical Association Journal* 116 (1977): 1369–70.

39 B. Brais, "Osler Society of McGill University: Report for the Academic Year 1982–83," *Osler Library Newsletter* 43 (1983): 1–2.

40 Department of Art History, Concordia University, "Luba Genush," http://art-history. concordia.ca/eea/artists/genush.html.

41 MNI, *MNI AR*, 1980–81, 47.

42 MNI, *MNI AR*, 1983–84, 45, 47.

43 Ibid., 8, 119.

44 Ibid., 43.

45 Ibid.

46 The keynote speakers were Joan Gilchrist, director of the School of Nursing at McGill University, and Josephine Flaherty, principal nursing officer, Department of National Health and Welfare, Ottawa. Joan Gilchrist presented "Education for Practice and for Health" and Josephine Flaherty's topic was "Nursing Today as the Beginning of the Future." Three seminars were held under the direction of the MNI nursing staff: Lucie Dalicandro and Felicia Skretkowicz, "Spinal Cord Lesions"; Marion Everett and Linda Robbins, "Cerebro-vascular Surgery," and Faye Belle and Sheila Koutsogiannopoulos, "Intracranial Pressure Monitoring." These activities were held in the presence of Eileen Flanagan, Bertha Cameron, Joy Hackwell, and Caroline Robertson, the four women who had guided nursing at the institute for five decades. This was followed by the distribution of awards to the stewards of the MNI employees union.

47 MNI, *MNI AR*, 1983–84, 48.

48 M.C. Preul, Z. Caramanos, D.L. Collins, J.G. Villemure, R. Leblanc, A. Olivier, R. Pokrupa, and D. Arnold, "Accurate, Noninvasive Diagnosis of Human Brain Tumors by Using Proton Magnetic Resonance Spectroscopy," *Nature Medicine* 2 (1996): 323–5.

49 Synapse 50 documents, MNI Archives.

50 Folder 28, box 48, Edward Archibald Fond, Osler Library of the History of Medicine, McGill University; J.P. Evans, "Exciting Beginnings," *Canadian Medical Association Journal* 116 (1977): 1367.

THEME ONE

1 This text is based on one written by William Feindel, 1 February 2014, with editorial work by Matthew Garsia. I acknowledge Matthew's contribution, as well as the assistance of Duncan Cowie and Leina Godin.

2 Penfield sent the sketch to Edward Archibald on 18 January 1929 with a letter that introduces the idea of building an institute: "The idea and the plans have been slowly taking form in my mind."

3 Correspondence over the summer of 1932 reveals discussion of three sites. The MNI's

eventual site was discussed in a 14 June 1932 letter from Penfield to Martin. In addition, a memo from the architects dated 13 July discusses the University Street site. Penfield, however, wrote to Currie on 24 August still pushing for the site "immediately back of the Ross Memorial Pavilion near the Ross Pavilion." Then in a 29 August letter to Penfield, Currie writes that the call for tenders would be made on 1 October, and that he hoped construction could begin 15 October. File A/N 1-1/4, WPA.

4   Arthur Currie to Allan Gregg, 27 November 1931, file 57, box 7, series 427.A, RG 1.1, Projects, Rockefeller Foundation Records, RAC.

5   At the time there was plenty of space available at the top of University Street. The only feature on the site was the McGill tennis courts, west of Molson Stadium, with the charming twin towers of Bellevue designed by Percy Nobbs.

6   Wilder Penfield, *The Significance of the Montreal Neurological Institute* (Oxford: Oxford University Press, 1934), 16.

7   In an unpublished draft of a book on the history of the MNI, which he intended to title *The Brain Doctors*, Dr Feindel wrote that Currie had made the opening of the Biological Building in 1922 a major McGill event, inviting two distinguished guest lecturers, Sir Charles Sherrington, President of the Royal Society of London, and Harvey Cushing, the leading neurosurgeon in the United States. (Both doctors had been valued teachers of Penfield.)

8   Annmarie Adams, *Medicine by Design: The Architect and the Modern Hospital, 1893–1943* (Minneapolis: University of Minnesota Press, 2008), 86–7.

9   Ibid., 71–86.

10 A detailed description of the scheme sited at the RVH can be found in "Montreal Neurological Institute," a twenty-four-page application to the Rockefeller Foundation, no date. See file A/N 2-3, WPA.

11 Currie tells Jaquays he received letters from Pitts, Little, Shorey, McDougall, Fetherstonhaugh, and others. 31 May 1932. See file 220 7E 1312, C 68, RG 2, MUA.

12 Arthur Currie to Homer January, 31 May 1932, ibid.

13 Penfield, *No Man Alone*, 381n61.

14 Later, at the official opening of the institute, Penfield would extol the work of Ross & Macdonald, as well as that of the builders and engineers, for their generous cooperation and unflagging interest. Not only were they able to reduce the building costs without too far exceeding the original financial estimates to meet Currie's insistence on keeping within the budget, but they incorporated historical features, at Penfield's suggestion, in bas-relief plaques on the facade of the edifice – ancient surgical trephines, the brain and spinal axis on the dedication plaque, the brain again beneath the Aesclepian staff and serpent on the lintel over the main entrance – that symbolize the function of the building as a place to teach and treat disorders of the brain and nerves. Penfield wrote, "Mr R.H. MacDonald [*sic*] is responsible for such virtue as may be found in this general conception of the building. He has allowed function to dictate form without loss of consideration for beauty." (Penfield, *The Significance of the Montreal Neurological Institute*, 4.) Later, he referred to MacDonald as "a creative genius": "When the architects were appointed, I discovered that we were most fortunate to have the enthusiastic cooperation of a clever architect, R.H.

MacDonald, who understood the need of accurate detail. He also had other talents that architects should have such as general knowledge, culture, independent resourcefulness and a sense of humor." (Penfield, *No Man Alone*, 313, 381.) The Scottish baronial style of the building followed that of the Royal Victoria Hospital (1894) and matched that of the Pathological Institute (1924) next door, designed by McGill's director of architecture, Percy Nobbs, who was also responsible for creating the elegant Osler Library (1929).

15 Evidence appears in several letters: Chenoweth to Holt, 17 November 1931; Holt to Beatty, 19 November 1931; Penfield to Gregg, 23 November 1931; Chenoweth to the RVH board, 26 November 1931; Currie to the RVH board, 26 November 1931; Currie to Gregg, 27 November 1931. See file 1309, C 68, RG 2, MUA; and file 57, box 7, series 427, RG 1.1, Projects, Rockefeller Foundation Records, RAC.

16 It should be pointed out that Chenoweth's dogged opposition to the creation of the MNI stemmed from a staunch sense of loyalty to the interests of the RVH. Whereas Currie saw great benefits that would come from Penfield's institute, Chenoweth, wary of change, erred on the side of caution, seeing the project instead as a potential drain on RVH resources.

17 Chenoweth estimated the costs to the RVH to be $325,000, with an annual upkeep of $19,000. In his letter to Holt, Chenoweth clearly viewed this ongoing expense as an unwanted burden to the RVH and argued that an endowment would have to be established in order to recover the losses.

18 Chenowith to Holt, 17 November 1931, file 1309, C 68 (1931–3), RG 2, MUA.

19 Holt to Beatty, 19 November 1931, file 1309, C 68 (1931–3), RG 2, MUA.

20 Ibid.

21 Gregg to Currie, 27 November 1931, file 57, box 7, series 427.A, RG 1.1, Projects, Rockefeller Foundation Records, RAC.

22 The full title of Currie's address was, "The Building of a Neuro-Surgical Institute by McGill University on Property Owned by the Royal Victoria Hospital, the Institute to Be Operated, Directed and Controlled by the University and the Royal Victoria Hospital."

23 Ibid.

24 Currie called Penfield one of "the most important saviours of human life," with a surgical success rate of 85 per cent: an impressive score, considering the often high-risk nature of the cases he treated. Penfield's success rate was, at that time, better than the average for many other simpler cures, such as kidney, stomach, lung, and heart disease. This note was written by Dr. Feindel, unknown source. file A/M 1-1/2 at the Osler.

25 Penfield, *No Man Alone*, 316.

26 Archives 1927–1933, Neurological Institute MUA.

27 See Currie to Penfield 17 August 1932; Penfield's four-page response; and Currie to Penfield, 29 August 1932. File 1309, C 68, RG 2, MUA.

28 Penfield, *No Man Alone*, 317.

29 Ibid.

30 Ibid., 318.

31 Penfield and his successors held to this statement that "the Institute will pay its way."
    Indeed, over the years, although it was a McGill building, the institute paid on its
    own for utilities such as heating and electricity supplied through McGill, unlike other
    university departments, where such costs were covered automatically by the McGill
    budget.

32 Penfield, *No Man Alone*, 317.

33 A pledge is made in Penfield to Currie, 22 January 1933 (see files A/N 1-1/5 and A/N
    1-1/7, that funds could be used from the Penfield Research Fund to cover cost over-
    runs, and that the fund could later be paid back). However, in a record of a "Tele-
    phone Conversation with Mr Glassco," 13 July 1933 (see A/N 1-2), Penfield states that
    Glassco wanted to know if the $10,000 in the Ottman Fund could be used to cover
    part of the deficit from construction. Penfield argued that "it could not inasmuch as
    the difference of $10,000.00 had been made by using steel instead of concrete [which
    presumably was Penfield's preferred more economical construction material] and I
    think it would be justifiable to use research money in order to get steel instead of
    concrete." Penfield goes on to explain that he also told Glassco that Rockefeller money
    could not be used to cover the budget shortfall, owing to the use of steel, because the
    university had made a commitment to the Rockefeller Foundation to spend the funds
    given in specific ways. Yet he then suggests that $10,000 could be donated from "this
    research fund" (presumably the Ottmann Fund) if it is "used as an inducement for
    other people to give the additional amount." In Penfield to George [presumably
    Robert] Macdonald, 7 February 1935 (see A/M 2-6/1), Penfield explains that he had
    just authorized "the payment of $22,449.24 from the Penfield Research Fund to make
    up for the over-expenditure for building the Institute."

34 Wilder Penfield, *The Significance of the Montreal Neurological Institute*, 4.

35 See H.S. Hayden, "A New Technique for Surgical Photography in the Operating
    Room," *Photographic Journal* 76, n.s. 60 (January–December 1936): 205–9.

36 When Feindel paid a short visit to the institute in 1942 to learn special techniques for
    the microscopic examination of peripheral nerves, I was assigned a cubicle with a
    fine Zeiss binocular microscope, on the base of which was a small metal plaque that
    read, "Gift of Madeline Ottmann."

37 Penfield, *Significance of the Montreal Neurological Institute*, 15.

38 The original bust of Jackson disappeared from its Queen Square setting. A replica of
    the Montreal copy was later commissioned by Fred Anderman and presented by the
    Neuro staff to the Queen Square Hospital at a symposium of the two institutes in
    the late 1990s. Michael R. Trimble, "Hughlings Jackson Comes Home," *Journal of the
    Royal Society of Medicine* 90 (1997): 350–1. There is much information on the statue
    in Penfield to Martin, 14 March 1933, AN 1-2/2.

39 The full name is Barnet Philips Company, Architectural Decorators from New York.
    There is a selection of his work from 1930 in New York State and Connecticut. He
    also decorated the Royal Bank of Canada Building in Montreal (York and Sawyer).

40 Penfield reports that he always longed for a copy of the statue and carried around a
    photograph of it in his pocket. See Penfield, *No Man Alone*, 314.

41 Penfield, *Significance of the Montreal Neurological Institute*, 8.

42 Penfield, *No Man Alone*, 319.

43 Penfield, *Significance of the Montreal Neurological Institute*, 16.

44 The firm was responsible for many of McGill's buildings during the interwar period: Divinity Hall (now the Birks Building) (1919–21), Douglas Hall (1936), and the Eaton Electronics Building (1950, demolished 1996).

THEME THREE

1 W. Penfield, "Oligodendroglia and Its Relation to Classical Neuroglia," *Brain* 47 (1924): 430–52; P. del Río-Hortega and W.G. Penfield, "Cerebral Cicatrix: The Reaction of Neuroglia and Microglia to Brain Wounds," *Bulletin of Johns Hopkins Hospital* 41 (1927): 278–303.

2 W.V. Cone, C. Russel, and R.U. Harwood, "Lead as a Possible Cause of Multiple Sclerosis," *Archives of Neurology and Psychiatry* 31 (1934): 236–69.

3 Among the neuropathology fellows in the 1940s was Murray Bornstein, who became a leader in understanding immune mediate injury of neural cells as applied to multiple sclerosis and pioneered glatiramer acetate therapy in North America.

4 Montreal was the site of the second organized Multiple Sclerosis Society in North America.

5 MNI, *MNI AR*, 1949–50, 29.

6 MNI, *MNI AR*, 1947–48, 25.

7 MNI, *MNI AR*, 1949–50, 24.

8 MNI, *MNI AR*, 1948–49, 44.

9 Ibid., 19. Dr Swank's initial support came from an anonymous donor, from the Multiple Sclerosis Society of Canada, and from a Dominion-Provincial Public Health Research Grant. See MNI, *MNI AR*, 1949–50, 7.

10 R.L. Swank, "Multiple Sclerosis: A Correlation of Its Incidence with Dietary Fat," *American Journal of Medical Sciences* 220 (1950): 421–30; R.L. Swank, O. Lerstad, A. Strom, and J. Barker, "Multiple Sclerosis in Rural Norway: Its Geographic and Occupational Incidence in Relation to Nutrition," *New England Journal of Medicine* 246 (1952): 721–8.

11 MNI, *MNI AR*, 1951–52, 31.

12 R.L. Swank, A.E. Franklin, and J.H. Quastel, "Effects of Fat Meals and Heparin on Blood Plasma Composition as Shown by Paper Chromatography," *Proceedings of the Society of Experimental Biology and Medicine* 75 (1950): 850–4; V. Wilmot and R.L. Swank, "The Influence of Low Fat Diet on Blood Lipid Levels in Health and in Multiple Sclerosis," *American Journal of Medical Sciences* 223 (1952): 25–34.

13 R.L. Swank, "Treatment of Multiple Sclerosis with Low-Fat Diet," *Archives of Neurology, Neurosurgery and Psychiatry* 69 (1953): 91–103.

14 MNI, *MNI AR*, 1953–54, 19.

15 B. Barry Arnason, personnal communication, 19 September 2014.

16 F. Andermann, J.B. Cosgrove, D. Lloyd-Smith, and A.M. Walters, "Paroxysmal Dysarthria and Ataxia in Multiple Sclerosis: A Report of Two Unusual Cases," *Neurology* 9 (1959): 211–15.

17   I. Grant, G.W. Brown, T. Harris, W.I. McDonald, T. Patterson, and M.R. Trimble, "Severely Threatening Events and Marked Life Difficulties Preceding Onset or Exacerbation of Multiple Sclerosis," *Journal of Neurology, Neurosurgery and Psychiatry* 52 (1989): 8–13; D.C. Mohr, D.E. Goodkin, P. Bacchetti, A.C. Boudewyn, L. Huang, P. Marrietta, P. Cheuk, and B. Dee, "Psychological Stress and the Subsequent Appearance of New Brain MRI lesions in MS," *Neurology* 55 (2000): 55–61.

18   A.L. Sherwin, "Immunochemical Studies of the Nervous System" (PhD diss., McGill University, 1965).

19   A.L. Sherwin, M. Richter J.B. Cosgrove, and B. Rose, "Myelin-Binding Antibodies in Experimental 'Allergic' Encephalomyelitis," *Science* 134 (1961): 1370–2; Sherwin, Richter, Cosgrove, and Rose, "Studies of the Blood–Cerebrospinal Fluid Barrier to Antibodies and Other Proteins," *Neurology* 13 (1963): 113–19; Sherwin, Richter, Cosgrove, and Rose, "Antibody Formation following Injection of Antigen into the Subarachnoid Space," *Neurology* 13 (1963): 703–7.

20   MNI, *MNI AR, 1983–84*, 55.

21   H. Link and R. Müller, "Immunoglobulins in Multiple Sclerosis and Infections of the Nervous System," *Archives of Neurology* 25 (1971): 326–44.

22   Ibid.

23   J. Allen, W.A. Sheremata, J.B.R. Cosgrove, and K. Osterland, "CSF T and B Lymphocyte Kinetics Related to Exacerbations of Multiple Sclerosis," *Neurology* 26 (1976): 579–83; W.A. Sheremata, J.B.R. Cosgrove, and H. Eylar, "Cellular Hypersensitivity to Basic Myelin (A1) Protein and Clinical Multiple Sclerosis," *New England Journal of Medicine* 291 (1974): 14–17; W.A. Sheremata, B. Younge, and J.B.R. Cosgrove, "Retrobulbar Neuritis: In Vitro Evidence of Sensitization to Myelin Basic Protein in Patients without Multiple Sclerosis," *Neurology* 27 (1977): 557–60; W.A. Sheremata, D.D. Wood, A.A. Moscarello, and J.B.R. Cosgrove, "Sensitization to Myelin Basic Protein in Attacks of Multiple Sclerosis," *Journal of the Neurological Sciences* 36 (1978): 165–70; W.A. Sheremata, D.D. Wood, and A.A. Moscarello, "Cellular and Humoral Responses to Myelin Basic Protein in Multiple Sclerosis: A Dichotomy," *Advances in Experimental Biology* 100 (1978): 501–11.

THEME FOUR

1   L. Horlick, *They Built Better Than They Knew: Saskatchewan's Royal University Hospital – A History, 1955–1992* (Saskatoon: Louis Horlick, 2001).

2   Ibid.; memorandum from W. Feindel, professor of neurosurgery, to J.W. Macleod, dean of medicine, College of Medicine, University of Saskatchewan, 3 February 1959, University Archives and Special Collections, University of Saskatchewan.

3   Ibid.

4   M. Riesberry, W. Feindel, and D.R. Fourney, "The History of Neurosurgery at the University of Saskatchewan, Canada" (unpublished, 2014).

5   Horlick, *They Built Better*; J.M. Findlay, "Neurosurgery at the Toronto General Hospital, 1924–1990: Part 1," *Canadian Journal of Neurological Sciences* 21 (1994): 146–58.

6   Riesberry, Feindel, and Fourney, "History of Neurosurgery."

7   Feindel to Macleod, 1 August 1955, University Archives and Special Collections, University of Saskatchewan.

8   Feindel to Macleod, 29 November 1955, University Archives and Special Collections, University of Saskatchewan; W. Feindel, Annual Report 1957, date stamped 11 June 1958, College of Medicine Fonds, Report to the President, 1963–64, Department of Neurosurgery, Ad 7-20a/3, University Archives and Special Collections, University of Saskatchewan.

9   W. Feindel to J. E. Merriman, secretary, Committee on Scientific Affairs, memorandum, 24 April 1959, Scientific Affairs (completed progress note forms) Faculty Committees – Scientific Affairs – Registration of Research Projects, 1957–60, College of Medicine Dean's Office Fonds, Ad. 8.2/7A – c.b.24, University Archives and Special Collections, University of Saskatchewan; Riesberry, Feindel, and Fourney, "History of Neurosurgery"; W. Feindel, C-109, MNI Archives.

10 W. Feindel and R. Schneider, "Closed Circuit Television in Electrocorticography," *Electroencephalography and Clinical Neurophysiology* 12 (1960): 925–27.

11 W. Feindel, C-109, MNI Archives.

12 W. Feindel, "Report to the President, 1963–64," College of Medicine Fonds, Ad 7-20a/3, Department of Neurosurgery, University Archives and Special Collections, University of Saskatchewan; W. Feindel, Addendum, Department of Surgery (Neurosurgery), 1957–1958, College of Medicine, University Archives and Special Collections, University of Saskatchewan.

13 Prior to this, only otolaryngologists had published on the use of the microscope in surgery.

14 Riesberry, Feindel, and Fourney, "History of Neurosurgery."

15 MNI, *MNI AR*, 1953–54, 17.

16 Riesberry, Feindel, and Fourney, "History of Neurosurgery."

17 W. Feindel and J. Stratford, "The Role of the Cubital Tunnel in Tardy Ulnar Palsy," *Canadian Journal of Surgery* 1 (1958): 287–300.

18 W. Reid and H. Johns, "An Automatic Brain Scanner," *International Journal of Applied Radiation and Isotopes* 3 (1958): 1–7; W. Feindel, J. Stratford, G.A.B. Cowan, and S. Fedoruk, "Radio-active Encephalography: Automatic Scanning Using Radioactive Iodinated Albumin," *Journal of Neurology, Neurosurgery and Psychiatry* 22 (1959): 342; G.A.B. Cowan, S. Fedoruk, W. Feindel, and J. Stratford, "Localization of Intracranial Lesions Using Radioactive Iodinated Human Serum Albumin and an Automatic Scanner," *Journal of the Canadian Asociation of Radiology* 11 (1960): 15–22.

19 W. Feindel, C-109, MNI Archives. (Added by R. LeBlanc)

20 W. Feindel and S. Fedoruk, "Measurement of Brain Circulation Time by Radio-active Iodinated Albumin," *Canadian Journal of Surgery* 3 (1960): 312–18.

21 W. Feindel, Addendum, *Annual Report of the Department of Surgery (Neurosurgery)*, 1957–1958.

22 W. Feindel, *Annual Report of the Department of Surgery (Neurosurgery) to the President*, 1958–1959.

23   W. Feindel to Dean J. W. Macleod, memorandum, 7 December 1955, file Ad. 7/20A-2/1, College of Medicine Fonds, University Archives and Special Collections, University of Saskatchewan.

24   Feindel, *Annual Report.*

25   Ibid.

26   W. Feindel, ed., *Memory, Learning and Language: The Physical Basis of Mind* (Toronto: University of Toronto Press, 1960).

27   Feindel, *Annual Report.*

28   J. Stratford, *Department of Surgery (Neurosurgery) Annual Report*, 1959–1960, 25 October, 1960, College of Medicine Fonds, file Ad. 7/20A - 3 -, University Archives and Special Collections, University of Saskatchewan.

29   J. Stratford, letter to D. Parkinson, 25 May 1962, Joseph Stratford Collection, Osler Library, MUA.

30   J. Stratford, *Department of Surgery (Neurosurgery) Annual Report*, 1959–1960.

Index

Aaron, B., 89
Aaron family, 87
Abbott, Maude, 113
Abel, John Jacob, 63
Abou-Madi, Mounir, 391
absinthe, 107
Academy of Medicine (Warsaw), 181
Academy of Sciences (Moscow, USSR), 311
Acadia University (Wolfville, NS), 439
acetylcholine, 128, 203, 256, 459, 461–4, 467, 475
Ach. *See* acetylcholine
Adam, Evelyn, 327
Adams, Annmarie, 441
Adams, Raymond D., 247, 249, 331
adenosine triphosphate, 466, 488
adrenochrome, 476
adrenocorticotropic hormone, 502
adrenoreceptor, 487
Adrian, Lord Edgar Douglas, 166, 287
Advance of Neurology, The (mural), 114, 121, 150, 205, 259, 262–3, 268
Aerts, J.B., 305
Agnew, M., 327
Aguayo, Albert, 505
Aguilar, Mary-Jane, 299–300
Ajmone-Marsan, Cosimo, 127, 240–1, 251–3, 316, 320, 332
Alajouanine, Théophile, 264
Albany Medical College, 59, 72
Albe-Fessard, Denise, 351
Albert Einstein College of Medicine (New York, NY), 337, 407, 481
Alexander Welsh Lecture, 332

Allan Memorial Institute, 129, 418, 482
Altenburger, H., 124
Alzheimer, Alois, 85, 105
Alzheimer's disease, 129, 235, 424, 472, 481
Ambulatory Daycare Centre, 402
American Academy of Neurological Surgeons, 418, 439
American Association for Research in Nervous and Mental Diseases, 104, 163
American Association of Neurological Surgeons, 92, 198, 313, 356, 439
American College of Surgeons, 439
American Epilepsy Foundation, 395–6
American Epilepsy Society, 122
American Neurological Association, 107, 122, 278, 290
amygdala, 41, 77, 222, 224, 226–8, 276, 289–1, 298–9, 362, 368, 396, 406, 430, 438
Amyot, Roma, 60, 94, 95, 98, 100, 129, 143, 259, 261
amyotrophic lateral sclerosis, 427
Anatomical Institute (University of Basel, Switzerland), 298
Anatomie des centres nerveux, 216, 218
Anatomy Lesson, 261
Andermann, Eva, 194, 393–4, 396, 477, 494
Andermann, Frederick, 114, 194, 362, 378–9, 393, 396–7, 477, 494
Andermann's syndrome, 393
Anderson, Evelyn, 106
Andrews, E., 405
aneurysm, 56, 69, 75, 117, 119–21,

198, 316, 319, 331, 351, 355–6, 395, 417, 508
angiography, 71, 115, 117–21, 123, 282, 358, 369, 395, 398–9, 429, 484
angular gyrus, 217–19
Animal Care Facility, 492
annex. *See* military annex
anoxia-ischemia. *See* ischemia: anoxia-ischemia
Antel, Jack, 300, 498, 505
aphasia, 35, 204, 213–15, 221, 248, 255, 294, 316, 319, 337
Appel, Stanley, 434
arachidonic acid, 474–7, 489
Archer, David, 489–90, 495
Archibald, Edward, 4, 16–20, 23–4, 40–2, 45, 146–7, 263, 341, 344, 435
Archibald, Sam, 42
architectonic, 132, 254, 317
area X, 212–13
Arfel-Capdevielle, Geneviève, 311
Armed Forces Institute of Pathology, 107, 113, 352
Armstrong, J., 378
Arnason, Barry, 408, 501–2
Arnold, Douglas, 431–2, 505
Arpin, Elaine Joy, 423, 425
arterial ligation, 106
arteriovenous malformation, 118–20, 255, 354–6, 359, 395, 408, 417, 510
Arts, Marcus, 347, 358
Arutiunov, O.I., 342
Association des neurochirurgiens du Québec, 440
Association pour les Épileptiques du Québec, 333
astrocyte, 77, 498
asymmetry, 336
ataxia-telangiectasia, 334
Atkinson, E.M., 101

Atkinson Morley's Hospital, 397
Atomic Energy of Canada, 97, 376, 420, 422
À tout prendre, 351
Aubé, Michel, 235, 396
Auer, J., 366
Augusta, George, 389
aura, 110–11, 131, 206, 228
Austin, George, 199, 201, 237, 301
automatism, 77
autonomic epilepsy, 63
autoradiography, 420
aviation medicine, 158
avitaminosis, 164
Avoli, Massimo, 426, 494

Babinski, Joseph, 30, 52, 95, 146, 180
Babkin, Boris Petrovitch, 159, 203–4, 231, 253, 350
"Baby Cyclotron," 420
Bacia, Tadeusz, 347
Bailey, A.A., 194
Bailey, Allan, 272
Bailey, O., 165
Bailey, Pearce, 250–2
Bailey, Percival, 53, 75, 166, 181, 280, 311, 516
Bain, Evelyn, 327
Baldwin, Maitland, 106, 198, 201, 222, 224, 226–7, 230, 250–3, 256
Banting Institute, 159
Barbeau, André, 129, 329, 382
Barbeau, Antonio, 95, 129, 233
Barber, Jesse Jr, 197–9, 313, 329
Bard, Philip, 166
Barnes, Jennifer, 391
Barnett, Henry, 418
Bar-Or, Amit, 505
Barr, Murray, 351
Barrias, Ernest, 454
Barrie, Sir James, 305
Barrowman, Elizabeth, 327, 381, 405, 409
Barrow Neurological Institute (Phoenix, AZ), 368, 391
basal ganglia, 178, 298, 315, 349
Basic Mechanisms of the Epilepsies, 128
Basingstoke, UK, 73, 144–56, 158, 160, 169, 171, 175
Bates, Donald, 351
Batten's disease, 393, 472, 479
Baxter, Donald, 401–2, 423, 482, 503, 505
Bazemore, Alva, 299, 469, 494
Bazett, H. Cuthbert, 12, 203

BCNU, 429
Beatty, Edward, 21, 81, 445
Beaudet, Alain, 425–6
Bechman, Fella, 53
Beck, Diana, 276
Bedam, Christine, 305
Beevor, Sir Charles, 146
Bégin, Monique, 416
Beijing Neurosurgical Institute, 342
Beit Memorial Fellowship for Medical Research, 12, 460
Bélanger, Gary, 399
Bell, George Maxwell, 390
Bell, James, 40
Bellevue Hospital, 16, 71
Bennett, T.S., 516
Benson-DeLemos, Maureen, 251–2
Bentley, D., 516
Berger, Emile, 313
Berger, Hans, 371–2
Bergeron, Irene, 409
Bergström, Sune K., 474
Bertrand, Claude, 160, 174, 194, 235, 259, 319, 408, 516
Bertrand, Gilles, 74, 127–8, 198, 233, 235–6, 270, 298–9, 310–1, 313, 315, 320, 325, 335, 348–9, 367, 369, 374, 377–9, 381–2, 391, 423, 425
Bessborough, Earl of. *See* Ponsonby, Vere Brabazon
Best, Charles H., 166
Beth Israel Hospital (Harvard University), 431
Bethune, Norman, 45, 192, 246, 341–4, 364
Bethune-Chao fellowships, 346, 417
BIC. *See* McConnell Brain Imaging Centre
Biltmore Hotel, 86, 441
Biochemical Institute (Cambridge University), 459
biology building (McGill), 443
Birkett, Herbert S., 20
Birks, Gerald, 167
Birmingham, Marion, 461, 494
bis-chloroethyl nitrosourea, 429
Bjorklund, Anders, 418
Black, Perry, 313
Blackcock, H., 70
Blackstock, Harriet, 279, 283
blast injury, 149
blood plasma, 71, 162
Blood Plasma for Great Britain Project, 162

Bloomer, Irene, 173
Blume, Howard, 418
Blundell, John, 298, 310–11, 313, 315, 325, 329
Bohr, Niels, 337
Boldrey, Edwin Barkley, 54, 100–2, 140, 142–3, 205, 212, 319, 322, 343
Bolis, Elana, 346
Bollard, Brenda, 469, 494
Bollock, T.H., 408
Bonhomme, Jean-Paul, 421
Bornstein, Murray, 158, 161, 504
Boski, Marina, 375–6
Bossy, Freda, 145, 150, 152–4, 156, 172
Boston Children's Hospital, 337
Boston City Hospital, 44, 66, 247, 402
Botterell, Harry, 147, 150, 164
Boucaud, J., 405
Bound, Verna, 433
Brain, Sir Russell, 264, 337
Brain and Conscious Experience, 371
Brain Babies. *See Children of the Brain, The* (sculpture)
brain edema. *See* edema: cerebral edema
Brain Electrolytes and Fluid Metabolism, 407, 481
brain injury, xiv, 14, 34, 40, 107, 164, 214–15, 287, 295, 300–1, 337–40, 368, 419, 461, 476, 482–4, 486–91
brain-mind, 242. *See also* mind
Brain Research Institute (Zurich), 425
brain swelling, 330, 461
brain trauma. *See* brain injury
brain tumour, 13, 18, 23, 41–2, 44, 50, 53, 60–2, 95, 104–5, 115–17, 140–1, 170, 198, 270, 316, 330–1, 336, 352–3, 365, 367, 399, 408, 434–5, 450–1, 470, 506; glioblastoma multiforme, 105, 330; glioma, 61, 104, 115, 197, 254, 280, 330, 355, 424, 429; hemangioma calcificans, 117; medulloblastoma, 140; oligodendroglioma, 60, 117, 141, 154, 280, 282, 334; spongioblastoma multiforme, 105
Branan, Richard, 417, 494
Branch, Charles Sr, 272, 294, 313, 315, 325, 330, 334, 336, 348–9, 418
Bray, Garth, 505
Breckenridge, Carol, 477, 494

Breslau, Germany, 29–30, 33, 37, 39–40, 46, 64, 181, 280
Brewer, Earle, 48, 57
Brewerton, D.A., 366
Brickner, Richard, 213, 282
bridge (MNI). *See* Bronfman Bridge
Bridge of Sighs (Cambridge), 456
Bridge of Sighs (Venice), 456
Brindle, G. Frederick, 325, 368–9, 374
British Expeditionary Force, 178
Broca, Pierre Paul, 85, 220–1, 230
Broca's area, 212, 214, 217–19, 289, 293
Brodal, Alf, 382
Brodkin, Elliott, 463
Bronfman Bridge, 59, 86–7, 89, 257, 449, 453, 455–6
Bronfman family, 87, 89, 240
Bronk, Detlev Wulf, 142, 166
Brookhaven National Laboratory (Upton, NY), 353, 419
Brooks, E.C., 98
Brophie, Maurice, 50
Brophy, Doris, 464–5
Browder, Jefferson, 322
Brown, James A., 48
Brown, Richard, 285
Brown, Warren, 322
Brown University (Providence, RI), 124
Bruce, Robert, 375
brutalism, 456–7
Buchthal, F., 408
Buckham, Lynn, 79, 321
Bucy, Paul C., 33–4, 74, 182, 289, 366
Buczek, Marek, 488, 495
Budden, Mrs, 469
Bulke, J., 378
Burdenko Institute of Neuro-surgery (Moscow), 277

Cairns, Sir Hugh, 49, 181, 221, 238, 244, 276, 438
Cajal, Santiago Ramón y, 14, 56, 84, 129, 317
calcium, 74, 462, 466–7, 490
calcium antagonism, 425
Calender, Helene, 173
California Institute of Technology (Pasadena), 336, 366, 407
Callahan, J., 475, 478, 494
callosotomy, 139
Cambridge University. *See* University of Cambridge

Cameron, Alice, 327–8, 381
Cameron, Bertha, 103–4, 324, 326–9, 374, 378–9
Cameron, Ewen, 163
Cameron, J., 103
Camp, J.B., 164
Campbell, B.A., 164
Canadian Association of Neurological Sciences, 417
Canadian Centre for Architecture, 442–4
Canadian Medical Hall of Fame, 440
Canadian Neurological Society, 95, 122, 203, 212, 511
Canadian Neurosurgical Society, 440
Cannon, Walter B., 166
Cantlie, Hortense Douglas, 101–2, 206, 258–60
Cardenas, Dr, 343
Carmen, Eleanor, 327
Carmichael, Edward Arnold, 150, 182–4
Carmichael, Leonard, 124
Carnegie Foundation, 5–6
Carney, Anne, 381, 405
Caron, Sylvio, 233
carotid cavernous fistula, 74
carotid occlusion, 248–9, 510
Carpenter, Malcolm B., 351
Carpenter, Stirling, 194, 300, 362–3, 365, 393–4, 407, 424, 427, 477, 494–5
Carvalho, Victor, 356
carving. *See* stone carving
Case Western Reserve University (Cleveland), 488
Cashman, Neil, 505
Casselman, M., 104
Castonguay, Claude, 377
CAT. *See* computed tomography
Catholic University of Louvain, 298, 313
Cavanaugh, Mary, 327–8, 381, 405, 409
Caveness, William F., 194, 252
cavernous angiomas, 117
cell-staining techniques, 13–14, 49, 60, 66, 107; gold cell-staining technique, xiv, 31, 37, 49, 85; silver cell-staining technique, xiv, 31, 37, 49, 62, 85, 90, 202
cellular immunology, 504
Center for Research in Behavioral Neurobiology (Concordia University, Montreal), 490

Centre d'études nucléaires (Paris), 425
centrencephalic integrating system, 63, 142, 212, 221, 265, 292–3, 316–17, 340, 414
ceramide trihexoside, 478
ceramide trihexosidosis, 478
cerebellum, 77, 85, 140, 230, 238, 383, 454, 474
cerebral blood flow, 66, 134–5, 137, 178, 352–3, 359, 408, 417, 419–20, 422, 426, 429, 439, 510
cerebral cortex, 31, 33–4, 38, 40, 52–4, 66, 68–9, 71, 74, 89, 102, 106, 110, 118, 124, 126, 128, 130–2, 135, 137–8, 140, 142, 159, 165, 167, 178, 200, 202–20, 223, 228, 230, 254, 258, 265–7, 270, 276, 287, 291–3, 298–9, 301, 316–17, 332, 334, 340, 350, 352, 355–7, 360, 366, 368, 371, 383, 396, 418–19, 426, 450, 461, 466–7, 470, 473, 475, 477–9, 489, 491, 507
"Cerebral Cortex and Consciousness, The," 142, 265
Cerebral Cortex of Man, The, 106, 203, 205–6, 208–9, 211–12, 323, 332
cerebral ischemia. *See* ischemia: cerebral ischemia
cerebral localization, 30–2, 34–6, 54, 72, 85, 124–6, 142, 168, 200, 204–20, 222–8, 264–7, 271, 317, 320, 332, 369, 430
cerebral metabolism, 276, 352, 359, 420, 435, 470, 476–7, 481–2, 484, 488–91
cerebral steal syndrome, 352, 355, 359, 369
cerebral trauma. *See* brain injury
cerebrovascular accidents, 476
cerebrovascular disease, 74, 246, 248, 331, 390, 425–6
cerebrovascular innervation, 67
cerebrovascular physiology, 32
cerebrovascular surgery, 434
ceroid lipofuscinoses. *See* Batten's disease
Chalk River, 97, 288
Chandi, Sushil, 196
Chandy, Jacob Jaya, 194, 196, 201, 319
Chandy, Mathew, 196
Chang, Fu Lien-, 343–4
Chao, Ke-ming, 346
Chao, Yi-cheng, 129, 159, 315, 342–3, 345–6
Charcot, Jean-Martin, 85, 109, 261

Charlevoix, Quebec, 393–4

Chateau Apartments (Montreal), 449

chemotherapy, 334

Chen, C.J., 194

Chenoweth, William, 442, 445, 447, 455

Chernikoff, Sainada, 409

Chiang Kai-shek, 175

Chiasson, Josephine, 500

Childe, Arthur E., 98, 100, 140, 143, 144–5, 171, 174, 177

Children of the Brain, The (sculpture), 257–9, 260, 457

China, 45, 129, 175, 299, 341–6, 431

China Medical Board, 299

Chinese Medical College, 343, 347, 470

Chong, G., 378

Chorobski, Jerzy Ludwik, 32, 49, 52–3, 57, 60–1, 63, 67–8, 138, 177–8, 180–6, 189, 221, 254, 311, 315–16, 320, 347, 369, 514

Chorobski, Victoria, 177, 185

Christian Medical College and Hospital (Vellore, India), 196

chronaxie, 124

Cipriani, André J., 97, 100, 137, 139, 143, 158, 174, 178, 343, 464

circle of Willis, 248

City Hospital (Moscow), 338, 339, 340

Clarke, Joe, 378, 393, 475, 478–9

Clarke, William, 13, 24

classification of brain tumours, 60–1, 104–5, 140–1

Clegg, Roberta, 381

Cleveland Clinic, 399

clinical staff, Montreal Neurological Institute, 27 September 1934 to 31 December 1935 (table), 98

clinical staff, 1960–61 (table), 325

closed-circuit television, 507

Cloward, Ralph, 74

Cobb, Stanley, 43–4, 52, 66–8, 95, 115, 166, 221, 249, 265, 300, 369

Coburn, Donald F., 92, 98, 101

Coceani, Flavio, 474–5, 494

collagen, 31

Collège de France (Paris), 351

College of the Medical Evangelist, 301. *See also* Loma Linda University

Collins, M., 103

Collip, Bertram, 238

Colombo Plan, 312, 344

Colpitts, Byron C., 103

Columbia University (New York), 13, 15, 213, 351, 382

Comar, Dominique, 433

Communist Party of Canada, 341

Complex Partial Seizures, 406

computed tomography, 108, 350, 365, 397–9, 419, 432, 439

Concordia University (Montreal), 490

concussion, 164

conditioned reflex, 140, 159, 203–4, 277, 298, 419

Cone, Avis, 305

Cone, William Vernon: *Advance of Neurology,* 263; American Association for Research in Nervous and Mental Diseases (1936), 104; Barber, Jesse, 198; Bertrand, Gilles, 235; Bossy, Freda, 156; brain abscesses, 318; Byron Pevehouse, 299; Cameron, Bertha, 326; cerebrovascular occlusion, 246; Chandy, Jacob, 196; Chorobski, Jerzy, 183; citizenship, 126; Currie, Sir Arthur, 445; Cushing, Harvey, 167; death, 302–6, 310, 511; demanding work schedule, 121; establishment of the MNI, 446; Feindel, William, 438; Feindel's departure for Saskatoon, 272, 273, 274; Fellows Lecture, 75; fellows reunion (1957), 300; Flanagan, Eileen, 244–5; First Foundation, 93; *Great Physician, Always Near,* 309; Greene, Clarence, 197; head of neurosurgery and neuropathology, 270; Hodge, Charles, 357; hydrocephalus, 317, 318; Inglis, Ruth, 280; memorial regarding his influence, 317; microgryia, 131–2; MNI staff 1936, 100; MNI staff 1938, 343; MNI staff, 1945–46, 194; Mrs Samuel Reitman Nursing Bursary, 329; multiple sclerosis, 498; Neuropathology Laboratory (RVH), 48–51, 59–62, 452; neurosurgical service, 272; Nichols, Martin, 180; nurses at Basingstoke, 172; papers on intervertebral discs, spinal fusion after discoidectomy, and complications from spinal cord injury 160; *Peter Pan* (statue), 305, 306; Peterson, Eric, 73; Presbyterian Hospital, 14–19, 24; Reitman, Ruth, 383; removal

of a ruptured cervical intervertebral disc, 107; Silver Anniversary discussions of Dr Cone, 317–18, 320; shortage of research space, 367; Swank, Roy, 500; Tarlov, Isadore, 53; wartime service, 143–5, 147–50, 152, 154, 170–2, 174–5

Cone-Barton tongs, 171

Cone Laboratory for Neurosurgical Research, 74, 135, 330, 349, 352, 354–6, 359–60, 369, 417, 419–20, 422, 425

Cone Professor of Neurosurgery, 236, 314–15, 378, 438, 453, 511

Conklin, Edwin Grant, 5, 7

consciousness, 12, 110–11, 142, 153, 200, 221, 238, 265–7, 292–3, 317, 332, 339–40, 371, 470

contour brain scanner, 330, 352

convolectomy, 163

coomasie blue dye, 355, 358

Cordeau, Jean-Pierre, 128, 362

Corkin, Suzanne H., 335, 337

Cornell University (Ithaca, NY), 399

Corner, George W., 372

cornerstone, 58, 81, 391

corpus callosum, 59, 126, 137, 139, 280, 283, 337, 393, 473

Corsi, Philip, 336

cortical ischemia. *See* ischemia: cortical ischemia

cortical mapping, 35–6, 38, 118–20, 142, 205–20, 255, 450–1

Cosgrove, J.B.R. "Bert," 325, 333, 349, 378–9, 499, 501–5

Countway Medical Library (Harvard University), 281

Courtois, Guy, 200–1

Couturier, Alphonse, 324

Crandall, Paul, 356

craniotomy, 32, 54, 64, 106, 222, 226, 356, 486, 507

cranio-vertebral junction, 236

creatine phosphokinase, 367

Critchley, McDonald, 268

Croft, Arlene, 256

Cronan, Dean, 405

Crossland, James, 467, 494–5

Crystals, K., 396

CT. *See* computed tomography

CTH. *See* ceramide trihexoside

Cuadrado, Luis, 391

cubital tunnel, 438, 508

Cure, C.W., 194

Currie, M., 104

Currie, Sir Arthur, 21–2, 93, 442–8
Curtis, R., 378
Cushing, Harvey, 9, 11–13, 18, 22, 42–4, 49, 51, 53, 55–6, 63, 67, 85, 93, 163, 166–8, 180, 280–1, 322, 331, 438
Cybernetics, 240, 316–17
cyclic adenosine monophosphate, 74
cyclic-AMP, 74
cyclotron, 420–1, 432
cytoarchitectonic, 37
Cytoarchitecture of the Human Brain Stem, 402
Cytology and Cellular Pathology of the Nervous System, 61

Dadoun, Ralph, 488, 495
Daigle, E., 378
Dale, Sir Henry, 203, 230
Dalhousie University (Halifax), 159, 174, 275, 312, 322, 356, 369, 438
Dalicandro, Lucy, 381, 402, 405, 416–17
Daly, David, 99, 320
Danaher, Helen, 327
Dandy, Walter, 13, 43, 282
Dart, Catherine, 50
Darville, Mabel, 173
Davidson, Elabel, 194, 236, 238, 499
da Vinci, Leonardo, 52
Davis, Loyal, 74, 181
Davison, Wilburt, 11
Dawson, Anne, 338
Dayes, Lloyd, 199, 483, 485, 495
de Guzman, M., 405
déjà vu, 430
Dejerine, Jules, 30, 94, 146, 214, 216–18, 295
Dejerine-Klumpke, Augusta, 95
Dejerine's area, 219. *See also* angular gyrus
Dekaban, Anatole S., 237, 251–2
del Carpio, Raquel, 423
Delmas, André, 235
del Río-Hortega, Pio, 31, 49, 60, 66, 107
de Martel, Thierry, 180, 189
Denis Mélançon Neuroradiology Conference and Annual Lecture, 427
Denny-Brown, Derek, 164, 259, 402
Denstedt, Orville F., 480
deoxyglucose, 420, 483, 487–8
deoxyribonucleic acid, 470

Department of Neuroanatomy (MNI), 230, 325, 425
Department of Neurochemistry (MNI), 199, 230, 255, 270, 330–1, 362, 426, 449, 459–95
Department of Neurology and Neurosurgery (McGill), 60, 61, 314, 330, 375, 400–2, 472, 481–2
Department of Neurophotography (MNI), 356–8, 484
Department of Neuropsychology (MNI), 279–96, 334–7, 403, 427
Department of Neuropsychology, 1962–63 (table), 337, 427
Department of Psychology (McGill University), 282, 286, 287
Department of Psychology (Université de Montréal), 288
Department of Social Services, 236, 333, 499–500
depth electrodes, 226–9, 395, 430
de Romer, Baroness Anna, 231
Derry, David, 473, 494
Desbiens, L., 417
Descartes, René, 238
de Toledo Morrell, Leyla, 430–1
dexamethasone, 367, 484, 486, 489
Diabetic Manual (Joslin), 244
diatrizoate, 399
dichotic listening test, 335
Dickey, Catherine, 495
Dickey, Kathy, 469
Dickson, I., 103
diencephalon, 61, 200, 203–4, 265, 292, 317
Diencephalon of the Cat, 332
Dieppe Raid, 144
dietary lipids, 500
Diksic, Mirko, 420, 429, 495
Dila, Carl J., 336, 368, 378, 424, 485, 487, 495
Diseases of the Nervous System (Walshe), 211, 264
Dixon, M., 459
Dobkin, A.B., 507
Dockrill, Edward, 50, 66–7
Dogali, Michael, 407
dolichols, 472, 477, 479
Donaghy, Peardon, 366
Donner, William Henry, 263, 465
Donner Canadian Foundation, 239, 449, 465, 481
Donner Laboratory of Experimental Neurochemistry, 239, 270, 331, 360, 367, 393, 465, 467, 469, 472, 481, 490, 493

Douglas, K., 405
Drager, Glenn, 250
Drake, Charles G., 56, 350, 425, 434
dreamy state, 146
Drew, Charles, 198
Droogleever-Fortuyn, Jan, 200, 316
Droz, Walter, 409
dual brain, 367
DuBoulay, George, 399
Dubuisson, David, 416, 431
Duchenne muscular dystrophy, 363, 427
Duchow, Sandra, 376
Duke University (Durham, NC), 73, 270, 318, 331
Dunkirk, France, 144, 178, 180
Duplessis, Maurice, 229, 245, 259, 263
Durham, Heather, 427
Durinian, Ruben Ashotovich, 347
Durnford, Galt, 257, 259, 456
Durnian, Ruben Ashotovich, 347
Dykes, Robert, 426
Dynamics of Brain Edema (Pappius and Feindel), 406
dyskinesia, 165, 298
Dyve, Suzan, 487, 490, 495

Earle, Kenneth, 222, 227, 237
Easter EEG Society Ski Meetings, 253
Eaton's department stores (Montreal and Toronto), 443
Eberle, H.M., 104
Eccles, Sir John Carew, 242–3, 383
Echlin, Francis Asbury, 69, 71–4, 135, 138, 143, 301, 314, 343
ECoG. *See* electrocorticogram
ECT. *See* electroconvulsive therapy
edema, 301, 482, 484, 486, 488; cerebral edema, 159–60, 254, 298, 330, 406–7, 465, 481–4, 486–9; vasogenic cerebral edema, 484
Edinburgh tradition of medical instruction, 9
Edinger, Ludwig, 258
Edwards, Rita, 173, 175
Edwin Smith papyrus, xiv
EEG. *See* electroencephalography
eicosanoids, 474, 477
Eileen Flanagan prize (nursing), 329
Eisen, Andrew, 194, 367, 378–9, 393, 407, 417, 423–4
Eisenhart, Louise, 166
Electrical Stimulation of the Brain, 332

Electric and Musical Industries Limited, 397
electroconvulsive therapy, 294
electroencephalography, 34, 87, 120–1, 123–7, 139, 158, 165, 177, 198, 201, 205–6, 209, 222–3, 241, 251–3, 261, 263, 293, 310–11, 315, 317, 320, 324, 335, 369, 371–2, 376, 383–5, 393, 395–6, 402, 410–11, 416, 432, 452, 484, 486, 507; and clinical neurophysiology, Montreal Neurological Institute, 1975–76 (table), 396
electromyography, 378, 424
electron microscope, 363, 394
electrophysiology, 97, 243
El Greco, 261
Elizabeth Kenny Foundation, 331
Elleker, George, 424
Elliott, Harold, 57, 160
Elliott, K.A.C., collaborators and students (table), 494
Elliott, Kenneth Allan Caldwell, 128–9, 160, 177, 194, 199, 239, 242, 253, 255–6, 263, 276, 299, 314, 325, 331, 346–7, 362, 369, 374, 420, 434, 459–62, 464–7, 469–71, 480, 482, 494–5
Elliott's solution, 160, 461, 465, 492
Ellis, Stanley, 174, 263
Ellwood & Henderson (architects), 456–7
Elsberg, Charles, 14–17
Elvidge, Arthur Roland, 48, 55–8, 61, 98–100, 104–5, 114–21, 123, 143, 194, 198, 253, 255, 263, 272–3, 299, 315, 325, 334, 343, 349, 374, 438, 514, 516
EMG. See electromyography
EMI. See Electric and Musical Industries Limited
EMI scanner, 397, 398, 399
endarteritis calcificans cerebri, 117
Engel, A.G., 408
Engel, King, 367
engram, 140, 286, 293
Epilepsies, The (volume of Vinken and Bruyn's Handbook of Clinical Neurology), 406
epilepsy, 13–14, 24–5, 29–31, 46–8, 61, 63, 68, 100, 105–6, 109–11, 122–3, 125–6, 128, 130, 138, 159, 163, 177, 194–5, 200–1, 205, 246, 253, 259–60, 264, 276, 289, 298, 311, 333, 354, 368, 383–4, 387, 390, 395–6, 406, 408, 416, 424, 430, 451, 461–2, 464, 470, 476; bitemporal

lobe epilepsy, 430; epilepsy and pregnancy, 394; experimental epilepsy, 56, 138; focal epilepsy, 32, 63–4, 66, 106, 126, 134, 222, 224, 256, 288, 369, 399; generalized epilepsy, 139, 384, 395; mesial temporal lobe epilepsy, 222; post-traumatic epilepsy, 32, 37, 64; psychomotor epilepsy, 227; temporal lobe epilepsy, 41, 106, 117, 133, 140, 146, 222–4, 226–9, 289, 290, 295, 332, 350–1, 396–7, 430, 438
Epilepsy and Cerebral Localization (Penfield and Erickson), 126, 163, 174, 205
"Epilepsy and Surgical Therapy" (Penfield), 105
Epilepsy and the Functional Anatomy of the Human Brain (Penfield), 122, 126, 133, 212, 264, 265–7, 437
epilepsy clinic, 236, 333
epilepsy surgery, 30–9, 105, 194, 222, 252–3, 367, 378, 387, 406, 452, 507
epileptic seizures, 30–1, 35, 39, 64–6, 69, 108, 110, 112, 122–3, 126, 134–5, 137–8, 140, 213, 276, 289, 335, 337, 352, 354, 395, 411, 414, 426, 430, 459
epileptogenesis, 66, 70, 130, 276, 430–1
Erb, Wilhelm, 85
Erb-Weishoff, Millie, 508
Erickson, Theodore Charles, 58, 60–1, 92, 100–1, 126, 135, 137–40, 143, 163, 165, 174, 230, 276, 285, 322
Ethier, Roméo, 108, 121, 325, 365, 378, 393, 397–9, 423
Evans, Alan C., 220, 422, 505
Evans, Joseph P., 48, 51, 57–8, 60–1, 63, 75, 100, 106, 138, 164, 247, 259, 279, 282, 286, 300, 301, 315, 319, 514
Everett, Marion, 381, 405
experiential phenomena, 349, 354, 430

F.C. (patient), 289–90
Fabry's disease, 393, 478–9
Factor I, 467, 469
Falconer, Murray, 351
Faulk, Murl, 278
Fedoruk, Sylvia, 353, 508–10
Feindel, Faith Lyman, 272, 302

Feindel, William Howard, 3, 18; Advance of Neurology, The, 264; amygdala, 438; amygdala and epilepsy, 222, 224, 227–9; appointments and departures under directorship, 424; as member of staff 1969–70, 378; as member of staff 1970–71, 379; as new director, 391, 407; Baby Cyclotron, 420; Barber, Jesse, 197–8; biography, 437–40; Bronfman bridge, 86; cerebral blood flow studies, 510; cerebral steal, 354–5; China, 346; Cone Laboratory, 330, 349, 352; Cone Professor of Neurosurgery, 438; Cone's death, 303; construction of Penfield Pavilion, 391, 397; contour brain scanner, 330; death, 437, 438, 439, 440; Electrical Stimulation of the Brain, 332; Elliott, K.A.C., 494; EMI CT scanner, 397; Fellows Society, 230; French-English relations, 370; Inglis, Ruth, 280; intracranial obliteration of an anterior circulation aneurysm, 120; international symposium on computerized axial tomography, 399; intraoperative cerebral blood flow, 353; Hughlings Jackson Memorial Lecture, 108; Leblanc, Richard, 74, 425; McConnell Brain Imaging Centre, 330, 432, 439; medical training, 49; Memory, Learning and Language, 511; mesial temporal structures and temporal lobe epilepsy, 146; MNI attending and house staff (1945–46), 193–4; MNI clinical staff (1960–61), 325; MNI Life Achievement Award, 482; MNI/MNH funding, 400–1; MNI neurosurgical staff (1964), 348–9; MNI staff photograph (1980), 423; neuroimaging, 439; neurosurgical service, 349; nominated as director, 390; on Francis McNaughton, 122; opening of Penfield Pavilion, 416; operating, 453; Penfield's death, 412; Peterson, Eric's junior resident, 73; PET scanner, 419–20; piano, 323; portrait, 389; radioisotope laboratory, 315; Rasmussen, 323; "Recent Research on the Cerebral Microcirculation" (symposium), 369; research fellow, 174,

201; research on cerebral edema, 160; research on vasoconstriction and epileptic seizures, 135; Saskatoon, 402, 438; Saskatoon (departure for), 270, 272–4; Saskatoon scanner, 508–9; Saskatoon (teaching), 510–11; Silver Anniversary, 319; skiing, 253; Steiner, Ursula, 404; symposium on Penfield's ninetieth birthday, 431; Synapse 50, 433; Theodore Rasmussen, 322; Third International Workshop on the Dynamic Aspects of Cerebral Edema, 481; Thomas Willis, 351; University of Saskatchewan, 506–8; Webster Pavilion, 432; wedding, 175; William Cone Professor, 314–15; *World of Neurology, The* (triptych), 387; Yamamoto, 353–4

Feindel Foyer. *See* foyer (MNI)
Feindel Lecture, 438
Feist, Ursula, 469
Fellows Day Lecturers, 1957–84 (table), 515
Fellows Lecture, 75, 270, 300, 318, 320, 331, 351, 383, 418, 434
Fellows Library, 177, 258, 375
Fellows Prize, 435
Fellows Society, 113, 230, 264, 320, 351, 368
Fenniak, Paul, 233
Fenwick, M., 103
Ferguson, Shirley, 276
Ferrier, David, 30, 34, 110, 146, 271
Ferrier Lecture, 203, 211
Fetherstonaugh, Durnford, Bolton, Chadwick (architects), 456, 457
Fewer, Derek, 378, 391–2
Filer, Mary, xv, 114, 121, 150, 169, 173, 205, 239, 259, 261–4, 268
Finesinger, Jacob, 67
Finney, John, 6–7, 11
First Foundation, 257
First International Symposium on Positron Emission Tomography, 419–20
Fisher, Charles Miller, 99, 103, 122, 178, 187–8, 190–1, 193–4, 201, 246–9, 316, 319, 408, 433–4
Fitzgerald, G., 417
Flanagan, Eileen Constance, 103–4, 194, 197, 243–6, 261, 304, 319, 326, 374, 435
Flanigin, Herman, 201, 224

Fleming, 99
Flexner, Abraham, 6
Florey, Elizabeth, 467, 469, 494
Florey, Ernst, 275, 299, 467, 469, 494
Florey, Howard, 69, 71
fluorescein angiogram, 347, 358
focal cerebral ischemia. *See* ischemia: focal cerebral ischemia
focus (of epileptic seizure), 31, 34–5, 37–8, 64, 66, 68, 124–6, 130, 135, 139, 206, 214, 222, 237, 278, 311, 368, 376, 395, 411, 430–1, 507
Foerster, Otfried, 25, 29–39, 42, 46, 63–4, 93, 109, 124, 181, 280, 338
folate, 490
Forbes, Henry, 52, 66, 95, 369
Forbes window, 66–7
Ford, Robert, 350
Foster Radiation Laboratory, 420
foyer (MNI), xii, xiv, 83–5, 105, 412, 451, 453–5
Frampton, Meredith, 305
Frampton, Sir George, 305
Francis, Gordon, 424, 505
Francis, William, 167
Franklin Institute, Biochemical Research Foundation (Philadelphia), 460
Frazier, Charles H., 13, 58
Freedman, Mark, 505
Freedmen's Hospital, 197–8
Freeman, Walter, 163
French, Lyle, 356
Frenkel, Heinrich, 30
Friedreich's ataxia, 393–4
frontal lobe, 25, 213–14, 277, 279–83, 286, 289, 336, 405, 408, 427
Front de libération du Québec, 370
Fu, Lien-Chang, 344
Fulton, John, 162–4
Furlong, P., 405
Fyles, Shirley, 313

GABA. *See* gamma amino butyric acid
Gage, Lyle Everett, 48, 53–4, 57, 60–1, 138, 315, 319, 322, 369, 514
Gage, Phineas, 281, 286–7
Gairdner Foundation, 108
Gajdusek, Carleton, 300
galactosidase, 478–9
Galahad School, 4, 7
Galen, xiii, xiv, 450
Galloway, Dan, 399
gamma amino butyric acid, 128, 299, 426, 467, 469

gangliosidosis, 472, 478
gap junction, 331
Garcia-Flores, E., 378
Garcin, Raymond, 235, 339–40
Garneau, Jean, 325
Garretson, Henry, 61, 313, 330, 348–9, 352, 354–6, 378–9, 391
Gasser, Herbert Spencer, 124, 300
Gates, Frederick, 20–1
Gauthier, Serge, 235, 375, 417, 424
Gendron, Daniel, 424
Genush, Luba, 77, 229, 307, 387, 432
Georgetown Medical Center (Washington, DC), 352
Geschwind, Norman, 336, 418
Geyelin, Rawle, 117
Giacomini, Paul, 505
Gibbs, Clarence F., 383
Gibson, William Carleton, 101, 112–13, 194, 202, 237, 431
Gilbert, Richard R., 325, 391
Gillespie, Isabel, 172
Gilliatt, R., 408
Gillies, Sir Harold, 158
Gindé, Ramchandra, 196
Gjedde, Albert, 487, 490, 495
Glaser, Gilbert, 383
Glen Eagles Apartments (Montreal), 449
glial cells. *See* neuroglial cells
Gliddon, W.O., 164
glioma. *See* brain tumour
gliosis, 31, 396
Globus, Joseph H., 105
Gloor, Pierre, 126, 228, 272, 276, 298–9, 310, 312, 315, 320, 325, 335, 350, 362, 367–8, 371–2, 376, 378, 384, 392–6, 406, 412, 416, 423, 426, 430, 481
glycolipid storage disorders, 472
glycoprotein, 472, 477
GM1-gangliosidosis, 478
Goad, George, 481
Goad Unit, 479, 481
Golden, Hughie, 7
Golgi, Camillo, 84, 454
Gordon, G., 103
Gordon-Taylor, Rear Admiral, 158
Gotman, Jean, 395–6
Gourday, 15
governor-general of Canada. *See* Buchan, John; Léger, Jules; and Ponsonby, Vere Brabazon
Gowers, Sir William, 40, 109, 146
graduate degrees awarded, Montreal Neurological Institute, 1950–51 (table), 237

graduate theses investigating a putative vascular mechanism in epilepsy (table), 138

Graham, Bernard, 122, 313, 325, 349, 378–9

Graham, William, 112

Granit, Ragnar, 243, 405, 408

Grant, D.M., 309

Grant, François Clark, 43

Grant, William, 56–7, 60–1, 98, 101, 112, 301

Graschenko, Propper, 129–30, 175, 338–40

Gratton, Lucien, 502–3

Graves, Robert W., 59–60

Great Physician, The (stained glass window), 309

Green, Cecil Howard, 202

Green, Janette, 493

Green, John, 368

Green College (University of British Columbia), 202

Green College (University of Oxford), 202

Greene, Clarence Jr, 198

Greene, Clarence Sumner Sr, 196–9

Greenfield, J. Godwin, 12, 93, 129, 230, 238, 438, 517

Gregg, Allan, 258, 263–4, 274, 284, 442–3

Grenier, Yannick, 300

Griffin, Cynthia, 333, 378

Griffith McConnell, Lily, 258, 263

Grimes, Evelyn, 145, 150

Guillain-Barré syndrome, 180, 424, 505

Guiot, Gérard, 339, 350

Guitton, Daniel, 426

Gulati, Des Raj, 329–30, 483, 495

Gurd, C., 378

Guy's Hospital (London), 243

Gybells, Jan, 298

H.M. (patient), 278, 290, 291, 335

Hackwell, Joy, 379–81, 402

Hackwood House, 73, 153

Haddad, Fuad, 319

Haggart, Margaret, 173

Hakim, Antoine, 426, 490, 495

Hall, C.W., 516

Hall, Louise, 327

Hall of Neurological Fame, 93, 454

Halpenny, Gerald W., 309

Halsted, William Stewart, 5, 11

Hamel, Edith, 425–6, 431

Hanbery, John, 201, 270

Handbook of Clinical Neurology, The (Vinken and Bruyn), 406

Hannah Institute for the History of Medicine, 440

Hansebout, Robert, 334, 376, 378, 379, 395, 402, 425, 485–6, 495

Hanson, Fred H., 143–5

Hardy, Jules, 313, 365

Harrower, Mary Molly Rachel, 143, 163, 165, 174, 282–7, 343

Harrower-Erickson, Mary Molly Rachel. *See* Harrower, Mary Molly Rachel

Hart, Geraldine, 381, 405

Harvard College (Harvard University), 197, 254

Harvard University, 7, 11, 43–4, 51–2, 57, 73, 95, 141, 144, 166, 194, 241, 249, 254, 281, 286, 300, 351, 355, 366, 385, 399, 401, 403, 416, 418, 431

Harvey, John, 324

Harvey, William, 9

Harvey Cushing Society, 197–8, 356

Harwood, Robert Unwin, 59–61, 498

Hasse, Sigurd, 469

Hassler, Rolf, 236, 378

Hastings, Ken, 363

Hayden, H.S., 90–2, 356, 450

Haymaker, Webb, 101, 106–7, 112–13, 316, 320, 352, 494

head injuries, 30, 42, 147, 159, 164, 176, 255, 331

head nurses, Montreal Neurological Institute, 1974–84 (table), 405

Heart of Spain, The (film), 344

Hebb, Donald Olding, 141–3, 221, 277, 282–9, 297, 300, 343, 369

Hebei Medical University (Shiji-azhuang, China), 417

Hecaen, Henri, 416

Heller, Irving, 270, 275–6, 325, 333, 349, 378–9, 465, 469–70, 491–2, 494

hemangioma calcificans. *See* brain tumour

hemispherectomy, 406

hemosiderosis, 406

Henderson, L., 378

Henderson, Nora, 461, 494

Henneman, Elwood, 73, 403, 408

Henry Ford Hospital, 13, 247, 301

Héon, Maurice, 275, 392

Herscovitch, Peter, 375, 420, 423–4, 426

Hertford Bridge (Oxford), 456

Hesse, Sigurd, 469

hypothalamus, 418

Hibben, John Grier, 6

higher level centres, 110

Hilal, S.K., 408

hippocampus, 41, 223–4, 226–8, 289–92, 295–6, 298, 315, 331, 336, 362, 397, 426, 430

Hippocrates, xiv, 29, 264, 268, 450

Hitzig, E., 110–11

HMS Voltaire, 187

Hobbiger, Franz, 469, 494

Hodge, Charles, 208, 325, 335, 355–8, 407, 484, 494–5

Hoen, Thomas I., 48, 55–7, 71, 165, 314

Hokkaido Imperial University (Sapporo, Japan), 294, 352

Holland, Paul, 427

Hollenberg, Robert, 378

Holman, Emile, 11

Holmberg, Rick, 418

Holmes, Sir Gordon, 12–13, 93, 146

Holmes Gold Medal, 58, 73

Holt, Sir Herbert, 86, 443–5, 450, 455

homunculus, 54, 100–2, 206–9, 211, 267

Hôpital de la Pitié (Paris), 188–9, 220, 311

Hôpital de la Salpêtrière (Paris), 96, 233, 235, 264

Hôpital de l'Enfant-Jésus, 233

Hôpital Foch (Suresnes, France), 339

Hôpital Hôtel-Dieu, 94, 233

Hôpital Notre-Dame, 94, 99, 329, 365, 382, 391

Hôpital Sacré-Coeur, 341

Hôpital Saint Luc, 56

Hopkins, Sir Frederick Gowland "Hoppy," 459–60

Horrax, Gilbert, 164

Horsley, Sir Victor, 12–13, 40, 84, 113, 146

Houde, Camillien, 82, 263

Hounsfield, Sir Godfrey, 350, 397–9

House, Arthur Maxwell, 312–13

house staff and fellows, Montreal Neurological Institute, 1934–35 (table), 101

Howard, Campbell, 20

Howard University (Washington, DC), 197–8, 329

Howe, H., 165

Howell, David, 325

Howell, William, 11
Howlett, M., 103
"How Your Brain Works" (Feindel), 511
Hubel, David, 121, 240–2, 264, 351, 366, 383, 416, 431
Hudson, Anna, 103, 145, 150, 172
Hughlings Jackson Amphitheatre, 108, 121, 271, 393, 405, 453–4
Hughlings Jackson lecturers, 1935–84 (table), 517–19
Hughlings Jackson Memorial Lecture, 108, 112, 124, 141–2, 166, 203, 230, 238, 241, 243, 264, 300, 317, 331, 351, 366, 369, 382, 405, 418–19, 431, 434
"Human Memory and the Medial Temporal Region of the Brain" (Corsi), 330
humid chamber, 461–2
Humphreys, Storer, 135, 138, 143, 144, 159
Hunter, John, 99, 200–1, 301, 329
Huntington Medical Research Institutes (Pasadena, CA), 301
Hurteau, Everett, 230
Hurtz, Mr, 160
Hyden, Holger S., 369
hydrocephalus, 50, 53, 301, 316–18, 398, 406, 424
Hyndman, Olan R., 59–61, 139
hyperventilation, 32, 64
hypothalamus, 77, 107, 368, 392
hypothermia, 418, 507
hypothyroidism, 409, 464

IBRO. See International Brain Research Organization
IgG. See immunoglobulin G
Illinois Neuropsychiatric Institute (Chicago), 73
image-guided neurosurgery, 236
Images of the Neuro (Feindel), 438
Imbeault, G., 417
immunoglobulin G, 504
immunosuppression, 502
incisura, 227
incisural sclerosis, 106, 133, 222, 227–8, 351, 397
Indiana University (Bloomington), 100
indomethacin, 476, 489
Inglis, Ruth, 53, 117, 141, 279–82
Ingraham, Frank, 165
Ingvar, David, 276, 300
Institute of Experimental Medicine (St Petersburg), 159

Institute of Physiology (Lund, Sweden), 300
insula, 228, 278, 350
insulin shock, 163, 467
intensive care unit, 366, 416–17, 506
International Brain Research Organization, 127–8, 311, 315
International Peace Hospital, 346
Interns Residence (RVH), 443
interpretive cortex, 292–3
interventional neuro-radiology, 427–9
intervertebral discs, 160, 165
intra-arterial chemotherapy, 330, 424, 429
intracranial hemorrhage, 60
intracranial tumour. See brain tumour
invited speakers, Second Foundation, 20 November 1953 (table), 259
IQ, 286
Isaacs, Norma, 404–5
ischemia, 71, 133, 227, 247, 324, 359, 369, 484; anoxia-ischemia, 133; cerebral ischemia, 63, 138, 246–7, 323, 367, 484; cortical ischemia, 71; focal cerebral ischemia, 31, 66
Island of Reil, 278
Istituto Superiore di Sanita (Rome), 351
Ivan, Leslie, 507
Ives, John, 376, 384–5, 395–6, 411
Izaak Walton Killam Memorial Endowment, 391

J.W. McConnell Ward, 86
Jackson, Ira, 301, 317–18, 320
Jackson, John Hughlings, 13, 64, 84, 86–7, 109–11, 113, 141, 146, 203, 317, 320
Jacksonian march, 35, 109, 130
Jacob, J.C., 196
Jacobsen, Carlyle, 282
James, Cyril, 245, 258, 263, 274
James Administration Building (McGill). See biology building (McGill)
Jane, John, 299, 313
Japan Chapter of the Montreal Neurological Institute, 1955–84 (table), 512–13
Jaquays, Homer M., 444
Jaskari, Shirley, 329
Jasper, Goldie, 127
Jasper, Herbert H., Advance of Neurology, The, 263–4; applica-

tion of electroencephalography to neurology, 123–7; Arfel-Capdevielle, Geneviève, 311; centrencephalic integrating system, 265–6, 293, 316, 413–14; cerebral edema, 160; citizenship, 242; coordination of filming of epileptic patients with their EEG tracing, 201; cortex and diencephalon interrelationship, 200; death of Wilder Penfield, 413; death of William Cone, 310, 317; departure, 360–2, 374; "Diencephalon of the Cat," 332; Elliott, K.A.C., 348, 460–1; Epilepsy and the Functional Anatomy of the Human Brain, 212, 264; Feindel's departure for Saskatoon, 273; Fellows Society president, 230; G-force experiments, 158, 161; Gybels, Jan, 298; Hubel, David, 240–1; International Brain Research Organization, 128–9, 315; introduction of electroencephalography at the MNI, 120–1, 124–7, 395; Journal of Electroencephalography and Clinical Neurophysiology, 128–9, 203; Li, Choh-luh, 254; "Localization of Epileptic Discharge in Temporal Lobe Automatism," 228; mesial temporal lobe epilepsy, 222, 224, 227–8; mesial temporal structures, 146, 200; MNI attending and house staff (1945–46), 194; MNI clinical staff (1960–61), 325; MNI fellows at the origin of the NINDB, 252–4; MNI Silver Anniversary, 317, 320; MNI staff (1938), 343; operating room gallery, 206, 209, 437; retirement of Wilder Penfield, 314–15; Rothballer, Alan, 337; sea sickness experiments, 158–9; Smirnov, Georgii Donatovich 311, 339; stereotaxic operations for Parkinson's disease, 349; Synapse 50, 434; Van Buren, John, 253–4; wartime role, 158–62, 174, 177
Jeanne Timmins Auditorium (MNI), 87, 415, 433
Jefferson, Sir Geoffrey, 178, 238, 259, 314
Jefferson Medical College (Philadelphia), 162, 329
Jerry Lewis MDA Telethon, 363–5
Jet Propulsion Laboratory, 384
Jewish General Hospital, 313

Johns, Harold, 508–9
Johns Hopkins Hospital (Baltimore, MD), 5–6, 9, 11, 20, 57, 167, 241
Johns Hopkins Institute of the History of Medicine, 351
Johns Hopkins University, 5–7, 11, 53, 55–6, 144, 146, 166, 194, 204, 241, 259, 408, 418, 506, 508
Johnson, Annie, 327, 381, 405
Johnson, Beatrice, 303
Johnson, Dorothy, 469, 494–5
Jones, Barbara, 425
Jones, Etta, 145, 150
Jones, Ottiwell, 49–51, 57, 183
Jones-Gotman, Marilyn, 289, 407
Joron, G.E., 194
Jotic, G., 405
Joubert syndrome, 394
Journal of Electroencephalography and Clinical Neurophysiology, 127, 203
Jouvet, Michel, 425
Jutra, Claude, 351

K. (patient), 35
K.A.C. Elliott Lecture, 431, 471
K.M. (patient), 277, 283, 286–7, 289
Kaada, Birger, 200
Kacprzak, Marcin, 186
Kahn, Edgar, 337
Kaiser Wilhelm Institute, 254. *See also* Max Planck Institute
Kapitsa, Pyotr, 337–8
Kapitza Institute for Physical Problems (Moscow), 338–9
Kaplan, Paige, 494
Karamchandani, Jason, 132
Karolinska Institute (Solna, Sweden), 422, 474
Karpati, George, 194, 312, 363–5, 367–9, 393, 407, 427, 477, 494
Katschurick, Simon, 409
Katzman, Robert, 407, 481, 495
Keilin, D., 459
Keith, Haddow M., 56–7, 60, 100, 107, 143
Kekesi, F., 378
Kelly, E., 104
Kelly, Howard, 5
Kendall, Helen, 145, 150–1, 172
Kennedy, Foster, 164
Kenyatta General Hospital (Nairobi, Kenya), 195
Kershman, John, 56–7, 60–1, 100–1, 126, 140, 143, 170, 174, 176–7, 194, 222, 227–8, 263, 343, 392, 395
ketanserin, 476, 489

Keynes, Sir Geoffrey, 276
Khan, Tariq, 469, 494
Khare, P., 378
Kidd, K., 104
Kiev Neurosurgical Institute (Kiev, USSR), 342
Killam Scholarships, 376, 391
Kimberley, Audrey, 327
Kimura, Doreen, 335, 337
kindling, 140, 276
King's County Hospital (Brooklyn, NY), 322
Kirkham, Trevor, 426
Klatzo, Igor, 37, 201, 237, 251–2, 254, 301, 320, 407, 434, 467, 482, 494–5
Klemperer, Wolfgang, 322, 343
Klingler, Joseph, 298
Kluver, Heinrich, 289
Kluver-Bucy syndrome, 74
Knighton, Robert, 301
Knowles, John, 416
Knowles, Stanley, 122
Kocher, Theodor, 11
Krabbe's disease, 393
Krause, Fedor, 64
Krayenbuhl, Hugo, 335
Kreiger, D., 408
Kristiansen, Kristian, 200–1, 259, 315, 319, 351, 514
Krnjevic, Krešimir, 366
Kryk, Helen, 327, 368, 381
Krysztofiak, B., 378
Kuchner, Eugene, 486, 495
Kuffler, Stephen, 241
Kuhl, David, 434
Kurnicki, Ania, 469, 494

L.B. (patient), 131–2
Laboratory services, Montreal Neurological Institute, 27 September to 31 December 1935 (table), 98
Lachrité, Marieleurrie, 173
Laidlaw, 15
Lamarre, Yves, 351
Lambertus, C., 103–4
Lambo, Thomas A., 408, 416
Landau, Lev Davidovich, 130, 311, 337–41, 350
Lane Medical Lectures (Stanford University), 203, 206, 209
Langevin, P., 378
Lapicque, Louis, 124
Lapierre, Yves, 505
Largo, Cecilia, 381, 405
Lashley, Karl, 141, 221, 286–7
Laurelli, H., 378

Lavigeur, J., 378
Laxer, Kenneth, 407
Lazure, Denis, 416
LCGU. *See* local cerebral glucose utilization
L-DOPA, 382, 395
Leacock, Stephen, 244
lead absorption, 464
LeBlanc, C.T., 103
LeBlanc, Francis, 235, 376–9, 392, 494
Leblanc, Richard, 73–4, 121, 135, 220, 223, 236, 247, 257, 347, 358, 366, 416, 418, 422–3, 425–6, 431
Lechter, M., 378
leech muscle bioassay, 462
Léger, Jules, 416
Legrand, Émile, 60, 94–5, 98, 100, 129, 234
Lehmann, Peter, 160, 173–5
Leksell, Lars, 311
Lende, Richard, 71, 72–3, 299, 324, 350
Lenin, Vladimir Ilyich, 29, 39, 291, 338
Leningrad Neurosurgical Institute (Leningrad, USSR), 298
Lenox Hill Hospital (New York), 71, 73
Leonard, G., 427
Leppik, Ilo, 399, 407
Lesage, Jean, 324
Levin, Emilio, 469, 494
Levine, Dr, 376
Levitsky, W., 336
Lewin, Marcial G., 378, 486, 495
Lewin, Revis, 230
Lewin, Walpole, 331
Lewis, Hope, 50
Lewis, Jerry, 363–4
Lewis, Shirley, 251–2, 256
Lewis-Baldwin, Shirley. *See* Lewis, Shirley
Li, Choh-luh, 201, 230, 237, 242, 251–2, 254, 437
Libman, Israel, 313
Lienard-Boisjoly, Margot, 492
Life of Sir William Osler (Cushing), 22
Lifshitz, Evgeny, 339
Lily Griffith McConnell Foundation for Neurological Research, 258
Lima, Almeida, 282
limbic system, 126, 331, 406
Lincoln University (Oxford, PA), 198

Lister Oration (Royal College of Surgeons of England), 238, 332
Lloyd-Smith, Donald, 122, 201, 246, 299, 310, 325, 349, 369, 378–9
lobby (MNI). *See* foyer (MNI)
lobotomy, 163, 290–1
local anaesthesia, 34
local cerebral glucose utilization, 487–9, 490–1
"Localization of Epileptic Discharge in Temporal Lobe Automatism" (Penfield and Jasper), 228
Loewi, Otto, 203
Loma Linda University (Loma Linda, CA), 199
London Hospital Medical College (London), 49, 57
Longo, V.G., 351
Lord, John, 251–2
Lord Camrose. *See* William Ewart Berry, 1st Viscount Camrose
"Loss of Recent Memory after Bilateral Hippocampal Lesions" (Scoville and Milner), 278
Lotspeich, Edward Jr, 301, 516
Lovell, Richard, 469, 494
Lowden, J.A. (Sandy), 469, 473, 494
Lubyanka Prison, 338
lucite calvarium, 162, 164
Lust, David, 488, 495
luxury perfusion syndrome, 354
Lyman, Faith. *See* Feindel, Faith Lyman

MacDonald, David Keith Chalmers, 331–2
MacDonald, Delta, 327, 381, 405, 409
Macdonald, Robert Henry, 443–4
MacDonald, Ruth, 508
MacKay, Allan, 58
MacKay, F.H., 60, 98, 100, 143
Mackay, Janet C., 145, 150
Mackenzie, Kenneth, 167, 417
Macklem, Peter T., 22
MacLennan, Hugh, 192
MacLeod, C., 103
MacLeod, J. Wendell, 272, 506
MacMillan, Irene, 381, 405
Madeleine Ehret Ottman Research Fellowship, 47–8, 51–2, 58, 180
Madrid cubicles, 50–1, 452–3
magnetic resonance imaging, 130, 140, 291, 295, 365, 429, 435, 439, 505
magnetic resonance spectroscopy, 439, 475, 505

Magnus, William, 201
Magoun, Horace, 73, 166, 267
Mailloux, Noël, 288
Majkowski, Jerzy, 298
Maleki, Mohammed, 418
Malloch, Archibald, 18, 43
Mallory, Frank Burr, 44, 49
Mallory, Joan, 409
Mammen, Elizabeth, 196
Manchen, M., 417
manipulation hemiplegia, 71, 324
Mao Zedong, 175, 341, 343–4
Marburg, Otto, 105–6
Marie, Pierre, 30, 146, 216
Markle Foundation, 256
Marlag und Milag, 187
Maroun, Falah, 312
Marshall, John, 331
Martell, Jerome, 192
Martin, Charles F., 19–20, 22–4, 45, 167
Martin, H. Newell, 5
Martin, Joseph B., 401–2
Martin, Paul, Sr, 229, 264
Massachusetts General Hospital (Boston), 227, 243, 276, 398, 504
Massachusetts Institute of Technology (Cambridge, MA), 331, 335, 366, 403, 405, 407
Massey, Vincent, 258
Masson, J., 59–60
Masson, Pierre, 202
materialism, 111, 221, 316, 371
Mathews, Brian, 501
Mathieson, Gordon, 292, 300, 314, 325, 363, 378, 396–7
Matson, Donald, 337
Matthew, Elizabeth, 424
Matthews, George, 368
Matthews, Marjorie, 161
Matthews, Paul, 505
Maudsley Hospital (London), 472
Max Planck Institute, 236, 378
Maxwell, Edward, 443, 458
Maxwell, William, 443, 458
Mayo Clinic, 56–7, 322, 398–9, 408, 506
Mazars, Gabriel, 201
McAlpine, Douglas, 501–2
McAlpine Multiple Sclerosis, 501
McArdle, Brian, 243
McAuley, Lillian, 327, 405, 409
MCC. *See* meningocerebral cicatrix
McCann, William, 484–6, 495
McCarter, J., 343
McCauley, Lillian, 381

McClure, G.Y., 143
McConnell, John Wilson, 230, 258, 263, 450
McConnell, L., 101
McConnell Brain Imaging Centre, 330, 359, 426, 432, 439, 505
McConnell Pavilion (MNI), 223, 239, 243, 257–60, 264, 367, 456–7, 465
McConnell Ward. *See* J.W. McConnell Ward
McConnell Wing. *See* McConnell Pavilion
McCormack, Flora, 381
McCouch, Grayson, 301
McCrae, John, 20
McCulloch, W., 165
McDonald, M., 103
McEachern, Donald, 60, 98, 100, 141, 143, 169, 174, 194, 202, 255, 261, 263, 343, 459–63, 465, 494, 500
McGill Chapel, 53
McGill hammer, 160
McGill Medical School, 8, 69, 73, 166, 193, 240, 320
McGill Surgical Unit, No. 3 Canadian General Hospital, 20
McGill University School of Architecture, 444
McGuire, N., 405
McHugh, Michael, 483, 487–8, 495
McIlwain, Henry, 470, 472
McIntosh, Maureen E., 327
McKenzie, Kenneth, 259
McKenzie Prize (Canadian Neurosurgical Society), 418
McKhann, G., 408
McLaughlin, R.S., 375
McLean Hospital (Boston), 331
McLennan, Hugh, 237, 275, 462, 467, 494
McLeod, Cora, 92, 104
McMaster University (Hamilton, ON), 334, 425
McMillan, Irene, 327
McMillan, Jean, 304
McNaughton, Francis Lothian, 100–1, 114, 121–3, 129, 138, 143, 177, 194, 197, 234–6, 246, 260–1, 270, 272, 309–10, 312, 319, 325, 333–4, 341–3, 346, 349, 374, 378–9, 383, 392, 417, 434, 516
McNichol, L., 104
McNichol, Margaret, 173
McQuarrie, I., 165
McRae, Donald L., 194, 263, 325, 369, 374, 434

McRae, Elizabeth, 173

MDA, 363. *See* Muscular Dystrophy Association

Meagher-Villemure, Kathleen, 424

Meakins, Jonathan, 20, 22–4, 50, 86, 367

Medical College of South Carolina, 334

Medical Research Council of Canada, 182, 361–2, 400–1, 425, 439, 472, 503

medulloblast, 140

Mélançon, Denis, 365, 399, 427–9

Melzak, Ronald, 376

Memorial University (St John's), 312

memory, 77, 238, 271, 278, 286, 289–93, 295–6, 298, 300, 311, 316, 331, 335–6, 355, 360, 369, 370, 397, 403, 407, 409, 430, 491

Memory, Learning and Language: The Physical Basis of Mind (ed. Feindel), 511

meningocerebral cicatrix, 14, 30–3, 37, 63–4, 66

meningomyelocele, 60

Mercer, David, 378, 486, 495

Merck, 469

Meredith, Sir Vincent, 23–4, 43

Mériel, Paul, 71

Merritt, H. Houston, 165, 382

Merton College, 7, 9, 438–9

mesial temporal lobe, 117, 146, 222, 227

mesial temporal lobe epilepsy. *See* epilepsy: mesial temporal lobe epilepsy

mesial temporal sclerosis, 140, 224, 227

metallic stain, 253

Mexican muralists, 259–61

Meyer, Ernst, 220, 411, 422, 425

Meyer, John Stirling, 99, 160, 194, 407–8

MGH. *See* Montreal General Hospital

microglia. *See* neuroglial cells

microgyria, 130–1, 133, 134

Middlesex Hospital (London), 276, 501

migraine, 122, 235, 408

Mikulicz-Radecki, Johann von, 32, 40

military annex, 125, 173, 176, 199–200, 228, 443–4, 456

Military Neurosurgery, 149

Millar, Ronald, 325, 374

Miller, H.Y., 408

Miller, Isabelle, 173

Millette-Stewart, Lucy, 103, 150, 154

Mills, W.H., 459

Milne, Alan Alexander (A.A.), 276

Milner, Brenda, 215, 219, 278, 286–96, 298, 325, 334–7, 349, 367, 378, 396–7, 403, 407, 416, 419

Milner, Peter, 285, 287

mind, 10, 111, 142, 203, 221, 230, 238, 242–3, 252, 265, 266, 277, 292–3, 300, 314, 337, 340, 348, 370–3, 414

Mini Cyclotron. *See* cyclotron

Miracle of the Empty Beds, 245

Mishkin, Mortimer, 403

MIT. *See* Massachusetts Institute of Technology

Mitchell, Silas Weir, 85

Mixter, William Jason, 44, 107, 227

MNI class of 1959 (table), 313

MNI South: MNI fellows at the origin of the National Institute of Neurological Diseases and Blindness (table), 252

Mob Quad (Merton College, University of Oxford), 9

Molaison, Henry Gustav. *See* H.M. (patient)

Molson, Hartland, 375

Moniz, António Egas, 115, 282

Monnier, Alexandre, 124

Monnier, Andrée, 124

Montes, José, 418

Montreal Children's Hospital, 311, 313, 328–9, 472

Montreal Declaration, 341–2

Montreal General Hospital, 8, 16–17, 56, 58–9, 99–100, 115, 160, 199, 240, 247–8, 251, 329, 350, 401, 438, 505, 511

Montreal General Hospital Research Institute, 418

Montreal Group for the Security of the People's Health, 341–2

Montreal Medico-Chirurgical Society, 99, 202

Montreal Neurological Institute, Royal Victoria Hospital, 1933 (table), 60

Montreal Neurological Institute nursing staff 1961–62 (table), 327

Montreal Neurological Society, 99, 230, 403, 440

Montreal Star, 190, 309

Moon, Virgil, 162, 164

Moris, A.A., 516

Morphy, A.G., 100, 143

Morrell, Frank, 276, 430–1

Morris, Arthur Allan, 165, 194, 230

Morton, Alan, 313, 334

Morton, Guy, 334, 516

Moscarello, Mario, 504

Mossakowski, Miroslaw, 298, 313

Mountcastle, Vernon, 418–19

Mount Royal Club, 23

Mount Royal Hotel (Montreal), 443

movement disorders, 236, 253, 298, 381–3

MRI. *See* magnetic resonance imaging

Mrs Samuel Reitman Nursing Bursary (nursing), 329

Mullan, Sean, 75

multiple sclerosis, 59, 95, 122, 129, 158, 230, 325, 395, 409, 417, 424, 498–505; malignant MS, 502

Multiple Sclerosis Clinic, 333, 501, 504–5

Multiple Sclerosis Society of Canada, 333–4, 470, 499–500, 503–4

Murphy, F., 405

Murray, Patricia, 329, 381

Murray, Patrick, 392

Murray, Robert, 508

muscular dystrophy, 363–5, 427

Muscular Dystrophy Association, 363, 365

Mushatt, C., 516

myasthenia gravis, 276, 366, 464

myelin basic protein, 504

myelocele, 60

myelotomy, 395

Myer, Ernst, 220, 411, 420, 422

Myles, Terry, 377, 392

Mystery of the Mind, The (Penfield), 142, 371–2, 414

Naffziger, Howard C., 49, 183

Nageotte, Jean, 454

Nangia, B., 378

NASA. *See* National Aeronautic and Space Administration (US)

Nashold, Blaine, 73, 270, 434

National Academy of Sciences (India), 312

National Academy of Sciences (US), 142, 166, 299, 407

National Aeronautic and Space Administration (US), 107, 113, 384, 385

National Film Board of Canada, 344

National Institute of Mental Health (US), 482, 488

National Institute of Neurological and Communicative Disorders and Stroke (US), 346

National Institute of Nervous Diseases and Blindness (US), 250–4, 256, 363

National Institute of Neurological Diseases and Stroke (US), 250, 251, 406, 420

National Institutes of Health (US), 194, 241, 249–50, 257, 297, 300–1, 367, 375, 396, 399, 403, 409, 420, 424, 434, 439

National Research Council of Canada, 14, 331, 376, 472

Natucci, B., 405

Nature se dévoilant devant la Science, La (statue), 83–5, 435, 454

Needham, Charles, 368

Nelson, James, 418

Nelson, Robert, 368

neuroanatomy, 12, 58, 95, 97, 103, 177, 252, 254, 271, 274, 320, 322, 351, 416, 438

Neuroanatomy, Department of (MNI), 230, 325, 425

Neuroanatomy Lecture, 271, 331, 351, 366, 368

neurochemistry, 230, 239, 252, 256, 330, 360, 362, 369, 416, 431, 459–95

Neurochemistry (ed. Elliott), 470

Neurochemistry, Department of (MNI), 199, 230, 255, 270, 330–1, 362, 426, 449, 459–95

Neurochemistry Laboratory, 199, 255, 449, 460, 464–5, 470, 492

neurofibrils, 62, 129

neurofibromatosis, 62

neurogenetics, 394

neuroglial cells, 13–14, 31, 49, 51, 61, 85, 107, 140, 298, 454, 470, 473, 481, 498; microglia, 50, 498; oligodendrocyte, 14, 498

Neurolinguistic Research Institute (Paris), 416

Neurological and Neurosurgical staff, MNI, 1963–64 (table), 349

Neurological Biographies and Addresses, xii, 56, 80, 93–4

Neurological Institute of New York, 14–17, 24, 43, 213, 337

Neurological Service, Montreal Neurological Institute, 1970–71 (table), 379

Neurology and Neurosurgery, Department of (McGill), 60, 61, 314, 330, 375, 400–2, 472, 481–2

neuromuscular disease, 250, 363, 367, 427, 464

Neuromuscular Research Group, 363, 427

Neuromuscular Research Laboratory, 427

Neuromuscular Research Laboratory (MNI), 312

neuronal ceroid-lipofucsinoses, 479

neuronal trophism, 367

neuro-oncology, 61, 440

neuropathology, 11–12, 14, 16–17, 49, 53, 60, 73, 97, 99, 106–7, 112, 129, 227, 230, 247, 252, 254, 259, 299–300, 318, 320, 362, 396, 399, 452, 473, 498

Neuropathology, Department of (Columbia University), 15

Neuropathology, Department of (MNI), 132, 174, 363, 424

Neuropathology, Laboratory of (RVH), 17, 49–50, 62

Neurophotography, Department of (MNI), 356–8, 484

neurophysiology, 35, 63, 69, 97, 103, 127, 203, 230, 235, 239–41, 252–3, 271, 298, 311, 360, 362, 396, 416, 426, 438, 451, 505

Neurophysiology, Department of (MNI), 107, 126, 200, 270, 276, 351, 362, 366, 376, 426, 486

Neuropsychology, Department of (MNI), 279–96, 334–7, 403, 427

Neuropsychology, Department of, 1962–63 (table), 337, 427,

Neuroscience Research Institute (University of Ottawa), 426

Neurosurgical Management of the Epilepsies, 406

Neurosurgical Service, Montreal Neurological Institute, 1970–71 (table), 379

Neurosurgical Training Program, 97–102

Newnham College (University of Cambridge), 287

New York Academy of Sciences, 368, 419

New York College of Physicians and Surgeons, 7, 13, 24

New York Medical College, 53, 56

New York University, 56, 71

Ng Ying Kin, N.M.K., 475, 477, 494

Nichols, W. Martin, 135, 137–8, 143–4, 178–80, 316, 319, 334

Nielsen, J.M., 204

NIH. *See* National Institutes of Health (US)

Nikkinen, Leo, 420

NINDB. *See* National Institute for Nervous Diseases and Blindness (US)

Nissen hut, 152–3

Nissl, Franz, 85, 105

NLD. *See* neuronal ceroid-lipofucsinoses

No. 1 Canadian General Hospital, 160

No. 1 Canadian Neurological Hospital, 73, 144–7, 152–3, 160, 171–2

No. 3 Canadian General Hospital, 146

Nobel Institute of Neurophysiology (Stockholm), 405–6

Nobel Prize, 36, 84, 108, 121, 124, 139, 166, 203, 208, 230, 240–3, 264, 282, 287, 300, 337, 366–7, 383, 397, 406, 418, 420, 431

nociferous cortex, 34, 286–7

non-war-related addresses given at the MNI during the Second World War (table), 165

Norcross, Nathan C., 101, 135, 137–8, 301

Norfolk and Norwich University Hospital (Norwich, UK), 431

Norman Bethune Exchange Professor, 470

Norman Bethune Foundation, 122, 342, 346

Norris, John W., 483–4, 495

Northwestern University, 166, 366

notable research fellows, 1945–49 (table), 201

notable speakers at the MNI, 1971–76 (table), 408–9

Nowik, J., 378

Nudleman, Kenneth, 417

Nuffield Orthopaedic Centre (Oxford), 230

nursing: Cone, 302–4; Cone, Elvidge, and Penfield, 121; design of the MNI, 88; No. 1 Neurological Hospital, 144, 150–6, 172; Nurses Ball, 435; operating room nursing, 45, 92, 104, 121, 172–3,

175, 251–2, 259, 263, 303–4, 327, 329, 381, 404–5, 437, 508, 510; provincial health insurance, 234; Royal University Hospital (Saskatoon), 508; specialized care, 402; training in neurological and neurosurgical nursing, 103, 170, 172–3, 245, 328–9, 368, 3/9, 380, 381; under Bertha Cameron, 326–9; under Caroline Robertson, 402–3; under Eileen Flanagan, 103–4, 243–6; under Joy Hackwell, 379–81

nursing administration, Montreal Neurological Institute, 1974–84 (table), 405

nursing staff, Montreal Neurological Institute, 1934–35 (table), 104

nursing staff, Montreal Neurological Institute, 1970–1971 (table), 381

Nutik, Stephen, 378, 392

Observations on the Pathology of Hydrocephalus, 50

OCBs, 504. *See* oligoclonal bands

occipital lobe, 53, 336, 483

Ochoa, J., 409

Ochs, Rachel, 423

Odom, Guy Leary, 73, 129, 143, 159, 230, 318, 320, 322, 331, 343, 409

Oeconomos, Doros, 319

Oertel, Horst, 23

Oh, J.H., 483, 495

Ojemann, George, 253

Oldendorf, W.H., 409

oligoclonal bands, 504

oligodendrocyte. *See* neuroglial cells: oligodendrocyte

oligodendroglioma. *See* brain tumour: oligodendroglioma

Olivier, André, 74, 236, 377–9, 381, 429

Olszewski, Jerzy, 37, 201, 230, 237, 242, 254, 263, 270, 273–4, 299, 316–17, 351, 402, 510

Ommaya, Ayoub, 399

operating room, 13, 34, 45, 88–91, 147, 169, 170, 172–3, 236, 359, 381, 410, 416, 443, 448, 450, 453, 461, 492, 507–8

operating room gallery. *See* operating room viewing gallery

operating room number one (MNI), 88–92, 208–9, 357, 416, 437, 450–3

operating room photography, 89–92, 209, 416–17, 450

operating room viewing gallery, 88–90, 92, 206, 208–9, 256–7, 416, 443, 450, 452–3, 506–7

Oppenheim, Hermann, 146

optic neuritis, 95, 505

Order of Canada, 440

Ordre national du Québec, 440

Orth, Johannes, 19

Ortiz-Galvan, A., 320

Osler, Lady, 8, 10, 12

Osler, Revere, 12

Osler, Sir William, 5–12, 18, 20–2, 40, 42–3, 146, 166, 261

Osler Library of the History of Medicine (McGill University), 167, 351, 440

Osler Society (McGill University), 431

Osterholm, Jewell, 313

Osterland, Kirk, 300, 502

Ottman, Madeleine Louise, 45–8, 448

Owens, Guy, 337

Owens, Trevor, 505

Oxford University. *See* University of Oxford

oxidative metabolism, 461

P.B. (patient), 289–90, 396

Pace-Asciak, Cecil, 378, 474–5, 494

Pace-Floridia, Albert, 377

Page, I.H., 470

pallidotomy, 311

Palma, Eduardo, 319

Palmer, Walter, 14

Panet-Raymond, Jean, 201

papaverine, 72

Pappius, Hania (Hanna) M., 239, 298, 325, 330, 367, 378, 406–7, 426, 459, 464–7, 469–70, 476, 481, 483, 487, 493–5

Pappius, Hanna collaborators and students (table), 495

Paquette, Albiny, 229

parietal lobe, 35, 106, 130, 214–15, 259

Parkinson's disease, 121, 128–9, 236, 298, 311, 329, 335, 349–50, 368, 382, 395, 410, 506

Pasquet, André, 275, 437

Pathological Institute (McGill University), 23, 254, 376, 442, 456

Pathology of Skeletal Muscle, 427

Pathology of Tumours of the Nerv-

ous System (Russell and Rubenstein), 50, 331

Patten, B.M., 165

Pavlov, Ivan, 85, 140, 159, 203–4, 231, 277–8, 298, 419

Pavrovsky, Josef, 99

PDP-12 (a Digital Equipment Corporation computer), 376, 381, 409–10

Peabody, Francis Weld, 43

Pearce, Richard, 21–2

Peden, J., 378

PEG. *See* pneumoencephalogram

Peking Institute of Neurosurgery, 342, 345–6

Peking Union Medical College (Beijing), 342

Pellerin, Luc, 475, 477, 494–5

Pena, Sergio, 427

Penfield, Charles Samuel, 4

Penfield, Helen Kermott, 3, 11–12, 344, 412

Penfield, Jean Jefferson, 3–4, 6–7, 31, 83, 206, 448

Penfield, Ruth. *See* Inglis, Ruth

Penfield, Wilder Graves: administration of MNI during wartime, 147, 152, 157–8, 170–1, 176; *Advance of Neurology* (triptych), 259–64; Baldwin, Maitland, 222, 224, 226, 252; Barber, Jesse, Jr, 198–9; Biltmore Hotel sketch of the MNI, 441–2; brain tumours, 104–5, 140–1; Cameron, Bertha, 326; centrencephalic integrating system, 142, 203–4, 221, 265–8, 292–3, 316–17, 340, 413–14; cerebral blood flow and metabolism affecting epilepsy, 134–7; *Cerebral Cortex of Man, The,* 205–12; Chandy, Jacob, 196; *Children of the Brain, The* (sculpture), 258–9; Chorobski's 1959 Montreal visit, 185–6; communication with/about Jerzy Chorobski, 177–8, 182–5; coronation of Queen Elizabeth II, 242; death of Collin Russel, 274; death of Harvey Cushing, 166–8; death of Wilder Penfield, 412–14; death of William Cone, 310; Elvidge, Arthur, 115, 117–21; epilepsy and surgical therapy, 105–6; *Epilepsy and the Functional Anatomy of the Human Brain,* 264–67; establishing the MNI, 71–3, 75, 79–80,

82–6, 93–6, 441–53, 455–6, 458; European research (1928), 29–39; *Evolution of Neurology, The* (sketch for), xv; Feindel's departure for Saskatoon 272–4; Fisher, Charles Miller, 247, 9; Flanagan, Eileen, 244–6; French-English scientific relations and the MNI, 232–5, 270, 370; frontal lobe and Ruth Inglis, 279–82; Greene, Clarence, 196–8; Harrower and Hebb, 282–5, 286–7, 297; Hodge, Charles, 357; Hughlings Jackson Amphitheatre (christening), 405; Hughlings Jackson Lecture, 108–12, 141–2; insular cortex resection, 350; Jasper, Herbert, 123–6; Johns Hopkins, 11; kindling and the spread of epileptic activity, 140; language/speech and the supplementary motor area, 212–19; Landau, Lev, 338–40; lobby, xiv; Mathieson, Gordon, 397; McConnell Pavilion (MNI), 228–30, 243, 257; McNaughton, Francis, 121–2; microgyria, 130–4; Milner, Brenda, 278, 287–93, 334, 396–7; mind/consciousness, 243, 292–3, 314, 332, 340, 371–3; MNI fellows (1934), 514; MNI staff photograph (1969–70), 378; MNI 25th anniversary, 315–17; move to Montreal 18, 23–5; multiple sclerosis, 498, 503; Nichols, Martin, 178–80; neocortical and limbic interaction, 430; neurochemistry, 460–1, 465, 492, 494; neurosurgery at University of Saskatchewan, 511; Oxford education, 7–10, 11–12; Percival Bailey and 1944 residents and staff of the MNI, 516; Perot, Phanor, 332, 354; portrait, 79; postwar administration of MNI, 199–200; postwar lectures, 203; postwar research, 176; postwar research on epileptic discharges in isolated cerebral cortex and cortical excision, 193, 200–1; Presbyterian Hospital, 13–17; pre-war research, conferences, other events, 106–8; Pribram, Karl, 271; Princeton, 4–7; Queens Square 12–13; Rasmussen, Theodore, 322–3; red cerebral veins, 352; research and fellows at the RVH (1928–34), 49–63; research on a vasomotor mechanism of focal epilepsy, 64–9; retirement announcement, 314–15; shortage of research space, 367; "Significance of the Montreal Neurological Institute, The," xii; Soviet-Western relations, 348; sub-department of neurosurgery (RVH), 40–9; Synapse 50, 435; temporal lobe epilepsy, 222–8, 350–1; Tower, Donald, 255–6; trip to China (1962), 175, 341–6; trip to USSR (1956), 277–8; trip to Warsaw, 182; Wada test, 293–5; wartime nursing, 153–4; wartime trip to China, 173; wartime trip to England, 149; wartime trip to USSR, 175; youth, 3–4; Zemskaya, Alexandra and Yuri Savchenko, 298

Penfield Award for Excellence, 368, 407, 418, 431
Penfield Pavilion, 366, 390, 401, 416, 471
penicillin epilepsy, 396
Pennsylvania Hospital (Philadelphia), 460
Pentland, Thomas Henry, 375
Percival Molson Stadium, 193, 322, 432, 442
peripheral nerve injuries, 53, 160
Perot, Phanor, 72, 313, 332, 334, 348–9, 354–5, 368, 418
Pertuiset, Bernard, 201
PET. *See* positron emission tomography
Peter Bent Brigham Hospital, 11, 43, 57, 167, 281
Peter Pan, 305–6
Peter Pan (statue), 305–6, 328
Peters, Terry, 423, 429
Petersen, J. Norman, 55–8, 60–1, 88, 98, 100, 104, 143, 176, 343
Peterson, Eric Weston, 73–4, 99, 158, 161–2, 193–4, 376, 425–6, 516
Petrides, Michael, 289, 427
Petrin, Barbara, 381, 405, 416–17
Pevehouse, Byron Cone, 298–9, 313
Pew, Paul, 399
PGD₂. *See* prostaglandin: prostaglandin D₂
PGE₁. *See* prostaglandin: prostaglandin E₁

PGE₂. *See* prostaglandin: prostaglandin E₂
PGF₂alpha. *See* prostaglandin: prostaglandin F₂alpha
Phénomène humain, 371
Phillips, Barnet, 454
Pietrowski, Zygmunt, 163
Pike, Bruce, 505
Pillar of Fire, 129
Pitié (hospital). *See* Hôpital de la Pitié (Paris)
Planques, Jean, 71
plasticity, 286, 298, 369
pneumoencephalogram, 23, 31, 64, 140, 216
pneumoencephalography, 31–2, 52, 115, 117, 139–40, 198, 398, 402, 476
Poirier, Louis, 236, 298, 369, 378
Pokrupa, Ronald, 426, 494–5
poliomyelitis, 95, 165, 202
Polish Academy of Sciences, 298, 313
Polish Institute of Arts and Sciences, 482
Pollock, L.J., 164
polymicrogyria, 133, 137; focal polymicrogyria, 130, 132. *See also* microgyria
Pomerat, Charles M., 243
Ponsonby, Vere Brabazon, 81
Pontifical Academy of Sciences, 371, 419
Pool, J. Lawrence, 337
Pope, A., 194, 494
Positome I scanner, 419
Positome II scanner, 420
Positome III scanner, 432
positron emission tomography, 220, 307, 355, 359, 375, 387, 419–20, 422, 424, 432, 435, 439
Post-Basic Nursing Program, 327
Postgraduate Institute for Medical Education and Research (Chandigarh, India), 330
post-traumatic headache, 122, 159
potassium, 461–2, 464, 466–7, 483, 486–8
Potts, Gordon, 399
POW. *See* prisoner of war
Prados, Miguel, 129, 160, 163, 202
Preminger, Otto, 189
Presbyterian Hospital (New York), 3, 13–5, 23–4, 117, 162, 167, 198, 246, 251
Prescott, L., 378

Pribram, Karl, 200, 271
Prince, David, 434
Princeton, 3–6
Princeton Tigers, 7
Principles and Practice of Medicine (Osler), 9, 20
prisoner of war, 144, 179–80, 187, 189–90, 248
Problèmes sociaux de l'épileptique. See Social Problems of the Epileptic Patient / Problèmes sociaux de l'épileptique
prostaglandin, 367, 431, 472, 474, 475, 476, 477, 489; prostaglandin D_2, 477; prostaglandin E_1, 474; prostaglandin E_2, 474, 475, 476, 477; prostaglandin F_{2alpha}, 474, 476, 477
psychical phenomena, 41, 226, 332, 430
Psychology, Department of (McGill University), 282, 286–7
Psychology, Department of (Université de Montréal), 288
psychomotor epilepsy. *See* epilepsy: psychomotor epilepsy
Ptito, A., 427
Pudenz, Robert H., 100, 131, 143, 159, 162, 164, 301, 316, 318–19, 322
Pudenz-Heyer shunt system, 316
Putnam, Tracy, 165

Quastel, J.H., 470
Quebec Association for Epileptics. *See* Association pour les Épileptiques du Québec
Quebec Health Insurance Plan. *See* Régie de l'assurance maladie du Québec
Quebec Hospital Act, 333
Quebec Hospital Insurance Plan, 324
Quebec Hospital Insurance Service, 334, 374
Quebec Nursing Act, 245
Queen Elizabeth Hospital (Birmingham, UK), 144
Queen Elizabeth II, 242, 397
Queen Mary Veterans Hospital, 156, 247, 248
Queen Square (London), 12–13, 40, 52, 72, 93, 96, 111, 115, 129, 146, 182, 230, 238, 250, 268, 331, 399, 438, 454, 506
Queen's University (Kingston, ON), 251, 402, 426
Quesney, Luis Felipe, 395, 416, 494

Quiet Revolution, 327, 329, 351

R.I. *See* Inglis, Ruth
Rabinovitch, Reuben, 122, 178, 188–94, 201, 221, 246, 325, 349, 374, 499
Radcliffe Infirmary (Oxford), 221, 331, 337
Radda, George, 432, 434–5
Raichle, Marcus, 420
Rainey, Rupert, 74
Ramamurthi, B., 196
Rand, Carl, 56
Ranson, Stephen Walter, 166
Rasminsky, Michael, 505
Rasmussen, Andrew T., 163, 165, 271
Rasmussen, Theodore Brown: *Advance of Neurology, The*, 263; amygdala and temporal lobe epilepsy, 228; Canadian Centennial, 366; *Cerebral Cortex of Man, The*, 106, 146, 203, 205–6, 208–9; "Clinical and Surgical Studies of the Cerebral Speech Areas in Man," 219; Cone, William, 198; cortical localization, 224; Congress of Neurological Surgeons (1968) 369; cortisone in post-operative brain swelling, 330; departures for Saskatchewan, 272–3; directorship, 321–4; EEG techniques for clinical applications 310; Erickson, Theodore, 163; Fellows Society president, 230; final annual report, 390; function of the insula, 350; funding concerns, 297; hemispheric dominance for speech, 334; hemosiderosis, 406; homunculus, 54; Jasper, Herbert (departure), 360; Leblanc, Richard, 74, 425; left-brain injury and speech lateralization, 419; MNI attending and house staff (1945–46), 193–4; MNI neurosurgical service (1963–64), 348, 349; MNI neurosurgical service (1969–71), 378–9; MNI Silver Anniversary, 315, 317–19; medicare, 377; neuropathology teaching session (1947), 99; Penfield, Wilder (retirement), 314, 315; "Penfield the Surgeon," 431; portrait, 321; proposed expansion of MNI, 374–5; Quebec Hospital Act, 325, 333; Rasmussen, Andrew T., 271; Ras-

mussen's syndrome (Rasmussen's encephalitis), 299–300; return to MNI (1954), 258, 259; tuberous sclerosis, 334; University of Chicago, 74–5, 196; Wada, Juhn, 294–5
Rasmussen's encephalitis, 299–300
Rasmussen's syndrome. *See* Rasmussen's encephalitis
Ratcliff, Graham, 336
Ravvin, L., 378
Rayport, Mark, 276
Recent Advances in Mycology, 407
Red Arrow Express, 277
red cerebral veins, 69, 135, 347, 352, 354, 369
Red Cross hospital, 10–11
Reeves, David L., 92, 100–1
Régie de l'assurance maladie du Québec, 377
Reid, Kenneth H., 347
Reid, M., 103
Reid, William Lister, 100–1, 130, 143, 508–9
Reitman, Ruth, 383
Reitman family dinner, 383
Rembrandt (Rembrandt Harmenszoon van Rijn), 261
Remillard, Guy, 397
residents and fellows, Sub-Department of Neurosurgery, Royal Victoria Hospital, 1928–32 (table), 57
reticular activating system, 337, 414
Rhoads, Cornelius Packard, 164
Rhodes Scholar, 4, 6–7, 10–11, 315
Rhodes Scholarship, 4, 6–8, 11–12, 438
Rhodes University College (South Africa), 459
"Richard Lende and Manipulation Hemiplegia," 71–2
Richard Lende Winter Neurosurgery Conference, 72
Richards, Hilda, 409
Richardson, F., 194
Richardson, J. Clifford, 368
Riesberry, Martha, 506
Riser, Marcel, 71
Roach, Mary, 45, 104, 145, 150, 172–3
Robb, J. Preston, 101, 115, 122, 176, 193–5, 213–15, 246–7, 263, 309, 324–5, 349, 374, 378–9, 383, 392, 401–2, 503, 516
Robbins, L., 405

Roberts, Lamar, 201, 213–19, 221, 230, 272, 293, 297–8, 319, 332, 437
Robertson, Caroline Elizabeth, 329, 381, 402–3, 405, 433
Robertson, David, 331
Robertson, J.S.M., 100
Robertson, Norman, 343
Robertson, Sloan, 319
Robichaud, L., 103
Robitaille, Yves, 300, 424
Rockefeller, Isabel Stillman, 14
Rockefeller, John D. Jr, 20–1
Rockefeller, John D., Sr, 6, 20–1, 30
Rockefeller Foundation, 20–2, 81, 104, 176, 183, 258, 264, 284, 299, 416, 444, 446–8, 450, 462
Rockefeller Institute, 6, 20, 300
Rockefeller-McGill program, 22
Rockefeller Pavilion (MNI), 86, 436, 459, 491
Rockefeller University (New York), 142
Roland, Per, 422
Roll, E., 405
Rosen, Harold, 99, 237
Rosenfeld, Michael, 466, 469, 494–5
Rosman, N.P., 409
Ross, Donald, 174, 516
Ross, George Allan, 443
Ross & Macdonald, Architects, 86, 436, 443–5, 447, 455, 457–8
Rossin-Arthiat, Estelle, 492
Ross Memorial Pavilion (RVH), 412, 442–3
Roswell Park Memorial Institute (Buffalo), 337
Roszkowski (dean, Academy of Medicine, Warsaw), 186
Rothballer, Alan, 337
Rouleau, Guy, 363, 401
Roussy, 105
Rovit, Richard, 310, 313, 325, 329, 352
Royal Architectural Institute of Canada Journal, 449
Royal College of Physicians and Surgeons of Canada, 439, 503, 508
Royal College of Surgeons of England, 238
Royal Red Cross medal, 150
Royal Society (London), 12, 22, 203, 211, 231, 331, 339, 403, 419
Royal Society of Canada, 331, 407, 439, 470, 472
Royal Society of Edinburgh, 331

Royal Society of New Zealand, 471
Royal University Hospital (Saskatoon), 506–9
Royal Victoria Hospital, 16–20, 22–4, 27, 40–3, 45–6, 48, 50, 52–3, 57–61, 64, 86–7, 89, 97, 146, 163, 172, 181, 183, 187–8, 190, 244–7, 250, 326–7, 329, 341, 344, 379, 392, 401, 412, 433, 438, 442–5, 447, 449, 455–6, 458–9, 472, 483, 492, 499, 503
Royal Victoria Women's Auxiliary, 271, 329
Royal York Hotel (Toronto), 443
Rubenstein, Lucien, 50, 331
Ruby Foo's Restaurant, 323
Rumer, Yuri, 338
Rush Presbyterian–St Luke Medical Center (Chicago), 430
Russel, Colin Kerr, 20, 40–1, 50, 56, 59, 61, 98, 100, 107, 109, 143–50, 171–2, 174, 194, 263, 274–5, 280, 343, 448, 498–9
Russell, Dorothy, 49–51, 57, 93, 105, 259, 276, 315, 318, 320, 331
Russell, Lord. *See* Russell, William Ritchie
Russell, William Ritchie, 221, 337
Russia, 85, 159, 175, 286, 311, 333
Rutherford, Sir Ernest, 338
RVH. *See* Royal Victoria Hospital

Saint Andrew's Church (Westmount, QC), 309
Saint George's Hospital (London), 350
Sala, Helen, 409
Salpêtrière. *See* Hôpital de la Salpêtrière (Paris)
Samson, J.E., 164
Sanchez-Perez, Jesus, 101, 107, 119
Sandhostel, 187
Sargent, Percy, 13
Sarojini, S., 196
Saskatoon scanner, 315, 330, 438, 508–10
Saucier, Jean, 60, 94–5, 98, 100, 129, 143, 261, 319, 341, 343, 374
Saumtally, A., 405
Saunders, Richard, 356
Savard, Ghislaine, 424
Savchenko, Yuri, 298
Savoy, George, 177
scalenus anticus syndrome, 163, 165
scar, 14, 30–2, 34, 37–8, 64, 66, 69, 106, 190, 223–4, 450

Schally, Andrew, 418
Schaul, Neil, 486, 495
Scheinberg, L.C., 409
Schiffer, I., 194
Schiller, Francis, 49, 220–1, 230
Schmidt-Lanterman clefts, 83
Schmitt, Francis O., 331
Schwartz, Myrtle, 154
sclerosis, 59, 95, 106, 122, 129, 133, 140, 158, 222–4, 227–8, 230, 249, 325, 334, 351, 395–7, 409, 417, 424, 427, 498–505
Scott, Evelyn, 103–4, 145, 150
Scotti, Giuseppe, 417
Scoville, William Beecher, 278, 290–1, 295, 334
Scudder, John, 162, 164
seasickness, 158–9
Sechenov, Ivan Mikhaylovich, 203
Second Foundation, 257–64
secondary epileptogenesis, 276, 430, 431. *See Social Problems of the Epileptic Patient / Problèmes sociaux de l'épileptique*
seizure focus, 31, 34–5, 37, 66, 124–5, 130, 135, 139, 206, 214, 222, 237, 278, 311, 368, 376, 395, 411, 430–1, 507
Seldin, Milton, 189–90
Selwyn College (University of Cambridge), 459–60
serotonin, 71, 425, 489–91
Sever, J., 409
Shanghai Neurological Institute, 346
Shankeweiler, Donald, 335, 337
Shanks, Helen, 145, 150
Sharpe, Miss, 172
Shaw, Mildred, 409
Sheremata, William, 498, 501, 503
Sherwin, Allan, 194, 330, 334, 349, 367, 378–9, 395–6, 399, 407, 503
Sherrington, Sir Charles, 8–12, 14, 22, 36, 69, 71, 84, 166, 202, 287
Sherwin, Allan, 194, 330, 334, 349, 367, 378–9, 395–6, 399, 407, 503
Shibata, Shobu, 495
Shih, Chung Jen, 299
shock, 32, 160, 162, 164
Shoubridge, Eric, 432
Shy, Milton, 221, 250–2, 320
Siddons-Grey, Norma, 409
Sidhu, R., 378
Silfvenius, Herbert, 350
Silver Anniversary Celebrations, 315–20
Silver Anniversary Celebrations, 5–8 October 1959 (table), 319–20
Simpson, John A., 365

Sir Herbert Holt Ward, 86
Sirois, Georges-Henri, 368
Sirois, Jean, 233
Sise, Hazen, 344
Skretkowicz, F., 405
Skuce, Douglas, 376
SMA. *See* supplementary motor area
Smeaton, M., 405
Smirnov, Georgii Donatovich, 311, 313, 339–40
Smith College (Northampton, MA), 284
Snell, Henry Saxon, 442–3, 458
Social Services, Department of (MNI), 236, 333, 377, 433, 499–500
Society of Neurological Surgeons, 42, 313, 440
sodium pump, 466
Sokoloff, Louis, 420, 482, 488, 495
Solomon, Mitty, 492
somatotopic organization, 40, 146, 209, 264, 417–18, 426, 490
Sorbonne, La (Paris), 124
soul, 200, 243, 372
Sourkes, Theodore, 350, 417
Soviet Academy of Science, 127–8, 311
Spaner, S., 516
Spanish Civil War, 341, 344
Spanish technique. *See* cell-staining techniques
speakers at the reunion in honour of William Cone, 28–29 April 1957 (table), 301
Speakman, Tom, 334
Speech and Brain Mechanisms, 214, 216–18, 222, 298, 332
Spence, Mathew, 473, 475, 494
Spencer, Herbert, 111
Sperry, Roger, 139, 242, 264, 336, 366–7, 407
Sperti, Luigi, 312
sphenoidal electrodes, 310, 395
Spielmeyer, Walther, 105–6, 129
spinal cord trauma, 53, 56, 160, 176, 188, 408, 418, 427, 486–7, 502
Sprong, Wilbur, 48, 56–7, 60–1
squash court, 91, 159, 199, 448–9, 464
SS *Sussex*, 10
SSPE. *See* subacute sclerosing panencephalomyelitis
Stadie-Riggs microtome, 461
Stalag 17, 189
Stalag 17 b, 189

Stalag Luft I, 179, 180
Stalag X b, 187, 188
Stalag XVII b. *See* Stalag 17 b
St Andrews College (Grahamstown, South Africa), 459
Stanford University (Stanford, CA), 270, 276
Stanley, Phoebe, 263, 327, 437
Starling, Ernest Henry, 159
St Augusta Hospital (Jerusalem), 313
Staunton, Thomas, 431
Stavraky, George W., 56–7, 60, 101, 107
Steelman, Harry, 99, 194, 201, 222–3, 224, 230, 368
Steiner, Matilda, 285
Steiner, Ursula, 381, 404–5
Stephens, G.F., 202
Stepien, Lucjan, 311, 313
stereotactic neurosurgery, 236, 298, 311, 349–50, 369, 381–2, 395, 408, 429–30
Stern, Karl, 129, 494, 516
Stevens, R.H., 143
Stevenson, Lloyd G., 271, 319
Stewart, James, 40–1
Stewart, John, 418
Stewart, Margaret, 150
Stewart, Oscar William, 5, 143–5, 149–50, 155–6, 343
stone carving, 93, 96, 257–60, 314, 412, 449–50, 457
Stookey, Byron, 16, 164
Store, Viola, 327
St Petersburg, 159, 254, 298
St Petersburg Academy (St Petersburg), 298
Straja, Alexander, 368
Strand, Paul, 344
Stratford, Joseph, 160, 201, 237, 274, 350, 402, 438, 507–8, 511
Strauss, Clara, 378
Strauss, Israel, 105
stream of consciousness, 292–3
Strother, Stephen, 435
Strowger, Berk, 160
Stuck, Ralph, 60–1
Stuck, Walter, 322
subacute sclerosing panencephalomyelitis, 505
subarachnoid hemorrhage, 69, 71
subarachnoid space, 71, 117, 429
Sub-Department of Neurosurgery (Department of Surgery, RVH), 40, 43, 45–9, 51, 57
Sub-Department of Neuro-

surgery, Royal Victoria Hospital, 1928–32 (table), 48
subdural hematoma, 49, 165, 398
sulfa drugs. *See* sulfonamide
sulfonamide, 147, 150, 160; sulfapyridine, 188
Summers, Mr, 305
Summers, Mrs, 305
Sunderland, Sydney, 331
superficial hemosiderosis, 406
supplementary motor area, 72, 209–10, 212–14, 216, 218–20, 228, 293, 299
Surgery of the Head (Cushing), 42
Surgical Affections and Wounds of the Head (Archibald), 42
Swank, Roy, 122, 129–30, 246–7, 462, 494, 498, 500–1
Swartz, Myrtle, 145, 150, 172
Swicker, K., 104
Symonds, Sir Charles, 238, 315, 331, 414, 438
Synapse 50, 433–4; lecturers (table), 434
syringomyelia, 236, 428
Szylinger, Hanna, 469, 488, 492, 495

tabes dorsalis, 30
Tampieri, Donatella, 429
Tandon, Prakah Narain, 312–13
Taori, G.M., 196
Tarazi, Anton, 313
tardy ulnar palsy, 438, 508
Tarlov, Isadore, 53, 57, 100–1, 140, 164, 486
Taschereau, Louis Alexandre, 82
Tatlow, William, 325
Taveras, Juan, 399
Taylor, James, 109
Taylor, Laughlin, 335–7, 367, 369, 378
Taylor, Saul, 399
Tay-Sachs disease, 478
Teilhard de Chardin, Pierre, 371
telemetry, 385, 411
temporal lobe, 41, 52, 75, 106, 117, 133, 140, 146, 214, 222–4, 226–9, 241, 253–4, 257, 266, 271, 286, 289–90, 292–3, 295, 310, 332, 335, 350–1, 354, 376, 396–7, 406, 409, 430–1, 438; mesial temporal structures, 41
Temporal Lobe and Limbic System (Gloor), 406
Terbrugge, Karel, 417
Teuber, Hans-Lukas, 335

Texas Instruments, 202

thalamotomy, 311, 382, 395

thalamus, 72, 107, 165, 236–7, 253, 264, 266, 270, 293–4, 315, 334, 349–50, 366–8, 371, 378, 382, 410

thermocouple, 137

Théron, Jacques, 429

thiamine, 331, 426, 470, 490

Third Foundation, 415, 439

Thomas, André, 94–5

Thomas, David, 391

Thomas, G.W., 194, 378

Thomas, Joan, 236, 238

Thomas Willis Lecture, 397, 418, 432, 434–5

Thompson, Christopher, 236, 376, 381, 385, 395–7, 399, 410–11, 420, 423

Thompson, Gordon, 276, 313

Thor (German ship), 187

thromboxane B$_2$, 475–7

Tianjin General Hospital, 342

Tianjin Neurological Institute, 346

Tilney, Frederick, 15

Timmins, Jeanne, 433

Tong-Ren Hospital, 342

Torkildsen, Arne, 52–4, 61, 177, 435

Tower, Donald Bailey, 122, 193, 201, 206, 211, 237, 246, 250–2, 254–6, 346, 383, 420, 431, 433, 463–4, 494

Trainor, Judith, 381

transient monocular blindness, 248

Tremblay, Monica, 508

trigeminal nerve, 165

trigeminal neuralgia, 122

Trinity College (Dublin), 243

Trop, Davy, 368, 391

Tulane University (New Orleans), 73, 354

Turnbull, Frank, 164

Tutt, Henry, 378, 495

Tweedsmuir, Baron. *See* Buchan, John

Tweedsmuir, Lady, 107

twist-drill, 170, 320

Tyler, H. Richard, 418

Tyler, Jane, 426, 429, 435

Ugolik, Claudia, 376

uncus, 224, 227, 290–1

Union Médicale du Canada, 94

Union of Soviet Socialist Republics, 29, 130, 159, 175, 184, 277–8, 337, 347. *See also* Russia

Università Vita-Salute San Raffaele (Milan), 417

Université catholique de Louvain (Louvain-la-Neuve, Belgium), 298, 313

Université de Montpellier (Montpellier, France), 95

Université de Montréal (Montreal), 94–5, 100, 128–9, 232, 234–6, 329, 333, 360–1, 368, 391, 403, 417, 424–5

Université de Paris (Paris), 94–5, 189, 235, 311

Université de Sherbrooke (Sherbrooke), 275, 368, 392

Université Laval (Quebec City), 232–3, 236, 368–9, 378

University Club (Montreal), 435

University College (University of Liverpool), 9

University College London (London), 300, 369, 403

University of Alberta (Edmonton), 75, 334, 424

University of British Columbia (Vancouver), 113, 202, 276, 369

University of Calgary (Calgary), 377, 418

University of California (San Diego, CA), 481

University of California (San Francisco, CA), 57, 202

University of California's Institute of Experimental Biology (Berkeley, CA), 106–7

University of Cambridge (Cambridge), 242, 287, 289, 335, 338, 366, 403, 456, 460, 470–1

University of Chicago (Chicago), 51, 53, 73–5, 181, 286, 300, 314, 324, 334, 390, 425, 502

University of Colorado (Boulder, CO), 72, 251

University of Delaware (Newark, DE), 425

University of Edinburgh (Edinburgh), 9 22, 144

University of Florida (Gainesville, FL), 285

University of Geneva (Geneva), 424

University of Glasgow (Glasgow, UK), 366

University of Illinois (Chicago), 73

University of Iowa (Iowa City), 124

University of Kansas (Lawrence), 92

University of Krakow (Krakow), 185

University of Lausanne (Lausanne), 424

University of Liverpool (Liverpool), 9

University of London (London), 284, 431

University of Louisville (Louisville, KY), 391

University of Lund (Lund, Sweden), 418

University of Miami (Miami), 376

University of Michigan (Ann Arbor, MI), 337

University of Minnesota (Minneapolis, MN), 163, 271

University of New Zealand (Christchurch), 471

University of Odessa (Odessa, Ukraine), 159

University of Oregon (Eugene), 72, 500

University of Oslo (Oslo), 52, 57

University of Ottawa (Ottawa), 73–4, 366, 376, 418, 425–6

University of Oxford (Oxford), 4, 6–13, 21, 43, 75, 85, 113, 146, 181, 202–3, 238, 276, 397, 403, 432, 434, 438, 456, 501

University of Pennsylvania (Philadelphia), 9, 57, 142, 251, 460

University of São Paulo (São Paulo, Brazil), 481

University of Saskatchewan (Saskatoon), 272–4, 438, 506

University of Southern California (Los Angeles), 74

University of St Andrews (St Andrews, UK), 467

University of Sydney (Australia), 202

University of Tehran (Tehran), 418

University of Texas (Galveston), 202, 243, 317, 332

University of Toledo (Toledo, OH), 276

University of Toronto (Toronto), 368, 417

University of Vermont (Burlington), 366

University of Warsaw (Warsaw), 52, 57, 181–2, 186

University of Western Ontario (London, ON), 56, 350–1, 418, 472

University of Wisconsin (Madison), 165, 285

University of Zurich (Zurich), 369
Up from Little Egypt (Bailey), 166

Van Buren, John, 201, 237, 251–3
Vancouver General Hospital, 276
Vane, John, 431
van Gelder, Nico, 469, 494
vascular malformation, 117, 336
vascular nerves, 66
vasoconstriction, 31, 66, 68–2, 135
vasodilator nerves, 32, 67–8, 138
vasogenic edema, 482, 484
vasomotor, 53, 64, 66, 69, 71, 108, 134, 138, 351
vasospasm, 69–5, 121, 359, 409, 425
ventricular shunt, 316–19
ventricular system, 52–3, 117
ventriculogram, 90, 115, 117, 170–1, 339–40, 429
Vera, Christian, 312, 486, 495
vertebral artery, 71, 118
Vézina, Jean, 365, 391
Victor, Maurice, 409
video-telemetry, 430
Villemure, Jean-Guy, 236, 407, 424, 429
Vincent, Clovis, 180, 188–9, 220
Vincent, George, 21
Vineberg, Harold, 158
Viner, Norman, 98, 100, 143, 343
Virtuti Militari Cross, 182
"Visual and Auditory Perception after Temporal-Lobe Damage" (Kimura), 335
vitamin B deficiency, 464
vitamin B12, 490
vitamin E, 464
Vogt, Cécile, 37, 201, 212, 230–1, 254
Vogt, Marthe, 230
Vogt, Oskar, 37, 201, 212, 230–1, 254, 291
von Monakow, Constantin, 85, 146
von Nida, Mrs, 374
von Recklinghausen's disease, 60, 62
von Santha, Kalman, 100, 135, 137
Vosic, Harry, 189–90

Wada, Juhn Atsushi, 276, 293–5
Wada test, 219, 293–5
Walberg, Fred, 368
Walker, A. Earl, 100–1, 164–5, 259, 409
Walker, Michael, 433
Walshe, Sir Francis, 112, 211–12, 221, 266–8

Walter Adams Bequests, 375
Walter Chamblet Adams Memorial Endowment, 334
Walter Reed Army Institute of Research, 241
Warburg apparatus, 461, 466
Ward, Arthur, 117, 164, 224, 254, 319, 516
Ward Laboratory, 464–5, 491–2
war-related addresses at the MNI (table), 164
Warren Anatomical Museum, 281
Warrington, Elizabeth, 403
wartime research, 158–66, 176
Washington State University (Pullman), 124
Washington University (St Louis, MO), 420
Wason, Winsome, 405
Watch That Ends the Night (MacLennan), 190, 192
Webb, Jim, 237, 461
Webb, Winifred, 409
Webster, Colin, 315, 432–3
Webster, Howard, 390, 397, 432–3
Webster, Senator Lorne C., 390
Webster Brain Research Fund, 390
Webster Pavilion (MNI), 432–3
Weir, Bryce, 75, 334, 392
Weiskrantz, Lawrence, 403
Welch, Keasley, 61, 99, 194, 201, 213, 230, 315, 319, 330, 409
Welch, William H., 5, 20–1
Wells, John, 418, 423, 425
Wernicke, Karl, 30
Wernicke's area, 214, 217–19, 293
Whipple, Allen, 13–14, 93, 165
White, James C., 243
white matter, 31, 131–2, 298, 393, 470, 483, 488
Wieland, Heinrich, 460
Wiener, Norbert, 240
Wiesel, Torsten Nils, 241–2, 366
Wigglesworth, Sir Vincent, 471
Wilder Penfield Archives, 440
Wilgress, Leolyn Dana, 184–5
Wilkinson, Elizabeth (Lisa), 391
William Cone Memorial Research Fund, 315
William Ewart Berry, 1st Viscount Camrose, 144, 152
William Feindel Chair of Neuro-Oncology, 440
Willis, Thomas, 9, 85, 351, 391
Windsor Station, 17, 23, 152, 244
Winnie the Pooh (Milne), 276
Winslow, Marjorie, 257, 259, 305

Winter, Constance, 145, 150, 172
Wolbach, S.B., 164
Wolfe, Leon collaborators and students (table), 494
Wolfe, Leonhard Scott, 325, 330–1, 362, 367, 393–4, 407, 469, 471–9, 481–2, 487, 489, 494–5
Wong, Eva Chong, 173
Woods, Ivan (John), 194, 378–9, 383, 385, 396
Woolsey, Clinton, 72, 165, 204, 299, 409
World Health Organization, 346, 439
World of Neurology, The (triptych), 77, 229, 307, 387, 431–2

X-ray-guided percutaneous cervical cord puncture, 427–9

Yakovlev, Paul, 331
Yale University (New Haven, CT), 163
Yamamoto, Yazokazu Lucas, 74, 135, 352–5, 378, 411, 419–20, 425–26, 494
Yang, Tian-zhu, 417
Yang, Yu-Jia, 487, 490, 495
Yanjing University (Peiping), 342
Yasargil, Gazi, 366, 369, 434
Yates, Alan, 488, 495
Yegorov, Boris Grigorevich, 338–40
Yokohama National University (Yokohama), 353
Yong, V. Wee, 505
Young, Arthur, 59–61, 98, 100, 143, 263, 343, 392, 499–500
Young, John Zachary, 103, 300, 369

Zangwill, Oliver, 287, 335, 403
Zatorre, Robert, 220, 332, 427
Zemskaya, Alexandra Georgievna, 298
Zervas, Nicholas, 276
Zifkin, Benjamin, 423, 494
Zülch, Klaus Joachim, 34
Zwicker-Grier, Kathleen, 45